MW00844146

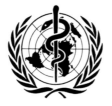

World Health Organization Classification of Tumours

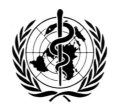

WHO   OMS

International Agency for Research on Cancer (IARC)

4th Edition

WHO Classification of
Tumours of Endocrine Organs

Edited by

Ricardo V. Lloyd

Robert Y. Osamura

Günter Klöppel

Juan Rosai

International Agency for Research on Cancer

Lyon, 2017

World Health Organization Classification of Tumours

Series Editors	Fred T. Bosman, MD PhD
	Elaine S. Jaffe, MD
	Sunil R. Lakhani, MD FRCPath
	Hiroko Ohgaki, DVM PhD

WHO Classification of Tumours of Endocrine Organs

Editors	Ricardo V. Lloyd, MD
	Robert Y. Osamura, MD
	Günter Klöppel, MD
	Juan Rosai, MD
Project Assistants	Asiedua Asante
	Anne-Sophie Hameau
Technical Editor	Jessica Cox
Database	Alberto Machado
	Delphine Nicolas
Layout	Anna Büsching
Printed by	Maestro
	38330 Saint-Ismier, France
Publisher	International Agency for Research on Cancer (IARC)
	69372 Lyon Cedex 08, France

The WHO Classification of Tumours of Endocrine Organs presented in this book reflects the views of a Working Group that convened for a Consensus and Editorial Meeting at the International Agency for Research on Cancer, Lyon, 26–28 April 2016.

Members of the Working Group are indicated in the list of contributors on pages 285–295.

Published by the International Agency for Research on Cancer (IARC),
150 Cours Albert Thomas, 69372 Lyon Cedex 08, France

Distributed by
WHO Press, World Health Organization, 20 Avenue Appia, 1211 Geneva 27, Switzerland
Tel.: +41 22 791 3264; Fax: +41 22 791 4857; email: bookorders@who.int

First print run (10 000 copies)

Format for bibliographic citations:
Lloyd RV, Osamura RY, Klöppel G, Rosai J, editors (2017).
WHO Classification of Tumours of Endocrine Organs (4th edition).
IARC: Lyon 2017

IARC Library Cataloguing in Publication Data

WHO classification of tumours of endocrine organs / edited by Ricardo V. Lloyd, Robert Y. Osamura, Günter Klöppel, Juan Rosai.
– 4th edition.

(World Health Organization classification of tumours)

1. Endocrine gland neoplasms – genetics   2. Endocrine gland neoplasms – pathology   3. Pituitary neoplasms
4. Thyroid neoplasms   5. Parathyroid neoplasms   6. Adrenal gland neoplasms
7. Pancreatic neoplasms   8. Neuroendocrine tumours   9. Neoplastic syndromes, hereditary

I. Lloyd, Ricardo V. II. Series

ISBN 978-92-832-4493-6   (NLM Classification: WK 145)

Contents

CHAPTER 1

Tumours of the pituitary gland

Pituitary adenoma

Pituitary carcinoma

Pituitary blastoma

Craniopharyngioma

Neuronal and paraneuronal tumours

Tumours of the posterior pituitary

Mesenchymal and stromal tumours

Haematolymphoid tumours

Germ cell tumours

Secondary tumours

WHO classification of tumours of the pituitary

Pituitary adenomas

Pituitary adenoma	8272/0
Somatotroph adenoma	8272/0
Lactotroph adenoma	8271/0
Thyrotroph adenoma	8272/0
Corticotroph adenoma	8272/0
Gonadotroph adenoma	8272/0
Null cell adenoma	8272/0
Plurihormonal and double adenomas	8272/0

Pituitary carcinoma	8272/3
Pituitary blastoma	8273/3*
Craniopharyngioma	9350/1
Adamantinomatous craniopharyngioma	9351/1
Papillary craniopharyngioma	9352/1

Neuronal and paraneuronal tumours

Gangliocytoma and mixed gangliocytoma-adenoma	9492/0
Neurocytoma	9506/1
Paraganglioma	8693/3
Neuroblastoma	9500/3

Tumours of the posterior pituitary

Pituicytoma	9432/1
Granular cell tumour of the sellar region	9582/0
Spindle cell oncocytoma	8290/0
Sellar ependymoma	9391/1*

Mesenchymal and stromal tumours

Meningioma	9530/0
Schwannoma	9560/0
Chordoma, NOS	9370/3
Chondroid chordoma	9371/3
Dedifferentiated chordoma	9372/3
Haemangiopericytoma/Solitary fibrous tumour	
Grade 1 HPC/SFT	8815/0
Grade 2 HPC/SFT	8815/1
Grade 3 HPC/SFT	8815/3

Haematolymphoid tumours

Germ cell tumours

Germinoma	9064/3
Yolk sac tumour	9071/3
Embryonal carcinoma	9070/3
Choriocarcinoma	9100/3
Teratoma, NOS	9080/1
Mature teratoma	9080/0
Immature teratoma	9080/3
Teratoma with malignant transformation	9084/3
Mixed germ cell tumour	9085/3

Secondary tumours

The morphology codes are from the International Classification of Diseases for Oncology (ICD-O) {898A}. Behaviour is coded /0 for benign tumours; /1 for unspecified, borderline, or uncertain behaviour; /2 for carcinoma in situ and grade III intraepithelial neoplasia; and /3 for malignant tumours. The classification is modified from the previous WHO classification, taking into account changes in our understanding of these lesions.
*These new codes were approved by the IARC/WHO Committee for ICD-O.

Introduction

Osamura R. Y.
Lopes M. B. S.
Grossman A.
Kontogeorgos G.
Trouillas J.

This chapter describes pituitary adenomas, pituitary carcinoma, and various other tumours occurring in the sellar and parasellar region of the pituitary gland. Pituitary adenomas, the most frequent tumours involving this region, are mostly benign tumours. Pituitary carcinoma is very rare, and because signs of histopathological malignancy are lacking, its diagnosis is only considered when metastases are present. A new entity, pituitary blastoma, is described in this chapter as part of a known genetic background (*DICER1* mutation). Also described in detail are tumours arising in the posterior pituitary, in particular those believed to be derived from pituicytes (the modified glial cells of the posterior pituitary), including pituicytoma, granular cell tumour of the posterior pituitary, and spindle cell oncocytoma. Although these tumours are very rare, their recognition is important because they are a crucial differential diagnosis for the most common adenoma; therefore, their accurate diagnosis has important therapeutic implications.

Other tumours arising in the sellar region that are reviewed in detail include craniopharyngioma (a non-rare tumour with a bimodal age distribution), mesenchymal tumours, and germ cell tumours.

New classification of pituitary adenomas

Terminology

Our improved understanding of the role of transcription factors in the differentiation of anterior pituitary cells and the regulation of specific pituitary hormones (e.g. PIT1, SF1, and TPIT) has changed our understanding of the presumed nature of the pituitary cells from which adenomas derive. In light of this new knowledge, the current classification focuses on pituitary-cell lineage for the designation of adenomas. For example, the new designation "somatotroph adenoma" defines a group of tumours that are derived from a PIT1 lineage and secrete growth hormone; this replaces the former term "growth hormone–producing adenoma". The new classification remains based on immunohistochemistry for the main secreting hormones. Other immunohistochemical markers, such as keratin, allow for differentiation between clinically relevant histological subtypes, such as densely and sparsely granulated somatotroph adenomas, which were previously identified on the basis of ultrastructural features. Electron microscopy is now rarely used to classify pituitary tumours.

Prognosis and prediction

Although most pituitary tumours behave benignly (i.e. do not metastasize) and are therefore called adenomas, they frequently invade into the adjacent structures, leading to recurrence. Therefore, clinical and pathological parameters for predicting such clinically aggressive behaviour are essential.

In the 2004 classification, the category of pituitary tumours was divided into three subcategories: typical adenoma, atypical adenoma, and carcinoma. Atypical adenomas were defined by a high mitotic index, a Ki-67 proliferation index > 3%, and strong nuclear p53 staining. With these criteria, the incidence of atypical adenoma was relatively variable (5–10%), and prognostic significance could not be established despite more than 10 years of research on the utility of this classification. Therefore, the term "atypical adenoma" is no longer recommended. However, we recommend the assessment of markers of tumour proliferation (i.e. mitotic count and Ki-67 proliferation index), in addition to other clinical parameters such as invasion assessed by MRI studies and/or intraoperative examination, for the evaluation of individual tumours that may behave in a more clinically aggressive manner. Adenoma invasion, as assessed by MRI studies and/or intraoperative examination, should be considered an important prognostic feature in these more clinically aggressive adenomas (see p. 17 {2814}).

Special adenoma subtypes that commonly show aggressive behaviour must also be taken into account. These include sparsely granulated somatotroph adenoma (see *Somatotroph adenoma*, p. 19), lactotroph adenomas in men (see *Lactotroph adenoma*, p. 24), Crooke cell adenoma and silent corticotroph adenoma (see *Corticotroph adenoma*, p. 30), and plurihormonal PIT1-positive adenoma (previously called silent subtype 3 adenoma; see *Plurihormonal and double adenomas*, p. 39).

Genetic profile and susceptibility

Although most adenomas are sporadic, certain familial syndromes are associated with pituitary adenomas, including multiple endocrine neoplasia type 1, multiple endocrine neoplasia type 4, Carney complex, familial isolated pituitary adenoma, McCune–Albright syndrome, SDH-related familial pituitary adenoma, neurofibromatosis type 1, von Hippel–Lindau syndrome, and *DICER1* syndrome (pituitary blastoma). Most of the tumours associated with familial syndromes secrete growth hormone and/or prolactin and suggest activation of the PIT1 transcription factor.

Pituitary adenoma

Osamura R.Y.   Lopes M.B.S.
Grossman A.   Matsuno A.
Korbonits M.   Trouillas J.
Kovacs K.

Definition
Pituitary adenoma is a neoplastic proliferation of anterior pituitary hormone–producing cells. The tumours are typically benign, but can be aggressive and invasive into adjacent structures.

ICD-O code   8272/0

Epidemiology
Pituitary adenomas constitute approximately 15% of all intracranial neoplasms. Most pituitary tumours are adenomas and are benign and non-invasive (i.e. confined to the sella turcica). But invasive adenomas are also frequent. Pituitary carcinomas are rare, accounting for only 0.1–0.2% of all pituitary endocrine tumours.

Etiology
Some cases arise due to known somatic mutations, but for a substantial proportion of pituitary adenomas the etiology is poorly understood. The findings of experimental studies suggest that the tumorigenic mechanisms involve the loss of antioncogenic factors or the overexpression of oncogenic factors, probably on or near the cell surface.

Localization
Most pituitary adenomas are localized to the sella turcica, but some occur in the sphenoidal sinus; these are called ectopic pituitary adenomas {2764}.

Clinical features
The signs and symptoms of pituitary adenomas include symptoms caused by the excess hormones produced by so-called functioning adenomas. Mass effects, such as bitemporal hemianopia, diplopia, and headache, are most commonly seen in clinically non-functioning adenomas. Symptoms of hypopituitarism can also occur: excess production of growth hormone (GH), prolactin, TSH, and ACTH, respectively, can cause acromegaly and gigantism, galactorrhoea and hypogonadism, hyperthyroidism, and Cushing disease. In such symptomatic cases, the corresponding serum hormone levels are elevated.

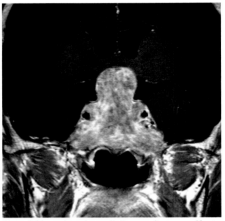

Fig. 1.01 Invasive pituitary adenoma, Knosp grade 4. Adenoma involving bilateral cavernous sinus surrounding carotid arteries.

Adenomas are termed silent when the patient shows no clinical signs and there is no hormonal elevation in the serum but the tumour demonstrates hormone production on immunohistochemistry {2914}. Recently, the term "aggressive" has been used by clinicians to designate radiologically invasive adenomas, which grow rapidly, tend to recur or progress, and are resistant to combined treatment including surgery and radiation {461,1742,1824, 2255}.

Imaging
On the basis of their largest dimension, adenomas are designated as micro-

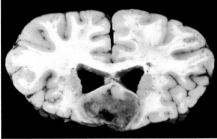

Fig. 1.02 Pituitary adenoma. Macroscopy.

adenomas (< 1 cm), macroadenomas (1–4 cm), or giant adenomas (> 4 cm). Many adenomas (35–45%) invade into adjacent structures {1799,3088}; macroadenomas and giant adenomas are particularly likely to invade into the cavernous sinus. Suprasellar and parasellar extensions can be distinguished from true invasion to the cavernous or sphenoidal sinus on the basis of anatomical studies {877} and imaging. On the basis of endoscopic verification, only grade 3 and 4 tumours according to the Knosp classification are now considered to be invasive into the cavernous sinus {461}.

Microscopy
Imprint cytology
For rapid intraoperative diagnosis, imprint specimens may be helpful for distinguishing between pituitary adenomas and other tumours, including malignant

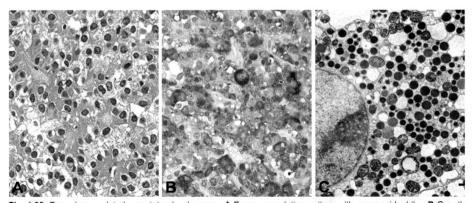

Fig. 1.03 Densely granulated somatotroph adenoma. **A** Dense granulation pattern with many acidophils. **B** Growth hormone immunohistochemistry showing strong cytoplasmic staining. **C** Electron microscopy showing many secretory granules (dense granulation).

lymphoma, astrocytoma, and secondary tumours {11,2192}.

Microscopy algorithm and protocol
Typically, on H&E staining, somatotrophs are eosinophilic and corticotrophs are basophilic. Gonadotrophs and thyrotrophs are usually chromophobic {1400, 1820,2029}.

Immunophenotype
Immunohistochemistry is the gold standard for the diagnosis of pituitary tumours and for their classification into seven main subtypes: somatotroph, lactotroph, thyrotroph, corticotroph, gonadotroph, null cell (immunonegative and transcription factor–negative), and plurihormonal. The great majority of tumours (except lactotroph adenomas) are strongly positive for synaptophysin and chromogranin A. Immunohistochemistry for the follow-ing hormones should be routinely performed: GH, prolactin, TSH-beta, ACTH, FSH-beta, LH-beta, and alpha subunit. Immunohistochemistry for transcription factors, including PIT1, SF1, and TPIT, may be useful for further classification, but the validity of these markers is still under investigation.

Immunohistochemical staining allows for the classification of pituitary adenomas according to their hormone content and distinguishes specific adenomas that could previously be described only on an ultrastructural basis. The density of secretory granules within a given cell and tumour can be determined based on the intensity and distribution of hormonal reactivity by immunohistochemistry. For example, densely granulated somatotroph adenomas are characterized by strong immunoreactivity for GH throughout the cytoplasm and by diffuse labelling of the majority of the adenoma cells, whereas sparsely granulated somatotroph adenomas (SGSA) show weaker and more focal GH immunoreactivity.

Immunoreactivity for low-molecular-weight cytokeratin, using CK7/8 (CAM5.2) or CK18 antibodies, may also facilitate additional discrimination of specific adenomas. Cytokeratin is diffusely and strongly positive in corticotroph adenomas. It can also distinguish SGSAs from their densely granulated counterparts: dot-like or globular cytokeratin reactivity is consistent with the presence of the fibrous bodies seen ultrastructurally in SGSAs. Ring-like cytokeratin immunostaining in normal and neoplastic corticotrophs is diagnostic of Crooke changes.

Antimitochondrial antibodies can be used to identify oncocytic changes. Therefore, many of these particular im-

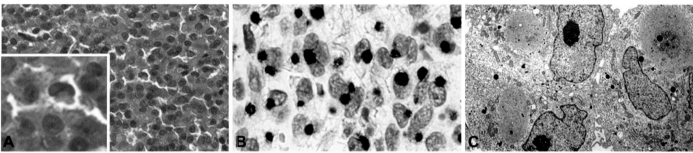
Fig. 1.04 Sparsely granulated somatotroph adenoma. **A** Sparse granulation pattern with a fibrous body. **B** Fibrous body with positive keratin staining. **C** Electron microscopy.

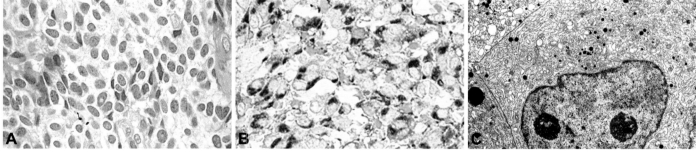
Fig. 1.05 Lactotroph adenoma. **A** Sparsely granulated type. **B** Prolactin staining reveals a Golgi pattern. **C** Electron microscopy.

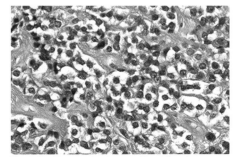
Fig. 1.06 Thyrotroph adenoma. Focal fibrosis.

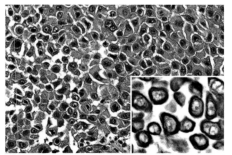
Fig. 1.07 Crooke cell adenoma. H&E staining and keratin staining (inset).

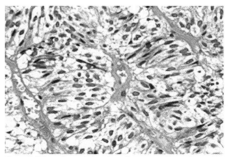
Fig. 1.08 Gonadotroph adenoma. Pseudorosette pattern.

munohistochemical patterns are suitable alternatives to ultrastructural studies. Proliferation is evaluated using the mitotic count and the Ki-67 proliferation index as determined using the MIB1 antibody {2390,2814}. Ki-67 commonly stains diffusely throughout the adenoma, with identifiable hotspots in only a few cases. When present, such hotspots should be used for the mitotic counts. The validity of p53 immunostaining for predicting behaviour is still controversial {2391,2814}. To facilitate therapeutic prediction, the expression of the somatostatin receptors SSTR2–5 {496} can be tested in somatotroph, corticotroph, and thyrotroph adenomas.

Ultrastructure
Electron microscopy is not necessary for the routine investigation of pituitary tumours. However, ultrastructural evaluation may be useful in the differential diagnosis of undifferentiated tumours and in a very limited number of adenoma subtypes, such as plurihormonal PIT1-positive adenoma.

Reporting
Classification of pituitary adenomas requires morphological and hormonal immunohistochemical assessment (see Table 1.01). The Ki-67 proliferation index can be used as a parameter for prognostic evaluation of individual adenomas {2390,2814}. Additional parameters that may be of prognostic significance in pituitary adenomas are listed in Table 1.02.

Prognosis
Certain subtypes of pituitary adenomas tend to show more-aggressive behaviour {461,1824}: SGSA, lactotroph macroadenoma in men, Crooke cell adenoma, silent corticotroph adenoma, and plurihormonal PIT1-positive adenoma (previously called silent subtype 3 adenoma). More-detailed discussion of these entities is included in the individual sections on each type.
In the 2004 classification, the category of pituitary tumours was divided into three subcategories: typical adenoma, atypical adenoma, and carcinoma. However, this division could not be clinically validated {2370,3088}. Nevertheless, some of the pathological parameters included in that classification do seem to be of value as prognostic markers, such as a high mitotic index and a high Ki-67 proliferation

Table 1.01 Morphofunctional classification of pituitary adenomas

Adenoma type	Immunophenotype	Transcription factors and other cofactors
Somatotroph adenoma		
Densely granulated somatotroph adenoma[a]	GH ± PRL ± alpha subunit LMWCK: perinuclear or diffuse	PIT1
Sparsely granulated somatotroph adenoma	GH ± PRL LMWCK: dot-like (fibrous bodies)	PIT1
Mammosomatotroph adenoma	GH + PRL (in same cell) ± alpha subunit	PIT1, ER-alpha
Mixed somatotroph and lactotroph adenoma	GH + PRL (in different cells) ± alpha subunit	PIT1, ER-alpha
Lactotroph adenoma		
Sparsely granulated lactotroph adenoma[a]	PRL	PIT1, ER-alpha
Densely granulated lactotroph adenoma	PRL	PIT1, ER-alpha
Acidophilic stem cell adenoma	PRL, GH (focal and inconstant) LMWCK: fibrous bodies (inconstant)	
Thyrotroph adenoma	TSH-beta, alpha subunit	PIT1, GATA2
Corticotroph adenoma		
Densely granulated corticotroph adenoma[a]	ACTH, LMWCK: diffuse pattern	TPIT
Sparsely granulated corticotroph adenoma	ACTH, LMWCK: diffuse pattern	TPIT
Crooke cell adenoma	ACTH, LMWCK: ring-like pattern	TPIT
Gonadotroph adenoma		
Sparsely granulated gonadotroph adenoma[a]	FSH-beta, LH-beta, alpha subunit (various combinations)	SF1, GATA2, ER-alpha (variable)
Null cell adenoma	No markers	None
Plurihormonal adenomas		
Plurihormonal PIT1-positive adenoma[b]	GH, PRL, TSH-beta ± alpha subunit	PIT1
Adenomas with unusual immunohistochemical combinations	Various combinations	Other transcription factors (variable)
Double adenomas		
Distinct adenomas	Usually PRL and ACTH, respectively	PIT1 and TPIT, respectively

ACTH, adrenocorticotropic hormone; FSH-beta, follicle-stimulating hormone subunit beta; GH, growth hormone; LH-beta, luteinizing hormone subunit beta; LMWCK, low-molecular-weight cytokeratin; PRL, prolactin; TSH-beta, thyroid-stimulating hormone subunit beta.
[a] Most common subtype.
[b] Previously called silent subtype 3 adenoma.

Table 1.02 Other parameters that may be of prognostic significance in pituitary adenomas in addition to the morphofunctional classification (see Table 1.01)

Tumour size (largest dimension): microadenoma (< 1 cm), macroadenoma (1–4 cm), or giant adenoma (> 4 cm)

Tumour's clinical presentation: clinically functioning, clinically non-functioning, or silent

Invasiveness on MRI (Knosp grade): non-invasive (grade 1 or 2) or invasive (grade 3 or 4)

Metastasis or spinal spread: carcinoma

Additional immunohistochemistry:
- Chromogranin A
- Low-molecular-weight cytokeratin: CK7/8 (CAM5.2), CK18
- Proliferation markers: Ki-67, p53 (in limited cases)
- Transcription factors and cofactors: PIT1, SF1, ER-alpha, TPIT, GATA2, NeuroD1
- Predictive markers: SSTR2, SSTR5, MGMT, MSH6

index (> 3%). Expression of p53 was also included in the previous classification, but it is unclear whether p53 expression is an independent factor.

More recent approaches for prognostication of pituitary adenomas have taken into account tumour invasion (evaluated by MRI and/or histology) in addition to the histopathological parameters discussed in the 2004 classification, with the addition of precise cut-off points for mitotic index and p53 immunoexpression {1835, 2814,3088}. In 2013, Trouillas et al. proposed a new clinicopathological classification with five grades based on invasion and proliferation, and demonstrated its prognostic value in a retrospective multicentric case–control study {2814}.

High-risk pituitary adenomas
Some pituitary adenomas show features that tend to predict recurrence and resistance to conventional therapy. These features include rapid growth, radiological invasion, and a high Ki-67 proliferation index. Tumours with these features are referred to by some as clinically aggressive adenomas. It is recommended that adenomas with the combination of these characteristics be investigated more intensively and followed up more closely.

Transcription factors for functional differentiation
The differentiation of pituitary cells depends on transcription factors. PIT1 is the transcription factor for somatotroph differentiation, PIT1 and ER-alpha for lactotroph differentiation, and PIT1 and GATA2 for thyrotroph differentiation. Corticotroph differentiation depends on TPIT and NeuroD1, and gonadotroph differentiation on SF1 and GATA2.
Immunohistochemistry for transcription factors can be used to subclassify

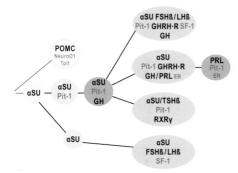

Fig. 1.09 Pituitary differentiation and transcription factors in the human pituitary gland. Adapted from: R Y Osamura et al. {2059A}.

pituitary adenomas, and is especially useful in immunonegative adenomas and plurihormonal adenomas such as plurihormonal PIT1-positive adenoma {1657, 1850,2007,2069,2412,2695,2839}.

Genetic profile
Genetic profiles have been established in order to clarify the tumorigenic process and facilitate prognostication of pituitary adenomas. Somatic mutations in *GNAS* have been identified in 40% of sporadic somatotroph adenomas, resulting in up-regulation of the cAMP pathway {1543}. Mutations in *USP8* have been identified in 36–62% of corticotroph adenomas, leading to upregulation of the EGFR pathway {1698,2150,2271}. Exome sequencing studies have not identified recurrent somatic mutations in non-functioning adenomas {1973} or somatotroph adenomas {2332,2845}. Whole-genome sequencing of somatotroph adenomas has identified copy-number losses in chromosomes 1, 6, 13, 14, 15, 16, 18, and 22, and copy-number gains in chromosomes 3, 7, 20, and X {2845}. Increasing evidence shows that certain genetic changes are related to aggressive behaviour in pituitary adenomas {461}. These changes include genomic imbalance (11q allelic loss); DNA aneuploidy; MYO5A expression (which is linked to invasiveness); germline mutations associated with multiple endocrine neoplasia type 1, multiple endocrine neoplasia type 4, Carney complex, familial isolated pituitary adenoma, and SDH-related familial pituitary adenoma; various microRNAs; loss of expression of p27; and overexpression of cyclin E (in corticotroph adenomas {1430,1452}).
Other changes that may be associated with aggressive behaviour include changes in senescence markers (p16, p21, beta-galactosidase), HEPN1 (which shows lower expression in aggressive somatotroph adenoma), growth factors (EGF, VEGF) and their receptors (EGFR, VEGFR), FGF2 and pituitary tumour–derived FGFR4, matrix metalloproteinases, CD56 (also called NCAM), and galectin 3 (in corticotroph and lactotroph adenomas) {2291}. Further analysis of these changes may facilitate the evaluation of prognosis and response to therapy. *TP53* mutations have occasionally been reported in pituitary adenomas, but may relate to malignant transformation of the adenomas {1597,2725}.

Table 1.03 Genetic predisposition to pituitary adenomas

Disease	Associated gene(s)
Syndromic diseases	
Multiple endocrine neoplasia type 1	*MEN1*
Multiple endocrine neoplasia type 4	*CDKN1B*
SDH-related familial paraganglioma and phaeochromocytoma syndromes	*SDHA, SDHB, SDHC, SDHD, SDHAF2*
Carney complex	*PRKAR1A, PRKACA*
McCune–Albright syndrome	Mosaic *GNAS*
Neurofibromatosis (very rare)	*NF1*
DICER1 syndrome	*DICER1*
Isolated pituitary disease	
Familial isolated pituitary adenoma (somatotroph)	*AIP*
X-linked acrogigantism syndrome	*GPR101*
Familial isolated pituitary adenoma	Unknown

Genetic susceptibility
Most pituitary adenomas are sporadic. However, a substantial minority (most commonly somatotroph and lactotroph adenomas) occur due to germline genetic abnormalities (see Table 1.03). Experimentally, *MEN1*, *PRKAR1A*, *CDKN1A*, *SDHB*, and *AIP* heterozygote knockout rodents develop pituitary adenomas {1451}.

Treatment and predictive factors
Therapies are directed at reduction of tumour volume, as well as against excessive hormone production in functioning adenomas. If the tumours are localized to the sella or are only mildly invasive, surgery (transsphenoidal, usually endoscopic) is the first choice; the exception is lactotroph adenomas, for which a dopamine agonist is the first choice of therapy even for large or giant adenomas. For invasive or aggressive pituitary adenomas or carcinomas, pharmacotherapies and various modalities of radiotherapy must be considered.

Surgery
Surgical resection is the mainstream option for managing pituitary tumours, and an endoscopic approach is the first choice for various pituitary adenomas. Surgery is indicated in the following

settings: (1) functioning tumours with acromegaly, Cushing disease, and thyrotroph adenoma; (2) mass effect due to tumour compression; (3) ineffective prior treatment such as pharmacotherapy.

Radiation therapy

Radiation therapy should be considered for residual or recurrent pituitary adenomas. Stereotactic radiotherapy and radiosurgery with a system such as Gamma Knife, CyberKnife, or a linear accelerator provide tumour and hormonal control comparable with that achieved by conventional radiotherapy {1852}, but the use of these systems is limited to zones away from the optic pathways.

Pharmacotherapy

Dopamine agonists. For lactotroph adenomas, dopamine agonists are the first choice, both for suppression of hormone secretion and for decreasing the tumour size. Some non-functioning adenomas also respond to dopamine agonists such as cabergoline.

Somatostatin analogues. Octreotide and lanreotide are used for the treatment of somatotroph and thyrotroph adenomas {1805,2919}; they bind to SSTR2, and the expression of SSTR2 on the cell membrane is essential for the therapeutic effects. Pasireotide has been used for the treatment of corticotroph adenomas that express SSTR5 {432}. Its indication in acromegaly was approved in Europe and the USA in 2014 {2404}. Occasional nonfunctioning tumours may also respond to somatostatin analogues.

Temozolomide for aggressive adenoma and carcinoma. Although there is a correlation between decreased MGMT expression and the likelihood of treatment response, many studies have also showed response with no correlation with MGMT expression or MGMT staining {210,353,1145,2257}. In aggressive tumours and carcinoma, the expression of DNA mismatch repair proteins, including MSH6, may correlate with temozolomide treatment effects {210,1145}.

Pituitary hyperplasia

Pituitary hyperplasia is a rare condition, accounting for < 1% of sellar surgical specimens. It has several etiologies and its diagnosis is difficult. Hyperplasia can occur secondary to hypersecretion of hypothalamic stimulating hormones through either physiological or pathological mechanisms.

Characteristic physiological examples are hypertrophy of the gland during puberty {87} and lactotroph hyperplasia due to estrogen stimulation during pregnancy {2455,2637}.

Pathological hyperplasia can be induced by excessive levels of hypophysiotropic hormones; for example, thyrotroph hyperplasia can occur due to untreated primary hypothyroidism {1592, 2452,3076}. Although rare, pathological pituitary hyperplasia may occur due to ectopic secretion of hypothalamic releasing hormones by neuroendocrine tumours. For example, pancreatic and pulmonary GHRH-secreting tumours can cause somatotroph hyperplasia {219,811,1007,1955,2410,2772}, and pulmonary CRH-secreting neuroendocrine tumours can cause corticotroph hyperplasia {2512}.

Mammosomatotroph hyperplasia (i.e. of immature acidophilic cells secreting both GH and prolactin) or somatotroph and lactotroph hyperplasia is seen in familial pituitary syndromes including Carney complex, McCune–Albright syndrome, and multiple endocrine neoplasia type 1 {36,2644,2813}, as well as in X-linked acrogigantism syndrome causing acromegaly and/or gigantism {1901,2312}.

It has been postulated that corticotroph hyperplasia associated with Cushing disease may rarely occur either alone or in association with corticotroph adenoma {1163,1683}. However, this hypothesis is controversial, and is not accepted by some investigators {2812}.

Microscopy

By MRI and on macroscopic examination, the pituitary gland is globally enlarged and lacks a well-defined lesion distinguishable from the surrounding gland.

Histologically, the gland shows unevenly enlarged acini composed mostly of a single cell type {1163}. Hyperplasia may be diffuse within the gland or focal with formation of nodules. Reticulin staining is essential for the diagnosis of hyperplasia; it demonstrates expanded acini but with preservation of the reticulin acinar pattern. Immunohistochemistry for pituitary hormones identifies the hyperplastic cell population intermixed with the normal pituitary cell components. Occasionally, mixed somatotroph and lactotroph hyperplasia is very difficult to differentiate from mixed somatotroph and lactotroph adenoma. The normal pituitary cell components of each type are strongly immunopositive and are dispersed throughout the whole fragments, which is not observed in pituitary adenoma.

Somatotroph adenoma

Mete O.
Korbonits M.
Osamura R. Y.
Trouillas J.
Yamada S.

Definition
Somatotroph adenoma is a pituitary adenoma that expresses mainly growth hormone (GH) and arises from PIT1-lineage cells. These tumours often result in GH excess, leading to gigantism and/or acromegaly. Pure somatotroph adenomas are divided into two clinically relevant histological subtypes: densely granulated somatotroph adenoma (DGSA) and sparsely granulated somatotroph adenoma (SGSA). Other adenomas leading to acromegaly and/or gigantism cosecrete GH and prolactin (PRL); these include mammosomatotroph adenomas, mixed somatotroph and lactotroph adenomas, and plurihormonal adenomas.

ICD-O code   8272/0

Synonyms
Somatotrope adenoma; somatotrophinoma; GH-producing adenoma; GH-secreting adenoma; GH-cell adenoma; GH adenoma

Epidemiology
Acromegaly and pituitary gigantism result from excess GH and IGF1; more than 95% of cases are associated with pituitary somatotroph adenomas. The reported prevalence of acromegaly is 125–137 cases per 1 million population {18,604,1043}. Gigantism due to GH excess is rare and typically occurs during childhood or puberty, before epiphyseal closure {800,1327}. Somatotroph adenomas can occur in patients of any age; the mean patient age at diagnosis is 47 years. There is an approximately equal sex distribution {1180}. Among young individuals, about 20% of paediatric gigantism cases and 8–11% of acromegaly cases have been associated with *AIP* mutation, and at least half of these patients have a family history of familial isolated pituitary adenoma {36,1137, 2199}. At least 80% of reported cases of very early onset paediatric gigantism (i. e. patient age < 5 years at diagnosis) have been associated with X-linked acrogigantism syndrome due to a microduplication involving the *GPR101* gene {1661, 2808}. GH excess can also occur in the setting of syndromic presentations, such as Carney complex, McCune–Albright syndrome (MAS), multiple endocrine neoplasia type 1 (MEN1), and multiple endocrine neoplasia type 4 (MEN4) {2348}. Somatotroph adenomas account for approximately 10–15% of all resected pituitary adenomas {31,99,2788}. DGSAs are the most common cause of acromegaly {99}. SGSAs are most frequent in younger females, whereas DGSAs more commonly occur in older patients {1551, 1802,2279,3036}. Mammosomatotroph adenomas are very frequent in young adults with acromegaly {99}. Plurihormonal adenomas are extremely rare {2148}.

Etiology
Genetic and epigenetic factors, hormonal stimulation, and growth factors and their receptors contribute to the tumorigenesis of pituitary somatotroph adenomas (see *Genetic susceptibility*).

Localization
Most somatotroph adenomas are intrasellar, but some are macroadenomas with or without cavernous sinus invasion. Ectopic presentations have also been reported {245,853,1857,2239}.

Clinical features
Clinical symptoms and signs
Most somatotroph adenomas are biochemically active, but rare silent forms have also been reported {94,961,2007}. The clinical diagnosis of acromegaly can be straightforward and is often made by various specialists dealing with the patient's symptoms {1802}. Despite the well-known clinical stigmata, diagnosis is often delayed, with a mean time to diagnosis from the onset of symptoms of 8 years (range: 4–10 years) {2235}.
Patients with mammosomatotroph adenomas and mixed somatotroph and lactotroph adenomas develop gigantism and/or acromegaly, along with amenorrhoea and galactorrhoea, due to cosecretion of GH and PRL. Multinodular goitre (with or without hyperthyroidism) is common in acromegaly {1327}. Rarely, central hyperthyroidism can occur due to TSH cosecretion, especially in plurihormonal adenomas {2148}.
Headache, visual field deficits, mild hyperprolactinaemia, hypopituitarism, and

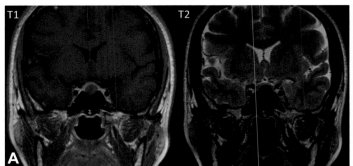
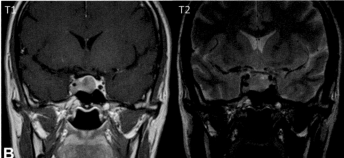

Fig. 1.10 Somatotroph adenomas. **A** T1- and T2-weighted MRI of a densely granulated somatotroph adenoma (DGSA). Most DGSAs are T2-hypointense and responsive to somatostatin analogues. **B** T1- and T2-weighted MRI of a sparsely granulated somatotroph adenoma (SGSA). Unlike DGSAs, most SGSAs are invasive macroadenomas that are usually T2-hyperintense.

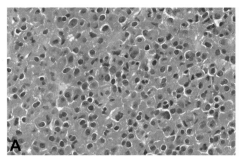  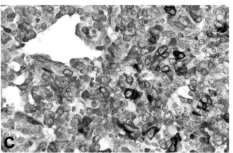

Fig. 1.11 Densely granulated somatotroph adenoma (DGSA). **A** DGSAs are characterized by eosinophilic (acidophilic) tumour cells. **B** Consistent with the high density of secretory granules, diffuse and strong growth hormone expression is noted in these tumours. **C** Most DGSAs also express alpha subunit.

pituitary apoplexy have been described in patients with invasive macroadenomas {1327,1804,1820,1853}. Symptomatic apoplexy is more common in *AIP*-mutated childhood cases {1137}.

Diagnostic tests
Virtually all patients with gigantism and/or acromegaly have increased serum concentrations of GH and IGF1. Serum IGF1 levels are stable, whereas GH concentrations fluctuate. Oral glucose intake suppresses GH secretion in healthy individuals, but patients with somatotroph adenomas do not show full suppression. Therefore, the biochemical diagnosis of GH hypersecretion is based on the finding of an IGF1 level above the age-specific normal range and confirmed by an oral glucose tolerance test in which the GH level is not suppressed to < 1 ng/mL {1327}. When an ectopic source of GHRH is a suspected cause of acromegaly, measurement of plasma GHRH using a cut-off point of 250–300 ng/L has been shown to have excellent specificity for the diagnosis of a GHRH-producing tumour {290,930}.

Imaging
Somatotroph adenomas are usually highly visible on MRI, but in rare instances small adenomas can be difficult to identify on conventional MRI {1667}. At diagnosis, most somatotroph adenomas are macroadenomas {414,2189}. DGSAs have been reported to be smaller, to less frequently invade the cavernous sinus, and to more rarely compress the optic chiasm compared with SGSAs {2189}. The T2 intensity of a somatotroph adenoma may be used to predict responsiveness to somatostatin analogues. Most DGSAs are T2-hypointense and responsive to somatostatin analogues {1120,2189}. Unlike DGSAs, most SGSAs are invasive macroadenomas that are

usually T2-hyperintense {1120,2189}. In the setting of a normal or bulky hyperplastic gland, GHRH measurement and a search for a GHRH-secreting tumour could lead to the correct diagnosis. In young patients with normal MRI findings and acromegaly, X-linked acrogigantism syndrome should be considered.

Macroscopy
Like other pituitary adenomas, somatotroph adenomas are soft and white to greyish-red. Macroadenomas often display invasion into adjacent structures {2005}. Tumours from patients with pituitary apoplexy contain haemorrhagic necrosis. Post-treatment adenomas may show fibrosis.

Microscopy
Acromegaly and/or gigantism occur due to somatotroph adenoma or somatotroph or mammosomatotroph hyperplasia. Exceptionally, ectopic GH-secreting neuroendocrine tumours have been seen {240,811,812,959,2209}. Therefore, histopathological assessment should start with confirmation of adenohypophyseal proliferation. Disruption of the reticulin framework distinguishes adenoma from hyperplasia that has an intact but expanded reticulin framework {1820}.
The identification of multifocal pituitary somatotroph adenoma or somatotroph adenoma in association with underlying somatotroph and/or mammosomatotroph hyperplasia raises the possibility of GHRH-secreting neoplasms, Carney complex, or MAS {1011,2209,2395,2396, 2902}. Recently, some cases associated with familial isolated pituitary adenoma {2879} and X-linked acrogigantism syndrome {2808} also showed a hyperplasia-to-neoplasia progression sequence in association with gigantism and acromegaly. Compared with somatotroph adenomas, somatotroph hyperplasia is

uncommon in MEN1-related pituitary disease, but most cases of MEN1-related pituitary hyperplasia are associated with GHRH-producing pancreatic neuroendocrine tumours {2813}. Somatotroph adenomas have also been reported in the context of double adenomas colliding with lactotroph, gonadotroph, or corticotroph adenomas {1209,1364,2414,2686, 3126}. SGSA with a ganglionic component has also been described in association with *AIP* mutation {2011} (see also the *Pituitary hyperplasia* subsection (p. 18) of *Pituitary adenoma*).
Adenomas causing only GH excess originate from somatotrophs. On the basis of their density of GH-containing secretory granules and their low-molecular-weight cytokeratin expression patterns, these tumours can be divided into two clinically relevant histological subtypes: DGSA and SGSA.

Densely granulated somatotroph adenomas are composed of tumour cells with eosinophilic cytoplasm, correlating with the high density of GH-containing secretory granules. These tumours are positive for PIT1, GH (diffusely and strongly), and alpha subunit. Low-molecular-weight cytokeratin (CAM5.2 or CK18) immunohistochemistry shows characteristic perinuclear staining {1011,1820,1823, 2042}. Ultrastructurally, the tumour cells contain abundant large secretory granules, measuring 400–600 nm {94}. These tumours are known to be responsive to somatostatin analogues {246,814,1551, 1820}, are associated with relatively high levels of GH and IGF1, are somewhat smaller and have a more benign clinical course than SGSAs, and are typically T2-hypointense or T2-isointense on MRI {871,1120,2189}.

Sparsely granulated somatotroph adenomas are composed of chromophobic to pale eosinophilic tumour cells that are positive for PIT1. Nuclear pleomorphism, including multinucleated bizarre cells, can be noted. Consistent with sparse granularity, positivity for GH is variable, with reactivity ranging from weak to focal or patchy. Unlike DGSAs, these tumours lack alpha subunit expression {149,1437, 1820}. Low-molecular-weight cytokeratin staining reveals characteristic fibrous bodies (called juxtanuclear keratin aggresomes) in the vast majority (> 70%) of the tumour cells {1011,1820,2042}. Fibrous bodies may also be recognizable on H&E-stained slides, because the nuclei are indented by these globular structures. Ultrastructurally, SGSAs contain sparse secretory granules, measuring 100–250 nm. Fibrous bodies occur as spherical aggregates of keratin filaments with trapped secretory granules and a variable amount of endoplasmic reticulum {94}. SGSAs are associated with poor response to somatostatin analogues {246,1011,1820,1823}, larger tumour size, lower levels of GH and IGF1, and T2-hyperintensity on MRI {871,1120,2189}. Rarely, gangliocytomas can be admixed with SGSAs {94,2011}.

The term "intermediate-type somatotroph adenoma" has been proposed for a subset of DGSAs displaying occasional fibrous bodies. Because such tumours have not been found to be biologically different from other DGSAs, most experts consider them to fall within the morphological spectrum of DGSA {1820,2042}.

Pituitary adenomas causing excess of both GH and PRL can be divided into three groups: mammosomatotroph adenoma, mixed somatotroph and lactotroph adenoma, and plurihormonal adenoma.

Mammosomatotroph adenomas consist predominantly of eosinophilic cells containing both GH-containing and PRL-containing secretory granules. Mammosomatotroph adenomas are positive for PIT1, GH, PRL, estrogen receptor, alpha subunit, and low-molecular-weight cytokeratin (which shows perinuclear staining) {1011,1820}. Ultrastructurally, these tumours are distinguished by the presence of pleomorphic and heterogeneous secretory granules measuring 150–1000 nm and by misplaced exocytosis (i.e. extrusion of secretory granules along the lateral cell surfaces), which is a hallmark of PRL secretion {94}.

Mixed somatotroph and lactotroph adenomas are composed of PIT1-expressing densely granulated somatotrophs (eosinophilic cells) and sparsely granulated lactotrophs (chromophobic cells) {1820}. Lactotrophs are typically positive for estrogen receptor and PRL (sparsely granulated lactotrophs show Golgi-type PRL staining; densely granulated lactotrophs show diffuse cytoplasmic PRL reactivity) and negative for alpha subunit. GH and alpha subunit expression depends

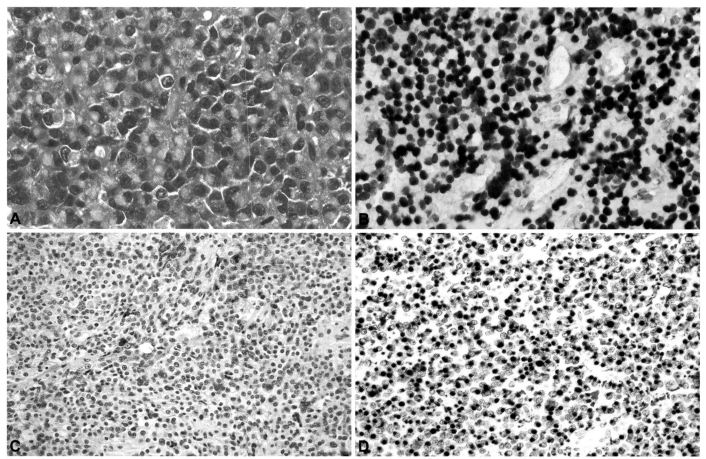

Fig. 1.12 Sparsely granulated somatotroph adenoma (SGSA). **A** SGSAs are typically composed of chromophobic to pale eosinophilic tumour cells. Fibrous bodies, a pathognomonic feature of these tumours, may be recognizable on H&E-stained slides, because the nuclei are indented by these globular structures. **B** Like densely granulated somatotroph adenomas (DGSAs), SGSAs are positive for PIT1. **C** Unlike in DGSAs, positivity for growth hormone in SGSAs is variable, with reactivity ranging from weak to focal or patchy. **D** Low-molecular-weight cytokeratin (CAM5.2) staining reveals characteristic fibrous bodies in the vast majority of the tumour cells.

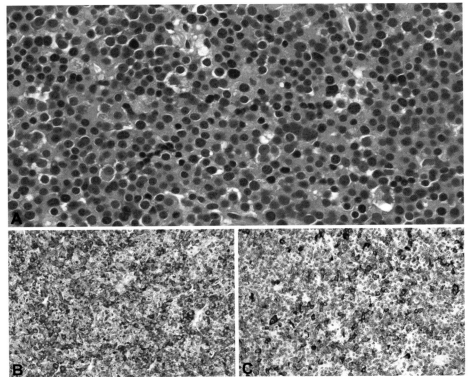

Fig. 1.13 Mammosomatotroph adenoma. **A** These tumours consist predominantly of eosinophilic cells. **B** Diffuse cytoplasmic growth hormone reactivity is noted in most of the tumour cells. **C** The extent of prolactin expression is often less than that of growth hormone expression, and diffuse staining throughout the tumour cell cytoplasm can be seen.

on the type of somatotroph. In some cases, the distinction of mammosomatotroph adenoma from mixed somatotroph and lactotroph adenoma may be difficult without ultrastructural examination {1011, 1820}. The presence of pleomorphic and heterogeneous secretory granules in a monomorphic cell population distinguishes mammosomatotroph adenomas from mixed somatotroph and lactotroph adenomas displaying the ultrastructural characteristics of two cell populations {1820}.

Plurihormonal adenomas causing clinical and/or biochemical evidence of GH excess are rare. GH-producing plurihormonal adenomas are typically classified within this group, but acidophil stem cell adenomas and plurihormonal PIT1-positive pituitary adenomas (previously called silent subtype 3 adenomas) can also present with signs and symptoms of acromegaly.

Growth hormone–producing plurihormonal adenomas consist mainly of DGSAs, with variable thyrotroph and mammosomatotroph differentiation. Positivity for PIT1, GH, and alpha subunit, along with

variable positivity for TSH-beta, PRL, estrogen receptor, and low-molecular-weight cytokeratin (perinuclear) is noted {1820}. The ultrastructural features are those of the various PIT1-lineage adenohypophyseal cells.

Drug effects in somatotroph adenomas
Increased numbers of lysosomes, enlargement of secretory granules, increased tumour cell apoptosis, and stromal fibrosis have been variably described in some tumours treated with somatostatin analogues {813,957,1442}. Data on the effects of cabergoline, pegvisomant, and temozolomide treatment are sparse.

Genetic profile
Somatic activating mutations (traditionally called gsp mutations) in *GNAS*, which encodes the G-protein alpha subunit (G$_s$-alpha), have been identified in as many as 40–60% of somatotroph adenomas, typically in adult cases and frequently in DGSAs {94,871,1551, 3053}. Postzygotic somatic activating *GNAS* mutations have also been implicated in pituitary disease related to MAS

{1011,1822,2395,2902}. These mutations result in constitutive activation of the cAMP / protein kinase A pathway, leading to increased intracytoplasmic cAMP levels, hypersecretion of GH, and expression of alpha subunit in somatotrophs. G protein–mediated high cAMP levels may explain the clinical responsiveness of DGSAs to somatostatin analogues, but not all DGSAs harbour these mutations. Therefore, the histological subtype of a somatotroph adenoma is a better predictor of somatostatin responsiveness than is the tumour's *GNAS* mutation status {1551}. Some authors have postulated that the differing somatostatin receptor expression profiles of DGSAs and SGSAs may affect the response to somatostatin analogues {1204,1774}. Somatic *GHR* mutations have been described in SGSAs altering GH autoregulation and STAT signalling {97,100}, but this finding has not been confirmed by others {1551}.

Genomic imbalances have been described at chromosomes 10q, 11q, and 13q {175,694,1438}. No recurring mutations have been found using whole-genome sequencing, but an enrichment of variants affecting the calcium-related and ATP-related pathways, as well as chromosomal losses in chromosomes 1, 6, 13, 14, 15, 16, 18, and 22 and chromosomal gains at chromosomes 12 and X have been {2845}. Whole-genome sequencing has not revealed a recurrent somatic mutation {2332,2845}.

Epigenetic alterations involving *CDKN2A* (also called *P16*), *RB1*, *DAPK1*, *GAD-D45G*, *RHBDD3* (also called *PTAG*), *THBS1* (also called *TSP1*), *RASSF1A*, *FGFR2*, *MGMT*, *CASP8*, *TP73*, and p14 have been described in somatotroph adenomas {2133}. However, most of these alterations are not specific to somatotroph adenomas {2133}. Downregulation of several microRNAs targeting *HMGA1*, *HMGA2*, and *E2F1* has also been identified {597}. *PTTG1* has been shown to have higher mRNA levels in somatotroph adenomas than in non-functioning adenomas {1196}. Subsequent studies demonstrated that expression of the *PTTG1* gene product was indeed higher in various hormone-secreting invasive adenomas {1824}.

Dysregulation of FGFRs has been reported by some authors to play a role in the tumorigenesis of pituitary adenomas {100,817,1824}. IKZF1, a chromatin-remodelling factor that plays an important role in hypothalamic GHRH neuronal development {815}, has been shown to target FGFR4 promoter activity in somatotrophs {816}. The FGFR4-R388 polymorphism has been found to be correlated with tumour size and hormone excess in somatotroph adenomas {2728}.

Genetic susceptibility
Pituitary adenomas are usually sporadic, but they can also arise due to genetic predisposition, either as part of a syndromic disease or as an isolated pituitary disease (see Table 1.03, p. 17). In a large cohort of patients with familial isolated pituitary adenoma, acromegaly was found to be the most common diagnosis {1137}. Acromegaly was also the most common diagnosis among young patients (< 30 years old at disease onset) with non-syndromic pituitary adenoma in which a genetic predisposition could be identified {1137}. Syndromic cases include both paediatric-onset pituitary gigantism and adult-onset acromegaly.

Multiple endocrine neoplasia type 1 and multiple endocrine neoplasia type 4
In older series, somatotroph adenomas were found to be the second most common pituitary manifestation of MEN1 (occurring in 25% of cases) {2746}, but more recent series including patients with regular screening have shown non-functioning adenomas to be far more common {631,1023}. Several acromegaly cases with adult or paediatric onset of disease have been described in MEN4.

SDH-related familial paraganglioma syndromes
SDH-related pituitary adenomas are rare {663,3019,3020}. They present with macroadenomas with characteristic intracytoplasmic vacuoles {663}. Acromegaly cases account for 27% of all described cases {2040}.

Carney complex
Patients with Carney complex have abnormal GH, PRL, and IGF1 levels in as many as 80% of cases, with about 10% presenting with symptomatic acromegaly {2396}. The mean patient age at onset is 36 years, but several paediatric-onset cases have been described. The histological picture is characterized by somatotroph and mammosomatotroph hyperplasia or single or multiple adenomas.

McCune–Albright syndrome
The clinical presentation of MAS is variable, due to the mosaic nature of the disease. The pituitary gland is affected, causing GH excess in 20–30% of cases {2396}, with accompanying hyperprolactinaemia in 80% of cases. The mean patient age at onset of acromegaly is 24.4 years (range: 3–64 years). Macroadenomas account for most of the cases, but microadenomas and hyperplasia have also been described. Immunostaining usually shows mixed somatotroph and lactotroph adenohypophyseal proliferations, but pure somatotroph and plurihormonal samples have also been described.

Neurofibromatosis type 1
Neurofibromatosis may cause optic gliomas with excess GH or possibly GHRH secretion.

Familial isolated pituitary adenoma
Twenty percent of familial isolated pituitary adenoma kindreds are associated with germline AIP mutations. Patient age at onset is in the second or third decade of life in most cases, with very few patients presenting before the age of 10 years {1137}. A substantial proportion of patients have gigantism, which is more common in males. Patients with AIP mutations most often have somatotroph adenomas. Mixed somatotroph and lactotroph adenomas are also common, as are pure lactotroph adenomas and plurihormonal adenomas. Clinically non-functioning pituitary adenomas often stain for GH and/or PRL, but corticotroph, thyrotroph, and gonadotroph adenomas are rare {193,1137}.

X-linked acrogigantism syndrome
Patients with germline or somatic GPR101 microduplication present before the age of 5 years {2808} with pituitary adenoma or pituitary hyperplasia (25% of cases). The majority of the patients have hyperprolactinaemia {2348}. Histological features include mixed somatotroph and lactotroph adenomas rather than mammosomatotroph adenomas {196}.

Prognosis and predictive factors
Uncontrolled GH or IGF1 secretion is associated with high morbidity and mortality. Surgery is the first-line treatment option for somatotroph adenomas {2005}; however, a cure cannot be achieved in all cases of invasive macroadenoma, in particular those associated with cavernous sinus invasion {2005}. Risk stratification is often based on a combination of parameters including histological subtype and tumour invasiveness, as well as the biomarker profile of the tumour, including the Ki-67 proliferation index {1011,1823, 1824}. The detailed histopathological classification of somatotroph adenoma is of clinical significance: SGSAs are less responsive to somatostatin antagonists and may require treatment with the GH receptor antagonist pegvisomant {1011, 1823}. In such cases, somatostatin receptor detection by immunohistochemistry may be a useful predictor of treatment response.

Lactotroph adenoma

Nosé V.
Grossman A.
Mete O.

Definition
Lactotroph adenoma is a pituitary adenoma that expresses mainly prolactin (PRL) and arises from PIT1-lineage adenohypophyseal cells. These tumours are classified into three distinct histological subtypes: sparsely granulated lactotroph adenoma (SGLA), densely granulated lactotroph adenoma (DGLA), and acidophil stem cell adenoma (ASCA).

ICD-O code   8271/0

Synonyms
PRL-producing adenoma; PRL-secreting adenoma; prolactinoma; lactotrope adenoma; lactotroph cell adenoma

Epidemiology
Lactotroph adenomas are the most common pituitary adenoma, accounting for approximately 30–50% of all pituitary adenomas in autopsy and prevalence series {604,1468,1820,2788}. SGLAs are

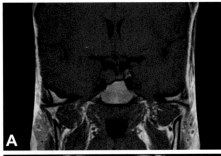
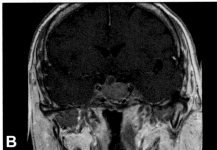

Fig. 1.14 Lactotroph adenoma. **A** Coronal T1-weighted MRI showing a small right-side lactotroph microadenoma in a 25-year-old woman who had an 18-month history of secondary amenorrhoea and a serum prolactin level of 100 g/L. **B** Post-gadolinium coronal T1-weighted MRI of a 50-year-old man with severe headaches and erectile failure; his serum prolactin level was 2500 mg/L.

the most common subtype {1820,1823}, but their incidence is very low in surgical series due to successful pharmacotherapy. Lactotroph adenomas have a female predominance and occur frequently in adults, with a peak incidence among patients aged 21–40 years. Most of these tumours are small in women, but in men they tend to present as invasive macroadenomas or giant adenomas (> 4 cm) {656,657}. Giant adenomas account for 2–3% of all lactotroph adenomas {656, 2811}. Lactotroph adenoma is also the most common pituitary adenoma in childhood and adolescence, with a frequency of 41.5% and 52%, respectively {1499,1640,2121}. Most pituitary carcinomas are lactotroph carcinomas.

Etiology
The etiology and pathogenesis of these adenomas are largely unknown in humans. Estrogens may play a role in the development of experimental lactotroph adenomas and during pregnancy.

Localization
Lactotroph microadenomas are localized in the lateral and posterior part of the anterior pituitary. Some tumours arise in ectopic locations. Ectopic presentations involving the sphenoidal sinus and parapharyngeal region {537,1356,1654,2245, 2529}, clivus, middle nasal meatus, temporal bone, hypothalamus, and third ventricle {74,1401,1627,1761,2245}, as well as parasellar and suprasellar compartments, have also been reported {731,1159}.

Clinical features
Clinical symptoms and signs
Lactotroph adenomas are a frequent cause of reproductive and sexual dysfunction, and the clinical manifestations differ depending on sex {217,2006,2811}. Serum PRL levels correspond approximately with tumour size {1696,2006}. Pretreatment serum PRL levels in men exceed those in women, at least in part because these neoplasms are usually larger in men {1696,2006}. Lactotroph adenomas < 10 mm in diameter are

usually classified as microadenomas. Patients with lactotroph microadenomas generally have serum PRL levels of 100–250 ng/mL. Women usually present at a younger age and tend to have microadenomas, whereas men have substantially larger tumours {656,1696,3015}. PRL levels above the upper limits of normal (25 ng/mL in women and 20 ng/mL in men) as high as 100 ng/mL (rarely, as high as 245 ng/mL) may be an effect of drugs or other causes. Serum PRL levels > 250 ng/mL typically indicate a lactotroph macroadenoma. Giant lactotroph adenomas (> 4 cm) tend to result in PRL levels > 1000 ng/mL {1633,1719}.

The most common symptoms in women with lactotroph adenoma are galactorrhoea, ovulatory disorders, and/or amenorrhoea. At younger ages, women with lactotroph adenoma tend to have microadenomas, due to the readily detected symptoms of galactorrhoea and amenorrhoea, and in general these rarely grow, even in the absence of treatment.

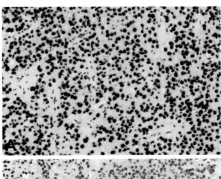
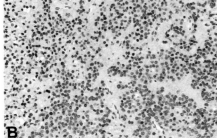

Fig. 1.15 Lactotroph lineage-specific features. Regardless of secretory phenotype and histological subtype, all lactotroph adenomas are positive for the nuclear transcription factor PIT1 (**A**) and estrogen receptor (**B**).

Lactotroph adenomas are less common in men; 80% of lactotroph adenomas in men are macroadenomas, which may present with mass effect symptoms such as visual field abnormalities, hypopituitarism, and sexual dysfunction {656,657}. Visual field defects occur in about 45% of patients with lactotroph macroadenomas, and hypopituitarism in about 35% {1314}; galactorrhoea is rare. In men, lactotroph adenoma symptoms, such as erectile dysfunction and decreased libido, can be more subtle, resulting in delayed intervention.

Lactotroph adenoma in youth usually causes primary amenorrhoea and delayed puberty. Approximately 60–80% of lactotroph adenomas in children present as macroadenomas with symptoms of mass effect {921,1208,1402,1640,2394}.

Unlike DGLAs and SGLAs, ASCAs often present with hyperprolactinaemia and mildly elevated serum growth hormone and IGF1 {1165,1618}.

Imaging
Microadenomas, with subtle radiological abnormalities, are common in women. High-resolution MRI reveals small tumours in most patients with hyperprolactinaemia. On pre-gadolinium coronal T1-weighted MRI, lactotroph microadenomas are generally hypointense relative to the surrounding pituitary; after gadolinium injection, they show early lack of enhancement, although enhancement appears later. Macroadenomas tend to have haemorrhagic features and show suprasellar extension, as well as downward invasion into sinuses and adjacent structures. Macroadenomas are generally characterized by robust contrast enhancement. Microcalcification is frequently observed in lactotroph adenomas.

Macroscopy
Microadenomas are expansile, compressive lesions; they can usually be distinguished from the normal anterior lobe by their soft consistency and their reddish-tan appearance, with a pseudocapsule. Some tumours are firm and greyish-white, containing abundant amyloid stroma. Some tumours have a microscopic invasive pattern. Macroadenomas are usually widely invasive into adjacent structures. Fibrosis, cystic changes, and calcification may be present in macroadenomas, as well as in previously treated tumours {2737}.

Microscopy
Lactotroph adenomas are classified into three clinically relevant histological subtypes: SGLA, DGLA, and ASCA.

Sparsely granulated lactotroph adenoma (SGLA) is composed of chromophobic tumour cells that give a negative periodic acid–Schiff (PAS) reaction. These tumours display a large variety of growth patterns, including diffuse, solid, trabecular, papillary, and pseudopapillary architecture. Elongated cells with indistinct cell membranes can also be encountered. Cellular or nuclear pleomorphism is generally uncommon. Psammoma bodies are occasionally seen. Interstitial fibrosis or amyloid of endocrine type that stains with Congo red and shows apple-green birefringence with polarized light may be present {2060,2638,2645}.

Non-tumorous lactotrophs of human anterior pituitary are sparsely granulated cells displaying characteristic perinuclear Golgi-type staining for PRL. This staining pattern is an important feature that distinguishes SGLAs from other lactotroph adenomas (i.e. DGLAs and ASCAs) {99,1011,1820,1823}. The tumour cells are also positive for PIT1 and estrogen

receptor (ER) {99,1011,1820,1823}. The Ki-67 proliferation index is usually low, but can be higher as a rebound effect in previously treated SGLAs and some aggressive tumours.

Ultrastructurally, the tumour cells display large euchromatic nuclei, prominent nucleoli, well-developed Golgi complexes and rough endoplasmic reticulum forming concentric whorls, and sparse secretory granules measuring 150–300 nm. The hallmark of all lactotroph adenomas is misplaced exocytosis (i.e. extrusion of secretory granules along the lateral cell surfaces) {94}.

Densely granulated lactotroph adenoma (DGLA) has an eosinophilic to acidophilic cytoplasm. DGLAs display strong and diffuse PRL expression throughout the cytoplasm {99,1011,1820,1823} and coexpress PIT1 and ER. Ultrastructurally, the tumour cells have less-abundant rough endoplasmic reticulum and abundant secretory granules as large as 700 nm. Misplaced exocytosis may be seen in this tumour type. DGLA is a rare and aggressive subtype of lactotroph adenoma {99,1011,1820,1823}.

Acidophil stem cell adenoma (ASCA) is composed of tumour cells with variable oncocytic features due to cytoplasmic eosinophilia, accompanied by clear vacuoles reflecting the accumulation of abnormal (often dilated) mitochondria in the cytoplasm {99,1820}. The tumours exhibit stromal fibrosis and nuclear pleomorphism {99,315,1011,2684}.

ASCAs present with hyperprolactinaemia and sometimes mild acromegaly {1165, 1618}. They express PRL (often showing diffuse cytoplasmic staining as seen in DGLAs), growth hormone (variably), PIT1, and ER {1820}. Occasional fibrous bodies can be identified by low-molecular-weight

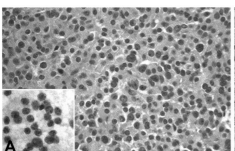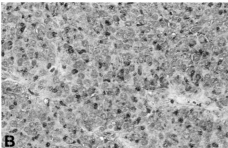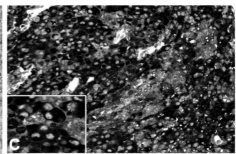

Fig. 1.16 Lactotroph adenoma. **A** Histology and imprint cytology (inset) of a sparsely granulated lactotroph adenoma (SGLA). Note the uniform tumour cells with chromophobic cytoplasm. **B** SGLAs display a characteristic perinuclear Golgi-type staining for prolactin. **C** Diffuse staining for prolactin is a feature of densely granulated lactotroph adenoma.

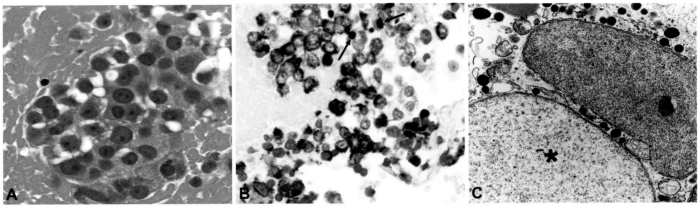

Fig. 1.17 Acidophil stem cell adenoma (ASCA): characteristic features. **A** These tumours are composed of eosinophilic so-called oncocytic cells that exhibit cytoplasmic vacuolization because of dilated and giant mitochondria. **B** Scattered fibrous bodies (arrows) are often identified. **C** Ultrastructural hallmark of ASCAs is the presence of giant mitochondria (asterisk) and dilated mitochondria.

cytokeratin immunostaining {1011,1820, 1823}. Ultrastructurally, the hallmark of these tumours is the presence of numerous dilated or giant mitochondria with loss of cristae {1165}.

Morphological effects of dopamine agonists. The use of dopamine agonists, such as bromocriptine and cabergoline, usually results in a rapid decrease in serum PRL followed by marked morphological changes. The cells become dramatically smaller, with cytoplasmic shrinkage and increased N:C ratios. The nuclei are hyperchromatic. In patients on long-term treatment, extensive perivascular fibrosis and interstitial fibrosis are common. Single-cell necrosis is rare. In some cases, PRL immunoreactivity is decreased and only some cells remain immunopositive. Ultrastructurally, the volumes of rough endoplasmic reticulum and Golgi complexes are markedly reduced. In some cases, a variable response is identified.

Perivascular fibrosis and evidence of prior haemorrhage are common {2638}. Morphologically, lactotroph adenomas with treatment effect may be mistaken for lymphomas, plasmacytomas, or other small round cell tumours. The demonstration of PRL, PIT1, and ER expression distinguishes these tumours.

The morphological alterations are usually rapidly reversible upon discontinuation of medication. Scattered cells can sometimes continue to show ongoing effects {2638}.

Genetic profile

Like other pituitary adenoma subtypes, lactotroph adenomas show abnormal expression of growth regulatory molecules and their receptors, intracellular signal transduction proteins, and cell cycle regulatory molecules. A variety of etiological factors have been implicated in the development of pituitary tumours {98, 99,810}. Epigenetic alterations involving

CDKN2A, *RB1*, *DAPK1*, *GADD45G*, *THBS1* (also called *TSP1*), *RASSF1A*, *FGFR2*, *MGMT*, *CASP8*, *TP73*, and p14 have also been described in lactotroph adenomas {591,2133}, but most of these alterations are not specific to lactotroph adenomas {2133}. Altered gene expression is uncommonly detected, but abnormal microRNAs and somatic mutations have been described. Loss of chromosome 11 has been described in two aggressive lactotroph adenomas and three carcinomas {2986}. Some sporadic lactotroph macroadenomas have also been reported in association with somatic *SDHA* mutations {979} and loss of heterozygosity of the *SDHD* locus {2091}.

Genetic susceptibility

A minority of pituitary adenomas are associated with familial predisposition. Approximately 5% of all pituitary adenomas have a genetic predisposition associated with multiple endocrine neoplasia

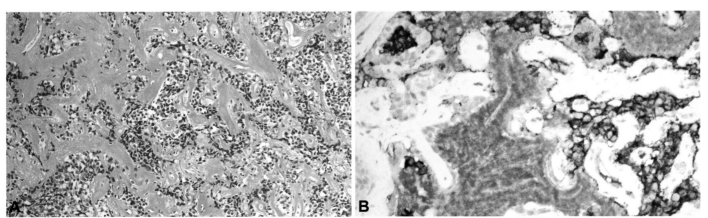

Fig. 1.18 Lactotroph adenoma. **A** Dopamine agonists produce cytoplasmic shrinkage and increased N:C ratios in tumour cells, along with stromal fibrosis, hyalinization, cystic changes, and haemorrhage. Lactotroph adenomas with treatment effect can be mistaken for lymphomas, plasmacytomas, and other small round cell tumours. The expression of PIT1, estrogen receptor, and prolactin (**B**) distinguishes these tumours.

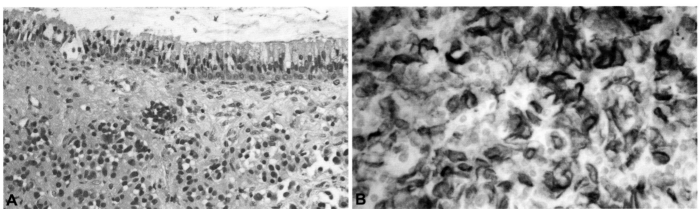

Fig. 1.19 Sinonasal lactotroph adenoma. **A** Respiratory mucosa overlying a monotonous proliferation of adenohypophyseal cells, which are positive for neuroendocrine markers and prolactin. **B** This sinonasal pituitary lactotroph adenoma stained exclusively for prolactin.

type 1 (MEN1) or multiple endocrine neoplasia type 4 (MEN4) {591,2745, 2813}, McCune–Albright syndrome, familial isolated pituitary adenoma {1137, 2868}, *GPR101* microduplication–related X-linked acrogigantism syndrome {196}, SDH-related familial paraganglioma and phaeochromocytoma syndromes {663}, or Carney complex {347,603,605,2027}. Familial pituitary lactotroph adenomas are most commonly associated with MEN1 {655,1747,2027,2865}. The reported prevalence of pituitary adenoma in MEN1 is 20–60% {655,1640}, depending on the study. The mean patient age at onset of pituitary adenoma is 38 ± 15 years, with rare occurrences in children aged < 5 years. About 70% of PRL-expressing pituitary adenomas associated with MEN1 present as either solitary or multicentric lactotroph adenomas {2027,2813}. Others have been shown to be plurihormonal {2813}.

Prognosis and predictive factors

Pharmacotherapy with dopamine agonists is the preferred treatment for lactotroph adenomas. Cabergoline is the main agent used for treating lactotroph adenomas, achieving normoprolactinaemia in > 80% of patients with lactotroph microadenomas and in 75–95% of those with lactotroph macroadenomas. Patients who have invasive macroadenomas with resistance to pharmacotherapy or who are intolerant to medications may require transsphenoidal surgery {2588}. The distinction of typical lactotroph adenoma from ASCA is of clinical significance because ASCAs tend to be more aggressive {99,1011,1820,1823}. Radiotherapy or (rarely) temozolomide may be considered for recurrent aggressive and invasive tumours that fail surgical and conventional pharmacotherapy.

Thyrotroph adenoma

Osamura R. Y.
Grossman A.
Nishioka H.
Trouillas J.

Definition
Thyrotroph adenoma expresses mainly TSH and arises from PIT1-lineage adeno-hypophyseal cells.

ICD-O code   8272/0

Synonyms
TSH-producing adenoma; thyrotropin-secreting adenoma; thyrotrope adenoma

Epidemiology
Thyrotroph adenomas are rare tumours that account for < 2% of all pituitary adenomas {191,192,3038}.

Etiology
As is the case with other types of pituitary adenoma, the etiology of most thyrotroph adenomas remains to be determined, except for a few cases of pituitary adenomas or hyperplasia developing in patients with hypothyroidism {237,1592, 3042} and in families with multiple endocrine neoplasia type 1 {114,555}.

Localization
Most cases are localized in the sella turcica {191,192,3038}. A few cases of

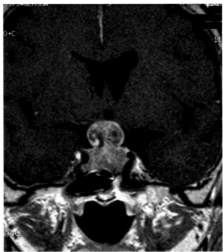

Fig. 1.20 Thyrotroph adenoma. These adenomas are most often macroadenomas and are frequently invasive.

ectopic thyrotroph adenoma in the nasopharynx have been reported {2611}.

Clinical features
Thyrotroph adenomas are a rare cause of hyperthyroidism. Recently developed ultrasensitive TSH immunometric assays have facilitated the diagnosis of this disease. Failure to recognize the presence

of this tumour may result in dramatic consequences, such as inappropriate thyroid ablation that may cause the pituitary volume to further expand. The diagnosis is made on the basis of clinical and biochemical thyrotoxicosis (elevated free thyroxine and triiodothyronine levels) in the presence of normal or high serum TSH. Unless there is evidence of interference with the TSH assay, the major differential diagnosis is the syndrome of thyroid hormone resistance. With thyrotroph adenomas, the ratio of alpha subunit to TSH is elevated and there is little or no TSH response to TRH.

Macroscopy
The tumours are frequently macroadenomas with extrasellar expansion and cavernous sinus invasion {2928,3038}. The average tumour size of clinically nonfunctioning (silent) thyrotroph adenomas has been found to be significantly larger than that of clinically functioning thyrotroph adenomas ($P < 0.05$). Invasiveness was detected in 33% of silent thyrotroph adenomas and 20% of functioning thyrotroph adenomas. In a series published by Saeger et al. {2370}, all cases of thyrotroph adenoma were invasive

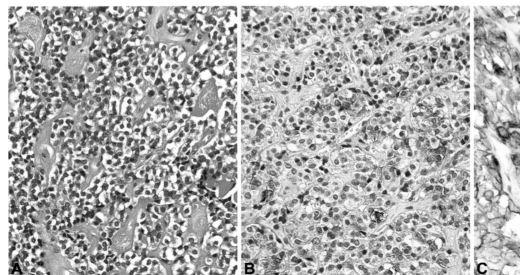
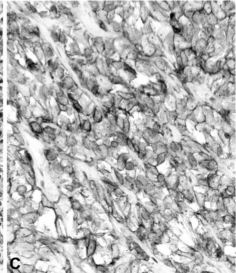

Fig. 1.21 Thyrotroph adenoma. **A** Chromophobic tumour cells, fibrosis, and hyalinization. **B** The tumour cells are immunopositive for TSH-beta. **C** Many tumour cells are immunopositive for SSTR2 on their cell membrane.

macroadenomas, but microadenomas have also been recognized.

Microscopy

The morphological features include chromophobic polygonal or short-spindled tumour cells with pleomorphic nuclei, usually arranged in a diffuse pattern and exhibiting a globoid or whorl-like appearance, with intertwined cytoplasmic processes. Stromal fibrosis and calcification are often noted.

In a given adenoma, the number of cells that are immunopositive for TSH-beta is highly variable {2928}. The tumour cells are frequently positive for both TSH-beta and alpha subunit by immunohistochemistry, suggesting the production and secretion of intact TSH from the tumour cells.

Thyrotroph adenomas frequently (i.e. in 84% of cases) coexpress growth hormone and prolactin without clinical manifestations {1391}. Both PIT1 and GATA2 are expressed in these adenomas. In most cases, the Ki-67 proliferation index is < 3% {3038}.

In most cases, the tumour cells are strongly positive for SSTR2. Membranous SSTR2A and SSTR5 immunoreactivity has been found in the vast majority of thyrotroph adenomas {2928}.

Genetic profile

In a series of sporadic tumours, loss of heterozygosity of 11q13 and inactivating mutations of the *MEN1* gene were described {114}.

Genetic susceptibility

Very occasionally, thyrotroph adenomas are a component of multiple endocrine neoplasia type 1 {1934}.

Prognosis and predictive factors

The Ki-67 proliferation index was found to be related to invasiveness and tumour size in one study {2928}, but was unrelated to tumour size or recurrence in others {620,1391}.

Surgery. With transsphenoidal surgery, total removal with endocrine remission was achieved in 84% of cases overall: in 100% of microadenomas, 81% of macroadenomas, and 38% of cases with cavernous sinus invasion. Of the 8 Knosp grade 4 tumours studied, none could be totally removed with endocrinological remission. Poor surgical outcome may be related to tumour fibrosis, cavernous sinus invasion, or large tumour size {3038}.

Pharmacotherapy. The great majority of cases are exquisitely sensitive to pharmacotherapy with somatostatin analogues such as octreotide or lanreotide, which are effective in reducing TSH secretion in > 90% of cases, with consequent normalization of free thyroxine and free triiodothyronine levels and restoration of the euthyroid state {189,190,192}.

Corticotroph adenoma

Mete O.
Grossman A.
Trouillas J.
Yamada S.

Definition

Corticotroph adenoma is a pituitary adenoma that expresses ACTH and other proopiomelanocortin-derived peptides and arises from TPIT-lineage adenohypophyseal cells. These neoplasms are histologically classified into three subtypes: densely granulated corticotroph adenoma, sparsely granulated corticotroph adenoma, and Crooke cell adenoma.

ICD-O code   8272/0

Synonyms

ACTH-producing adenoma; ACTH-secreting adenoma; corticotropinoma; corticotropic adenoma; corticotrope adenoma

Epidemiology

Cushing syndrome is the constellation of symptoms and signs produced by excess glucocorticoid activity {1983}. If the syndrome occurs secondary to a corticotroph adenoma (or to corticotroph hyperplasia, although this is very rare), it is referred to as Cushing disease {707, 1983}. The annual incidence of Cushing disease is 3–10 cases per 1 million population {2801}. This figure may well be an underestimate, because many cases of mild subclinical Cushing disease may go undiagnosed. Corticotroph adenomas account for approximately 15% of all pituitary adenomas {1820}. The peak incidence is in patients aged 30–50 years. There is a male predominance among prepubertal patients, whereas a female preponderance is seen in adults {1708, 2652,2653}. In the paediatric population, corticotroph adenomas account for approximately 55% of all pituitary adenomas in children aged < 11 years {1499} and 75% of all cases with Cushing syndrome in children aged > 5 years {2653}. The most common histological subtype is densely granulated corticotroph adenoma {1820}.

Etiology

Genetic and epigenetic factors, hormonal stimulation, and growth factors and

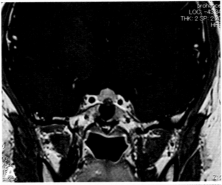
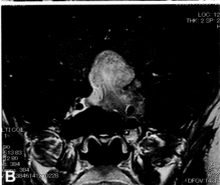

Fig. 1.22 Cushing disease. **A** Most patients with pituitary-dependent Cushing syndrome (i.e. Cushing disease) present with densely granulated corticotroph adenomas (DGCAs), which are usually determined to be microadenomas on MRI. **B** Most sparsely granulated corticotroph adenomas and Crooke cell adenomas and almost all silent corticotroph adenomas (unlike DGCAs) present as invasive macroadenomas. Cavernous sinus invasion is a frequent feature of silent corticotroph adenomas.

their receptors contribute to the tumorigenesis of corticotroph adenomas (see also *Genetic profile*).

Corticotroph adenomas show normal expression of stimulatory CRH and vasopressin (ADH) receptors, normal glucocorticoid receptor expression, and slightly diminished ACTH feedback receptor expression, with no mutations commonly found; the ratio of 11-beta-dehydrogenase isoenzymes 1 and 2 is altered, resulting in deranged cortisol feedback, but this is not specific to corticotroph tumours. The expression of cyclins, cyclin-dependent kinases, and their regulators is altered; the specific alterations in corticotroph adenomas are greatly reduced

expression of p27 and increased expression of cyclin E, and there are also changes in the feedback transcription factors SMARCA4 (also called BRG1) and HDAC2 {253}. Like other pituitary tumours, corticotroph adenomas show increased activity of the pro-proliferative signalling pathways based on PI3K/mTOR and MAPK {730,3018}.

Corticotroph hyperplasia has been reported as a cause of Cushing disease {2015}, although some doubt its existence {2812}. Corticotroph hyperplasia is an extremely rare condition often characterized by diffuse corticotroph proliferation due to either ectopic CRH-secreting tumours (gangliocytoma, neuroendocrine carcinoma, or paraganglioma) {183,691, 875,1822,2034,2442} or untreated Addison disease (also called primary adrenal insufficiency and hypocortisolism) {823, 1822,2994}.

There is evidence of a corticotroph hyperplasia-to-neoplasia progression sequence in the setting of both long-standing untreated Addison disease and prolonged stimulation of ectopic CRH by gangliocytomas {823,1822,2210,2371, 2994}.

Localization

Most corticotroph adenomas are located in the pituitary gland; however, ectopic presentations in the nasal cavity, sphenoidal sinus, cavernous sinus, orbit, clivus, and suprasellar region have also been reported {1055,1271,2501,2509}.

Clinical features

Clinical symptoms and signs

Most corticotroph adenomas are biochemically functioning; however, 20% of corticotroph adenomas lack clinical and biochemical evidence of ACTH and cortisol excess {35,554,1011,1162,2449}. These tumours, called silent corticotroph adenomas, are often detected as incidentalomas or when the tumour causes neurological or ophthalmic symptoms, including acute haemorrhagic necrosis leading to apoplexy {35,1011,1671,1820}. The diagnosis of Cushing disease can be

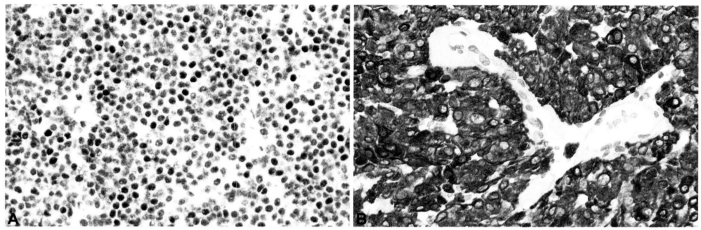

Fig. 1.23 Corticotroph lineage-specific features. **A** Regardless of secretory phenotype and histological subtype, all corticotroph adenomas are positive for the nuclear transcription factor TPIT and (**B**) keratin (CAM5.2).

very difficult without a comprehensive endocrine work-up. Many of the symptoms and signs, such as insulin resistance and diabetes, depression, obesity, and

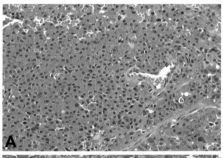

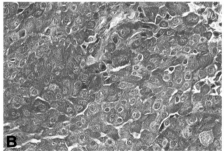

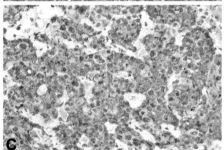

Fig. 1.24 Densely granulated corticotroph adenoma. **A** The tumour cells typically have a basophilic appearance. **B** Tumours are rich in secretory granules that give a positive periodic acid–Schiff (PAS) reaction. **C** Tumour cells show dense granulation on ACTH immunohistochemistry.

hypertension, are common in the general population, whereas Cushing disease is relatively rare. In children, weight gain with growth failure, due in part to inhibition of growth hormone release, is characteristic {707}. Complicating the diagnosis further, there are pseudo-Cushing states (i.e. morbid obesity, depression, anxiety, alcoholism, pregnancy, and certain medication effects) that are also associated with variable degrees of hypercortisolism, simulating Cushing syndrome {707,1820,1983}. Severe Cushing disease and Nelson syndrome (rapid enlargement of corticotroph adenoma with hyperpigmentation and muscle weakness following bilateral adrenalectomy) may cause hyperpigmentation due to overproduction of proopiomelanocortin-derived peptides.

Diagnostic tests
The principal diagnostic tests rely on the autonomous nature of cortisol release in Cushing syndrome, and are based on the failure of normal feedback and loss of circadian rhythmicity. If the disorder is ACTH-dependent, this is usually due to pituitary-dependent Cushing syndrome (i.e. Cushing disease), the diagnosis of which may require confirmation using bilateral inferior petrosal sinus sampling.

Imaging
Most pituitary lesions associated with Cushing disease are solitary microadenomas; 5–10% are macroadenomas {3006}. The ideal diagnostic circumstances are bilateral inferior petrosal sinus sampling indicative of a central source together with a compatible MRI scan. Even when there is clinical and

biochemical evidence of pituitary-dependent Cushing syndrome, failure to localize a lesion is not uncommon; for example, about 10% of Cushing disease cases diagnosed on the basis of endocrine tests were associated with no visible pituitary mass on MRI, even high-definition 3 Tesla MRI {3038A}. Silent corticotroph adenomas tend to present as macroadenomas invading the cavernous sinuses {35,554,1242,3040}.

Macroscopy
Like other pituitary adenomas, corticotroph adenomas are soft and white to greyish-red.

Microscopy
The histopathological correlates of Cushing disease include corticotroph adenoma and carcinoma.

Corticotroph adenomas have a basophilic appearance and give a positive periodic acid–Schiff (PAS) reaction {1011, 1820}. Regardless of the secretory phenotype and histological subtype, corticotroph adenomas are diffusely positive for TPIT, NeuroD1, and low-molecular-weight cytokeratin (CAM5.2) {1011,1820, 1823}.

Densely granulated corticotroph adenomas are composed of basophilic PAS-positive cells that are diffusely and strongly positive for ACTH, consistent with the abundance of secretory granules seen at the ultrastructural level {1011, 1820,1823}.

Sparsely granulated corticotroph adenomas are composed of faintly basophilic or chromophobic PAS-positive cells

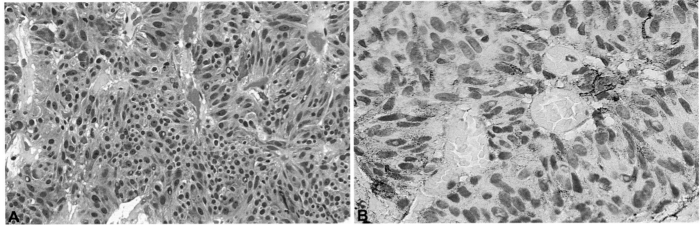

Fig. 1.25 Sparsely granulated corticotroph adenoma (SGCA). **A** Unlike densely granulated corticotroph adenomas, SGCAs are composed of lightly basophilic or chromophobic cells. **B** Positivity for ACTH is often variable, with weak and patchy staining.

with weak or patchy positivity for ACTH, consistent with the scant, small secretory granules seen ultrastructurally {1011, 1820,1823,2007}.

Crooke cell adenomas are composed of tumour cells with Crooke hyaline change. Ring-like cytokeratin expression is typical of these neoplasms {1011,1820,1823}; ACTH expression is dislocated to the cell periphery and juxtanuclear region. Ultrastructurally, intermediate filaments are arranged in a ring-like pattern.

Silent corticotroph adenomas (i. e. clinically non-functioning tumours) are classified into two subtypes: type 1 (densely granulated tumours) and type 2 (sparsely granulated tumours) {35,1820,2449}. Compared with type 1 tumours, type 2 silent corticotroph adenomas have a higher expression of biomarkers of cell invasion, migration, and proliferation, including FGFR4, MMP1, and CD29 (also known as integrin beta-1) {1826}. Rarely, some adenomas lack ACTH expression but express TPIT {2007}.

The proliferative activity of corticotroph adenoma is variable. Reduced p27 expression is common in these tumours {600,1430,1637,2500}. Unlike in functioning tumours, galectin 3 expression has been reported to be weak or absent in silent corticotroph adenomas {2758}. Another study identified galectin 3 expression in aggressive corticotroph adenomas {2291}.

Corticotroph adenomas are the main cause of Cushing disease; the extremely rare diagnosis of carcinoma can only be made when metastasis or cerebrospinal spread occurs. Most corticotroph adenomas are solitary lesions; however, some are a component of double adenoma {808,1800,1810} and others are intermingled with a gangliocytoma {2210, 2371} or adrenal cortical choristoma {49, 538,1828}.

The assessment of the surrounding anterior pituitary is clinically important, to identify Crooke hyaline change of corticotrophs. This morphological change reflects hypercortisolism on the hypothalamic–pituitary–adrenal axis, and is not seen in patients with pseudo-Cushing states or silent corticotroph adenomas {1011,1820,1823}.

Because ACTH expression can also be seen in other sellar neoplasms, including paragangliomas and metastatic neuroendocrine tumours, TPIT positivity is used to confirm corticotroph origin, and is also critical in the diagnosis of metastatic corticotroph carcinoma.

Genetic profile

Many somatic abnormalities have been described in pituitary tumours {730, 2500}, but few are specific to corticotroph adenomas. Recent studies have highlighted the role of the EGFR signalling pathway in the pathogenesis of corticotroph adenomas by revealing activating somatic mutations clustered in the *USP8* gene in approximately 40–60% of corticotroph adenomas {1698,2150, 2271}. *USP8* mutations result in increased mRNA levels of proopiomelanocortin and increased EGFR expression {1698,2150, 2271,2753}. Genotype–phenotype correlations suggest that *USP8* mutations are absent in silent corticotroph adenomas, and most *USP8*-mutant tumours present as small functioning corticotroph

adenomas at earlier patient ages than do wildtype tumours {1698,2150}. A recent study showed that *USP8*-driven corticotroph adenomas also have higher

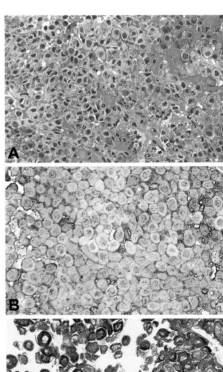

Fig. 1.26 Crooke cell adenoma. **A** These tumours are composed of corticotrophs with Crooke hyaline change. **B** Relocation of secretory granules in Crooke cells can be highlighted using ACTH immunohistochemistry. **C** Staining for keratin (CAM5.2) typically reveals ring-like expression (inset).

expression levels of SSTR5 and MGMT than do those not harbouring *USP8* mutations {1111}. Thus, the *USP8* mutation status may be predictive of responsiveness to pasireotide {1111}. PRKCD silencing results in increased EGFR expression. Recently, PRKCD was found to restrain growth in corticotroph adenomas {953}. miR-26a and PRKCD have been shown to play important roles in cell cycle control of corticotroph adenomas {954}.

Genetic susceptibility

Only very few cases of Cushing disease have been reported in familial isolated pituitary adenoma {2660}, multiple endocrine neoplasia type 1 (*MEN1*) {2566}, or multiple endocrine neoplasia type 4 (*CDKN1B*) {3018}. There have been two reported cases in patients with tuberous sclerosis (*TSC1/2*) {1952,2777} and one in a patient with multiple endocrine neoplasia type 2 {1962}. To date, no germline mutations in *USP8*, *PRKAR1A*, or *GNAS* have been reported in Cushing disease {730,2753,3018}. Germline *DICER1* mutations have been described in pituitary blastoma, a rare cause of infantile-onset Cushing disease {626,2376,2447,2450}.

Prognosis and predictive factors

Persistent Cushing disease is lethal {2182}. Surgery is the treatment of choice and is often curative for microadenomas. For certain tumours, particularly macroadenomas, the cure rate after surgery is lower. Silent corticotroph adenomas and Crooke cell adenomas show a clinically more aggressive behaviour {2449,3030}. Clinically aggressive corticotroph adenomas with low or absent MGMT expression have been reported to respond to temozolomide treatment {85,2393}. Prophylactic radiotherapy at the time of bilateral adrenalectomy may reduce the incidence of Nelson syndrome, but is no longer routine in most centres {2126}.

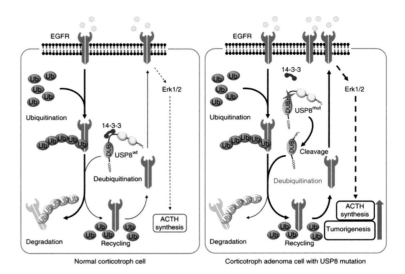

Fig. 1.27 *USP8* mutations in corticotroph adenoma. Schematic representation showing the proposed mechanisms through which *USP8* mutations lead to increased ACTH secretion and tumorigenesis in corticotrophs. Reprinted with permission from Reincke M et al. {2271}.

Gonadotroph adenoma

Yamada S.
Osamura R. Y.
Righi A.
Trouillas J.

Definition
Gonadotroph adenoma produces FSH-beta, LH-beta, and/or alpha subunit and arises from SF1-lineage adenohypophyseal cells. The most relevant criteria for the diagnosis of gonadotroph adenoma are immunohistochemical findings.

ICD-O code   8272/0

Synonyms
Gonadotropin-producing adenoma; gonadotropin-secreting adenoma; gonadotroph cell adenoma; gonadotrope adenoma; gonadotropinoma

Epidemiology
The incidence and prevalence rates of gonadotroph adenomas are difficult to estimate, and depend on the method of surveillance. In pathological studies of surgically removed pituitary adenomas, 25–29% were diagnosed as clinically non-functioning adenomas {2370,2914}, and 43–64% were classified as gonadotroph adenomas {2007,2370,3040}. Gonadotroph adenomas usually occur in middle-aged and older people, with a slight male preponderance, and are rare among individuals aged < 25 years {3043}. Gonadotroph carcinomas are exceptional {188,2328}.

Etiology
Gonadotroph adenomas are generally believed to arise spontaneously. Several case reports have suggested that some gonadotroph adenomas may be secondary to longstanding primary hypogonadism {1465,1980}.

Localization
Gonadotroph adenomas usually occur as macroadenomas. They often present with suprasellar and parasellar extension, with cavernous sinus invasion, or with a multilobulated configuration of the suprasellar portion.

Clinical features
Most gonadotroph adenomas are clinically non-functioning, with a history of

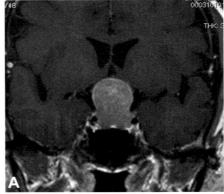
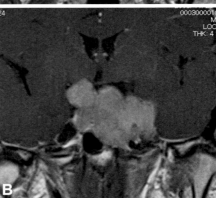

Fig. 1.28 Gonadotroph adenoma. These tumours are usually non-functioning adenomas and therefore often found as macroadenomas. Most are non-invasive (**A**), but some are invasive giant adenomas (**B**), as seen here on enhanced coronal T1-weighted MRI.

normal pubertal development and fertility. The tumours usually come to medical attention due to symptoms related to mass effects, such as visual disturbances, headaches, and hypopituitarism. Diminished libido and/or impotence are present in most male patients, and various degrees of other anterior pituitary hormone deficiencies occur. Among premenopausal women, menstrual disturbances and/or galactorrhoea are seen in many patients, whereas in postmenopausal women the most common clinical manifestations are related to mass effects. In rare cases, pituitary apoplexy can be the presenting symptom. However, with the widespread use of CT and MRI examination, the number of patients

in whom gonadotroph adenomas are found as pituitary incidentalomas is increasing {797}. Serum LH and FSH levels are usually not elevated by clinically non-functioning adenomas. Mild hyperprolactinaemia (usually of < 100 ng/mL) is often found.

Ntali et al. {2031} reviewed the clinical characteristics of clinically functioning gonadotroph adenomas and found that most cases are macroadenomas, constituting a rare clinical entity with distinctive manifestations (mainly menstrual irregularity and ovarian hyperstimulation syndrome in premenopausal females and adolescent girls, testicular enlargement in males, and isosexual precocious puberty in children). Premenopausal women with clinically functioning gonadotroph adenomas show normal or elevated FSH levels, suppressed LH levels, elevated estradiol levels, supranormal concentrations of prolactin, and evidence of ovarian hyperstimulation syndrome; in men, supranormal FSH concentrations may occur in association with testicular enlargement. In children, these tumours may cause precocious puberty {2031}.

On MRI, most gonadotroph adenomas can be identified as non-invasive, with

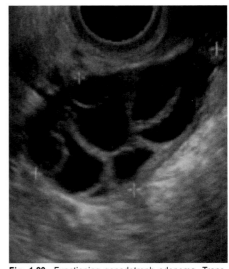

Fig. 1.29 Functioning gonadotroph adenoma. Transvaginal ultrasonography in a 32-year-old woman with ovarian hyperstimulation syndrome shows an enlarged polycystic right ovary.

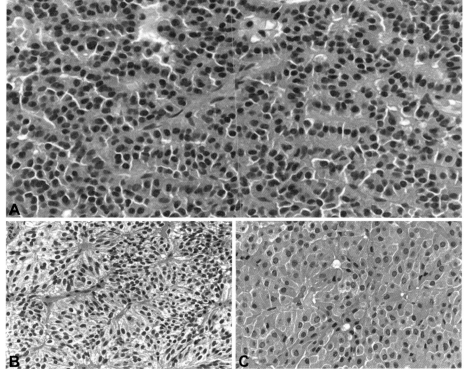

Fig. 1.30 Gonadotroph adenoma. **A** These tumours consist of chromophobic cells with prominent sinusoidal, trabecular, or tubular architecture along the blood vessels, which (**B**) often show markedly elongated cells arranged in a papillary (pseudorosette) pattern. **C** The tumours also show a diffuse pattern in some parts, and these polygonal cells possess abundant eosinophilic cytoplasm due to mitochondria accumulation (oncocytic change). No cellular or nuclear pleomorphism is noted in these tumours.

suprasellar or infrasellar tumour extension. Giant adenomas and marked cavernous sinus invasion are seen less commonly than in other silent adenomas {2008}.

Surgery is the primary treatment for gonadotroph adenomas. Postoperative radiation therapy may be indicated in cases with a large postoperative remnant or regrowth; pharmacotherapy seems to be of limited value in gonadotroph adenomas but may occasionally be effective {426, 1038}.

Macroscopy

Gonadotroph adenomas are usually large, with substantial suprasellar or infrasellar extension associated with sellar enlargement or destruction. They are well-vascularized, soft, tan to dark-brown tumours. They rarely appear as cystic adenomas and often contain areas of necrosis or haemorrhage. Some are invasive to the surrounding tissues.

Microscopy

Light microscopy shows that gonadotroph adenomas are chromophobic and give a negative periodic acid–Schiff (PAS) reaction, although they may have weak, minimal cytoplasmic PAS positivity. Variable oncocytic change may be seen. A distinctive perivascular papillary (pseudorosette) arrangement is a consistent and prominent histological feature of gonadotroph adenomas, but diffuse and sinusoidal arrangements are also seen. The tumour cells are small to medium-sized and polygonal. They exhibit marked polarity, with elongated cell processes in the areas of pseudorosette formation, a feature suggestive of gonadotroph differentiation {1439}. Nuclear pleomorphism is not marked, and mitoses are rare.

Diffuse and strong immunopositivity for FSH-beta, LH-beta, or alpha subunit is rare. Instead, most adenomas are immunopositive for one or more gonadotropin subunits. The type and proportion of immunopositive cells vary from adenoma to adenoma and from one area to another within the same tumour. These variations reflect cellular heterogeneity or may be due to differences in fixation, in the specificity of the antibodies, in antigen retrieval or signal amplification techniques {2411}, or in the methods of immunohistochemistry (automation platforms, manual technique, etc.) {1444}. Due to these technical issues, the great majority of tumours diagnosed as null cell adenomas or immunonegative adenomas are in fact gonadotroph adenomas {1439}. In one series, the proportion of tumours identified as immunonegative decreased from 10% to 1% with the use of an automated method {426,2411}.

The most common immunohistochemical type is the FSH-beta type or FSH-beta / alpha subunit type; the LH-beta type is the least common. In the great majority of tumours, the immunopositive cells are scattered throughout the fragments, but are often clustered; some fragments can be completely immunonegative. A high proportion of immunopositive cells may be observed, especially in clinically functioning gonadotroph adenomas. The immunoreactivity is strong within the cytoplasmic processes in polar cells, where accumulation of secretory granules is prominent, whereas the granules are diffuse in non-polar cells. However, from a practical standpoint, it is usually unnecessary to take into account such immunohistochemical heterogeneity within an individual tumour when diagnosing a clinically non-functioning adenoma as gonadotroph adenoma {3041}. Recently, it was reported that the SF1 transcription factor may play a complementary role in hormone-negative tumours {2007}.

Gonadotroph adenomas are also immunopositive for synaptophysin, chromogranin A, inhibin, and activin. They also express SSTR2 and SSTR5 {496, 2238}.

Genetic profile

Whole-exome sequencing studies of sporadic clinically non-functioning gonadotroph adenomas have shown that the somatic mutation rate is lower than in other tumour types. Genetic events (e.g. epigenetic changes and copy-number variations) other than a recurring somatic mutation are likely responsible for the pathogenesis of most gonadotroph adenomas {1973}. Cell proliferation may be controlled by the interplay between proliferative PTTG1, antiproliferative cell-specific FOXL2, and clusterin {478,738}. Silencing of the *DLK1-MEG3* locus on chromosome 14q32 was found to play an important role in the development of

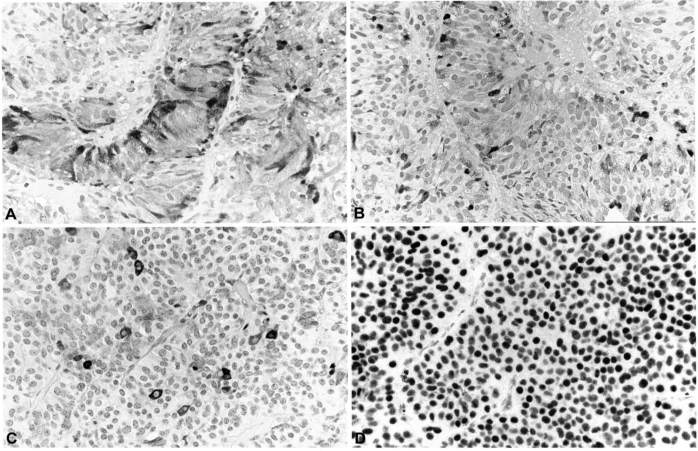

Fig. 1.31 Gonadotroph adenoma. **A** This tumour shows strong immunopositivity for FSH-beta and (**B**) less-intense reactivity for LH-beta. **C** In some tumours, only scattered cells are immunopositive for gonadotropin subunits; FSH-beta in this case. **D** The vast majority of the tumour cell nuclei are immunopositive for SF1.

human non-functioning adenomas (most of which were gonadotroph adenomas). The tumour suppressor function of this locus is at least in part attributed to the antiproliferative function of several genes within the locus, including *MEG3* and *MIR134* {489}.

Hypermethylation of the *CDKN2A* gene and loss of p16 protein are associated with clinically non-functioning adenomas, including gonadotroph adenomas {2358, 2567}.

Genetic susceptibility

Studies investigating germline or somatic mutations involving genes associated with hereditary pituitary adenomas (e.g. *AIP*, *MEN1*, *CDKN1B*, and *PRKAR1A*)

or activating mutations in *GNAS* have reported that these mutations are rarely observed in clinically non-functioning pituitary adenomas, including gonadotroph adenomas {1803}. However, gonadotroph adenomas have been rarely reported in patients with multiple endocrine neoplasia type 1 or familial isolated pituitary adenoma {2254,2689}.

Prognosis and predictive factors

In general, patient age, patient sex, and tumour size at diagnosis are not predictive factors for recurrence {710,2264}. Tumour invasion, especially in the cavernous sinus, is the major risk factor for incomplete removal and tumour recurrence {327,562}. Complete tumour

resection, as assessed by postoperative MRI, is associated with lower recurrence rates (10–20% at 5 years and 30% at 10 years) than is partial tumour removal (25–40% at 5 years and > 50% at 10 years) {562}.

No single biomarker has been found to independently predict aggressive behaviour in gonadotroph adenomas {920, 1820,2256}.

The Ki-67 proliferation index has been shown to be the most reliable marker of biological behaviour in non-functioning adenomas {2238,2390,2814}. Ki-67 labelling may be not predictive of recurrence risk, but could be a useful predictor of progression risk in tumour remnants.

Null cell adenoma

Nishioka H.
Kontogeorgos G.
Lloyd R. V.
Lopes M. B. S.
Mete O.
Nosé V.

Definition
Null cell adenoma is an adenoma composed of adenohypophyseal cells that show no evidence of cell-type–specific differentiation by immunohistochemistry for pituitary hormones and transcription factors.

Most of the data discussed in this section refer to the previous definition of null cell adenoma as a hormone-immunonegative adenoma. The data on null cell adenoma as it is currently defined are limited {2007, 2238}.

ICD-O code   8272/0

Synonyms
Hormone-immunonegative adenoma; transcription factor–immunonegative adenoma

Epidemiology
Null cell adenomas usually develop in elderly individuals, with a slight male preponderance {148,3039}. At the time of surgical intervention, most patients with null cell adenoma are in their sixth decade of life, although oncocytic null cell adenomas are common in the seventh decade of life {2007,2009,3037}. Hormone-immunonegative adenomas account for 5–30% of all surgically removed adenohypophyseal tumours {1439, 1444}. Hormone-negative and transcription factor-negative null cell tumours constitute < 5% of clinically non-functioning adenomas {2007}.

Localization
Null cell adenomas develop from the anterior pituitary; however, rare ectopic presentations have been reported.

Clinical features
Patients with null cell adenomas usually present with symptoms of mass effects, including visual disturbance, headaches, and various degree of hypopituitarism. They show no clinical symptoms of hormonal excess apart from occasional mild hyperprolactinaemia due to stalk section effect. A few cases are detected due to

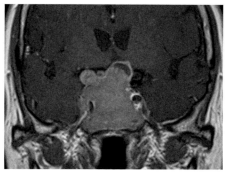

Fig. 1.32 Null cell adenoma. Gadolinium-enhanced coronal MRI showing a large macroadenoma with right cavernous sinus invasion and multilobulated growth of the suprasellar portion.

a neurological deterioration associated with pituitary apoplexy; others are diagnosed as incidentalomas on imaging studies {1886}.

Null cell adenomas are mostly macroadenomas with suprasellar extension. They often show cavernous sinus invasion and/or sphenoidal sinus extension. They are mostly solid tumours; however, cystic change or haemorrhagic components can occasionally be identified.

Macroscopy
The tumours are usually grey or yellowish-tan and soft.

Microscopy
Null cell adenomas are typically composed of chromophobic or weakly acidophilic round to polyhedral tumour cells that give a negative periodic acid–Schiff (PAS) reaction and are arranged in diffuse or sheet-like patterns. Unlike in gonadotroph adenomas, papillary and pseudopapillary growth patterns are less common. Oncocytic null cell adenomas are referred to as pituitary oncocytomas {3037}. Pleomorphic nuclei and mitotic figures are uncommon.

Ultrastructure
Ultrastructurally, null cell adenomas are composed of small or polyhedral cells with poorly developed Golgi complexes and scattered rough endoplasmic reticulum. A few small secretory granules

can be identified {1466}. Tumours with oncocytic change display abundant mitochondria {3037}.

Immunophenotype
Null cell adenomas are immunonegative for adenohypophyseal hormones (i.e. ACTH, GH, prolactin, TSH-beta, FSH-beta, LH-beta, and alpha subunit) and transcription factors (i.e. TPIT, PIT1, SF1, and GATA2) {1466,1820,2007}. Anti-mitochondrial antibody demonstrates the mitochondrial accumulation in the cytoplasm, which is in keeping with the electron microscopic findings {2009}. Null cell adenomas express chromogranin A and synaptophysin, and may be negative for cytokeratin. They may have a higher Ki-67 proliferation index than do gonadotroph adenomas {148}.

Variability in staining results may be due to technical differences in fixation, specificity and sensitivity of the antibodies, antigen retrieval, and signal amplification techniques {2411}, or in the methods of immunohistochemistry (automation platforms, manual technique, etc.) {1444}.

Differential diagnosis
Because the term "null cell adenoma" is restricted to pituitary adenoma that has no morphological, immunohistochemical, or ultrastructural evidence of any adenohypophyseal cell differentiation, the diagnosis of null cell adenomas is a diagnosis of exclusion from neuroendocrine proliferations in the sellar region. Immunohistochemistry for pituitary

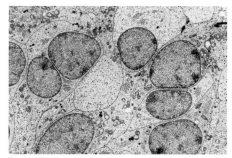

Fig. 1.33 Null cell adenoma. Ultrastructure of a case showing poorly developed cytoplasmic organelles and a few small secretory granules.

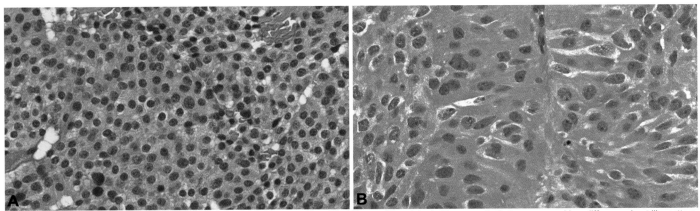

Fig. 1.34 A Null cell adenoma, typically composed of chromophobic or weakly acidophilic round to polyhedral tumour cells that are arranged in a diffuse or sheet-like pattern. **B** Oncocytic null cell adenoma. These tumours are composed of tumour cells with bright eosinophilic cytoplasm.

transcription factors is crucial, to prevent hormone-immunonegative adenomas from being mistakenly diagnosed as null cell adenoma {1820,2007}. A substantial proportion of gonadotroph adenomas are hormone-immunonegative, and can only be distinguished by their SF1 and ER-alpha immunoreactivity {1820}. Both null cell adenomas and gonadotroph adenomas are immunonegative for PIT1. When diagnosing keratin-negative and transcription factor–negative endocrine tumours, the possibility of pituitary paraganglioma should also be investigated. Positivity for tyrosine hydroxylase, which is the rate-limiting enzyme in catecholamine synthesis, confirms the diagnosis of pituitary paraganglioma {1820}. Metastatic neuroendocrine neoplasm should also be considered in the differential diagnosis of null cell adenoma. Whereas most metastatic tumours have more proliferative features compared with null cell adenomas, positivity for TTF1, CDX2, ISL1, and PDX1 in a sellar neuroendocrine tumour supports the diagnosis of metastatic neuroendocrine tumour {1820}.

Genetic profile

Comparative genomic hybridization studies of pituitary tumours (including null cell adenomas) comparing primary and recurrent tumours have shown that chromosomal imbalances are more common in recurrent adenomas {2285}. In null cell adenomas, methylation has been reported in the promoter region of multiple genes, including *LGALS3* (the gene encoding galectin 3) {2357}, *PLAGL1* (also known as *ZAC*) {2080}, the long noncoding RNA *MEG3a* {950}, and *WIF1* {767}. Several of these genes have antiproliferative or tumour suppressor functions, and promoter methylation lowers the expression of several of these genes. Recent studies have characterized a gene designated *ENC1*, which plays an important role in invasion in null cell adenomas {843}.

Genetic susceptibility

Patients with multiple endocrine neoplasia type 1 have an increased susceptibility to the development of pituitary tumours, including null cell adenomas. In a recent study of patients with multiple endocrine neoplasia type 1 and pituitary adenomas, 3% of the patients in the series had immunonegative adenomas {2813}. In patients with familial isolated pituitary adenoma, 13% of adenomas were immunonegative adenomas {195}.

Prognosis and predictive factors

The prognosis of null cell adenoma after complete surgical excision is good. The most significant factor associated with recurrence is extent of surgical resection. Complete resection is difficult in cases with a giant invasive tumour with extrasellar extension. Radiotherapy is beneficial for residual tumours. The Ki-67 proliferation index may be another useful prognostic marker.

Plurihormonal and double adenomas

Kontogeorgos G.
Kovacs K.
Lloyd R.V.
Righi A.

Definition

Plurihormonal adenomas are adenohypophyseal tumours that produce more than one hormone. They can be monomorphous, consisting of a single cell type producing two (or rarely more) hormones, or plurimorphous, consisting of two or more different cell lineages. Plurihormonal adenomas include plurihormonal PIT1-positive adenoma (previously called silent subtype 3 adenoma) {782,1166,1167,1820}, clinically functioning adenomas such as growth hormone (GH) / prolactin (PRL) / TSH–producing adenomas with acromegaly and thyroid dysfunction, and adenomas with unusual immunohistochemical combinations that cannot be explained by cytodifferentiation {1776,1800,2353,2878}. Adenomas that produce combinations of GH and PRL, or FSH and LH, are not considered plurihormonal in this sense.

Double adenomas are composed of two separate tumours with two different cell types in the same gland {1443}. More than two tumours can also coexist (multiple adenomas) {1015,1440}.

ICD-O code   8272/0

Synonyms

Polyhormonal adenomas; multiple adenomas

Epidemiology

Plurihormonal PIT1-positive adenoma is estimated to account for 0.9% of all adenomas {782}. Other plurihormonal adenomas with unusual combinations are also rare. Plurihormonal PIT1-positive adenomas have a slight female predilection and a substantial preponderance in younger patients {782,3040}.

The reported incidence rates of double adenomas are 0.4–1.3% in surgical series {1443,1877} and 0.9–1.85% in autopsy material {1015,1440}.

Etiology

The etiology remains uncertain. Adenomas belonging to two different cytogenetic lineages might originate from the incidental occurrence of two monoclonal components of transformed adenohypophyseal cells. Alternatively, they might be derived from clonal expansions of uncommitted cells having undergone multidirectional differentiation {1443}.

Localization

The tumours are located in the pituitary, with no reports of ectopic adenomas.

Clinical features

Most plurihormonal PIT1-positive adenomas are silent, although some patients do present with acromegaly, hyperprolactinaemia, or hyperthyroidism {782, 1166,1820}.

Double adenomas are synchronously diagnosed, although asynchronous development has been reported {1440,1443, 2759}. Most multiple adenomas are found incidentally in autopsy material {1015, 1440}. Triple adenomas are rare in surgical series {2086,2248}. They may also coexist with other pituitary tumours or tumour-like lesions {1461,3071}. Double

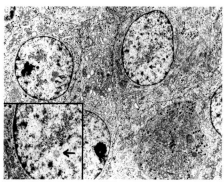

Fig. 1.36 Plurihormonal PIT1-positive adenoma. Typical ultrastructural features include large cells with irregular nuclei, nuclear spheridia (arrows), and prominent Golgi complexes.

and other unusual plurihormonal adenomas may be associated with endocrine symptoms due to hormone production by one or both adenomas {1290,2791}, or may be non-functioning {1443}. Imaging may identify two separate adenomas preoperatively {635,1364,2549}.

Due to the combined hormone secretion by functioning plurihormonal or double adenomas, clinical diagnosis is difficult. Double adenomas may be the reason for surgical failure in cases in which only one adenoma is removed and the other is left behind {1440,2791}.

Macroscopy

Most plurihormonal adenomas present as macroadenomas, whereas most double adenomas are microadenomas {782, 1167,1440}.

Microscopy

Plurihormonal PIT1-positive adenomas are chromophobic and give a negative periodic acid–Schiff (PAS) reaction. They are variably positive for GH, PRL, TSH-beta, alpha subunit, and ACTH, and show extensive nuclear PIT1 expression {782,1166,1820,1825}. Electron microscopy may be useful for the confirmation of this diagnosis, revealing abundant nuclear spheridia and sparse secretory granules measuring 50–250 nm {782, 1825}. Some tumours show glycoprotein hormone cell differentiation {782}.

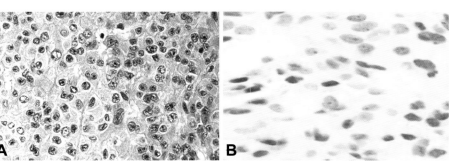

Fig. 1.35 Plurihormonal PIT1-positive adenoma. **A** Many tumour cells contain eosinophilic cytoplasm and markedly atypical nuclei with two nucleoli. **B** Many tumour cells contain PIT1-positive nuclei.

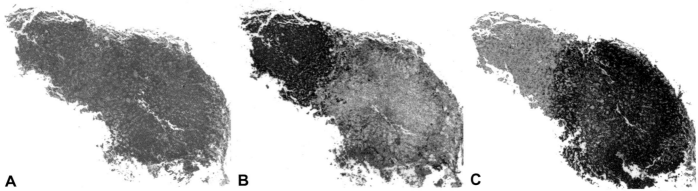

Fig. 1.37 Double pituitary adenoma. **A** A fragment including two clearly separated adenomas: in the upper part an acidophilic growth hormone–producing adenoma (**B**) and in the lower a chromophobic prolactin-producing adenoma (**C**).

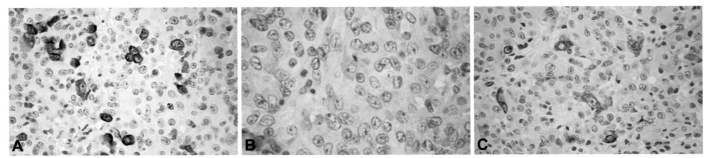

Fig. 1.38 Plurihormonal PIT1-positive adenoma. **A** Growth hormone–positive. **B** Prolactin-positive. **C** TSH-positive tumour cells.

Other plurihormonal adenomas include GH/ACTH-secreting adenomas {89,1776, 2236}, PRL/ACTH-secreting adenomas {808,1290,1800}, GH/PRL/TSH-secreting adenomas, and other (less common) combinations {808,2246,2878}.

Of the double adenomas, silent lactotroph adenomas with other adenoma types are the most frequent in autopsy series, whereas functioning somatotroph adenomas are most common in surgical series {1440,2248,2414}. Transsphenoidally removed double adenomas with the same immunoprofile cannot be recognized as separate tumours {1443}. Immunohistochemistry with transcription factors such as PIT1, TPIT, and SF1 can identify the divergent lineages of cytodifferentiation in double adenomas {1250}.

Genetic susceptibility

Few cases of double adenomas and plurihormonal PIT1-positive adenomas are associated with multiple endocrine neoplasia type 1 {2813} or familial pituitary adenoma unrelated to multiple endocrine neoplasia type 1 {782,1310,2414}.

Prognosis and predictive factors

Plurihormonal PIT1-positive adenomas are aggressive in terms of their size, growth rate, and invasiveness, with cavernous sinus invasion occurring in 67% of cases. They also have a 59% rate of persistent tumour and a 29–31% rate of recurrence {782,1166,3040}. Plurihormonal PIT1-positive carcinomas have also been reported {2330}. Some plurihormonal PIT1-positive adenomas express somatostatin receptors and respond well to treatment with long-acting somatostatin analogues {1166}. *MGMT* promoter methylation was noted in 42% and 33% of plurihormonal PIT1-positive adenomas and carcinomas, respectively. Low or negative immunohistochemical MGMT expression may predict response to temozolomide {2392}.

Pituitary carcinoma

Roncaroli F.
Kovacs K.
Lloyd R. V.
Matsuno A.
Righi A.

Definition

Pituitary carcinoma is strictly defined as a tumour of adenohypophyseal cells that metastasizes craniospinally or is associated with systemic metastasis. The definition is independent of the histological appearance.

ICD-O code   8272/3

Epidemiology

Pituitary carcinoma is uncommon. It accounts for about 0.12% of the adenohypophyseal tumours in the German Pituitary Tumour Registry {2370} and 6% of the invasive adenomas in the SEER database (although this figure is probably an overestimate) {1080}. The population-based RARECARE project, focused on rare cancers in Europe, estimated the annual incidence of endocrine carcinomas in Europe to be < 0.1 cases per 100 000 population {2846}; however, the fact that clinically silent metastases are sometimes discovered only at autopsy suggests that the reported incidence and prevalence rates of pituitary carcinoma could be underestimated {1301}. Pituitary carcinomas in children are exceptional {1187}. A slight female predominance is observed in the SEER database, with a female-to-male ratio of 1.33:1. The median patient age at diagnosis is in the sixth decade of life (range: 12 to > 70 years). More than 70% of reported cases are lactotroph and corticotroph carcinomas. Clinically non-functioning carcinomas present at a younger patient age than do their benign counterparts.

Etiology

The etiology of pituitary carcinoma is still unclear. No environmental or predisposing factors seem to increase the risk of developing metastases in patients with adenoma. Radiotherapy is not a risk factor for the progression of a pituitary adenoma to carcinoma {1851}. A stepwise process of transformation from a slow-growing adenoma into an invasive adenoma and eventually into a carcinoma, and much less frequently, the de novo development of carcinoma from either a normal gland or a conventional adenoma have been suggested {676}. In a single case report, the evidence of a loss-to-retention pattern in metastatic deposits compared with the pre-metastatic adenoma suggested at least two clones in the primary tumour, one of which gave rise to metastases {341}.

Localization

The primary lesion is located in the sellar region. There have been only two reported cases of ectopic adenomas that developed multiple metastases to the subarachnoid space and brain {1169,1306}. Metastases frequently occur within the craniospinal axis as the result of dissemination in the subarachnoid space {2153}; deep deposits in the brain parenchyma more often affect the cortex and cerebellum {1301}. Systemic metastases are most frequent in the bone, lymph nodes, liver, and lungs {2153}; unusual sites include the heart {914}, pancreas {914}, orbit {1527}, ovary and myometrium {2153}, middle ear {2993}, and endolymphatic sac {137}. Haematogenous dissemination can occur via the petrosal sinus. Because the pituitary gland has no lymphatic vessels, spread to lymph nodes may result from invasion of the skull and soft tissue {2446}. Tissue manipulation during surgery is unlikely to contribute to dissemination.

Clinical features

Like conventional adenomas, pre-metastatic lesions and metastases can be hormonally active or clinically non-functioning; endocrinologically active carcinomas are considerably more common {2231}. There are no clinical or biochemical features specific to an adenoma that will metastasize. Metastases from hormonally active primary tumours usually remain active and often sustain the endocrine syndrome when the sellar lesion is removed {1118}. Diabetes insipidus is uncommon. Progression to carcinoma has been documented in patients with Nelson syndrome {1343}. Persistence

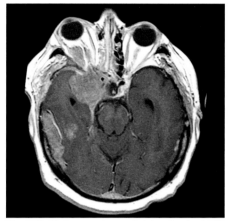

Fig. 1.39 Pituitary carcinoma. Axial postcontrast MRI shows multiple dural and intra-axial metastatic deposits from a pituitary corticotroph carcinoma.

of elevated hormone concentration after extensive or gross total removal of a functioning adenoma should prompt a search for metastases. The signs and symptoms of hormonally inactive metastases depend on the site of the deposit. Pain and fractures typically occur when the bone is involved. Metastases from clinically non-functioning tumours can remain asymptomatic for a long time, and may be found only at postmortem examination {1301}. Pre-metastatic lactotroph carcinomas and metastases typically develop resistance to dopamine agonists {1118}. Resistance can be present at onset or can be acquired during the course of treatment {2159}.

Macroscopy

Primary lesions usually present as invasive macroadenomas. Only a few microadenomas and lesions confined to the sella have been reported. The gross appearance of a pituitary carcinoma may be the same as that of any usual adenoma. Intra-axial and systemic metastases are indistinguishable from deposits of other solid cancers. Dural metastases can be indistinguishable from meningioma, particularly when slow-growing. Neuroimaging features of the primary lesion and metastases are the same as those of conventional adenomas {1760}.

Microscopy

There are no histological criteria that allow for the distinction between a locally invasive adenoma and an adenoma that will progress to carcinoma {1301}. For a diagnosis of pituitary carcinoma to be rendered, the following criteria must be met: (1) the primary lesion must be a histologically proven adenohypophyseal tumour; (2) an alternative primary lesion must be excluded; (3) there must be discontinuous spread in the craniospinal axis; and (4) the pathological features of metastases should be similar to those of the primary pituitary tumour. Neuronal differentiation is a rare event in pituitary carcinoma {2448}.

Extra-CNS metastases are often amenable to fine-needle aspiration, with a diagnostic accuracy believed to be comparable to that of frozen sections {3034}. The features seen on smears and imprints are those of a neuroendocrine carcinoma, and vary from bland to overtly malignant. Cytological appearances are often similar to those of the primary or recurrent sellar lesions.

About 60% of primary tumours have features of a conventional adenoma, but they may show more-proliferative features when they recur. Such tumours are usually associated with prolonged survival. Metastases often have more-abnormal histological features than the primary tumour, including abnormal mitotic figures, a high Ki-67 proliferation index, and vascular invasion. Less commonly, metastatic deposits retain the original benign appearance.

Immunophenotype

Both primary and metastatic tumours express markers of neuroendocrine differentiation, such as chromogranin A and synaptophysin. As is the case in conventional adenomas, expression of pituitary hormones is variable. Lactotroph carcinomas are the most common, followed by corticotroph carcinomas, including silent tumours {2331}, Crooke cell carcinomas {1463}, and carcinomas occurring in Nelson syndrome {916}. Carcinomas of the remaining adenoma subtypes, including somatotroph, thyrotroph, gonadotroph, and null cell adenomas, have mostly been reported in small series or individual case reports {1585,1786,1858,2231, 2328,2330,2451,2741}, and account for < 30% of cases overall. Rare examples of corticotroph carcinoma cosecrete ACTH,

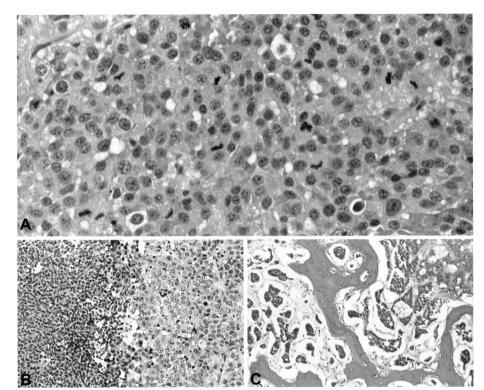

Fig. 1.40 Pituitary carcinoma. **A** This primary sellar lesion of a lactotroph carcinoma shows brisk mitotic activity. **B** In this sellar recurrence of a lactotroph carcinoma, features of conventional adenoma are juxtaposed with a distinct population of larger cells with atypical nuclei and prominent nucleoli. **C** This bone deposit from a silent corticotroph carcinoma shows the histopathological features of conventional adenoma.

CRH, and proopiomelanocortin {1961}.
The expression of several proteins, including BCL2 {1488}, topoisomerase 2-alpha {2875}, cyclooxygenase-2 {2874}, galectin 3 {2304}, and VEGF {1658}, has been reported to be higher in pituitary carcinomas than in adenomas. Other proteins, such as beta-catenin {2834} and p27 (also called p27^Kip1) {1614,2446}, are less expressed in pituitary carcinomas. In one reported case of pituitary carcinoma, menin was undetectable {2752}.

In both primary lesions and metastatic deposits, the Ki-67 proliferation index is higher in pituitary carcinomas than in conventional adenomas, with values as high as 45% reported in metastatic deposits {2331}. In primary lesions, values ≥ 10% have been associated with aggressive behaviour, and may suggest a diagnosis of carcinoma for the primary tumour {1301}. However, there is considerable overlap between indolent adenomas and lesions that metastasize.

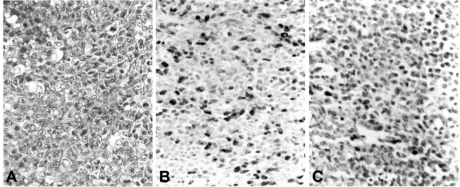

Fig. 1.41 Pituitary carcinoma. **A** This primary lesion of null cell carcinoma features nuclear atypia, mitotic activity and (**B**) a high Ki-67 proliferation index (MIB1). **C** Overexpression of p53 is limited to a few tumour cells (anti-p53 antibody).

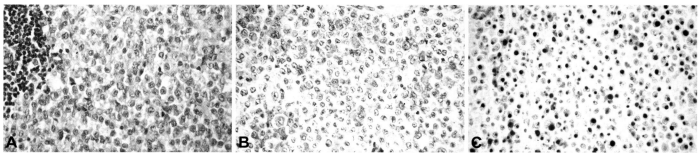

Fig. 1.42 Pituitary carcinoma. **A** Laterocervical lymph node metastasis from a sparsely granulated somatotroph adenoma. **B** Expression of growth hormone is weak to moderate. **C** Immunostaining for cytokeratin (CAM5.2) highlights fibrous bodies.

Primary lesions and metastases often show intense nuclear expression of p53 {2750}. Overexpression of p53 may be an indication of malignancy in both primary lesions and metastases {2330}. However, p53 can sometimes be undetectable in primary lesions and metastases {1492}.

Microvascular density is not usually increased in pituitary carcinoma compared with conventional and locally invasive adenomas, unless quantification is limited to the regions of higher vascular density {2876}. Matrix metalloproteinases are increased in most pituitary carcinomas, causing degradation of the extracellular matrix and consequent angiogenesis and invasion {2832}.

Expression of the enzyme MGMT can routinely be assessed by immunohistochemistry. MGMT is part of the DNA repair system, which is an important mechanism of resistance to the alkylating agent temozolomide, via repair of the alkylated guanine. Most pituitary carcinomas show < 10% MGMT-positive cells, and expression levels often remain similar in recurrent lesions. Low MGMT expression is common in lactotroph carcinomas, whereas corticotroph carcinomas often show moderate to high expression {1559}. Low immunoexpression may help to predict the response to temozolomide {1469,2520}, often correlating with a favourable response {2257,2687}, but this correlation is not absolute, and response is not always concordant with methylation of the *MGMT* gene promoter {2392}.

A national study by the Japanese Society for Hypothalamic and Pituitary Tumors showed that nuclear immunoexpression of the DNA mismatch repair protein MSH6 correlates significantly with response to temozolomide {1145, 1762,1932}. In the mismatch repair pathway, base mismatches are detected by heterodimers of MSH2 and MSH6, which assist another heterodimeric complex (of MLH1 and PMS2) {2650}. This pathway activates the G2-M DNA damage checkpoint and stimulates apoptosis during DNA synthesis. Pituitary carcinomas can express somatostatin receptors {1197}.

As is the case with conventional adenomas, electron microscopy contributes to defining the type and subtype of the primary lesion and metastases, but does not provide any information about aggressive behaviour or the potential to spread {2445}.

Genetic profile

Several genetic and molecular defects have been documented in pituitary carcinoma metastases and primary lesions, but there are no conclusive data on the genetic profile of pituitary carcinoma.

Point mutations in *HRAS* have been found in metastatic deposits but not in the premetastatic lesions, and may therefore be relevant to the formation and/or growth of metastases {2136}. Involvement of the *RB1* gene in pituitary carcinoma has been suggested based on a case in which a patient had a benign corticotroph adenoma and an adjacent and histologically distinct ACTH-positive carcinoma that metastasized, with the *RB1* gene expressed in the adenoma but not in the carcinoma {1144}.

Increased telomerase activity and TERT expression was observed in the metastasis of a lactotroph carcinoma {1090}. Overexpression of ERBB2 (also known as HER2/neu) was documented in one of two reported cases of gonadotroph carcinoma, and low-level gene amplification was found in the local recurrence and metastasis, suggesting an association between ERBB2 and more-aggressive behaviour {2328}.

Studies using comparative genomic hybridization in pituitary carcinomas have identified an average of 8.3 chromosomal imbalances per tumour: 7 gains and 1.3 losses {2286}. Gains of chromosomes 5, 7p, and 14q are the most common somatic imbalances, followed by gains of 13q22 and 14q and on 1q, 3p, 7, 8, 9p, and 21q. Loss of heterozygosity of 1p, 3p, 10q26, 11q13, and 22q12 was found in the metastasis of a pituitary corticotroph carcinoma compared with the sellar recurrence {1961}. Allelic loss in chromosome 11q was found in three lactotroph carcinomas, with loss of a common region spanning 139 coding genes. Five genes (*CD44*, *TSG101*, *DGKZ*, *HTATIP2*, and *GTF2H1*) were suggested to drive the aggressive behaviour {2986}. *TP53* mutations are rare; in one series, they were found in 2 of 6 cases {2725}. No studies have investigated *USP8* mutations in corticotroph carcinoma {2753}. Failure of mechanisms that regulate cell senescence has also been suggested to explain uncontrolled proliferation of neoplastic cells {54}. An expression microarray study {2359} identified genes overexpressed in carcinomas compared with adenomas, as well as a set of genes that were differentially expressed between corticotroph and lactotroph carcinomas. Another study, on lactotroph carcinoma, identified a total of 61 and 89 differentially expressed genes in invasive and aggressive–invasive lesions, respectively, compared with non-invasive samples; four genes (*SLC2A11*, *TENM1*, *IPO7*, and *CHGB*) were coexpressed, indicating their possible association with malignant progression {3104}. A role played by microRNAs, including miR-122, miR-20a, miR-106b, and miR-175p, has also been proposed {2647,2960}.

Genetic susceptibility

A higher risk of developing aggressive adenoma, as well as one case of pituitary carcinoma, has been reported in the

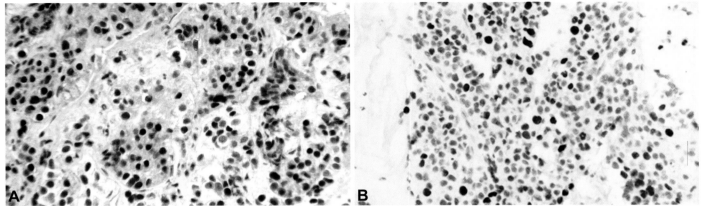

Fig. 1.43 Pituitary carcinoma. **A** MGMT-positive pituitary carcinoma. **B** Temozolomide-resistant pituitary carcinoma that shows nuclear expression of MSH6.

setting of multiple endocrine neoplasia type 1 {1017,2451}, but there is insufficient evidence to support an association between multiple endocrine neoplasia type 1 and pituitary carcinoma {590}. A case of SDH-mutated metastatic gonadotroph carcinoma was recently encountered, but the other genes mutated in pituitary adenomas, including *AIP* and *GPR101*, have not been associated with pituitary carcinoma.

Prognosis and predictive factors

The overall prognosis of patients with pituitary carcinoma is poor. About 80% of patients die of disease-related causes. Data from the SEER database indicate overall survival rates at 1, 2, 5, and 10 years of 57.1%, 28.6%, 28.6%, and 28.6%, respectively, with statistically significant differences in survival rates between invasive adenoma and carcinoma at 1, 2, and 5 years but not at 10 years {1080}. Multiple local recurrences are typical before metastasis. The reported time between onset and first recurrence varies greatly: from weeks to almost 3 decades. The reported latency period between diagnosis of the primary sellar tumour and metastasis also varies, from weeks {1216} to 38 years {1343}, although dissemination often occurs within the first 10 years after diagnosis of the sellar lesion. Metastases rarely present at early stages, and are almost never the first manifestation of the disease {338,1695}. Once metastases develop, the mean survival time is < 4 years. Patients with CNS metastases seem to live longer than those with systemic metastases, and patients with corticotroph carcinomas have the shortest survival {1301}. Several carcinomas have been reported in patients with Nelson syndrome, but the role of adrenalectomy in promoting progression is unclear; the prognosis of patients with silent corticotroph carcinomas is similar to that of patients with hormonally active corticotroph carcinomas {1909,2331}. Several reports of long-term survival after therapy have been published {1301,1544, 2454}. Sudden and marked elevation of hormones should alert the clinician of tumour recurrence or the presence of new metastases.

The data on outcomes and pathological features suggest two behaviourally distinct types of pituitary carcinoma {1301}. Tumours of the first type account for the majority of cases and behave like any other invasive adenoma, except that metastatic spread usually occurs after several sellar recurrences. The survival of patients with this type of pituitary carcinoma is prolonged. The second and less common type presents as a malignant-appearing lesion. Recurrences are multiple and occur within a short period of time. Metastases develop early and patients experience rapidly fatal progression, often with a survival time < 1 year.

PET imaging with radiolabelled octreotide has been suggested for the detection and monitoring of metastases {936, 2799}. Other PET modalities, including FDG-PET and ^{68}Ga-DOTATATE PET, can also reveal metastases, particularly those that are clinically non-functioning {1301}.

Most pituitary carcinomas are refractory to conventional therapies. Mainstream treatment includes surgery, radiotherapy, and adjuvant pharmacotherapy. Patients may succumb to complications related to hormonal excess rather than the mass effect of metastases {1117}. Therefore, treatment is aimed at both reducing the effects of hormone hypersecretion and slowing or stopping tumour growth, which can also reduce hormone levels. Several authors have advocated the use of temozolomide to control invasive adenomas and carcinomas, on the basis of reports of tumour response to the drug {1619}.

Pituitary blastoma

Rotondo F.
Syro L.V.
Lloyd R.V.
Foulkes W.D.
Kovacs K.

Definition
Pituitary blastoma (PitB) is a rare developmental early childhood neoplasm, arising within the fetal anterior pituitary. It consists of cells resembling primordial Rathke epithelium, small folliculostellate cells, and a limited range of partially differentiated secretory adenohypophyseal cells. Pituitary blastoma is usually associated with Cushing disease.

ICD-O code   8273/3

Synonym
Embryoma

Epidemiology
Pituitary tumours in the neonatal period or early childhood are rare, and the true incidence rate and epidemiology of pituitary blastoma is unknown {2447,2450, 3085}. Among pathologically proven cases, nearly half of the patients died. Death could be attributed to increased intracranial pressure and damage to the surrounding tissue or to the consequences of hypercortisolism {626}.

Etiology
All pituitary blastomas appear to have a single genetic cause: mutations in *DICER1*. In all cases for which constitutional DNA has been available, germline mutations in *DICER1* were present, usually accompanied by a somatic mutation in exons encoding the RNase IIIb domain or (more rarely) by loss of heterozygosity of the wildtype allele. It is possible that some cases have two somatic *DICER1* mutations rather than one germline and one somatic mutation {626,2376,2483}.

Localization
Pituitary blastoma is localized in the sellar and parasellar region.

Clinical features
Patients present with features of Cushing disease, with elevated blood ACTH levels and hypercortisolism. Ophthalmoplegia is also a frequent symptom. On imaging, the tumour usually presents as a lobulated, partly cystic, contrast-enhancing lesion extending into the sellar, suprasellar, and parasellar regions. Pituitary blastoma may also coexist with pleuropulmonary blastoma and cystic nephroma {626,2376,2447,2450,3085}.

Microscopy
All pituitary blastoma cases studied to date have had similar histopathology. The tumours are composed of three types of cells, present in varying proportions: (1) small, chromophobic, and undifferentiated blastema-like cells appearing unremarkable on light microscopy; (2) larger, patternless secretory epithelial cells characterized by round to oval nuclei containing inconspicuous nucleoli with abundant cytoplasm; and (3) cuboidal or columnar cells that make up

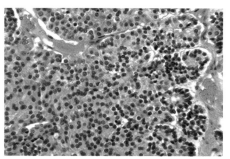

Fig. 1.44 Pituitary blastoma. The tumours are composed of three types of cell structures, present in varying proportions: (1) small, chromophobic, and undifferentiated blastema-like cells appearing unremarkable on light microscopy; (2) larger, patternless secretory epithelial cells characterized by round to oval nuclei containing inconspicuous nucleoli with abundant cytoplasm; and (3) cuboidal or columnar cells that make up glandular-like structures.

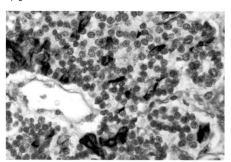

Fig. 1.45 Pituitary blastoma. This photomicrograph illustrates ACTH expression in several cells.

glandular-like structures. Normal anterior pituitary has not been identified in any of the cases.

Tumours containing large, polygonal, amphophilic cells that give a positive periodic acid–Schiff (PAS) reaction are immunoreactive for ACTH. Acidophilic cells, which are less common, are immunopositive for growth hormone. All tumours studied to date have been immunonegative for prolactin, TSH, FSH, LH, and alpha subunit. The Ki-67 proliferation index is higher in the follicular cells than in the hormone-producing cells, and its marked variation between cases indicates that pituitary blastomas occur in both low-grade and higher-grade types {626,2447,2450}.

Ultrastructure
The tumours resemble fetal pituitary of 10–12 weeks' gestation and contain fully differentiated corticotrophs and somatotrophs, scant cells of glycoprotein hormone–producing type with small secretory granules, and glandular epithelial cells consistent with mostly undifferentiated Rathke-type epithelium forming small rosettes to sizeable glands. In all tumours studied, the ultrastructural features of folliculostellate cells were also conspicuous {626,2447,2450}.

Genetic profile
In all fully analysed cases, at least one *DICER1* mutation (usually germline) has been identified, often accompanied by a somatic mutation affecting the RNase IIIb domain of *DICER1* {626,2376,2483}.

Genetic susceptibility
Pituitary blastoma is part of *DICER1* syndrome {626,2376,2483}; see *DICER1 syndrome* (p. 280) for more details.

Prognosis and predictive factors
The overall prognosis is poor. Patients should be regularly monitored by routine clinical examination, including endocrine profiling and serial MRI of the brain {2447, 2450,3085}.

Craniopharyngioma

Tihan T.
Lopes M. B. S.
Nishioka H.
Nosé V.
Yamada S.

Definition

Adamantinomatous craniopharyngioma (ACP) is a low-grade neoplasm composed of distinctive epithelium that forms stellate reticulum and basal palisading, as well as eosinophilic keratinous material (so-called wet keratin).

Papillary craniopharyngioma (PCP) is a low-grade neoplasm resembling squamous papilloma composed of non-keratinizing epithelium and fibrovascular cores.

ICD-O codes

Craniopharyngioma	9350/1
Adamantinomatous craniopharyngioma	9351/1
Papillary craniopharyngioma	9352/1

Epidemiology

The average age-adjusted annual incidence rate of craniopharyngioma in the USA in 2008–2012 was 0.18 cases per 100 000 population {2064}. A recent study estimated annual incidence rates in Denmark of 1.86 cases per 1 million population overall and 2.14 cases per 1 million children aged < 15 years, as well as a worldwide annual incidence of 1.34 cases per 1 million population overall {1982}. ACP shows a bimodal age distribution and no sex predilection. Rare congenital craniopharyngioma can be very large and may be life-threatening {476}.

The incidence of PCP is unknown. The tumours occur exclusively in adults, with a median patient age of 40–50 years {2139}. PCP shows no obvious sex predilection.

Localization

Craniopharyngioma is localized in the suprasellar region, sella turcica, third ventricle, and (rarely) sphenoidal sinus or posterior fossa.

Clinical features

The clinical features often relate to mass effect of the sellar or suprasellar mass. Visual disturbance, headache, endocrine deficiencies (in particular diabetes insipidus), and obesity are common, especially in children. Cognitive impairment or personality changes are observed in about half of all patients.

Macroscopy

Macroscopy shows a lobulated, solid–cystic mass with a spongy quality, which is often well defined. The cysts of ACP contain a dark, greenish-brown fluid resembling machine oil. Calcifications can be recognized in ACP. Cysts and calcification are often absent in PCP.

Microscopy

Adamantinomatous craniopharyngioma (ACP) has characteristic epithelium that creates a palisaded arrangement and loose background known as stellate reticulum. The epithelium can have cords, trabeculae, whorls, and nests of cells with squamous differentiation. So-called wet keratin and ghost cells are eosinophilic keratinous material typical of ACP. Tumours can have granulomatous inflammation, cholesterol clefts, gliosis, and Rosenthal fibres when infiltrating brain. They bear a striking resemblance to ameloblastoma and express enamel proteins {2499}. Tumours with frank squamous anaplasia, abundant mitoses, and necrosis are considered malignant. Primary suprasellar malignant odontogenic tumour {2010} may constitute a malignant variant of ACP. A rare form of ACP has overlapping features with PCP. Nuclear beta-catenin positivity in cell clusters has been reported as a reliable marker for ACP {1154}. CK7, CK8, and CK14 are variably positive {2729}.

Papillary craniopharyngioma (PCP) is a compact squamous papilloma with well-developed fibrovascular cores and non-keratinizing squamous epithelium. Rare goblet cells and ciliated cells can be recognized. A spectrum including Rathke cleft cyst with extensive squamous metaplasia and PCP has been suggested, although the molecular features of the two lesions are distinct. Features of ACP such as wet keratin are not observed in PCP. Mitoses are rare. The tumours are positive for V600E-mutated BRAF, claudin 1,

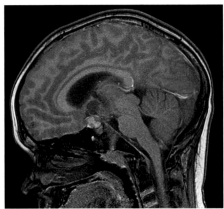

Fig. 1.46 Adamantinomatous craniopharyngioma. Sagittal contrast-enhanced T1-weighted MRI shows a partially cystic and partially enhancing sellar/suprasellar mass.

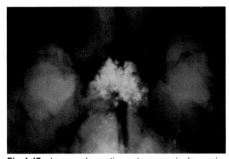

Fig. 1.47 Large adamantinomatous craniopharyngioma. Extending into the third ventricle. Postmortem X-ray shows extensive calcification.

and p63. It has been suggested that the staining patterns of claudin 1 and p63 differ in ACP and PCP {2628}.

Genetic profile

Mutations in *CTNNB1* (located on chromosome 3) are present in the great majority of ACPs. Most such mutations affect exon 3. *CTNNB1* mutation results in nuclear accumulation of beta-catenin and in WNT pathway activation. Rare ACPs have been found to harbour both *BRAF* V600E and *CTNNB1* mutations {1552}.

BRAF V600E mutations have been reported as the principal oncogenic driver of PCP {314}. PCP may respond to BRAF inhibitors {120,313}.

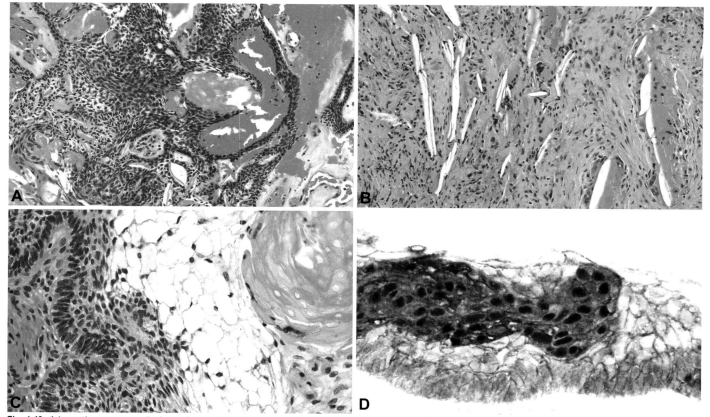

Fig. 1.48 Adamantinomatous craniopharyngioma. **A** Medium magnification of tumour composed of epithelial cells with basal palisading and wet keratin in a haemorrhagic background. **B** Cholesterol clefts and a giant cell granulomatous reaction are occasionally the only findings on biopsies of sellar craniopharyngiomas. **C** The characteristic stellate reticulum, palisading epithelial cells, and wet keratin can be recognized in this high-magnification image. **D** Beta-catenin staining.

Prognosis and predictive factors

For ACP, extent of resection is the most critical prognostic factor. Large tumours have a less favourable prognosis, in part due to a lesser extent of resection. Cases with malignant transformation have dismal prognosis.

Extent of resection is also the most critical prognostic factor for PCP. Patients with subtotal resection may benefit from radiotherapy {581}. The overall prognosis is favourable.

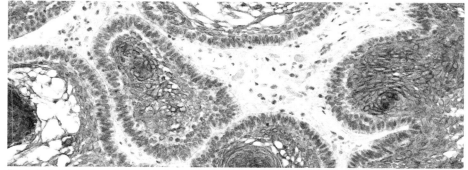

Fig. 1.48 E Adamantinomatous craniopharyngioma. Immunohistochemical staining with CAM5.2 antibody showing intense staining of the epithelium.

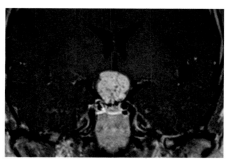

Fig. 1.49 Papillary craniopharyngioma. Coronal T1-weighted contrast-enhanced image shows predominantly a solid and homogeneously enhancing suprasellar mass.

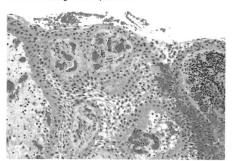

Fig. 1.50 Papillary craniopharyngioma. Well-differentiated squamous epithelium, fibrovascular cores, and scattered inflammatory cells are typical.

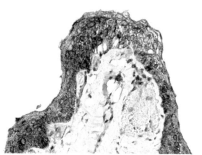

Fig. 1.51 Papillary craniopharyngioma. Immunohistochemical staining for V600E-mutated BRAF is often diffusely positive, with varying staining intensity.

Neuronal and paraneuronal tumours

Gangliocytoma and mixed gangliocytoma–adenoma

Osamura R. Y.
Lloyd R. V.
Tihan T.
Trouillas J.

Definition
Gangliocytoma and mixed gangliocytoma–adenoma is a pituitary (intrasellar) tumour that contains ganglion (neuronal) cells, which are frequently mixed with pituitary adenoma or hyperplasia.

ICD-O code   9492/0

Synonyms
Pituitary adenoma–neuronal choristoma; mixed gangliocytoma–adenoma; pituitary adenoma with gangliocytic component {135}

Epidemiology
Gangliocytic neoplasms are usually associated with pituitary adenomas; isolated cases are extremely rare {1764, 2218,3120}. Gangliocytoma and mixed gangliocytoma–adenoma accounts for 0.25–1.26% of all sellar tumours {1461, 1502}. There is a marked female preponderance {1502}.

Etiology
Three hypotheses regarding etiology have been proposed: (1) most gangliocytic tumours arise as a result of neuronal differentiation within conventional pituitary adenomas, mainly sparsely granulated somatotroph adenoma {1164, 1441,1764,2806}; (2) the primary gangliocytoma, which produces GHRH, stimulates the adenomatous transformation of the adjacent normal pituitary gland {1502,1764}; and (3) the tumour cells may constitute a spectrum of neurosecretory cells with features of adenomatous and gangliocytic cells. The third hypothesis is supported by the presence of NFP in pituitary adenomas, suggesting neuronal differentiation {1441}.

Table 1.04 The differential diagnosis of neuroendocrine/neuroectodermal neoplasms of the sinonasal tract {1895}

Neuroendocrine carcinoma
Well-differentiated (carcinoid)
Moderately differentiated (atypical carcinoid)
Poorly differentiated (small cell carcinoma or large cell neuroendocrine carcinoma)
Olfactory neuroblastoma/aesthesioneuroblastoma
Malignant melanoma
Ewing family of tumours (Ewing sarcoma / primitive neuroectodermal tumour)
Paraganglioma
Pituitary adenoma

Localization
These tumours are located in the sella turcica and parasellar region, with no connection with the hypothalamus.

Clinical features
Most mixed gangliocytic and adenomatous tumours occur in association with somatotroph adenoma presenting with acromegaly {1502,2218}. They occur less often with corticotroph adenomas with clinical presentation of Cushing disease {1602,1764,2210,2371}. Mixed tumours that produce prolactin {1842} or prolactin and ACTH {1395} have also been described.

Macroscopy
These tumours cannot be differentiated from usual adenomas by imaging or gross appearance.

Microscopy
Histologically, the tumours are composed of mature ganglionic cells (with or without admixed pituitary adenoma cells) and intermediate cells (with features intermediate between those of adenoma cells and ganglion cells) {946,1441,1502, 2218}. The adenomatous component is positive for growth hormone in the great majority of combined tumours, with other cases found to be positive for prolactin and ACTH {322,1764,1842}.

Intrasellar GHRH-secreting gangliocytomas (without adenoma) are extremely

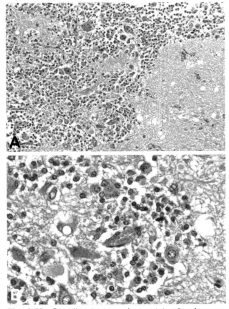

Fig. 1.52 Gangliocytoma and somatotroph adenoma. **A** Sparsely granulated somatotroph adenoma with fibrous bodies. **B** At higher magnification.

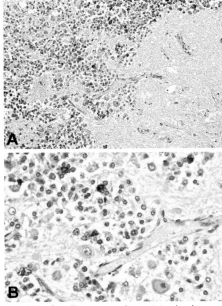

Fig. 1.53 Gangliocytoma and somatotroph adenoma. In the same case shown in Fig. 1.52, the adenoma cells are positive for growth hormone (**A**), whereas the ganglion cells are negative (**B**).

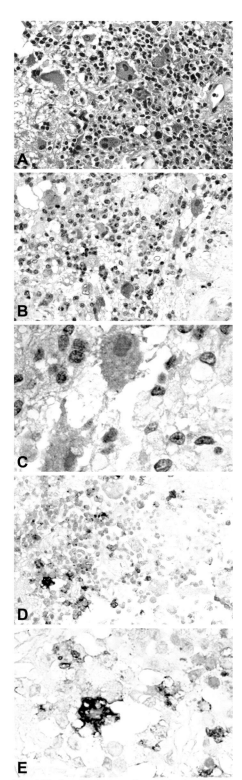

Fig. 1.54 Gangliocytoma and somatotroph adenoma. The ganglion cells are positive for GHRH and negative for growth hormone (GH). The adenoma cells are positive for GH. **A** H&E staining. **B,C** GHRH immunochemistry. **D,E** GH immunochemistry.

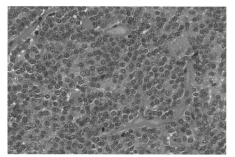

Fig. 1.55 Sellar neurocytoma. The tumour is composed of monotonous round cells with salt-and-pepper nuclei.

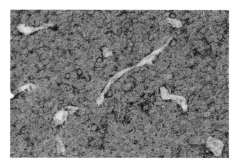

Fig. 1.56 Sellar neurocytoma. Neurocytomas express neuronal/neuroendocrine markers. This tumour shows neuron-specific enolase expression.

rare; only a few well-documented cases have been reported {103,582,1224}. A single case of pituitary gangliocytoma expressing both ACTH and CRH resulting in pituitary ACTH cell hyperplasia and Cushing disease has been reported {691}.

Prognosis and predictive factors
Information on prognosis and treatment is limited. Of 23 cases of intrasellar gangliocytomas associated with pituitary adenoma reported by Qiao et al. in 2014 {2218}, one case recurred 5 years after tumour resection. The surgical results and prognoses of the gangliocytomas were comparable to those of pituitary adenomas. In 2012, Crowley et al. {582} reported 2 cases of acromegaly with sellar gangliocytomas immunopositive for GHRH in which persistent growth hormone hypersecretion was successfully suppressed by a somatostatin analogue.

Neurocytoma

Mete O.
Kovacs K.
Lopes M.B.S.

Definition
Sellar neurocytoma is an extraventricular neurocytoma (WHO grade II) of the hypothalamic–pituitary area.

ICD-O code   9506/1

Synonyms
Extraventricular neurocytoma of the sellar region; hypothalamic neurocytoma; neurocytoma of the pituitary gland

Epidemiology
The incidence of these rare neoplasms is unknown. Sellar neurocytomas have been reported in adults aged 23–56 years {1332,1709,2146,2944,2946,3052}.

Localization
Neurocytomas can occur throughout the neuraxis; this section focuses on those of the hypothalamic–pituitary region.

Clinical features
Visual field deficit unassociated with substantial hypothalamic–pituitary dysfunction has been reported in all known cases {1332,1709,2146,2944,2946,3052}. Mildly elevated plasma prolactin levels have been noted {2944,2946}. This neoplasm usually presents as a non-calcified heterogeneously enhancing sellar and suprasellar mass resembling a pituitary macroadenoma {1709,2146,2944,2946}.

Microscopy
These tumours are composed of monotonous round cells with neuronal differentiation, in a background of fibrillary and vascular stroma. The cells contain nuclei with salt-and-pepper chromatin. Variable ganglion or smaller ganglioid cells can be identified {1709,2684}. Atypical histological features associated with adverse outcome in extraventricular neurocytomas include necrosis, microvascular proliferation, and increased mitotic activity (≥ 3 mitoses per 10 high-power fields) or an elevated Ki-67 proliferation index (> 3%) as determined using the MIB1 antibody {315}. The tumour cells express neuronal/neuroendocrine markers, synaptophysin, NeuN, chromogranin A (reported only in one case) {2146}, CD56, and neuron-specific enolase. They are negative for adenohypophyseal hormones and transcription factors, cytokeratins, glial markers (GFAP, S100

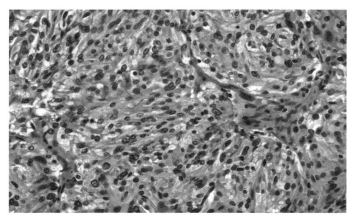

Fig. 1.57 Pituitary paraganglioma. Many eosinophilic cells with Zellballen formation.

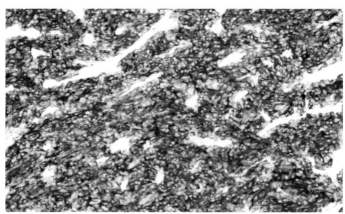

Fig. 1.58 Pituitary paraganglioma. Many tumour cells contain abundant cytoplasm, which is strongly positive for chromogranin A by immunohistochemistry.

protein, nestin, and OLIG2), neurofibromin, and EMA {1332,1709,2146,2946, 3052}. Positivity for vasopressin (ADH) has been reported in a single case {1709}. Ultrastructural examination confirms neuronal differentiation by revealing microtubules, neurosecretory granules, and synapses. The differential diagnosis of sellar neurocytoma includes pituitary paraganglioma, gangliocytoma, neuroblastoma, and pituicytoma.

Genetic profile
Unlike in other extraventricular neurocytomas, the genetic profile of sellar neurocytomas has not been investigated.

Prognosis and predictive factors
A better prognosis is associated with more complete resection and the absence of atypical features {1309,2684}. These neoplasms are sensitive to radiotherapy. Given the occurrence of late craniospinal dissemination, long-term follow-up is recommended {1332}.

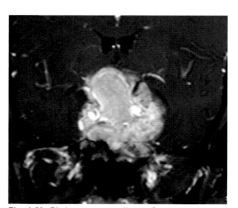

Fig. 1.59 Pituitary paraganglioma. Contrast-enhanced MRI reveals marked suprasellar extension of the tumour.

Paraganglioma

Osamura R. Y.
Kovacs K.
Lopes M. B. S.
Mete O.
Nishioka H.

Definition
Pituitary paraganglioma is a tumour arising from chief cells of the dispersed paraganglia of the sellar region.

ICD-O code   8693/3

Synonym
Sellar paraganglioma

Epidemiology
Paragangliomas at this site are extremely rare. Only about 10 sellar {268,1093, 1881,2073,2389,2403,2453} and 3 parasellar {463,2634} paragangliomas have been reported.

Etiology
Two hypotheses regarding etiology have been proposed: (1) the tumours derive from remnants of neural crest in the pituitary {250} and (2) they result from aberrant migration of glossopharyngeal nerve to the pituitary {1148,2634}.

Localization
Most are localized in the sella turcica, but some extend to suprasellar areas and cavernous sinus, mimicking pituitary macroadenomas {268,463,1881,2403}.

Clinical features
Clinical features include visual disturbances, headaches, and various signs of hypopituitarism {268}.

Microscopy
Like paragangliomas in other locations, the tumour shows many polyhedral chief cells, with ovoid hyperchromatic nuclei and pink to pale cytoplasm, arranged in a nested pattern forming Zellballen. Necrosis and mitoses are rare. The tumour cells are immunopositive for chromogranin A and synaptophysin and immunonegative for keratin, EMA, anterior pituitary hormones, and transcription factors {1829}. The sustentacular cells are positive for S100 protein and GFAP. Positivity for tyrosine hydroxylase distinguishes paragangliomas from null cell adenoma {748}. Immunohistochemistry for SDHB should be considered as genetic testing {748}. The differential diagnosis with sinonasal and nasopharyngeal tumours is summarized elsewhere {1896}.

Genetic susceptibility
Only a single case associated with von Hippel–Lindau syndrome has been reported {2453}.

Prognosis and predictive factors
Postoperative irradiation may be required due to the difficulty of achieving adequate removal of the tumour by transsphenoidal approach {1148,2073,2453, 2634}. No distant metastases have been reported.

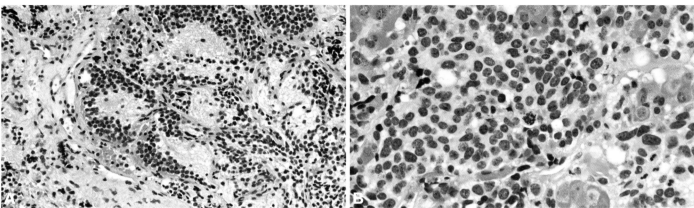

Fig. 1.60 Sellar neuroblastoma. **A** Neuroblastomas can contain anucleate areas with a neuropil-like matrix. **B** Neuroblastomas are highly cellular tumours composed of small cells with hyperchromatic nuclei. The tumour cells may diffusely infiltrate the adenohypophyseal parenchyma.

Neuroblastoma

Lopes M. B. S.
Lloyd R. V.
Roncaroli F.
Tihan T.

Definition
Sellar neuroblastoma is a neuroectodermal tumour similar to olfactory neuroblastoma.

ICD-O code   9500/3

Synonym
Sellar aesthesioneuroblastoma

Epidemiology
The incidence is unknown. For the < 20 cases that have been reported, the female-to-male ratio is 1.7:1, and the mean patient age is 40 years (range: 1.4–57 years) {718,1623,2070,2463}.

Localization
Suprasellar extension is common {1517, 2230}.

Clinical features
Visual deficits (occurring in 81% of cases) and pituitary endocrine disorders are common {718,2230,2463}. Neuroimaging findings are indistinguishable from those seen with adenomas.

Microscopy
The tumours show diffuse or lobular patterns with a rich vascular network and are composed of uniform populations of small cells with scant cytoplasm and dispersed chromatin. Neurofibrillary matrix areas are present; pseudorosettes and Homer Wright rosettes are rare. Most cases are low-grade tumours {2230}. The mitotic index is low and the Ki-67 proliferation index varies (from 1% to 30%), showing no correlation with tumour behaviour {718,2070,2230}. Ultrastructurally, dense-core membrane-bound neurosecretory granules can be seen {2230,2355}. The tumours express neuronal and neuroendocrine markers. S100 protein and GFAP label sustentacular cells. Pituitary hormones are absent. One tumour with vasopressin (ADH) immunopositivity was reported in a patient with syndrome of inappropriate antidiuretic hormone secretion (SIADH) {2230}. Differential diagnosis with null cell adenoma and metastatic neuroendocrine carcinoma can be challenging.

Prognosis and predictive factors
Due to the rarity of sellar neuroblastoma, prognostic factors are unknown. Surgery is the first-line treatment; adjuvant radiotherapy has been used in subtotally resected tumours. Recurrence is rare {2070,2710}. One patient developed multiple local recurrences and subsequently bone metastases {2070}. In the single reported paediatric case, the patient died with CNS and cervical lymph node metastases {2710}.

Tumours of the posterior pituitary

Mete O.
Lopes M. B. S.
Roncaroli F.
Tihan T.
Yamada S.

Definition

Tumours of the posterior pituitary are a distinct group of low-grade neoplasms of the sellar region, most likely constituting a morphological spectrum of a single nosological entity. They include pituicytoma, granular cell tumour of the sellar region, spindle cell oncocytoma and sellar ependymoma. All of these tumours are believed to derive from pituicytes, the specialized glia of the posterior pituitary.

ICD-O codes

Pituicytoma	9432/1
Granular cell tumour of the sellar region	9582/0
Spindle cell oncocytoma	8290/0
Sellar ependymoma	9391/1

Synonyms, histogenesis, and historical background

Historically, the term "pituicytoma" has been applied to a variety of neoplasms, including pilocytic astrocytomas and granular cell tumours involving the sellar/suprasellar region. The terms "posterior pituitary astrocytoma" and "infundibuloma" have also been used for pituicytomas {1674}. The detailed morphological and clinical features of a series of 9 pituicytomas were reported by Brat et al. in 2000 {316}. Subsequently, the 2007

WHO classification of tumours of the central nervous system adopted the term "pituicytoma" to define a distinct low-grade glioma originating from pituicytes, the specialized glia of the posterior pituitary {1674}.

Granular cell tumours of the sellar region are considered to be distinct due to their pituicyte origin {1399,1827,2168, 2456}. Many terms, including "Abrikossoff tumour", "choristoma", "granular cell myoblastoma", "granular cell neuroma", "granular pituicytoma", and "granular cell schwannoma", have been used for what is now recognized as granular cell tumour of the sellar region {1399,2168}.

In 2002, Roncaroli et al. {2329} reported 5 distinct non-endocrine pituitary neoplasms consisting of mitochondria-rich spindle to epithelioid cells. They introduced the descriptive term "spindle cell oncocytoma of the adenohypophysis" and suggested an origin from folliculo-stellate cells of the anterior pituitary gland {2329}.

In 2009, Scheithauer et al. {2456} proposed a pituicyte origin for sellar ependymomas and considered them a variant of pituicytoma based on ultrastructural similarities with ependymal pituicytes.

In 2009, Lee et al. {1570} demonstrated that pituicytes, pituicytoma, granular cell

tumours of the sella, and spindle cell oncocytomas express TTF1, whereas adenohypophyseal cells and folliculostellate cells are negative for TTF1. In light of these findings, the authors suggested a common pituicyte-lineage derivation of these neoplasms {1570}.

In 2013, Mete et al. {1827} confirmed the evidence of TTF1 expression in pituicytomas, spindle cell oncocytoma, and granular cell tumours. These authors also suggested an analogy between the ultrastructural variants of pituicytes and pituicytomas (i.e. dark and light pituicytes), granular cell tumours (granular pituicytes), and spindle cell oncocytomas (oncocytic pituicytes) {1827}. Given these findings, the authors proposed that spindle cell oncocytomas and granular cell tumours are variants of pituicytomas {1827}.

The advances made in our understanding of this distinct group of neoplasms suggest that these tumours most likely constitute a morphological spectrum of a single nosological entity. However, the concept of pituicyte origin is still evolving, and additional studies are required to refine the classification of these rare tumours.

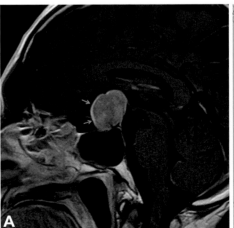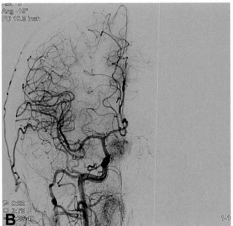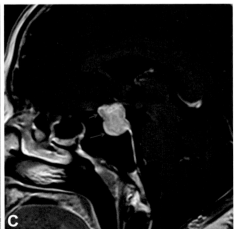

Fig. 1.61 Tumours of the posterior pituitary. **A** The imaging characteristics of this group of non-neuroendocrine tumours are indistinguishable from those of non-functioning pituitary macroadenomas. Enhanced anterior pituitary gland, which is usually displaced posterosuperiorly in pituitary macroadenomas, is often displaced anteriorly (arrows) in these tumours. This image shows a granular cell tumour of the sellar region. **B** Spindle cell oncocytomas, pituicytomas, and granular cell tumours of the sellar region are highly vascular lesions, as shown in this angiogram. **C** Pituicytoma. The anterior pituitary gland is displaced anteriorly (arrows).

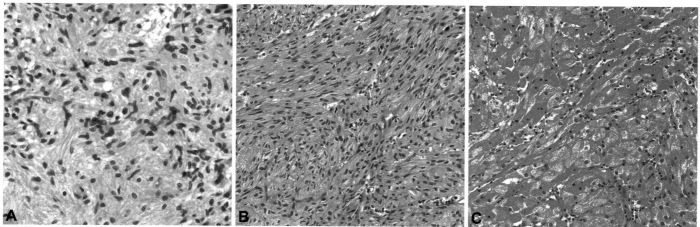

Fig. 1.62 Tumours of the posterior pituitary. **A** Pituicytomas are composed of solid sheets of elongated bipolar spindle cells that are typically arranged in short fascicles or a storiform pattern. **B** Spindle cell oncocytomas are composed of spindle to epithelioid tumour cells forming poorly defined lobules and interlacing fascicles. **C** Granular cell tumours of the sellar region are characterized by large polygonal cells with distinct eosinophilic granular cytoplasm.

Epidemiology

These pituitary non-neuroendocrine tumours are rare neoplasms; their true incidence in the general population is unknown. Within the large German Pituitary Tumour Registry, pituicytomas account for < 0.1% of all recorded sellar tumours {2370}. At one institution, spindle cell oncocytomas were found to account for 0.4% of all sellar tumours {2329}. Clinically detected (i.e. symptomatic) granular cell tumours of the pituitary gland have been estimated to account for < 0.5% of all sellar neoplasms {2443}; however, incidental microscopic granular cell tumours, also known as granular cell tumourlets, were identified in 17% of cases in a single series of adult autopsy studies {270}. Ependymomas are the least common, with only 7 documented cases {2112,2456}.

Most reported pituicytomas have occurred in adults, with a median patient age at onset in the fourth to sixth decade of life {572,2112}. Only a few pituicytomas and granular cell tumours have been described in children {211,363,442,1368}.

Granular cell tumours are more commonly seen in females {572}, whereas pituicytomas and sellar ependymomas are more frequent in males {572,2112,2456}. Spindle cell oncocytomas are slightly more common in females {572,1922}.

Etiology

The etiology of these rare tumours is still unclear. A pituicyte-derived origin has been proposed by some {1570,1827}.

Localization

Pure intrasellar, pure suprasellar, and mixed sellar/suprasellar presentations have been described {316,572,1399, 3127}. Most granular cell tumours are exclusively suprasellar, whereas all reported spindle cell oncocytomas have been infiltrative sellar and suprasellar tumours. Pituicytomas are most frequently either suprasellar or mixed sellar/suprasellar neoplasms, followed by pure sellar presentations {572}. Sellar ependymomas may extend to the suprasellar region {2112,2456}.

Clinical features

Clinical symptoms and signs

The manifestations of these tumours are indistinguishable from those of clinically non-functioning pituitary macroadenomas, which often present with symptoms and signs related to compression of the pituitary stalk and adjacent structures {572,1399}. Visual field defects have been the most common presenting symptoms, reported in > 50% of all cases {572,1399, 2456}. Mild hyperprolactinaemia due to pituitary stalk compression, hypopituitarism, fatigue, decreased libido, amenorrhoea, headache, nausea, and vomiting have been variably reported {572, 1399,2112,2456}. Panhypopituitarism is thought to possibly be more common in spindle cell oncocytomas {572}, which has been attributed to the infiltrative nature of these tumours compared with pituicytomas {572,3127}. However, the data should be interpreted with caution given the small number of cases reported to date. Diabetes insipidus is a rare

manifestation of sellar ependymomas, granular cell tumours, and pituicytomas {572,1924,2771,3127}. Isolated cases of thyroid carcinoma, goitre, pituitary adenoma, and parathyroid adenoma have been reported in patients with pituicytoma {363,1399,2481}. Granular cell tumour has been reported in a patient with multiple endocrine neoplasia type 2 {594}.

Imaging

Preoperatively, the overall imaging findings do not seem to allow for reliable distinction of tumours of the posterior pituitary, and overlap with the imaging findings seen in non-functioning pituitary macroadenomas. About 80% of tumours of the posterior pituitary are isointense on T1-weighted MRI and show either homogeneous or heterogeneous enhancement {572}. It has been suggested that the finding of hyperattenuated, well-circumscribed, pure suprasellar lesions on CT may suggest granular cell tumour, and that infiltrative mixed sellar/suprasellar lesions indistinguishable from the pituitary gland are likely to be spindle cell oncocytomas {572}. Cystic change and calcification have been described infrequently {1399,2112,2443}.

Macroscopy

Spindle cell oncocytomas, pituicytomas, and granular cell tumours of the sellar region can be highly vascular lesions with a propensity to bleed {288,901,1326, 2443}. Some lesions are easily resectable; others (especially spindle cell oncocytomas) are firm and infiltrative, making

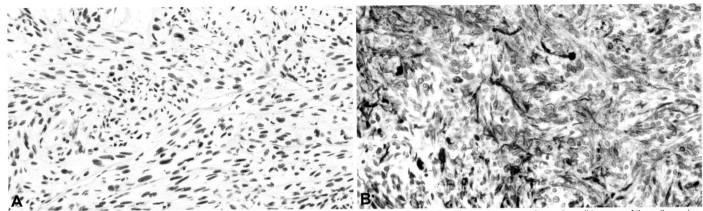

Fig. 1.63 Tumours of the posterior pituitary. **A** Nuclear TTF1 expression is a hallmark of pituicytomas, spindle cell oncocytomas, and granular cell tumours of the sellar region. The TTF1 expression profile of sellar ependymomas is largely unknown. This photomicrograph shows TTF1 positivity in a spindle cell oncocytoma. **B** These tumours are variably positive for GFAP, S100, vimentin, and EMA. This photomicrograph shows variable GFAP expression in a pituicytoma.

it difficult to achieve complete resection {3127}. Granular cell tumours have been described as firm tan to grey lesions {572,1399}.

Microscopy

Pituicytomas are composed of solid sheets of elongated bipolar spindle cells that are typically arranged in short fascicles or a storiform pattern {316}. Spindle cell oncocytomas are characterized by interlacing fascicles and poorly defined lobules of spindle to epithelioid tumour cells with variable eosinophilic or oncocytic cytoplasm {2329}. Granular cell tumours are composed of large polygonal cells with eccentric nuclei and distinct eosinophilic granular cytoplasm. The granules give a diastase-resistant positive periodic acid–Schiff (PAS) reaction {1399}. Sellar ependymomas are characterized by broad fascicles of bipolar cells displaying round to oval nuclei and scant cytoplasm. They are distinguished by their typical ependymal features, including perivascular pseudorosettes and true ependymal rosettes {2112,2456}.

Nuclear TTF1 expression is a hallmark of pituicytomas, spindle cell oncocytomas, and granular cell tumours of the sellar region {1570,1827}. TTF1 expression has also been noted in ependymomas of the third ventricle {3090} and in unusual pituicytomas with an ependymoma-like component {2369}; however, the TTF1 expression profile of sellar ependymomas is largely unknown. All tumours of the posterior pituitary are negative for chromogranin A, synaptophysin, adenohypophyseal hormones, and NFP, and

variably positive for GFAP, S100, vimentin, and EMA {1827,2112,2456}. Keratin expression can be focally positive in ependymomas, whereas it is negative in the other tumours of this group. Variable CD68 expression has been reported in pituicytomas, granular cell tumours, and spindle cell oncocytomas {1399, 1827}. Granular cell tumours are negative for CD56, BCL2, and galectin 3, whereas some pituicytomas and spindle cell oncocytomas express these markers {1827}. Antimitochondrial antibody highlights abundant mitochondria in spindle cell oncocytomas {2327,2329}. CD44 and nestin were reported in a single case of spindle cell oncocytoma {55}, and alpha-B-crystallin expression was noted in another case {2844}. The Ki-67 proliferation index (as determined using the MIB1 antibody) is generally low, but some recurrent spindle cell oncocytomas have a Ki-67 proliferation index of about 20% {1419}.

Tumours of the posterior pituitary reflect the five ultrastructural variants of pituicytes as described by Takei et al. {2699}. Like most light and dark pituicytes, pituicytoma tumour cells contain cytoplasmic intermediate filaments and a variable number of mitochondria, along with lysosomes and few short desmosome-like intermediate junctions {1827}. Like granular pituicytes, the tumour cells of granular cell tumours are rich in membrane-bound, electron-dense vacuoles consistent with lysosomes {1827}. Like oncocytic pituicytes, spindle cell oncocytoma tumour cells are spindle-shaped or polygonal, with variably well-formed desmosomes

and intermediate filaments, as well as cytoplasm filled with mitochondria {1827}. Like ependymal pituicytes, sellar ependymoma tumour cells contain a moderate number of intermediate filaments, occasional mitochondria, lysosomes, and lipid droplets, along with intracellular and intercellular lumina displaying microvilli, cilia, and desmosomal junctions {2456}. Isolated cases featuring oncocytic change along with ependymal differentiation or ependymoma-like features have also been described {2369,2844,3075}.

Genetic profile

The genetic profile of these tumours is largely unknown. Genomic copy-number imbalances, including losses on chromosome arms 1p, 14q, and 22q and gains on 5p, have been identified in pituicytomas {2164}. No *BRAF* V600E mutations or *BRAF*-KIAA fusions have been detected in pituicytomas, granular cell tumours, or spindle cell oncocytomas {1827}. These tumours have also been found to be immunonegative for R132H-mutated IDH1 {1827}.

Prognosis and predictive factors

Most pituicyte-derived tumours are associated with a favourable outcome. Recurrences have been linked to incomplete tumour resection. Recurrent tumours can have a more aggressive course, with an increased Ki-67 proliferation index (as determined using the MIB1 antibody) and necrosis {289,1419,1922}. To date, no distant metastases have been reported.

Mesenchymal and stromal tumours

Lopes M. B. S.
Kontogeorgos G.
Lloyd R.V.
Tihan T.

Definition
A variety of primary mesenchymal tumours can develop in the pituitary region; the most prevalent are meningiomas, but rare lesions with histological features corresponding to benign and malignant soft tissue tumours also occur (Table 1.05).
In this section, only the most relevant mesenchymal tumours are discussed.

Synonyms
The nomenclature and classification of mesenchymal tumours involving the pituitary region are those of the corresponding CNS and soft tissue tumours as described in the respective WHO classification volumes.

Epidemiology
Primary mesenchymal tumours of the pituitary region constitute a minority of the tumours involving this region. Meningiomas, which are the most common mesenchymal tumour of the region, account for approximately 5% of all sellar neoplasms {836,2370}; chordomas and chondrosarcomas collectively account for 0.5–2% {836,2370}. The incidence of other sellar mesenchymal tumours is uncertain; most of them are reported as individual cases {101,1077}. Primary sarcomas of the sellar region are extremely rare {1607,1669}. The great majority of sarcomas are associated with previous radiation therapy {223,2493}, including fibrosarcoma {19}, malignant fibrous histiocytoma {1501}, chondrosarcoma {2956}, and undifferentiated sarcoma {2422}. The reported latency periods between irradiation and development of sarcoma varies tremendously, from 2 to 27 years {1669}.

Meningioma

Definition
Meningioma is typically a slow-growing tumour attached to the dura mater and composed of neoplastic arachnoid cells.

ICD-O codes
See Table 1.06, p. 56.

Synonyms
Tuberculum sellae meningioma; diaphragma sellae meningioma; suprasellar meningioma

Epidemiology
Meningiomas account for about 5% of all sellar neoplasms {836,2370} and are the second most common suprasellar neoplasm in adults {836,1388}. The peak incidence occurs among patients in their fifth or sixth decade of life, and there is a female predominance {172,2065,2228, 2431}.

Etiology
Meningiomas are believed to originate from arachnoid cells.

Localization
Most tumours are suprasellar; they can originate in the planum sphenoidale, tuberculum sellae, and diaphragma sellae {33}. Intrasellar meningiomas, which are rare, are derived from the inferior leaf of the diaphragma sellae {1388}.

Clinical features
Visual deficits and headaches are the most common presentation {172,822, 1639,2228}. Endocrine hormonal abnormality is uncommon {1388,1639,2431}. Cranial nerve palsies may be seen in cases with cavernous sinus invasion {172}.
On imaging, the tumours are typically well-circumscribed, homogeneous, isodense or hyperdense masses, with diffuse enhancement on CT. The tumours are isointense to grey matter on T1-weighted MRI, but variable on T2-weighted images, with most being T2-hyperintense {388}. Contrast enhancement is strong and uniform, allowing most meningiomas to be distinguished from adenomas {388,2732}.

Macroscopy
Meningiomas are typically solid and firm lesions with a whorled or lobulated appearance; psammomatous variants may have a gritty appearance. Invasion of the dura and cavernous sinus is common.

Microscopy
Meningiomas have several histopathological appearances, varying in grade and biological behaviour. The most common subtypes are meningothelial, fibrous (fibroblastic), and transitional (mixed). Broad epithelioid cells with meningothelial whorl formation are seen in most of the subtypes. The distinctive cytological appearance of the nucleus includes well-distributed chromatin with nuclear

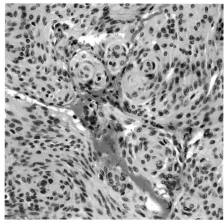

Fig. 1.64 Sellar meningothelial meningioma with prominent whorl formation.

Table 1.05 Mesenchymal tumours reported in the sellar region

Benign tumours
Chondroma
Chordoma
Fibroma
Glomangioma
Haemangioblastoma
Lipoma
Myxoma
Malignant tumours
Chondrosarcoma
Fibrosarcoma
Haemangiopericytoma / solitary fibrous tumour
Leiomyosarcoma
Osteosarcoma
Rhabdomyosarcoma

Meningioma variant	WHO grade	ICD-O code
Meningiomas with low risk of recurrence and aggressive behaviour:		
Meningothelial meningioma	I	9531/0
Fibrous (fibroblastic) meningioma	I	9532/0
Transitional (mixed) meningioma	I	9537/0
Psammomatous meningioma	I	9533/0
Angiomatous meningioma	I	9534/0
Microcystic meningioma	I	9530/0
Secretory meningioma	I	9530/0
Lymphoplasmacyte-rich meningioma	I	9530/0
Metaplastic meningioma	I	9530/0
Meningiomas with greater likelihood of recurrence and/or aggressive behaviour:		
Chordoid meningioma	II	9538/1
Clear cell meningioma	II	9538/1
Atypical meningioma	II	9539/1
Papillary meningioma	III	9538/3
Rhabdoid meningioma	III	9538/3
Anaplastic meningioma	III	9530/3
Meningiomas (of any subtype) with a high proliferation index		

clearing and nuclear pseudoinclusions. Mitotic activity and the Ki-67 proliferation index increase proportionally to tumour grade.

Atypical meningiomas are characterized by increased mitotic activity (≥ 4 mitoses per 10 high-power fields) or any three of the following features: increased cellularity, loss of pattern or sheet-like growth, small cells with a high N:C ratio, prominent nucleoli, and foci of necrosis.

Anaplastic meningiomas are distinct from meningeal sarcomas. Despite their high degree of nuclear and/or cellular anaplasia, increased mitotic activity (≥ 20 mitoses per 10 high-power fields), and extensive necrosis, these tumours retain histological features of meningiomas.

Meningiomas are immunoreactive for vimentin and EMA. S100 protein reactivity is variable. Progesterone receptor is expressed in most meningiomas, whereas estrogen receptor is less common. SSTR2A is strongly expressed in most meningiomas, including anaplastic tumours {1812}. Ultrastructural features include complex interdigitating cellular processes, abundant intermediate filaments, and desmosomal junctions.

The WHO grading system for meningiomas designates the tumours as benign (grade I), atypical (grade II), or anaplastic (grade III) according to specific histopathological criteria (above). Recognized histological variants with greater likelihood of recurrence and/or aggressive behaviour include chordoid and clear cell meningiomas (grade II) and papillary and rhabdoid meningiomas (grade III).

Genetic profile and susceptibility

A detailed discussion of the molecular genetics and genetic susceptibility of meningiomas is provided in the 2016 *WHO classification of tumours of the central nervous system* {1674,1674A}.

Prognosis and predictive factors

Prognosis depends on clinical factors, tumour histopathology, and tumour grade. Outcomes are favourable in patients aged < 50 years and patients with clinical presentation for < 1 year {820}. Surgical extension is strongly associated with recurrence rate {172,820,1506}. Surgical mortality rates are low {172}, but postoperative persistence of disease and endocrine disturbances is not uncommon {2431}. WHO grade, as described above, is a predictor for tumour recurrence.

Schwannoma

Definition

Schwannoma is a benign, commonly encapsulated nerve sheath tumour composed of well-differentiated Schwann cells.

ICD-O code   9560/0

Synonyms

Neurilemmoma; neurinoma

Epidemiology

Sellar schwannomas are extremely rare, with only about 20 reported cases {587,1462,1699}. Most tumours occur in adults, with a median patient age of 45 years (range: 33–73 years) {587} and no sex predilection. One case associated with a somatotroph adenoma has been reported {1462}.

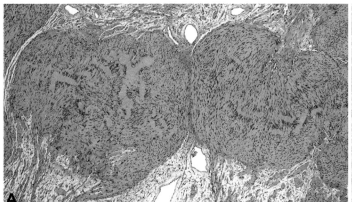
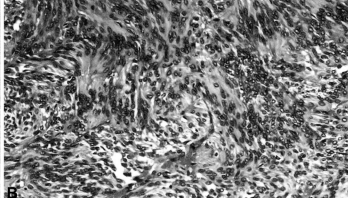

Fig. 1.65 Schwannoma. **A** Low-magnification view showing distinct Verocay body formations. **B** Spindle cells with elongated nuclei arranged in an Antoni A pattern.

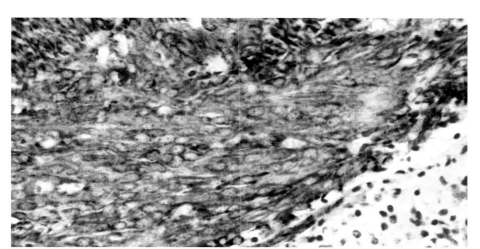

Fig. 1.66 Schwannoma. These tumours are strongly and diffusely immunoreactive for S100 protein. Note in contrast the negative stain of the surrounding anterior pituitary gland.

Etiology

The etiology is unknown. Because the pituitary is deprived of nerves, three possible geneses have been proposed: (1) the lateral sellar nerve plexus, (2) perivascular or ectopic Schwann cells, and (3) small sensory nerve twigs of the dura {1001,1699,2154}. Some authors favour the third hypothesis due to the tumoural dense adhesion to the dura {1699,2113}.

Localization

Purely intrasellar tumours are a minority {587}; most are sellar/suprasellar or parasellar tumours with extension into the sella {1699}.

Clinical features

Schwannomas are indistinguishable from non-functioning adenomas on a clinical or neuroradiological basis. Visual deficits and pituitary endocrine disturbances, including hypopituitarism and mild hyperprolactinaemia, are the most common symptoms {587,1699}. Increased intracranial pressure has been reported in association with tumours extending into the third ventricle {794,2113}.

Macroscopy

Most schwannomas are well-circumscribed, pseudoencapsulated masses with a glistening cut surface. Schwannomas are firmer and more vascular than are adenomas {587}.

Microscopy

Schwannomas are moderately cellular tumours composed of sheets of spindle-shaped cells arranged in fascicles that show distinct densely packed spindle-cell areas (Antoni A regions) and loosely arranged hypocellular areas with myxoid changes (Antoni B regions). The cells contain an elongated nucleus with dense chromatin. Palisaded rows (Verocay bodies) may be present. Tumoural vessels may show hyalinization, fibrinoid deposition, and thrombosis. Mitoses are inconspicuous. Neoplastic cells are diffusely and strongly immunoreactive for S100 protein and SOX10 {2020}. The differential diagnosis includes meningioma (fibroblastic), haemangiopericytoma/solitary fibrous tumour, and pituicytoma. Appropriate immunohistochemical stains are mostly diagnostic.

Genetic profile and susceptibility

Most schwannomas are sporadic. Inactivating mutations in the *NF2* tumour suppressor gene have been implicated in the tumorigenesis of sporadic schwannomas {1239}. Multiple schwannomas are associated with two genetic syndromes: neurofibromatosis type 2 and schwannomatosis. See the 2016 *WHO classification of tumours of the central nervous system* {1674,1674A} for detailed information about the genetic profile and susceptibility of schwannomas.

Prognosis and predictive factors

With the exception of a single case report with malignant progression to malignant peripheral nerve sheath tumour {1475}, all reported cases have had a benign course. Total surgical resection seems to be the best predictor of outcome {587}.

Chordoma

Definition

Chordoma is an aggressive tumour showing notochordal differentiation.

ICD-O codes

Chordoma, NOS   9370/3
Chondroid chordoma   9371/3
Dedifferentiated chordoma   9372/3

Epidemiology

Chordomas account for < 1% of CNS tumours. About 32% of chordomas are cranial tumours and a third of those are sellar lesions {1792,1979,2559}. The age-adjusted annual incidence rate in the USA is 0.08 cases per 100 000 population. These tumours are more common in males and in White populations {1792}. Chordomas occur in patients of all ages, with a peak incidence among patients in their fourth to fifth decade of life; < 5% of cases arise in children {251,501,1979}.

Etiology

Chordomas are believed to originate from persisting remnants of the embryonic notochord.

Localization

Most chordomas are parasellar or suprasellar; entirely intrasellar lesions are rare, with < 40 cases reported {1960,2760}. One case of a collision tumour of chordoma and lactotroph adenoma has been reported {1101}.

Clinical features

Headaches and visual deficits are typical {251,1241}, and cranial nerve palsies may be present {251,1241,2760}. Chordomas can also mimic non-functioning pituitary adenomas {1289,2760,3011}.

Chordomas are hyperintense on T2-weighted MRI sequences, with variable contrast enhancement, and show lower T1-weighted signal intensity than the clivus fat. Calcifications and sella and/or clival lytic bone destruction are frequently seen on CT {779}.

Macroscopy

Chordomas appear myxoid or gelatinous, with a multilocular appearance. Haemorrhages are frequent.

Microscopy

Chordomas are composed of cords of physaliphorous cells intermixed with smaller, partially stellate cells immersed within a rich extracellular myxoid and mucinous matrix. Chondroid chordomas have also been reported {3011}.

Chordomas express S100 protein, epithelial markers (EMA and cytokeratin), and vimentin {1021}. Brachyury is a highly specific marker for chordoma {1979, 2909} and helps to distinguish these tumours from chondrosarcoma and chordoid meningioma. The distinction between chordoma and chondrosarcoma has important therapeutic implications {1191}.

Genetic profile
The *T* gene (6q27), which encodes the protein brachyury, has been implicated in the pathogenesis of chordomas {2909}. Chromosomal gains of 7q and losses of 1p and 3p are other prominent alterations {1979}. Candidate regions for chordoma development on 1p36.13 and 7q33 have also been identified {1964}.

Genetic susceptibility
A germline alteration at the *T* locus has been associated with familial chordoma, and its amplification is present in about 5% of sporadic chordomas {1340,2201, 3055}.

Prognosis and predictive factors
Chordomas are aggressive tumours with a strong tendency towards local recurrence and invasiveness. The median survival time is about 7 years, with 5-year and 10-year survival rates of 67.6% and 39.9%, respectively {1792}. Tumour location (lower clivus) and extent of resection are important factors for recurrence {1241}. Several modalities of radiation therapy have been applied as adjuvant treatment for residual and/or recurrent tumours {251,1191,1226,1241}.

Haemangiopericytoma/ solitary fibrous tumour

Definition
Haemangiopericytoma (HPC) / solitary fibrous tumour (SFT) is a mesenchymal tumour of fibroblastic type encompassing a histological spectrum of tumours previously classified as meningeal SFT and HPC.

ICD-O codes
Grade 1 HPC/SFT   8815/0
Grade 2 HPC/SFT   8815/1
Grade 3 HPC/SFT   8815/3

Synonyms
Haemangiopericytoma; solitary fibrous tumour

Epidemiology
HPC/SFT is rare, accounting for < 1% of primary CNS tumours. About 20 cases in the sellar region have been reported {255,612,1274,3116}. The tumours affect adults in the fourth to sixth decade of life and show no sex predilection.

Localization
The tumours are mostly sellar, with parasellar and/or suprasellar extension {255, 422,1659}.

Clinical features
Signs and symptoms of mass effect, clinically mimicking a non-functioning pituitary adenoma, are common {1274,3016, 3066}. Tumour-related hypoglycaemia (paraneoplastic syndrome) has been described in one patient {3066}.

Macroscopy
The tumours are usually well-circumscribed, firm, tan to brown masses, depending on the degree of collagenous stroma. Variable myxoid or haemorrhagic changes can be seen. Dural attachment is common, but the tumours occasionally show an infiltrative growth {255}.

Microscopy
The histological spectrum encompasses two main morphological variants. The SFT phenotype is characterized by a patternless architecture with alternating hypocellular and hypercellular areas of fusiform cells with thick bands of collagen. The HPC phenotype is characterized by highly cellular tumour tissue composed of plump ovoid cells and a delicate, rich network of thin-walled, branching, staghorn-like vessels. Cases with hybrid or intermediate morphology are also seen.
Mitotic activity varies: SFT areas have a low mitotic index, whereas HPC areas have higher mitotic activity. Necrosis is common in HPC areas.
HPC/SFTs are diffusely positive for vimentin, CD34, CD99, and BCL2, but none of these markers is specific for the diagnosis. Strong nuclear STAT6 expression is highly specific and should be used for confirmation of the diagnosis (see below). Other markers, including EMA, progesterone receptor, cytokeratin, desmin, and SMA, can be focally positive. The tumours may also be positive for IGF2, which may explain the paraneoplastic hypoglycaemia associated with some cases {1064}.
The grading of these tumours has therapeutic implications. Although grading is

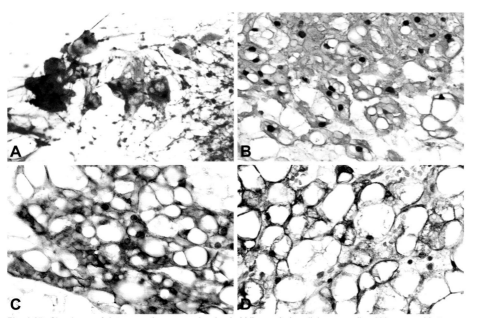

Fig. 1.67 Chordoma. A Intraoperative smear showing bubbling and physaliphorous cells within a myxoid stroma. **B** Chords of tumour cells displaying the classic bubbly cytoplasm. Chordomas are immunoreactive for EMA (**C**) and S100 protein (**D**).

Secondary tumours

Osamura R. Y.
Grossman A.
Kontogeorgos G.
Lloyd R. V.

Definition
Secondary tumours of the pituitary gland are tumours metastatic to the pituitary gland.

Synonym
Metastatic pituitary tumours

Epidemiology
Large autopsy series have shown that pituitary metastasis occurs in 1–3.6% of malignant tumour cases {310,832,1464, 1765}. Pituitary metastasis is an infrequent clinical occurrence, accounting for only 0.14–28.1% of all brain metastases in autopsy series {493,1784,2579}. Over the past few decades, pituitary metastases have been noted with increasing frequency, as a result of improved cancer survival rates and the development of more-sensitive imaging techniques {1433,1906,2360}. Examination of 190 symptomatic cases of pituitary metastasis showed the primary tumour to be latent at presentation in 43.7%. In 7–57.1% of the cases, the pituitary was reported to be the only site of metastasis {1433}. About 1% of pituitary tumours are metastatic lesions.

The primary neoplasms that metastasize to the pituitary most commonly are breast and lung cancers. Pituitary metastases are most often part of a generalized metastatic spread, usually occurring along with other metastases, most commonly to the bone. Pituitary metastases typically occur in patients in their sixth or seventh decade of life, and have no clear sex predominance {1433}.

Localization
Teears and Silverman {832,2734} reported that 57% of these lesions were localized to the posterior pituitary alone, 13% to the anterior pituitary alone, and 12% to both lobes, with the remainder localized to the capsule or stalk. Metastatic tumours located in the stalk can cause visual disturbances {1706}. It has been hypothesized that the posterior pituitary, because it receives a direct arterial blood supply, is more likely to develop metastases than is the anterior pituitary, which receives its principal blood supply from the hypophyseal portal system.

Clinical features
The findings in early autopsy series indicate that most pituitary metastases are clinically silent. According to Teears and Silverman {2734}, only 7% of pituitary metastases are symptomatic. Among the more commonly reported symptoms are diabetes insipidus, ophthalmoplegia, headache/pain, visual field defects, and anterior pituitary dysfunction {832}. Morita et al. {1906} noted that diabetes insipidus is more common in patients with symptomatic pituitary metastases than in those with symptomatic adenomas, in whom it is exceptionally rare. Approximately 60% of the patients treated for pituitary metastases had diabetes insipidus, whereas < 1% of patients with adenoma present with this condition. It has also been reported that 14–20% of patients presenting with diabetes insipidus have pituitary metastases {832,1173, 1370}.

Because of their invasiveness, tumours that metastasize to the pituitary are also likely to produce visual deficits as a result of suprasellar extension and painful ophthalmoplegia due to invasion of the cavernous sinus. Metastatic tumours can result in anterior pituitary hormone dysfunction {832}. It has also been reported that in a substantial proportion (56–64%) of symptomatic patients, pituitary symptoms were the initial presentation of malignant disease {311,1906}.

Imaging
Radiological evaluation has generally not been particularly helpful in distinguishing pituitary metastases from pituitary adenomas. A rapid increase in the size of a sellar tumour along with aggressive infiltration of adjacent tissue and the presence of diabetes insipidus should raise suspicion of pituitary metastasis.

Microscopy
The histopathological appearance of pituitary metastases depends on the histology of the primary sites. Because most metastatic tumours are located in the posterior lobe, it is essential to make

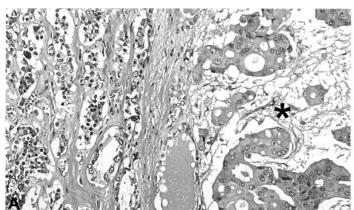
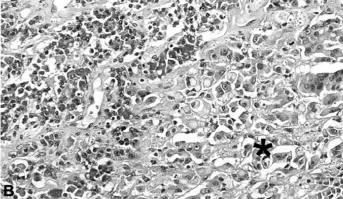

Fig. 1.73 Pituitary metastasis of lung adenocarcinoma. Metastases (asterisks) in the (**A**) posterior and (**B**) anterior lobe.

sections with an ample amount of posterior lobe tissue in addition to anterior lobe.

Diabetes insipidus is present in most cases of pituitary metastasis, due to the frequent localization of the metastatic tumours in the posterior lobe. Histological examinations of pituitary glands obtained during hypophysectomy for palliation in end-stage breast cancer and in autopsy series have revealed pituitary metastases in 6–29% of breast cancer patients {832}. Rare primary tumours that metastasize to the pituitary include hepatocellular carcinoma {2717}, differentiated (papillary) thyroid carcinoma {494}, and lung neuroendocrine carcinoma {637}. On very rare occasions, some cancers (including lung cancer) can metastasize to pituitary adenomas {899,1152}. In 1997, Sanno et al. {2410} reported that a metastatic GHRH-producing pancreatic neuroendocrine tumour induced somatotroph hyperplasia in the pituitary gland, resulting in acromegaly.

Some metastatic tumours mimic pituitary adenomas {1,2030}.

Prognosis and predictive factors

The prognosis of patients with pituitary metastases is poor, not due to the location per se, but because of the aggressiveness of the primary neoplasms {647, 1433}.

Predictive factors depend on the biological nature of the primary tumour and the extent of disease spread in the body. Pituitary metastases can be treated with multiple modalities, including resection, radiation therapy, and chemotherapy {832}. If the metastasis is confined in the sella turcica, patients may show improvement (particularly in visual defects) following transsphenoidal surgery. Theoretically, molecular targeted cancer therapies may be useful to suppress pituitary metastases. Therapeutic biomarkers such as overexpression of ERBB2 (also known as HER2), *EGFR* mutation, and RAS gene mutations may indicate the appropriate target therapy {2117}.

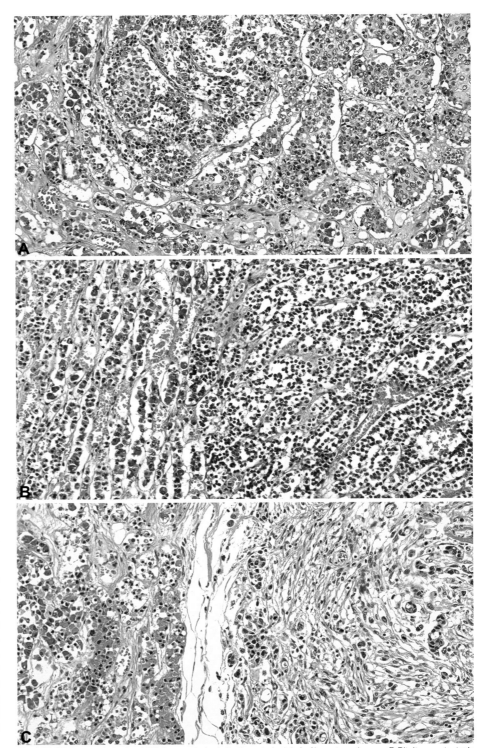

Fig. 1.74 Pituitary metastasis. **A** Pituitary metastasis (in the anterior lobe) of breast carcinoma. **B** Pituitary metastasis (in the anterior lobe) of small cell lung carcinoma. **C** Pituitary metastasis (in the posterior lobe) of hepatobiliary adenocarcinoma.

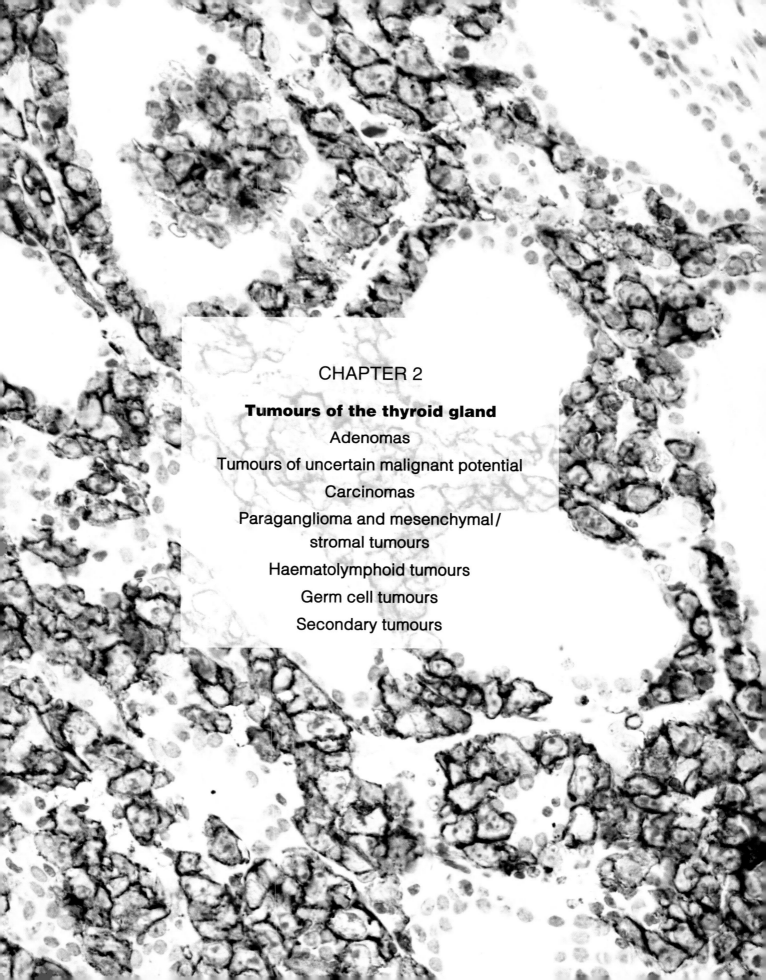

CHAPTER 2

Tumours of the thyroid gland
Adenomas
Tumours of uncertain malignant potential
Carcinomas
Paraganglioma and mesenchymal/
stromal tumours
Haematolymphoid tumours
Germ cell tumours
Secondary tumours

WHO classification of tumours of the thyroid gland

Follicular adenoma	8330/0
Hyalinizing trabecular tumour	8336/1*

Other encapsulated follicular-patterned thyroid tumours

Follicular tumour of uncertain malignant potential	8335/1*
Well-differentiated tumour of uncertain malignant potential	8348/1*
Non-invasive follicular thyroid neoplasm with papillary-like nuclear features	8349/1*

Papillary thyroid carcinoma (PTC)

Papillary carcinoma	8260/3
Follicular variant of PTC	8340/3
Encapsulated variant of PTC	8343/3
Papillary microcarcinoma	8341/3
Columnar cell variant of PTC	8344/3
Oncocytic variant of PTC	8342/3

Follicular thyroid carcinoma (FTC), NOS 8330/3

FTC, minimally invasive	8335/3
FTC, encapsulated angioinvasive	8339/3*
FTC, widely invasive	8330/3

Hürthle (oncocytic) cell tumours

Hürthle cell adenoma	8290/0
Hürthle cell carcinoma	8290/3

Poorly differentiated thyroid carcinoma	8337/3
Anaplastic thyroid carcinoma	8020/3
Squamous cell carcinoma	8070/3
Medullary thyroid carcinoma	8345/3
Mixed medullary and follicular thyroid carcinoma	8346/3
Mucoepidermoid carcinoma	8430/3
Sclerosing mucoepidermoid carcinoma with eosinophilia	8430/3
Mucinous carcinoma	8480/3

Ectopic thymoma	8580/3
Spindle epithelial tumour with thymus-like differentiation	8588/3
Intrathyroid thymic carcinoma	8589/3

Paraganglioma and mesenchymal/stromal tumours

Paraganglioma	8693/3
Peripheral nerve sheath tumours (PNSTs)	
Schwannoma	9560/0
Malignant PNST	9540/3
Benign vascular tumours	
Haemangioma	9120/0
Cavernous haemangioma	9121/0
Lymphangioma	9170/0
Angiosarcoma	9120/3
Smooth muscle tumours	
Leiomyoma	8890/0
Leiomyosarcoma	8890/3
Solitary fibrous tumour	8815/1

Haematolymphoid tumours

Langerhans cell histiocytosis	9751/3
Rosai-Dorfman disease	
Follicular dendritic cell sarcoma	9758/3
Primary thyroid lymphoma	

Germ cell tumours

Benign teratoma (grade 0 or 1)	9080/0
Immature teratoma (grade 2)	9080/1
Malignant teratoma (grade 3)	9080/3

Secondary tumours

The morphology codes are from the International Classification of Diseases for Oncology (ICD-O) {898A}. Behaviour is coded /0 for benign tumours; /1 for unspecified, borderline, or uncertain behaviour; /2 for carcinoma in situ and grade III intraepithelial neoplasia; and /3 for malignant tumours. The classification is modified from the previous WHO classification, taking into account changes in our understanding of these lesions.

*These new codes were approved by the IARC/WHO Committee for ICD-O.

TNM classification of tumours of the thyroid gland

T – Primary Tumour*

TX   Primary tumour cannot be assessed

T0   No evidence of primary tumour

T1   Tumour 2 cm or less in greatest dimension, limited to the thyroid

T1a   Tumour 1 cm or less in greatest dimension, limited to the thyroid

T1b   Tumour more than 1 cm but not more than 2 cm in greatest dimension, limited to the thyroid

T2   Tumour more than 2 cm but not more than 4 cm in greatest dimension, limited to the thyroid

T3   Tumour more than 4 cm in greatest dimension, limited to the thyroid or with gross extrathyroidal extension invading only strap muscles (sternohyoid, sternothyroid, or omohyoid muscles)

T3a   Tumour more than 4 cm in greatest dimension, limited to the thyroid

T3b   Tumour of any size with gross extrathyroidal extension invading only strap muscles (sternohyoid, sternothyroid, or omohyoid muscles)

T4a   Tumour extends beyond the thyroid capsule and invades any of the following: subcutaneous soft tissues, larynx, trachea, oesophagus, recurrent laryngeal nerve

T4b   Tumour invades prevertebral fascia or mediastinal vessels, or encases carotid artery

N – Regional Lymph Nodes

NX   Regional lymph nodes cannot be assessed

N0   No regional lymph node metastasis

N1   Regional lymph node metastasis

N1a   Metastasis in Level VI (pretracheal, paratracheal, and prelaryngeal/Delphian lymph nodes) or upper/superior mediastinum lymph nodes

N1b   Metastasis in other unilateral, bilateral or contralateral cervical (Levels I, II, III, IV, or V) or retropharyngeal lymph nodes

M – Distant Metastasis

M0   No distant metastasis

M1   Distant metastasis

Stage

Separate stages are recommended for papillary and follicular (differentiated) carcinomas, including Hürthle cell carcinomas, poorly differentiated, medullary, and anaplastic (undifferentiated) carcinomas:

Papillary and follicular (including Hürthle cell and poorly differentiated carcinomas); < 55 years

Stage I	Any T	Any N	M0
Stage II	Any T	Any N	M1

Papillary and follicular; ≥ 55 years

Stage I	T1a,T1b,T2	N0	M0
Stage II	T3	N0	M0
	T1,T2,T3	N1	M0
Stage III	T4a	Any N	M0
Stage IVA	T4b	Any N	M0
Stage IVB	Any T	Any N	M1

Medullary

Stage I	T1a, T1b	N0	M0
Stage II	T2, T3	N0	M0
Stage III	T1, T2, T3	N1a	M0
Stage IVA	T1, T2, T3	N1b	M0
	T4a	Any N	M0
Stage IVB	T4b	Any N	M0
Stage IVC	Any T	Any N	M1

Anaplastic

Stage IVA	T1,T2,T3a	N0	M0
Stage IVB	T1,T2,T3a	N1	M0
	T3b,T4a,T4b	N0,N1	M0
Stage IVC	Any T	Any N	M1

---

* Including papillary, follicular, poorly differentiated, Hürthle cell, medullary, and anaplastic carcinomas.

Adapted from: TNM Classification of Malignant Tumours, 8th Edition (2016). {323}

Introduction

Rosai J.

There have been several major developments in our knowledge of thyroid tumours since the publication of the third edition of the WHO classification of tumours of endocrine organs in 2004, reinforcing the long-held impression that the accurate classification of this family of neoplasms is an arduous and sometimes treacherous exercise. In 1970, the legendary French-Canadian pathologist Pierre Masson expressed this sentiment in his classic book *Human tumors* {1751A}, stating that "No classification is more difficult to establish than that of thyroid [carcinomas]", and adding that, as a consequence, "Of all cancers, they teach, perhaps, the greatest lessons of humility to histopathologists."

Arguably, the most important development in the field since the previous edition of the WHO classification has been the molecular-genetic characterization of well-differentiated follicular-patterned thyroid tumours composed of follicular cells. Our improved understanding of these tumours has impacted their time-honoured categorization into papillary versus follicular and benign versus malignant types.

Several new variants of papillary carcinoma have been identified, and the relative value of papillary formations versus a set of distinctive nuclear changes in the differential diagnosis remains a controversial subject.

Capsular and/or vascular invasion has remained the main criterion for the diagnosis of malignancy in encapsulated, well-differentiated tumours, and stricter criteria for the recognition of such tumours have been established. However, previously undervalued morphological features such as necrosis and mitotic activity have been found to have a level of prognostic significance that matches and in some cases surpasses that of the classic criterion of capsular and/or vascular invasion.

By far the most controversial issue that has impacted the field in recent years has been the proposed introduction into the classification of well-differentiated follicular tumours of a group of neoplasms (intermediate, borderline, etc., accompanied by several imaginative acronyms) that are morphologically and behaviourally intermediate between follicular adenoma and follicular carcinoma/the follicular variant of papillary carcinoma. These neoplasms can be considered the thyroid representatives of a group of tumours that have recently been described in a wide variety of organs, referred to as tumours of uncertain malignant potential. The crucial question of whether these tumours constitute distinct entities (and if so, whether they qualify as carcinomas/ neoplasms with low malignant potential) is currently the subject of discussion (see the *Introduction* subsection, p. 75, of *Other encapsulated follicular-patterned thyroid tumours*).

Poorly differentiated carcinoma and oncocytoma, members of two complex families of neoplasms, have been recognized as distinct entities, and the criteria for their diagnosis have been established. Various correlations between the molecular-genetic profile and the morphology of these tumours have been documented, although much work remains to be done in this area.

Issues concerning the relationship between anaplastic and squamous cell carcinoma, as well as the identification of a family of tumours equivalent in most respects to the similarly named neoplasms of the salivary glands, thymus, and other branchial arch derivatives, are less important from a practical standpoint due to their rarity, but are nevertheless of biological interest.

Follicular adenoma

Nikiforov Y.E.
Baloch Z.W.
Belge G.
Chan J.K.C.
Derwahl K.M.
Evans H.L.
Fagin J.A.

Ghossein R.A.
Lloyd R.V.
Oriola J.
Osamura R.Y.
Paschke R.
Sobrinho Simões M.

Definition
Follicular adenoma is a benign, encapsulated, non-invasive neoplasm showing evidence of thyroid follicular cell differentiation, without nuclear features of papillary thyroid carcinoma.

ICD-O code   8330/0

Epidemiology
The epidemiology of follicular adenoma is difficult to investigate due to the lack of reproducible histopathological criteria for distinguishing hyperplastic nodules from adenomas. Many pathologists do not make the diagnosis of adenoma in a multinodular gland, preferring to designate all lesions as hyperplastic nodules provided there is no evidence of malignancy. Biologically, follicular adenoma is a neoplasm and therefore has a clonal origin. This distinguishes follicular adenomas from hyperplastic nodules, which have a polyclonal origin. Without molecular analysis, it may not always be possible to distinguish follicular adenomas from hyperplastic nodules.
Based on data from autopsy series, the incidence of follicular adenomas in adults is estimated at 3–5% {118,259,2562}. This estimate correlates with the prevalence of thyroid nodules detectable by palpation. Palpable thyroid nodules are found in 3–7% of adults living in iodine-sufficient areas; three quarters of those nodules are found to be solitary on palpation and may be adenomas {553,1409}. The incidence of follicular adenoma is higher in iodine-deficient areas. Follicular adenomas more frequently affect females. They occur in all age groups, but most patients present during their fifth or sixth decade of life.

Etiology
Most follicular adenomas are sporadic. Radiation exposure and iodine deficiency are known risk factors. Radiation exposure during childhood and adolescence multiplies the risk of follicular adenoma by as much as 15 times {4,2555,3086}. Follicular adenomas typically have a longer latency period than do papillary carcinomas. They develop 10–15 years after exposure, with elevated risk persisting for ≥ 50 years. Follicular adenomas associated with radiation exposure are usually solitary and of the conventional type {4}. Palpable thyroid nodules are 2–3 times as frequent in areas of low iodine consumption as they are in iodine-sufficient areas, and a substantial proportion of palpable thyroid nodules are adenomas {203,204}. Some evidence points to a role of oxidative stress, excessive DNA damage, and increased mutagenesis within the thyroid gland in the formation of thyroid nodules {1313,1479}. Follicular adenomas can develop in patients with *PTEN* hamartoma tumour syndrome (in particular, Cowden syndrome) {772,1087,1157} or Carney complex {1393,2656}. Individuals with familial adenomatous polyposis have a high risk of papillary thyroid carcinoma, and also frequently present with multiple benign nodules, at least some of which are likely to be adenomas {844,2640}.

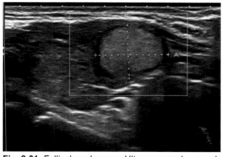

Fig. 2.01 Follicular adenoma. Ultrasonography reveals a distinct ovoid hypoechoic mass with smooth margins.

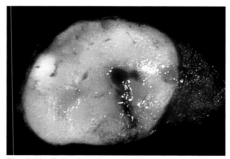

Fig. 2.02 Follicular adenoma. The tumour has a homogeneous light-tan cut surface and is well demarcated from the adjacent normal-looking thyroid tissue. A haemorrhagic needle tract is present.

Localization
Follicular adenoma can arise in the normal thyroid gland as well as in ectopic thyroid tissues and struma ovarii {2243}.

Clinical features
Thyroid adenoma typically presents as a painless thyroid nodule discovered incidentally by palpation or during thyroid imaging. Most adenomas are asymptomatic, although large tumours can cause difficulty in swallowing and other local symptoms. Haemorrhage into an adenoma, which can occur spontaneously or following vigorous neck palpation or fine-needle aspiration, can result in acute pain and tumour enlargement. On ultrasound, adenoma typically appears as a solid, well-demarcated, homogeneous mass that is hypoechoic or isoechoic. Most patients have a normally functioning thyroid gland. On radionuclide scan, most adenomas appear as so-called cold nodules, with the exception of hyperfunctioning (so-called hot) adenomas and nodules with normal uptake. Patients with hyperfunctioning adenomas may present with hyperthyroidism {168,2571}.

Macroscopy
Follicular adenoma is usually a solitary round or oval nodule surrounded by a capsule. Multiple adenomas are rare and should raise the possibility of an inherited disease. The tumours usually measure 1–3 cm, but can be much larger. The capsule can be thin or thick. The cut surface shows homogeneous greyish-white, tan, or brown fleshy tumour. Generally, tumours that are greyish-white are more cellular and have a solid or trabecular growth pattern, whereas tan to brown tumours have well-developed follicles with substantial colloid. Secondary changes such as haemorrhage and cystic degeneration may be present.

Microscopy
Follicular adenomas have a fibrous cap-

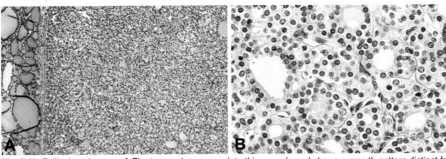

Fig. 2.03 Follicular adenoma. **A** The tumour has a complete thin capsule and shows a growth pattern distinct from that of the adjacent normal thyroid. **B** The cells have round, dark, uniform nuclei.

sule, which is typically thin or moderately thick. By definition, capsular and vascular invasion is absent. The architectural and cytological features of the tumour are different from those of the surrounding thyroid parenchyma. Follicular adenomas show a variety of architectural growth patterns: normofollicular, macrofollicular, microfollicular, solid, and trabecular. More than one pattern may be seen in a single nodule. Rarely, follicular adenomas show a papillary or insular growth pattern. The tumour cells are cuboidal or polygonal. In hyperfunctioning adenomas, tall cells are seen. The cytoplasm is moderately abundant and pale eosinophilic to amphophilic. The nuclei are basally located and round, with smooth contours and uniform chromatin distribution. Follicular adenoma with lipid-rich cells is composed of cells that have abundant cytoplasm full of vacuoles containing lipid {479,2478,2804}. The vacuoles are small or large in size, and have a clear or finely granular appearance. Some variability of the nuclear shape, size, and chromatin texture may be seen. Mitotic figures are rare. The stromal component of the tumour is typically scant. Some adenomas have abundant oedematous, mucinous, or hyalinized stroma, with hyalinized stroma being more pronounced in the central portion of the nodule. Secondary changes such as stromal fibrosis, hyalinization, haemorrhage, oedema, cystic degeneration, calcification, and osseous or cartilaginous metaplasia may be seen.

The distinction between follicular adenoma and hyperplastic nodule on microscopic examination is straightforward when follicular adenoma is solitary, has a well-defined fibrous capsule, and shows a uniform growth pattern that is markedly different from the surrounding normal-appearing thyroid parenchyma. However, the distinction is arbitrary when only some of these features are present and mutation status of the nodule is not available.

The only histological features that reliably distinguish follicular carcinoma from follicular adenoma are vascular invasion and capsular invasion, underscoring the importance of adequate sampling of the tumour–capsule interface to search for invasion. With grossly encapsulated nodules, submission of the entire capsule is recommended.

Immunophenotype
Follicular adenomas are immunoreactive for cytokeratins, thyroglobulin, TTF1, and PAX8, but not for calcitonin, CEA, or neuroendocrine markers. The Ki-67 proliferation index is typically < 5% {1942}. Immunoreactivity for galectin 3, HBME1, and CITED1 is rare {1942,2372,2488}.

Immunohistochemistry for thyroglobulin and calcitonin is helpful for excluding medullary carcinoma in tumours with a solid or trabecular growth pattern. Parathyroid adenoma arising within the thyroid gland can mimic follicular adenoma of the microfollicular, clear cell, or oncocytic type. The correct diagnosis can be established using immunostaining for thyroglobulin, TTF1, parathyroid hormone, and chromogranin.

Hyperfunctioning (so-called toxic or hot) adenoma
This variant is associated with biochemical or clinical evidence of hyperthyroidism due to autonomous production of thyroxine by the tumour cells. Histologically, these tumours can resemble conventional follicular adenomas, or the follicles can be lined by columnar cells, often with delicate papillary projections within the lumina. The cells have abundant, frequently vacuolated cytoplasm and round, uniform, basally located nuclei. The colloid is bubbly, with peripheral scalloping. The shape of the cells and papillary formations can rarely mimic the appearance of the tall cell variant of papillary carcinoma, but the absence of fibrovascular cores of papillary structures and lack of characteristic nuclear features of papillary carcinoma distinguishes hyperfunctioning adenoma. Molecular analysis may also help: *BRAF* V600E mutation is characteristic of the tall cell variant of papillary thyroid carcinoma, whereas *TSHR* and *GNAS* mutations are typically found in hyperfunctioning follicular adenomas {2119,2817}.

Follicular adenoma with papillary hyperplasia
This variant occurs predominantly in children and young adults and is characterized by a thick capsule, pronounced cystic changes, and predominantly

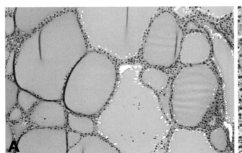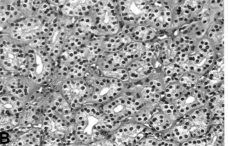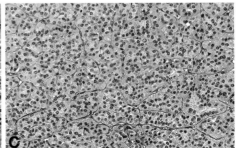

Fig. 2.04 Follicular adenoma. **A** Macrofollicular growth pattern. **B** Microfollicular growth pattern. **C** Solid growth pattern.

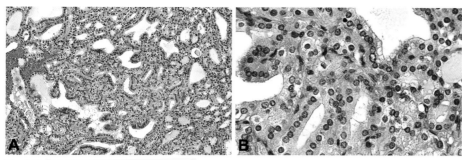

Fig. 2.05 Hyperfunctioning follicular adenoma. **A** Many follicles are irregularly shaped, are devoid of colloid, and have delicate papillary infoldings. **B** The follicular cells are tall, with basally located nuclei and vacuolated cytoplasm.

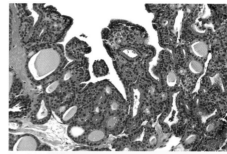

Fig. 2.06 Follicular adenoma with papillary hyperplasia. The papillary structures are non-arborizing and have a loose, oedematous stroma containing small follicles.

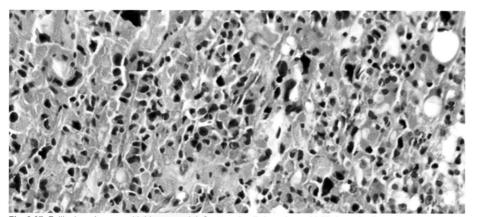

Fig. 2.07 Follicular adenoma with bizarre nuclei. Scattered cells have huge, highly irregular, hyperchromatic nuclei.

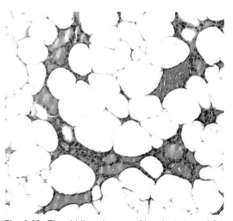

Fig. 2.08 Thyroid lipoadenoma. Abundant stromal fat cells intermixed with thyroid follicles.

papillary architecture {806,1716,2877}. The papillae are delicate and typically non-branching, and frequently have oedematous hypocellular cores, which may contain follicles. The tumour cells have a cuboidal to columnar shape and contain uniform, round, dark nuclei regularly aligned at the base. By definition, nuclear features of papillary thyroid carcinoma are absent. Some tumours show evidence of thyroid hyperfunction.

Lipoadenoma (also called adenolipoma)
In this variant, mature adipose cells are interspersed throughout the tumour {1362,1866,2477}. Variable proportions of adipose cells and follicular structures can be seen microscopically. Lipoadenomas have been reported in patients with Cowden syndrome {365,1087} and following exposure to radiation {998}.

Follicular adenoma with bizarre nuclei
This variant is characterized by isolated or small groups of highly atypical tumour cells with very large, irregularly shaped hyperchromatic nuclei within an otherwise typical follicular adenoma. These cells are more commonly seen in oncocytic adenomas and in patients treated with radioactive iodine {1032}. Mitotic figures are rare, and tumour necrosis is absent.

Signet-ring cell follicular adenoma
This variant is composed of cells containing a discrete cytoplasmic vacuole that displaces the nucleus to the periphery, producing a signet-ring appearance {754,962,1807}. The vacuoles are immunoreactive for thyroglobulin, and often stain positively for mucin. Ultrastructurally, the vacuoles appear as intracellular lumina lined by microvilli {2474}.

Clear cell follicular adenoma
This variant is characterized by cells with clear cytoplasm, which can be a result of ballooning of mitochondria, accumulation of lipid or glycogen, or deposition

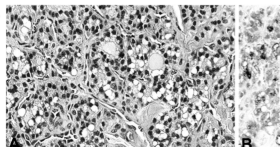
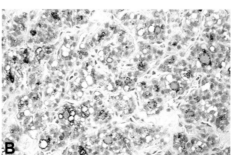
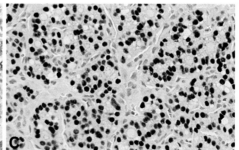

Fig. 2.09 Follicular adenoma with signet-ring cells. **A** Tumour cells show large cytoplasmic vacuoles that displace the nuclei to the periphery of the cells. **B,C** The cells demonstrate immunoreactivity for thyroglobulin (**B**) and TTF1 (**C**), confirming thyroid follicular cell origin.

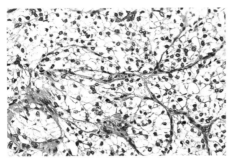

Fig. 2.10 Follicular adenoma with clear cells. The cells have water-clear cytoplasm. The main differential diagnosis is with metastatic renal cell carcinoma.

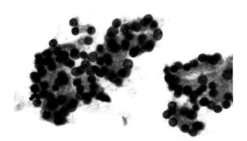

Fig. 2.11 Follicular adenoma. Fine-needle aspiration biopsy reveals cohesive microfollicular structures composed of a monotonous population of cells with round nuclei and uniform chromatin distribution. The specimen was diagnosed as follicular adenoma after excision.

of thyroglobulin {392}. As is the case in clear cell follicular carcinoma, immunoreactivity for thyroglobulin and TTF1 is useful for distinguishing this entity from metastatic renal cell carcinoma.

Spindle cell follicular adenoma
In rare cases, follicular adenoma can be composed predominantly of spindle cells. Immunoreactivity for cytokeratin, thyroglobulin, and TTF1 and negativity for calcitonin confirms the follicular thyroid cell origin of these tumours.

Black follicular adenoma
So-called black adenomas can be seen in patients treated with minocycline {1453}. The tumours have black discolouration visible on macroscopic examination and cytoplasmic accumulation of black pigment, with an appearance and staining qualities similar to those of minocycline-induced black thyroid.

Cytology
Aspirates of follicular adenomas are usually cellular, with numerous follicular cells and little or no colloid; deposits of thick colloid may be seen. Most often, the follicular cells are both dissociated and arranged in clusters with microfollicle formation. Microfollicles consist of groups of 6–12 nuclei in a small circle, sometimes with a small amount of thick luminal colloid. Macrofollicular adenomas demonstrate abundant colloid, with follicular cells arranged in monolayer sheets. This appearance is similar to that of hyperplastic nodules. The distinction of follicular adenomas from carcinomas is not possible in cytological preparations.

Genetic profile
Clonality
Follicular adenomas have a monoclonal origin (i.e. they arise from a single cell). Clonality assays based on the assessment of randomness of inactivation of X chromosomes in female tissue have confirmed the clonal origin of most follicular adenomas {1140,1949}. The clonal origin of a given tumour can also be established through the detection of an oncogenic mutation or cytogenetic abnormality in a large proportion of the lesional cells {1478,1480}.

Cytogenetics and loss of heterozygosity
Clonal cytogenetic aberrations are detectable in about half of all follicular adenomas {206,2742}. Most of these aberrations are numerical chromosome changes, typically whole-chromosome gains involving one or several chromosomes. Trisomy 7 (alone or with other trisomies) is the most common, followed by gains of chromosomes 12 and 5. Translocations involving the chromosomal regions 19q13.4 and 2p21 are frequent structural chromosomal changes {392, 2478}. Both breakpoint regions have been characterized, and candidate genes have been identified: *ZNF331* for 19q13.4 and *THADA* for 2p21 {205,2301, 2303}. However, these candidate genes have not yet been definitively proven to be the target of translocations. Two microRNA gene clusters, C19MC and miR-371-3, have been located in the breakpoint region 19q13.4 {215}. The translocations in the chromosomal region 19q13.4 seem to lead to the upregulation of genes encoding microRNAs of these clusters {2302}. On average, follicular adenomas have a 6% rate of loss of heterozygosity per chromosome arm {2947}.

Somatic mutations
Mutations of the RAS genes occur in

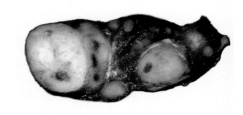

Fig. 2.12 Multiple follicular thyroid adenomas in a patient with *PTEN* hamartoma tumour syndrome.

about 30% of follicular adenomas {792, 1257,1586,1950}. The most commonly affected hotspot is codon 61 of *NRAS*, followed by codon 61 of *HRAS*, whereas *KRAS* is the least frequently involved gene. *PAX8/PPARG* rearrangements, a feature of follicular thyroid carcinomas, are found in about 8% of follicular adenomas {492,729,893,1257,1995}. Many of these tumours are cellular and have a thick capsule, but do not demonstrate invasion. Isolated cases of follicular adenoma carrying *BRAF* K601E mutation have been reported {8,2593}. *TSHR* and *GNAS* mutations are found in most hyperfunctioning thyroid adenomas {2119, 2817}; they are activating mutations in the functionally important domains of both genes, and cause increased thyroid function and iodine uptake. *PIK3CA* and *PTEN* mutations occur in about 5% of follicular adenomas {1171,1990}.

Genetic susceptibility
Patients with *PTEN* hamartoma tumour syndrome (in particular Cowden syndrome) and Carney complex are susceptible to the development of follicular adenomas. Carney complex is caused by germline *PRKAR1A* mutations and may be associated with follicular adenomas, which are often multiple and may have oncocytic features {1393,2656}. *PTEN* hamartoma tumour syndrome is caused by a germline inactivating mutation in *PTEN* {365,772,1157,1963}. Follicular adenomas in *PTEN* hamartoma tumour syndrome develop in younger patients and are multiple and bilateral. They are typically of the conventional histological type, but oncocytic adenoma, clear cell adenoma, and lipoadenoma can be also seen.

Prognosis and predictive factors
Completely removed follicular adenomas pose no further risk.

Hyalinizing trabecular tumour

Papotti M.
Volante M.

Definition

Hyalinizing trabecular tumour (HTT) is a follicular-derived neoplasm composed of large trabeculae of elongated or polygonal cells admixed with variable amounts of intratrabecular and intertrabecular hyaline material.

ICD-O code

8336/1

Synonyms

Hyalinizing trabecular neoplasm; hyalinizing trabecular adenoma

Epidemiology

HTT occurs predominantly in females. The mean patient age is 50 years (range: 21–79 years). The single reported malignant case occurred in a 28-year-old man {403,1026}.

Etiology

No etiological or risk factors are known, although previous radiation exposure has been occasionally reported.

Localization

HTT has a slight predilection for the right lobe {403}.

Clinical features

Most patients are asymptomatic. HTT shares ultrasonographic features with follicular adenoma and the follicular variant of papillary thyroid carcinoma, including solid texture, oval or round shape, well-defined borders, and hypoechogenicity {1578}. On scintigraphy, so-called cold nodules are seen {403}. The tumour is sometimes discovered during routine clinical examination or as an otherwise incidental finding.

Macroscopy

HTT is generally a well-circumscribed or encapsulated, single, solid neoplasm with a round or oval shape, a firm to soft consistency, a lobulated appearance on cut surface, and a white to yellow colour. The size ranges from 0.5 to 7.5 cm {403}; about half of all cases measure < 3 cm {403}. The single reported malignant case measured 3 cm and had capsular penetration {1026}.

Microscopy

HTT is a solid, well-circumscribed tumour without capsular, vascular, or thyroid parenchymal invasion (except for a single reported invasive case) {1026}. The tumours are composed of wide trabeculae or more rarely of small nests of cells delimited by thin stromal bundles conferring a Zellballen or lobulated appearance. The tumour cells are generally large or medium-sized (with a small-cell component in 11% of cases) {403} and polygonal or elongated. The cytoplasm is variably eosinophilic, finely granular, and occasionally clear, with perinuclear, sometimes yellow bodies {2352}. The nuclei are vesicular and round, and contain grooves, vacuoles, and membrane irregularities. Mitoses are rare, except in the single reported malignant case. Within the trabeculae, a variably abundant hyaline amorphous material (resembling amyloid but Congo red–negative) is present, sometimes enveloping tumour cells. This material is eosinophilic, gives a diastase-resistant positive periodic acid–Schiff (PAS) reaction, is mostly of the basal membrane type, and is partially related to colloid. The intertrabecular stroma is generally inconspicuous, with fine capillaries; it sometimes merges with the trabecular hyaline material. Stromal lymphocytic infiltration can occur. Calcium deposits are reported within the trabeculae or the stroma in 43% of cases {403}, occurring as round laminated structures of the psammoma-body type. HTT can be associated with chronic lymphocytic thyroiditis, nodular goitre, or papillary carcinoma.

Immunophenotype

HTT cells express thyroglobulin and TTF1 but not calcitonin. The expression of malignancy-related markers of follicular cells, such as HBME1, galectin 3, and CK19, is irregular, occurring in 0–50% of cases {403,917,919,1589}. The hyaline material is positive for collagen IV {403, 1603,2048,2102}. Ki-67 cell membrane reactivity is unique to HTT {419,1146}, but this characteristic non-nuclear staining occurs only when the MIB1 monoclonal antibody against Ki-67 is used, and only at room temperature {1590}.

Cytology

In fine-needle aspirates, cytological features (e.g. nuclear grooves, pseudoinclusions, and irregular borders) may suggest papillary carcinoma (in one study, this was seen in 33 of 55 cases) or medullary thyroid carcinoma {403,504}.

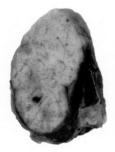
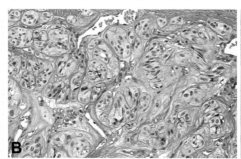
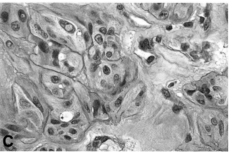

Fig. 2.13 Hyalinizing trabecular tumour. **A** Gross appearance of an encapsulated tumour. **B** The tumour has a peripheral capsule and large trabeculae, with intratrabecular hyalinization. **C** The tumour featured polygonal or elongated cells with papillary carcinoma–type nuclei. Note the prominent nuclear pseudoinclusions.

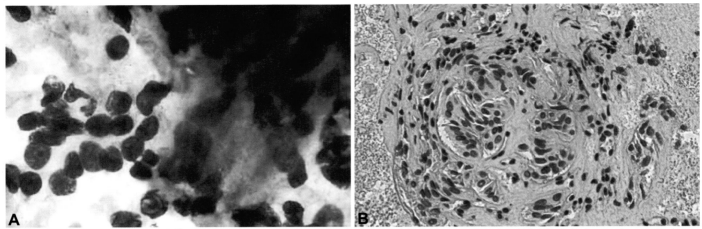

Fig. 2.14 Hyalinizing trabecular tumour. **A** Fine-needle aspiration specimen containing hyaline material in the tumour cell clusters. **B** Cell block of a fine-needle aspiration biopsy, with trabecular architecture and nuclear irregularities and vacuoles.

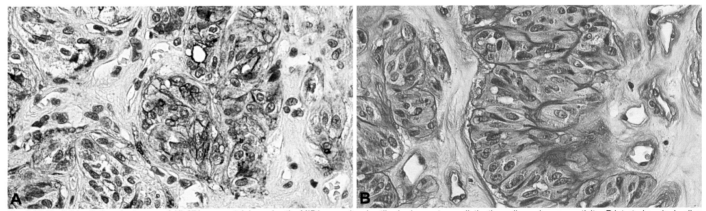

Fig. 2.15 Hyalinizing trabecular tumour. **A** Ki-67 immunostaining using the MIB1 monoclonal antibody shows strong, distinctive cell membrane reactivity. **B** Intratrabecular hyaline material that gives a positive periodic acid–Schiff (PAS) reaction is present in association with tumour cells.

These tumours are usually classified as indeterminate/suspicious; i. e. as category Thy3–5 in the British Thyroid Association (BTA) system or category IV–VI in the Bethesda system. Diagnostic clues favouring HTT include hyaline or amyloid-like material, loosely cohesive groups of tumour cells with a trabecular or syncytial pattern radiating outwards from a hyaline core, abundant cytoplasm, lack of papillae, and calcifications {134,420, 1366,1710}.

Genetic profile

The relationship between HTT and papillary thyroid carcinoma was originally suggested by the detection of *RET*/PTC1 rearrangements and RET immunoreactivity in approximately half of HTT cases {486,2107,2397}. However, neither RAS nor *BRAF* mutations have been detected in HTT {2397}. Limited microRNA profiling does not support the proposed link between HTT and papillary carcinoma {2537}.

Prognosis and predictive factors

The prognosis is extremely good, with only one documented case of distant metastasis in a series of 119 cases {403}; the patient developed pulmonary metastases, but was alive 5 years after diagnosis {1026}. Most cases in the series followed a benign course after surgery, with follow-up as long as 48 years {403}. Lymph node metastases are rarely observed {1782}.

Other encapsulated follicular-patterned thyroid tumours

Introduction

Chan J.K.C.
Nikiforov Y.E.
Tallini G.

Some encapsulated follicular-patterned neoplasms of the thyroid pose diagnostic difficulties due to uncertainty as to whether the nuclear changes are sufficient to justify a diagnosis of papillary thyroid carcinoma (PTC), or due to uncertainty about the presence of capsular or vascular invasion.

Encapsulated follicular-patterned tumours indeterminate between follicular adenoma and follicular carcinoma

For an encapsulated follicular-patterned tumour lacking nuclear features of PTC, capsular invasion can be equivocal, rendering it difficult to determine with certainty whether this represents follicular adenoma or follicular carcinoma. The Chernobyl Pathologists Group proposes calling this group of tumours "follicular tumour of uncertain malignant potential" {2989}. The current WHO classification retains this terminology, but with the scope expanded to include cases with equivocal vascular invasion.

Encapsulated or well-circumscribed follicular-patterned tumours with well-developed or equivocal nuclear features of papillary thyroid carcinoma

Because nuclear morphology takes precedence over architecture and other histological features in the diagnosis of PTC, a diagnosis of cancer, i.e. the follicular variant of PTC (FVPTC), can be made in an encapsulated or well-circumscribed follicular-patterned tumour as long as the nuclear features are compatible with PTC, irrespective of the presence or absence of capsular or vascular invasion. However, the assessment of nuclear features is highly subjective, and the threshold for rendering a diagnosis of FVPTC varies greatly among pathologists, resulting in poor interobserver concordance

Table 2.01 2014 Armed Forces Institute of Pathology (AFIP) fascicle on tumours of the thyroid and parathyroid glands: recommended nomenclature for encapsulated well-differentiated follicular-patterned tumours on the basis of the presence or absence of nuclear features of papillary thyroid carcinoma (PTC) and capsular invasion. Modified from Rosai J et al. {2340}

		Capsular invasion		
		Present	**Questionable**	**Absent**
Nuclear features of PTC	**Present**	Follicular variant of PTC		
	Questionable	Well-differentiated carcinoma, NOS	Well-differentiated tumour of uncertain malignant potential	
	Absent	Follicular carcinoma	Follicular tumour of uncertain malignant potential	Follicular adenoma

Table 2.02 2017 WHO classification: recommended nomenclature for encapsulated follicular-patterned tumours on the basis of the presence or absence of nuclear features of papillary thyroid carcinoma (PTC) and capsular or vascular invasion.

		Capsular or vascular invasion		
		Present	**Questionable**	**Absent**
Nuclear features of PTC	**Present**	Invasive encapsulated follicular variant of PTC	Well-differentiated tumour of uncertain malignant potential	Non-invasive follicular thyroid neoplasm with papillary-like nuclear features
	Questionable	Well-differentiated carcinoma, NOS		
	Absent	Follicular carcinoma	Follicular tumour of uncertain malignant potential	Follicular adenoma

in the diagnosis of encapsulated FVPTC {445,766,1655,2275}. The Chernobyl Pathologists Group considers it more appropriate to acknowledge this grey area in pathological diagnosis than to arbitrarily categorize well-differentiated encapsulated tumours with a follicular architecture and incompletely developed nuclear features of PTC as either definitely malignant or definitely benign {2989}. The term "well-differentiated tumour of uncertain malignant potential" has been proposed for cases with questionable PTC-type nuclear changes and no or questionable invasion, and this is also the term used in the 2014 Armed Forces Institute of Pathology (AFIP) fascicle on tumours of the thyroid and parathyroid glands (see Table 2.01) {2340}.

Many studies have demonstrated that non-invasive encapsulated FVPTC is associated with an excellent prognosis and has molecular features more similar to those of follicular adenoma/carcinoma than to those of conventional PTC {375, 428,925,1178,1293,1994,2307,2338}. An international Endocrine Pathology Society working group has proposed renaming the aforementioned non-invasive tumours with well-developed to incompletely developed nuclear features of PTC and no vascular or capsular invasion "non-invasive follicular thyroid neoplasm with papillary-like nuclear features", removing the word "carcinoma" from the nomenclature in an attempt to reduce overtreatment of this indolent tumour {1994}. Therefore, in the current WHO classification, the term "non-invasive follicular thyroid neoplasm with papillary-like nuclear features" encompasses non-invasive encapsulated follicular-patterned tumours previously called encapsulated FVPTC as well as well-differentiated tumour of uncertain

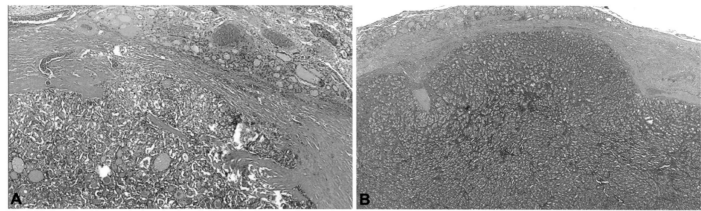

Fig. 2.16 Questionable capsular invasion in well differentiated tumour of uncertain malignant potential. **A** Hook-like protrusion of tumour cells deeply into but not completely through the capsule. **B** Broad-based bulge of tumour cells into the capsule that does not extend beyond its outer contour.

malignant potential. The term "well-differentiated tumour of uncertain malignant potential" is reserved in this classification for tumours with well-developed to incompletely developed PTC-type nuclei and questionable invasion (see Table 2.02, p. 75).

Tumours of uncertain malignant potential

Chan J.K.C.
Tallini G.

Definition

Thyroid tumours of uncertain malignant potential are encapsulated or well-circumscribed follicular-patterned thyroid tumours with questionable capsular or vascular invasion, irrespective of the presence or absence of papillary carcinoma–type nuclear features. Two types

are recognized: follicular tumour of uncertain malignant potential (FT-UMP) and well-differentiated tumour of uncertain malignant potential (WDT-UMP) {2989}.

Follicular tumour of uncertain malignant potential is an encapsulated or well-circumscribed tumour composed of well-differentiated follicular cells with no nuclear features of papillary thyroid carcinoma (PTC) and with questionable capsular or vascular invasion. That is, this is a tumour indeterminate between follicular adenoma and follicular carcinoma.

Well-differentiated tumour of uncertain malignant potential is an encapsulated or well-circumscribed tumour composed of well-differentiated follicular cells with well-developed or partially developed PTC-type nuclear changes and with questionable capsular or vascular invasion. WDT-UMPs in which capsular or vascular invasion has been excluded by

all means are called non-invasive follicular thyroid neoplasm with papillary-like nuclear features (see *Non-invasive follicular thyroid neoplasm with papillary-like nuclear features*, p. 78).

ICD-O codes
Follicular tumour of uncertain
  malignant potential   8335/1
Well-differentiated tumour of
  uncertain malignant potential   8348/1

Synonyms
Atypical adenoma (adenoma with atypia) {1547}; well-differentiated tumour of uncertain behaviour {1293}

Epidemiology
Reported prevalence rates are summarized in Table 2.03.

Localization
The tumour arises in the thyroid gland {1153}.

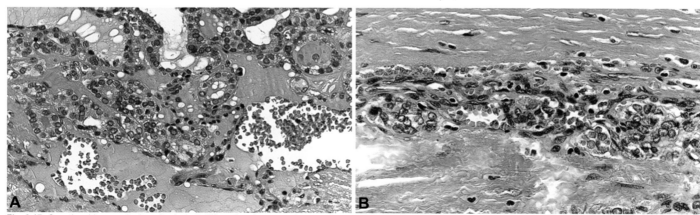

Fig. 2.17 Questionable vascular invasion in well-differentiated tumour of uncertain malignant potential. **A** Irregular outgrowth of neoplastic cells within vascular spaces of the tumour capsule. **B** Tumour cells closely intermixed with vascular spaces of the tumour capsule.

Table 2.03 Prevalence of tumours of uncertain malignant potential: well-differentiated tumour of uncertain malignant potential (WDT-UMP) and follicular tumour of uncertain malignant potential (FT-UMP) {1153,1644,2165}

Country	Thyroidectomy specimens analysed	Thyroid carcinomas	WDT-UMP[a]	FT-UMP[a]	Period examined
Italy	Not available	1020	5 (0.5%)	6 (0.6%)	1979–2004
France	1078	166	16 (8.1%)	15 (7.6%)	2004–2008
Japan	2648	501[b]	30 (5.6%)	Not available	1990–2009

[a] Listed in parenthesis: the proportion of the total number of possible malignant diagnoses (i.e. carcinomas plus tumours of uncertain malignant potential).
[b] Papillary thyroid carcinomas only.

Clinical features

Tumours of uncertain malignant potential present as thyroid nodules, usually single nodules.

Macroscopy

The general appearance is similar to that of follicular adenoma or hyperplastic nodule. The size is variable, with most cases measuring 1–3 cm and few cases > 4 cm {1153,1644}. Hyperplastic nodules in the surrounding parenchyma have been reported in approximately 40% of cases, and lymphocytic thyroiditis in 10–15% {1153}.

Microscopy

FT-UMP and WDT-UMP are pure follicular-patterned thyroid tumours that exhibit equivocal tumour capsular or vascular invasion after thorough sampling and exhaustive examination {1153,2989}. In FT-UMP, the tumour cells have round nuclei that lack the nuclear features of PTC {2989}. In WDT-UMP, there are well-developed to equivocal PTC-type nuclear alterations, with variable changes in nuclear size and shape (enlargement, overlapping, crowding, and elongation), nuclear membrane irregularities (irregular contours, grooves, and pseudoinclusions), and chromatin features (clearing) {445,2337,2989}. The PTC-type nuclear alterations of WDT-UMP overlap with those of non-invasive follicular thyroid neoplasm with papillary-like nuclear features (see *Non-invasive follicular thyroid neoplasm with papillary-like nuclear features*, p. 78).

Tumour capsular penetration is questionable when cells connected with the main tumour nodule invade into but not completely through the capsule (with or without mushrooming into it) or are identified as isolated nests confined within the fibrous stroma. These findings are of particular concern when the capsule is thick and irregular {805,2337}. Capsular invasion must be distinguished from reactive changes in the capsule induced by fine-needle aspiration procedures and from herniation of tumour cells due to cutting of the specimen prior to fixation {2337}.

Vascular invasion is considered questionable when a smooth-contoured tumour cell nest located within a vascular space of the tumour capsule lacks endothelial covering and associated thrombus, or when a tumour nest in the fibrous capsule abuts a blood vessel, eliciting consideration of early vascular invasion versus mere colocalization of the tumour nest and the blood vessel.

Immunophenotype

The immunohistochemical features of FT-UMP are similar to those of follicular adenoma, hyperplastic nodule, and minimally invasive follicular carcinoma. WDT-UMP may be positive for HBME1, galectin 3, and CK19, but these markers have limited diagnostic utility. The expression profile of WDT-UMP for these three markers is different from that of follicular adenoma but similar to that of the follicular variant of PTC, suggesting a pathogenetic link {1153,1644,2103,2488}.

Cytology

WDT-UMP shows enlarged nuclei and a few nuclear grooves, but usually no pseudoinclusions; the tumours generally fall into one of the indeterminate diagnostic categories (atypia of undetermined significance, follicular neoplasm, suspicious for papillary carcinoma) {1153,2001}. FT-UMP shows cytological features of follicular neoplasms (follicular adenoma/carcinoma).

Genetic profile

The genetic alterations reported in tumours of uncertain malignant potential are summarized in Table 2.04 {93,867, 1153,1644}. The presence of RAS family mutations and lack of *BRAF* V600E mutation are similar to the genetic profile of follicular neoplasms (i.e. follicular adenoma and follicular carcinoma). *RET/PTC1* rearrangements have been identified in approximately 10% of WDT-UMPs, possibly as subclonal events {911}. The gene expression pattern {93,867} and microRNA profile {474,1556} are heterogeneous, with features intermediate between benign follicular nodules and papillary carcinoma.

Prognosis and predictive factors

With encapsulated follicular-patterned tumours in which invasion of the tumour capsule and/or PTC-type nuclear alterations are the only histological evidence of malignancy, the risk of recurrence or metastasis is very low {925,1292,1632,2165, 2596,2769,2848,2984}.

Specific data on the long-term outcome of tumours of uncertain malignant potential (FT-UMP and WDT-UMP) are limited. Several studies have reported no nodal or distant metastases, tumour recurrence, or tumour-related deaths {93, 1644,2165,2596}. In one retrospective study of 2978 cases originally diagnosed as benign thyroid nodule/tumour, 5 cases were found to later develop distant metastases: 2 of these cases qualify as FT-UMP (one with questionable vascular invasion and the other with questionable invasion of the thyroid parenchyma) {1292}.

Table 2.04 Genetic alterations reported in tumours of uncertain malignant potential: well-differentiated tumour of uncertain malignant potential (WDT-UMP) and follicular tumour of uncertain malignant potential (FT-UMP) {93,867,1153,1644}

Alteration	Positive cases WDT-UMP	Positive cases FT-UMP
NRAS mutation	3/21 (14.3%)	2/15 (13.3%)
HRAS mutation	0/16 (0%)	1/15 (6.6%)
KRAS mutation	0/16 (0%)	0/15 (0%)
PAX8-PPARG	0/16 (0%)	1/15 (6.6%)
RET/PTC1	5/51 (9.8%)	0/15 (0%)
RET/PTC3	0/21 (0%)	0/15 (0%)
BRAF	0/66 (0%)	0/15 (0%)

Non-invasive follicular thyroid neoplasm with papillary-like nuclear features

(NIFTP)

Nikiforov Y.E.
Ghossein R.A.
Kakudo K.
LiVolsi V.
Papotti M.
Randolph G.W.
Tallini G.
Thompson L.D.R.
Tuttle R.M.

Definition

Non-invasive follicular thyroid neoplasm with papillary-like nuclear features (NIFTP) is a non-invasive neoplasm of thyroid follicular cells with a follicular growth pattern and nuclear features of papillary thyroid carcinoma (PTC) that has an extremely low malignant potential (see *Tumours of uncertain malignant potential*, p. 76).

ICD-O code   8349/1

Epidemiology

Tumours currently classified as NIFTP were formerly classified as the non-invasive encapsulated follicular variant of PTC (FVPTC) or well-differentiated tumour of uncertain malignant potential. Based on previously reported prevalence rates of non-invasive encapsulated FVPTC in several European countries and North America, NIFTPs are estimated to constitute 10–20% of all thyroid cancers in these regions {1281,1691}, with possibly lower prevalence in Asia {1644}. The female-to-male ratio is 3–4:1. These tumours have a wide patient age range, but most patients present during their fourth to sixth decade of life {1994,2762}.

Localization

These tumours can arise in either lobe of the thyroid or in the isthmus.

Clinical features

NIFTP typically presents as a painless, asymptomatic, mobile thyroid nodule, although large tumours may cause compression and other local symptoms. Patients are typically euthyroid. On ultrasound, there is a solid, well-demarcated, homogeneous mass, which is frequently hypoechoic.

Macroscopy

NIFTP is a solitary, well-demarcated nodule, typically with a thin to moderately thick capsule. Occasionally, the nodules may have a thick fibrous capsule. The cut surface is a homogeneous whitish-tan to fleshy-brown colour. Colloid-rich tumours may show a dark-brown cut surface resembling normal thyroid. Spontaneous secondary changes are rare; focal haemorrhage or cystic degeneration is typically the result of previous fine-needle aspiration. The tumours are usually 2–4 cm in size, but can be much larger {1994,2762}.

Microscopy

Four histological features are required for the diagnosis of NIFTP: (1) a complete capsule or clear demarcation of the tumour from adjacent thyroid tissue, (2) the absence of invasion, (3) a follicular growth pattern, and (4) nuclear features of papillary carcinoma. The capsule is often thin but is complete, although partial encapsulation or a smooth border with clear demarcation of the tumour from adjacent thyroid tissue may be seen. Thorough examination of the tumour capsule interface is required to exclude tumour capsular or lymphovascular invasion. The growth pattern is follicular (micro-, normo-, or macrofollicular), frequently with a mixture of follicles

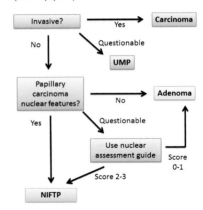

Fig. 2.20 Algorithm for the evaluation of encapsulated follicular lesions, including evaluation for invasion and evaluation of nuclear features. The use of the 3-point scoring scheme for degree of nuclear changes (nuclear score) {1994} facilitates the diagnosis of non-invasive follicular thyroid neoplasm with papillary-like nuclear features (NIFTP). UMP, tumour of unknown malignant potential.

of various sizes. Colloid is present and may be copious in tumours composed of large follicles. Simple papillary infoldings or abortive papillary structures may be seen, but true papillae with fibrovascular cores are absent, as are psammoma bodies. Exclusion features include a component of solid, trabecular, or insular growth accounting for > 30% of the tumour; high mitotic activity (≥ 3 mitoses per 10 high-power fields); and tumour necrosis. These are features of either the solid variant of papillary carcinoma or poorly differentiated thyroid carcinoma. The nuclear features of papillary carcinoma seen in NIFTP are separated into three categories: (1) size and shape (enlargement, overlapping, crowding, and elongation), (2) membrane irregularities (irregular contours, grooves, folds,

Table 2.05 Diagnostic criteria for non-invasive follicular thyroid neoplasm with papillary-like nuclear features {1994}

1. Encapsulation or clear demarcation
2. Follicular growth pattern with all of the following:
   < 1% papillae
   No psammoma bodies
   < 30% solid, trabecular, or insular growth pattern
3. Nuclear features of papillary carcinoma (i.e. nuclear score of 2–3)
4. No lympho-vascular or capsular invasion
5. No tumour necrosis
6. No high mitotic activity (< 3 mitoses per 10 high-power fields)

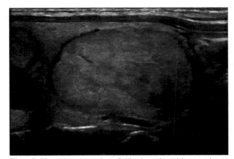

Fig. 2.18 Non-invasive follicular thyroid neoplasm with papillary-like nuclear features. Sagittal ultrasound image showing a well-delineated solid isoechoic mass with smooth margins.

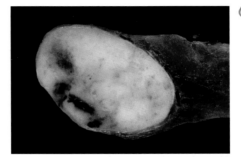

Fig. 2.19 Non-invasive follicular thyroid neoplasm with papillary-like nuclear features. Macroscopically, the tumour has smooth contours, a thin capsule, and a homogeneous tan-yellow cut surface with focal haemorrhage.

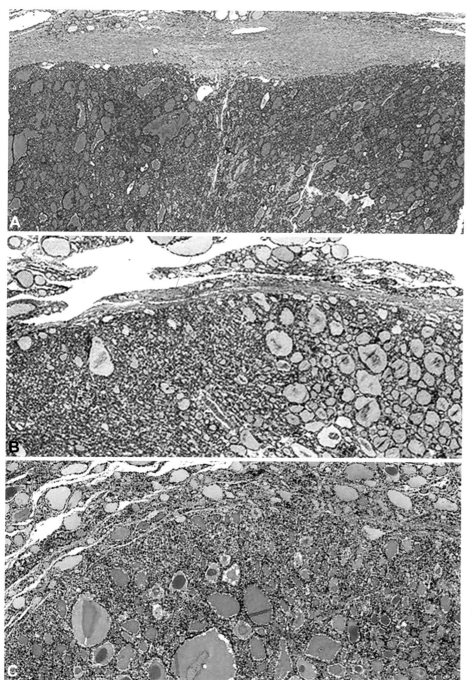

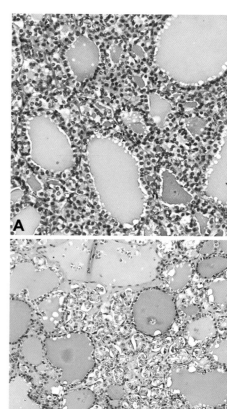

Fig. 2.22 Non-invasive follicular thyroid neoplasm with papillary-like nuclear features. **A** This tumour shows a mixture of small and larger-sized follicles and diffusely present papillary carcinoma–like nuclear features. **B** This tumour shows focal areas with microfollicular architecture and papillary carcinoma–like nuclear features interspersed with larger follicles lined by normal-appearing cells.

Fig. 2.21 Non-invasive follicular thyroid neoplasm with papillary-like nuclear features. The tumour can have a thick capsule (**A**) or a thin capsule (**B**), or it can have no capsule but be sharply demarcated from the adjacent normal thyroid parenchyma (**C**).

and pseudoinclusions), and (3) chromatin characteristics (clearing with margination, glassy nuclei). For a tumour to qualify as NIFTP, nuclear features from at least two of these three categories must be expressed to a substantial degree. Specifically following a 3-point scoring scheme in which each category of nuclear features is assigned a score of either 0 or 1, yielding a summation nuclear score of 0–3, a score of 2–3 is required for diagnosis {1994}. The nuclear features may be focal, patchy, or diffuse, reminiscent of the so-called sprinkling sign described in FVPTC {2853}.

NIFTP is distinguished from follicular adenoma and hyperplastic nodules by the presence of nuclear features of papillary carcinoma, from conventional PTC by the absence of papillae, and from invasive encapsulated FVPTC by the absence of capsular or vascular invasion.

Cytology
Fine-needle aspirates are usually cellular, with some colloid and variably expressed nuclear features of papillary carcinoma. Three-dimensional groups of follicular cells and microfollicles can be seen. About half of all NIFTPs are cytologically diagnosed as follicular neoplasms (Bethesda category IV); most of the remaining cases are diagnosed as either category V (suspicious for malignancy) or category III (atypia of undetermined significance or follicular lesion of undetermined significance) {1724}. In rare cases, a diagnosis of PTC is rendered. A reliable

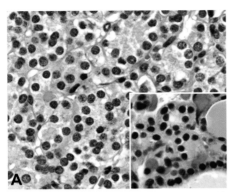 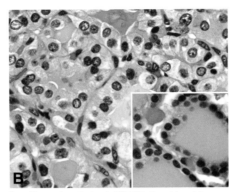 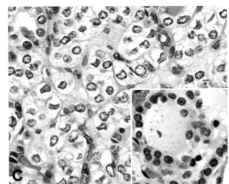

Fig. 2.23 Non-invasive follicular thyroid neoplasm with papillary-like nuclear features (NIFTP): thyroid nodules composed of cells showing different nuclear scores. **A** Nuclear score of 1: The cells of this lesion have enlarged nuclei as compared with the adjacent normal thyroid parenchyma (inset), but show no substantial irregularity of the nuclear membrane and no chromatin clearing. These features are insufficient for a diagnosis of NIFTP. **B** Nuclear score of 2: These cells have enlarged nuclei as compared with the adjacent normal thyroid parenchyma (inset) and show substantial irregularity of the nuclear contours, but no chromatin clearing. This meets the criteria for NIFTP. **C** Nuclear score of 3: These cells show enlarged nuclei as compared with the adjacent normal thyroid parenchyma (inset), pronounced irregularity of the nuclear contours, and chromatin clearing. This meets the criteria for NIFTP.

distinction between NIFTP and PTC cannot be made in cytological preparations. In some cases with indeterminate cytopathological aspirates, the possibility that these findings ultimately represent an entity now considered to be non-malignant (NIFTP) may shift the surgical recommendation from total thyroidectomy to hemithyroidectomy. The exact extent of this surgical clinical impact is yet to be determined {825}.

Genetic profile

NIFTPs share molecular alterations with other follicular-patterned thyroid tumours and have a high prevalence of RAS family mutations and sometimes *PPARG* and *THADA* gene fusions {375,1994, 2307,3024}. *BRAF* K601E mutations can also be present, but *BRAF* V600E mutations and *RET* fusions (characteristic of conventional PTC) are absent.

Prognosis and predictive factors

Provided the tumour is completely removed and careful examination of the tumour capsule interface reveals no capsular or lympho-vascular invasion, the risk of recurrence or other adverse events is extremely low: < 1% within the first 15 years after resection {1994}. Incomplete excision, with positive resection margins, may lead to tumour recurrence {2884}. NIFTP can be treated with lobectomy, allowing patients to avoid complete thyroidectomy and radioactive iodine therapy.

Papillary thyroid carcinoma

Rosai J.
Albores Saavedra J.
Asioli S.
Baloch Z. W.
Bogdanova T.
Chen H.
DeLellis R. A.
Erickson L. A.

Fagin J. A.
Franssila K. O.
Giordano T. J.
Hay I. D.
Katoh R.
Lloyd R. V.
Mete O.
Nikiforov Y. E.

Piana S.
Prasad M. L.
Sadow P.
Schneider A. B.
Soares P.
Sobrinho Simões M.
Vielh P.
Wenig B. M.

Definition
Papillary thyroid carcinoma (PTC) is a malignant epithelial tumour showing evidence of follicular cell differentiation and a set of distinctive nuclear features. PTC is usually invasive. Papillae, invasion or cytological features of papillary thyroid carcinoma are required.

ICD-O codes
Papillary carcinoma	8260/3
Follicular variant of PTC	8340/3
Encapsulated variant of PTC	8343/3
Papillary microcarcinoma	8341/3
Columnar cell variant of PTC	8344/3
Oncocytic variant of PTC	8342/3

Synonym
Papillary thyroid adenocarcinoma

Epidemiology
Age and sex distribution
PTC is the predominant form of thyroid cancer in both adults and children. It accounts for about 65% of cases in Ireland, 86.2% in the USA, and 93% in Japan and the Republic of Korea {869}. In the USA, the median patient age at diagnosis is 50 years, with 91% of patients diagnosed at an age of 20–74 years {1179}. The incidence rate in women is about 3 times the rate in men, but this disparity decreases with increasing patient age.

Incidence
In 2008–2012, the average annual incidence of thyroid cancer in the USA was 13.5 cases per 100 000 population. There has been a dramatic global increase in the reported incidence of thyroid cancer since the introduction of new, high-resolution imaging techniques (e.g. thyroid ultrasonography) into clinical practice {1516,2842}. In the USA, the incidence rate tripled over a 30-year period. Almost all of the tumours accounting for this recent increase are of the papillary type. Death due to PTC is uncommon, and despite the increasing incidence, mortality rates have either remained unchanged or decreased in most countries. In the USA, SEER data indicate that mortality remained stable between 2003 and 2012, and the 5-year survival rate was 97.9% {1179}. In 2012 in the USA, an estimated 600 000 people were living with or had a history of thyroid cancer. The increase in PTC incidence rates comprises an increase in both ultrasound-detected cases and larger, potentially palpable cases. This finding raises the possibility that there are other factors at play beyond improved imaging techniques {2842}.

Etiology
The best-documented environmental cause of PTC is exposure to ionizing radiation. Many other risk factors have also been identified, including reproductive factors, obesity, diabetes, smoking, alcohol consumption, dietary nitrates, dietary iodine excess, and genetic factors {616}. However, the relationship between these factors and PTC is not entirely clear.

Localization
PTC can arise in either lobe or in the isthmus of the normally situated gland, as well as anywhere that ectopic thyroid tissue may be present, such as in a thyroglossal cyst or struma ovarii.

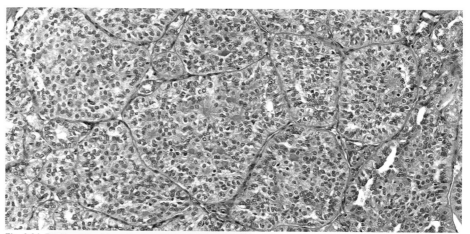
Fig. 2.24 Papillary thyroid carcinoma with a solid growth pattern. Mitoses were scant and necrosis was absent.

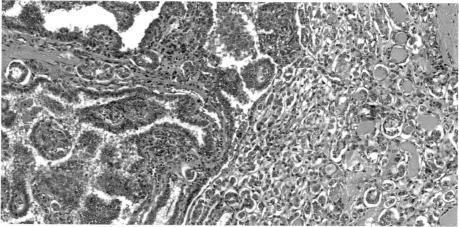
Fig. 2.25 Conventional papillary thyroid carcinoma with merging of papillary and follicular patterns.

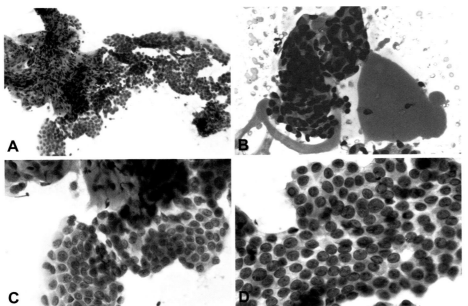

Fig. 2.26 Papillary thyroid carcinoma. FNAB of classic variant. **A** Tumour cells are arranged in complex papillary fragment. **B** The colloid is thick and ropy (so-called bubble gum colloid). **C** The tumour cells show elongated nuclei and demonstrate prominent "whorling" within groups. **D** Individual tumour cells demonstrate elongated nuclei with powdery chromatin, eccentrically placed inconspicuous micro-nucleoli, thickened nuclear membranes, intranuclear grooves and pseudo-inclusions.

Clinical features

Clinical symptoms and signs

PTC usually presents as an asymptomatic (painless) thyroid mass with or without enlargement of regional (cervical) lymph nodes {393}. Hoarseness and dysphagia occur in approximately 20% of cases {1193}, signalling recurrent laryngeal nerve involvement with vocal cord paralysis or tracheal compression. Nodal metastases in the lateral neck are reported in 27% of patients at presentation {1193}, most often originating from tumours in the ipsilateral thyroid lobe. Thyroid function testing has limited utility in the diagnosis of PTC because most patients have normal thyroid function.

Imaging

On thyroid scan (^{123}I), PTCs typically appear as cold (i.e. hypofunctioning) nodules, but rarely can appear as hot (i.e. hyperfunctioning) nodules {1367,1867}. Ultrasound examination is the imaging modality of choice for PTC. Sonographic features include a hypoechoic or isoechoic solid nodule with irregular or poorly defined margins, microcalcifications, taller-than-wide shape, and disorganized internal vascularity {1280, 1360}.

Ultrasound findings are also invaluable for guiding fine-needle aspiration biopsy of abnormal nodes. Other imaging modalities, including CT, MRI, and FDG-PET/CT, may be needed to assess the extent of extrathyroidal extension, to evaluate the presence of substernal masses, to detect recurrent tumour, and to improve diagnostic accuracy in iodine-negative differentiated thyroid carcinoma {1568,2083}.

Cystic change may be present. These sonographic findings may be very suggestive of PTC, but only fine-needle aspiration biopsy allows for a preoperative diagnosis.

Tumour spread and staging

In most series, approximately 20% of PTCs are multifocal {393}, but higher incidences have also been reported {1324, 1339,2362}, a finding that appears to correlate with the extent of sampling. Multifocal PTCs often constitute separate primary tumours, but intraglandular spread via lymph vessels also occurs {152,1486, 2116,2941}. Due to this tendency for lymphatic spread, metastasis to regional lymph nodes, including lateral neck and midline nodes (central compartment levels VI and VII), is common. Spread via blood vessels also occurs but is rare; it most frequently involves the lungs.

Macroscopy

Grossly, PTC typically presents as an invasive neoplasm with poorly defined margins, a firm consistency, and a granular white cut surface. Calcifications may be apparent. The size is widely variable, with a mean diameter of 2–3 cm {1104}. The proportion of tumours measuring ≤ 1.5 cm in diameter ranges across series from 13.7% {2824} to 64% {889}.

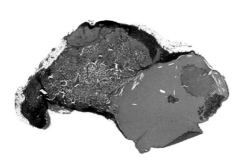

Fig. 2.27 Papillary thyroid carcinoma (PTC). A cystic metastasis from a conventional PTC is present in this lymph node.

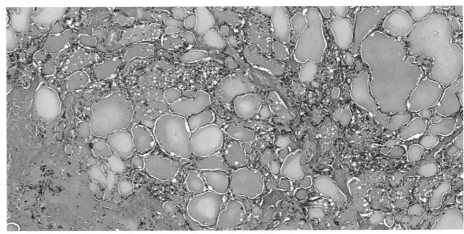

Fig. 2.28 Papillary thyroid carcinoma showing the so-called sprinkling sign.

Most of the variations in the gross appearance of PTC are related to its variants, and are discussed with them.

Tumour necrosis is unusual in PTC. Its detection in the absence of previous fine-needle aspiration should suggest an alternative diagnosis or the emergence of a more aggressive (i.e. poorly differentiated or undifferentiated) component within the tumour.

Microscopy

The two cardinal morphological features of conventional (classic) PTC are the papillae and the nuclear changes. The papillae are composed of a central fibrovascular stalk covered by a neoplastic epithelial lining. The papillae may be long, straight, or arborizing; arranged in a parallel, regimented fashion; short and stubby; or tightly packed. The thickness and composition of the papillary stalk is variable. The stalk is usually made up of loose connective tissue and variously sized thin-walled vessels. In its most characteristic form, PTC shows a great predominance of papillary structures throughout the tumour. However, it is very rare for the tumours to be composed exclusively of papillae {1645}. In most cases, the papillae are interspersed with neoplastic follicles that have similar nuclear features.

The nuclei of the cells of PTC display a characteristic set of abnormalities, which can be grouped into three categories: (1) changes in size and shape, (2) irregularities of the membrane, and (3) chromatin characteristics {1994}. Changes in nuclear size and shape include nuclear enlargement and often overlapping, as well as nuclear elongation {1033}. Such changes are best appreciated by comparing the nuclei of the tumour cells at the edge of the tumour with those of adjacent normal thyroid tissue. The nuclei of PTC are typically characterized by marked remodelling of the nuclear envelope, with highly irregular nuclear contours and nuclear pseudoinclusions or prominent longitudinal grooves {858}. The pseudoinclusions, which constitute deep cytoplasmic invaginations into the nucleus, appear as acidophilic, inclusion-like round structures, sharply outlined and slightly eccentric, with a crescent-shaped rim of compressed chromatin on one side {449,2490}. The other consistent feature of PTC nuclei is an empty appearance of the nucleoplasm {144}. The

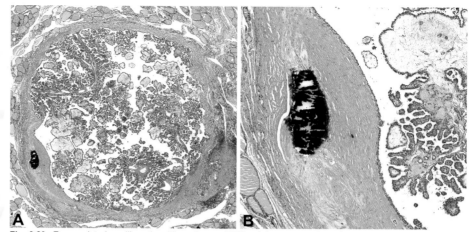

Fig. 2.29 Encapsulated papillary thyroid carcinoma (PTC). **A** Low-power view of an encapsulated conventional PTC. **B** High-power view of the same PTC shows the classic growth pattern. Calcification is apparent in the capsule.

inner aspect of the nuclear membrane is irregularly thickened by the apposition of chromatin material. These nuclei have been variously described as optically clear and resembling ground glass {648}. The ground-glass appearance is evident in fixed, paraffin-embedded material but is inconspicuous or absent in frozen sections from the same cases {395,1219}.

The cytoplasm of PTC cells is generally slightly eosinophilic. Mitotic figures are rare or absent in conventional PTC. The exception to this may occur after fine-needle aspiration. In addition to papillary and follicular patterns, PTC can grow in solid or trabecular formations {886}; this usually occurs as a focal change, but it can also involve most or all of the neoplasm.

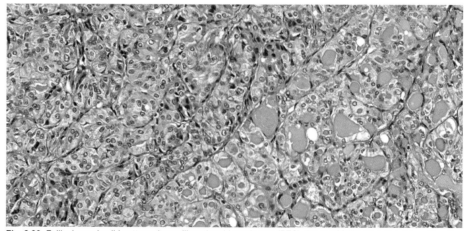

Fig. 2.30 Follicular and solid patterns in papillary thyroid carcinoma (PTC). Areas of follicular and solid proliferation merge in this PTC.

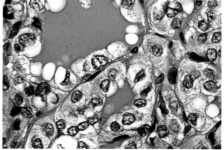

Fig. 2.31 Follicular variant of papillary thyroid carcinoma (PTC). Typical nuclear features of PTC are present. Note the darkly staining colloid.

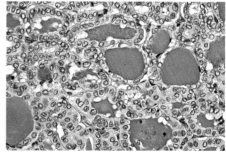

Fig. 2.32 Follicular variant of papillary thyroid carcinoma. Typical low-power appearance.

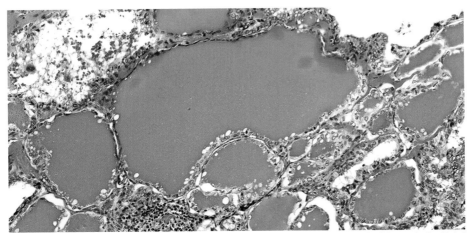

Fig. 2.33 Macrofollicular variant of papillary thyroid carcinoma. This variant is characterized by cystically dilated macrofollicles.

This should not be considered evidence that the tumour has become undifferentiated or poorly differentiated, providing the typical nuclear features of PTC persist. Structures classically associated with PTC are psammoma bodies, which are round calcific concretions that exhibit concentric lamination. Psammoma bodies are found in about 50% of cases overall and are particularly common in tumours with a predominantly papillary growth pattern {1267,2830}. True psammoma bodies are found within the stroma or in lymphatic channels. Psammoma body–like formations located within the lumina of follicles should be disregarded; in most instances, they are the result of inspissated secretion and are more commonly seen in connection with oncocytic neoplasms. Focal or extensive squamous metaplasia is also common in PTC, reported in 20–40% of cases {393,886}. An abundant fibrous stroma is a common feature of PTC and is particularly evident at the advancing edge {1645}. Some of

this stromal reaction has a very cellular (desmoplastic) appearance {1449}. Occasionally, it acquires morphological qualities consistent with fibromatosis, nodular fasciitis, or inflammatory myofibroblastic tumour, to the point of obscuring the neoplastic component {447,1863}. Scattered multinucleated giant cells of non-neoplastic histiocytic nature are often present, and are particularly conspicuous in cytological preparations {1047}. Secondary cystic changes are common. Most of these cysts are lined by papillary formations diagnostic of the entity, but others are covered by a much attenuated, single-layered, flat epithelium with a deceptively benign appearance. Blood vessel invasion is not as common as in follicular carcinoma, but it certainly does occur {393}. Invasion of lymph vessels is a much more common phenomenon, but is not always easy to detect. The vast majority of PTCs have the nuclear and architectural features already described {29,2308,2595}.

Immunophenotype
PTC cells are immunoreactive for thyroglobulin, TTF1, PAX8, and cytokeratins (pancytokeratin, CK7, CAM5.2, and AE1/AE3) {202,343,1132,2152,2630}. They are negative for CK20, calcitonin, and neuroendocrine markers. Contrary to common belief, traditional mucin stains are positive in a considerable number of PTCs {451,607}. Galectin 3, HBME1, CK19, and CITED1 immunostains may help to distinguish between PTC and benign lesions, but they should be interpreted in conjunction with microscopic features. Membranous HBME1 staining is most specific; it is typically seen in conventional PTC and with lower frequency in the follicular variant {418,2802}. Galectin 3 staining should be both nuclear and cytoplasmic; it is seen in most conventional PTCs, but can also be found in benign reactive cells such as in Hashimoto thyroiditis {163,1942,2488}. CK19 is the least specific marker of malignancy {2380}.

Variants
Papillary microcarcinoma
Tumours of this variant measure ≤ 1 cm in diameter. This variant has also been called occult sclerosing carcinoma, occult papillary carcinoma, and non-encapsulated sclerosing tumour {1113, 1190,1408}. More recently, a proposal has been advanced to call it papillary microtumour {2343}. In various series, the reported incidence in autopsy material is 5.6–35.6%. The prevalence of this tumour increases steeply from birth to adulthood and remains relatively constant afterwards. Due to their small size, these lesions can easily be missed on gross examination {1546,2186,3044}. Microscopically, the prototypical example of this variant has an irregular, scar-like configuration. The neoplastic elements predominate at the periphery, whereas other elements are entrapped in the centre. Some tumours are totally surrounded by an extremely thick fibrous capsule, which may be focally calcified. The general attributes of PTC are present, including typical nuclear changes, fibrosis, psammoma bodies, and occasional well-formed papillae. Overall, the prognosis of papillary microcarcinoma is excellent. In one series, 93% of the patients were free of disease on follow-up, and there were no instances of distant metastasis {393,2343}. However, the fact that these

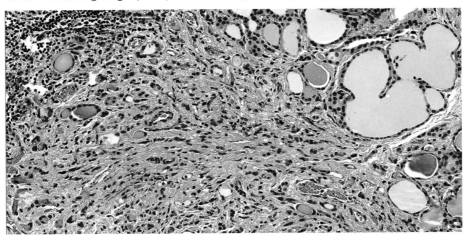

Fig. 2.34 Multifocal sclerosing thyroiditis. This benign lesion can simulate a papillary microcarcinoma.

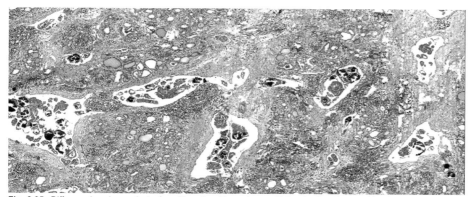

Fig. 2.35 Diffuse sclerosing variant of papillary thyroid carcinoma. Extensive lymph vessel involvement and dense fibrosis are evident.

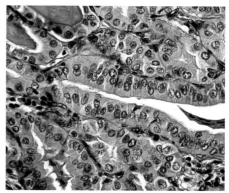

Fig. 2.36 Tall cell variant of papillary thyroid carcinoma (PTC). Nuclear features typical of PTC in cells with an abundant eosinophilic (tall) cytoplasm.

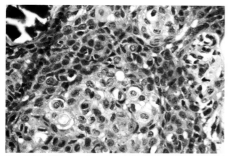

Fig. 2.37 Diffuse sclerosing variant of papillary thyroid carcinoma. Extensive squamous metaplasia and psammoma bodies are evident.

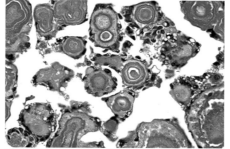

Fig. 2.38 Papillary thyroid carcinoma. Numerous psammoma bodies in various stages of formation.

lesions can exhibit malignant behaviour has been proven by several authors {269, 972,1814}, especially in cases with *BRAF* mutation {226}.

Encapsulated variant

This variant is a type of architecturally and cytologically typical PTC that is totally surrounded by a fibrous capsule, which may be intact or only focally infiltrated by tumour growth. The encapsulated variant accounts for about 10% of all cases of PTC {393,806,2476}. Encapsulated PTC has an excellent prognosis. Regional nodal metastases may be present, but bloodborne metastases are rare, and the

survival rate is nearly 100% {762,806, 2476}. The main differential diagnosis is with follicular adenoma with papillary hyperplasia, which lacks PTC-type nuclear changes {450}.

Follicular variant

This variant has an exclusively or almost exclusively follicular growth pattern {1054,2344,2948}. There are two main subtypes: infiltrative and encapsulated with invasion. In its most typical form (the infiltrative subtype), this variant shares many features with conventional PTC. Most importantly, the nuclei of the cells lining the follicles have features of

conventional PTC. The colloid within the lumina of the neoplastic follicles often has a strong and homogeneous eosinophilic quality. There are also some unusual variations of the follicular variant of PTC (FVPTC): rare cases in which the neoplastic follicles are cystically dilated, simulating nodular hyperplasia (macrofollicular variant) {41,1687,1943}; cases in which minute neoplastic follicles are scattered in a background of normal follicles (the so-called sprinkling sign) {2853}; and even rarer cases in which there is diffuse tumour involvement of the whole thyroid gland, without formation of grossly discernible nodules (diffuse or multinodular follicular variant) {1235,1870,2591}. The hypothesis that (unencapsulated) FVPTC belongs to the papillary family of thyroid neoplasms is supported by several findings: (1) some of these tumours are accompanied by multicentric foci within the thyroid that have a conventional papillary architecture {2344}; (2) the natural history of these tumours closely matches that of conventional PTC, particularly in regard to the high incidence of cervical lymph node involvement {393,805,3125}; (3) these nodal metastases often have a papillary configuration {393,464}; and (4) the types of keratin expressed by the tumour cells match those expressed by papillary rather than follicular carcinoma {140,1837}.

Diffuse sclerosing variant

This uncommon variant occurs more commonly in women, most frequently in the second or third decade of life {390, 2591}. The clinical presentation typically includes diffuse enlargement of the thyroid gland. Elevated serum antithyroglobulin and antimicrosomal antibodies may mimic Hashimoto thyroiditis {452,900,

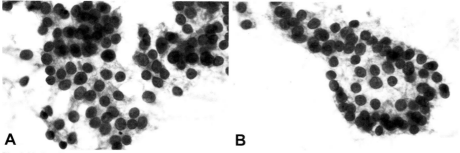

Fig. 2.39 Papillary thyroid carcinoma. FNAB of follicular variant **A** Tumour cells are arranged in follicular groups. **B** The individual tumour cells show elongated nuclei with powdery chromatin, delicate intranuclear grooves and eccentrically placed micronucleoli. Intranuclear inclusions are not common; therefore most cases are diagnosed as "suspicious for papillary carcinoma".

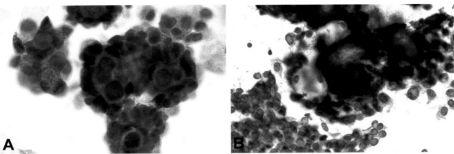

Fig. 2.40 Papillary thyroid carcinoma. FNAB of sclerosing variant. **A, B** Tumour cells with nuclear features of papillary carcinoma arranged in nests and numerous psammoma bodies or coarse calcification.

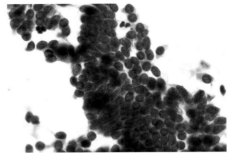

Fig. 2.41 Papillary thyroid carcinoma. FNAB of columnar cell variant. Tumour cells arranged in cohesive groups with prominent nuclear elongation and stratification. The tumour cell nuclei are elongated; however, the chromatin is coarser than in aspirates of classic papillary thyroid carcinoma.

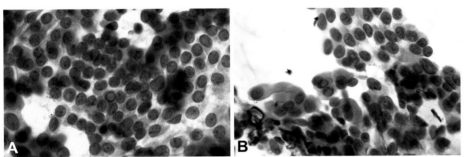

Fig. 2.42 Papillary thyroid carcinoma. FNAB of tall cell variant. **A, B** The tumour cells are tall in shape and demonstrate ample oncocytic cytoplasm with readily evident nuclear features of papillary thyroid carcinoma.

2910}, and a hard so-called woody gland may mimic Riedel thyroiditis {2920}. Histologically, there is diffuse involvement of a single lobe or the entire gland, characterized by dense sclerosis, numerous psammoma bodies, and background changes of chronic lymphocytic thyroiditis. Tumour nests appear solid, with associated squamous metaplasia, including squamous morules. The tumour cells have a propensity to invade intrathyroidal lymphatic spaces and a tendency to show extrathyroidal extension. They are variably reactive for thyroglobulin, TTF1, and cytokeratins (CK19) {1447,2768}. *RET*/PTC rearrangement is frequently found, but *BRAF* mutation is rare {6,1273, 2536}. Compared with conventional PTC,

the diffuse sclerosing variant is associated with a higher incidence of extrathyroidal extension; of cervical lymph node metastasis (both unilateral and bilateral); and of distant metastasis (which occurs in ~10–15% of cases), primarily to the lung. The diffuse sclerosing variant is also associated with a shorter disease-free survival {905,1446,2266}. However, the mortality rates are comparable to those of conventional PTC {25,509}, possibly due to the favourable effect of a younger patient age, with a 93% 10-year disease-specific survival rate {1528}.

Tall cell variant *— aggressive*

By definition, this variant is composed of cells that are two to three times as tall as

they are wide, and that show abundant eosinophilic (oncocytic-like) cytoplasm. Typical nuclear features of papillary carcinoma are present, and nuclear pseudoinclusions are usually easily found. Because tall-cell areas are frequently present in otherwise conventional papillary carcinomas, tall cells must account for ≥ 30% of all tumour cells for the diagnosis of the tall cell variant {923,966}. The tall cell variant of PTC occurs at an older patient age and is considered an aggressive variant, because the tumours show extrathyroidal extension and metastatic disease more frequently than do conventional papillary carcinomas {1907}. The prognosis remains less favourable in cases with no extrathyroidal extension {968} or with only tall-cell areas {923}. The tall cell variant of PTC accounts for a substantial proportion of radioiodine-refractory thyroid carcinomas {2306}. *BRAF* mutations are present in the vast majority of tall-cell-variant tumours. *TERT* promoter mutations are frequently found in the tall cell variant of PTC, as is the case with other aggressive variants {1638}.

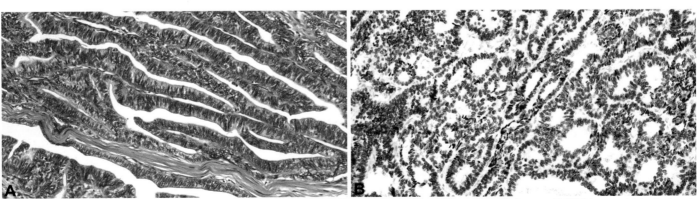

Fig. 2.43 Columnar cell variant of papillary thyroid carcinoma. **A** Long, slender papillae are arranged in parallel pseudostratified arrays. **B** CDX2 immunostaining is strongly positive.

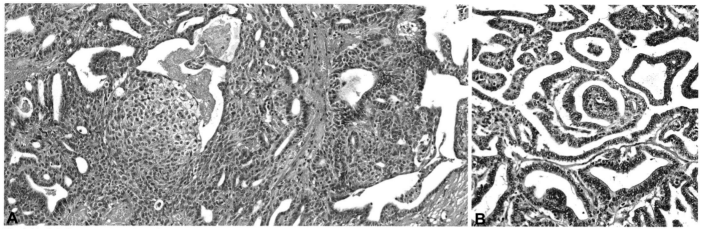

Fig. 2.44 Cribriform-morular variant of papillary thyroid carcinoma. **A** Prominent squamous metaplasia with morule formation. **B** Blending of cribriform and glandular patterns of growth.

Columnar cell variant

This rare variant is composed of columnar cells with prominent pseudostratification. Unlike in the tall cell variant, the cells lack the conventional nuclear features of PTC {2981}. Papillary thyroid tumours of the columnar cell variant are typically hypercellular neoplasms showing thin papillae or glandular-like spaces lined by pseudostratified epithelium, which can also be seen in fine-needle aspirates. The neoplastic cells show occasional subnuclear vacuolization or even clear cytoplasm reminiscent of an endometrioid or intestinal adenocarcinoma. The frequent immunoreactivity of the columnar cell variant with CDX2 {281}, a putative feature of intestinal-type differentiation, can be a confusing factor in differentiating this variant from a colonic metastatic carcinoma; however, TTF1 is invariably positive {2675}. The prognosis depends more on the encapsulation or infiltrative architecture than on the cytological features. Circumscribed tumours tend to have an indolent biological behaviour, whereas those with extensive extrathyroidal extension have a less favourable prognosis {471}.

Cribriform-morular variant

This variant is considered by some to constitute a distinct category of thyroid carcinoma. It can occur in a sporadic form or as a manifestation of familial adenomatous polyposis {364,1089,2618}. It occurs almost exclusively in females. Sporadic cases are usually solitary, whereas cases associated with familial adenomatous polyposis are often multifocal. The tumour is usually encapsulated and shows an intimate admixture of cribriform, follicular, papillary, trabecular, and solid growth patterns, with round squamoid structures called morules. Capsular and/or vascular invasion are usually present. The papillae are lined by cells of columnar shape, and intraluminal colloid is absent. The nuclei are not particularly clear, but they have varying numbers of grooves and pseudoinclusions. The morules contain optically clear nuclei that are different from those of conventional PTC but similar to those seen in morule-containing tumours of other sites {369}. They result from the accumulation of biotin, which can contribute to false immunostaining results {1303,1945}. TTF1 is often patchily positive. Thyroglobulin staining is often focal and weak. Nuclear beta-catenin is a characteristic finding in this variant {364}. Focal neuroendocrine differentiation has been described in one case {369}.

Hobnail variant – *aggressive*

This rare variant is defined by > 30% of cells with hobnail features {66,107,1292,1629,1915}. Histologically, it exhibits complex papillary and micropapillary structures, which are covered with follicular cells containing eosinophilic cytoplasm and apically located nuclei with prominent nucleoli that have a decreased N:C ratio and loss of cellular cohesion {108}. This distinctive hobnail feature can be associated with a follicular or clustered pattern of growth. Psammoma bodies are present but not numerous {108}. Necrosis, mitoses (including atypical forms), angiolymphatic invasion, and extrathyroidal extension are common. Recurrence and metastasis to lymph nodes and distant organs are frequent {107,108,3083}.

The neoplastic cells have the same immunohistochemical profile as conventional PTC: they are typically positive for TTF1 and variably positive for thyroglobulin, and > 25% of the nuclei are positive for p53 {108}. The neoplastic cells have a mean Ki-67 proliferation index (as determined using the MIB1 antibody) of 10% {108}. *BRAF* V600E mutations are by far the most common genetic alterations in this variant, followed by deleterious *TP53* mutations {109,207,1679}.

Papillary thyroid carcinoma with fibromatosis/fasciitis-like stroma

In rare cases, the stroma of PTC is so abundant and cellular that the tumour resembles nodular fasciitis, fibromatosis, or other proliferative myofibroblastic processes {447,983,1939}.

Solid/trabecular variant

It is not unusual for PTC to exhibit foci of solid and/or trabecular growth. This

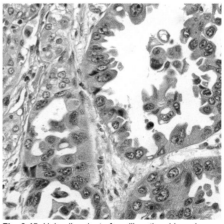

Fig. 2.45 Hobnail variant of papillary thyroid carcinoma. Hobnail cells display large nuclei and prominent nucleoli.

pattern is more common in paediatric tumours. The term "solid variant" should be used when all or nearly all of a tumour not belonging to any of the other variants has a solid, trabecular, or nested (insular) appearance. The solid variant constitutes 1–3% of adult papillary carcinomas {1529,1991}; it is more common in young patients and in patients with a history of exposure to ionizing radiation {1989, 2809}. These tumours appear to be more frequently associated with lung metastases and may confer a slightly higher mortality rate (of ~10%) in adults {1868, 1991}. This variant is frequently associated with *RET*/PTC3 fusions in paediatric and radiation-related cases {1993}, but not in tumours from the general, mostly adult population {1991}. This PTC variant should be distinguished from poorly differentiated thyroid carcinoma, which has the same growth pattern but is characterized by cells that lack the nuclear features of PTC and/or that show tumour necrosis and high mitotic activity {2891}. Some studies indicate that solid variant–predominant PTC in adults has a slightly more aggressive prognosis than does conventional PTC {2438,2561}; however, other studies have not found this tumour to be aggressive in behaviour {542}.

Oncocytic variant

In its pure form, this variant is extremely rare. Examples include papillary tumours that are often encapsulated but invasive and that have oncocytic cell cytology throughout {222,680,1717,1897}. This variant must be distinguished from the tall cell variant of PTC.

Spindle cell variant

Occasionally, PTC shows focal areas of spindle cell metaplasia. These areas may constitute from < 5% to > 95% of the

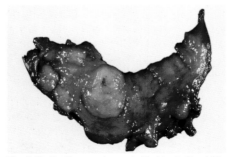

Fig. 2.46 Papillary carcinoma in Hashimoto thyroiditis. The largest nodule is a papillary carcinoma arising against a background of Hashimoto thyroiditis.

tumour {559,1697,2999}. These cells are epithelial in nature, as proven by staining for cytokeratin and TTF1. The spindle cells are not associated with haemorrhage or haemosiderin, and these areas are not geographical in there configuration, which distinguishes true spindle cell foci in PTC from post–fine-needle aspiration reactive change. Features that distinguish the spindle cell variant of PTC from anaplastic carcinoma include bland spindle cell cytology and the absence of mitoses and necrosis.

Clear cell variant

This variant is extremely unusual and is often seen in combination with oncocytic cytology of some of the tumour cells {680,1174,1574}. This variant must be distinguished from clear cell medullary carcinoma, intrathyroidal parathyroid proliferations, and metastatic renal cell carcinoma. Helpful immunostains include TTF1 and neuroendocrine markers such as chromogranin and synaptophysin, as well

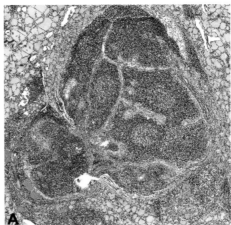 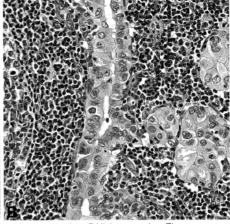

Fig. 2.47 Warthin-like variant of papillary thyroid carcinoma. **A** Low-power view. **B** High-power view. The appearance is very similar to that of the salivary-gland homologue.

as EMA and renal cell carcinoma antigen.

Warthin-like variant

This variant, which is usually circumscribed and rarely encapsulated, shares histological features with Warthin tumour of salivary-gland origin. The tumour cells lining the papillae are eosinophilic and large, and the cores of the papillae contain a prominent lymphoplasmacytic infiltrate. Often, the background thyroid shows chronic lymphocytic thyroiditis (Hashimoto thyroiditis); this may cause the tumour to be overlooked microscopically. Some of these tumours are centrally cystic. This pattern is recapitulated in metastatic lymph nodes. The prognosis of this tumour type is similar to that of conventional PTC of similar size and stage {142,1279,1684,3064}.

Cytology

Fine-needle aspiration specimens from conventional PTC are usually cellular and may demonstrate papillary structures,

Table 2.06 Summary of the most relevant genetic alterations in papillary thyroid carcinoma (PTC), with prevalence estimates from the literature.

PTC histotype	BRAF	RET	RAS	TERT promoter	ALK
All histotypes	30–90%	5–35%[a]	0–35%	5–25%	0–5%
Conventional PTC	45–80% {375,1600,2592}	5–25% {169,2613}	0–15% {375}	5–15% {1806,2217}	Not determined
Follicular variant	5–25% {375,1600,2592}	5–25% {169,2613}	15–35% {375,428}	5–15% {1806,2217}	Not determined
Tall cell variant	60–95% {375,673,1600}	35% {169,2613}	0% {375}	5–30% {673,1638}	Not determined

[a] Sporadic PTC.

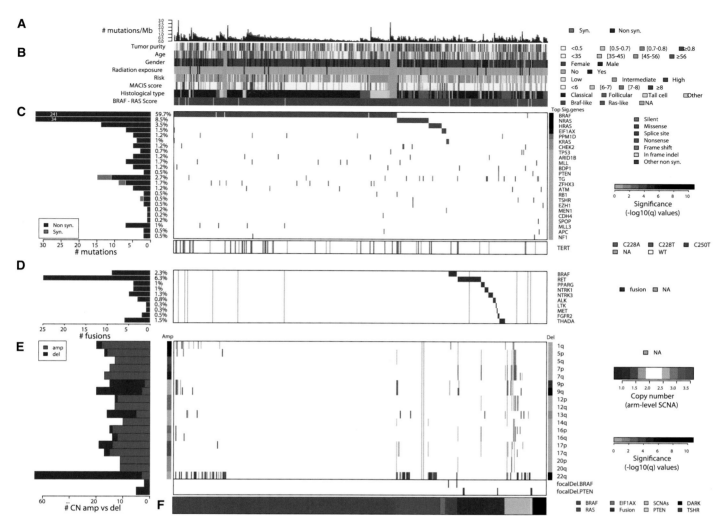

Fig. 2.48 Landscape of genomic alterations in 402 papillary thyroid carcinomas. **A** Mutation density (mutations/Mb) across the cohort. **B** Tumour purity, patient age, sex, history of radiation exposure, risk of recurrence, MACIS score, histological type, and *BRAF*-RAS score. **C** Number and frequency of recurrent mutations in genes (left) ranked by MutSig significance (right), and gene-sample matrix of mutations (centre) with *TERT* promoter mutations (bottom). **D** Number and frequency of fusion events (left), and gene-sample matrix of fusions across the cohort (centre). **E** Number and frequency of somatic copy number alterations (SCNAs, left), chromosome-sample matrix of SCNAs across the cohort (centre) with focal deletions in *BRAF* and *PTEN* (bottom), and GISTIC2 significance (right). **F** Driving variant types across the cohort. Samples were sorted by driving variant type, with dark matter (DARK) on the left. Abbreviations: amp, amplification; CN, copy number; del, deletion; MACIS, metastases, patient age, completeness of resection, local invasion, tumour size; NA, not applicable; Non syn., non-synonymous; Syn., synonymous; WT, wildtype. Reprinted from The Cancer Genome Atlas (TCGA) Research Network {375}.

monolayer sheets, and 3D groups in a background of watery or thick so-called ropy colloid, nuclear or calcific debris, macrophages, and stromal fragments. The individual tumour cells are enlarged, elongated, or oval, with eosinophilic cytoplasm. The nuclei show elongation, membrane thickening, chromatin clearing, grooves, and pseudoinclusions. The nucleoli are usually small and eccentrically located. The cytological interpretation of FVPTC can be challenging due to the paucity of diagnostic nuclear features. These tumours usually show enlarged follicular cells arranged in monolayer sheets and follicular groups in a background of thin and thick colloid. The

intranuclear grooves in FVPTC are delicate and do not traverse the entire length of the nucleus; however, intranuclear pseudoinclusions are very scarce. Cytological samples from the tall cell variant of PTC contain elongated cells with sharp cytoplasmic borders, granular eosinophilic cytoplasm, and variably sized nuclei. The diagnostic nuclear features of PTC are readily found in aspirates of this variant. Intranuclear pseudoinclusions can be multiple within the same nucleus, giving rise to a soap-bubble appearance. Fine-needle aspirates of the diffuse sclerosing variant show tumour cells with nuclear features of PTC arranged in nests and numerous psammoma bodies

or coarse calcification. Some cases also demonstrate a brisk lymphocytic infiltrate around the tumour cell groups and in the background. Squamous metaplasia is commonly seen in aspirates of the diffuse sclerosing variant. Fine-needle aspirates of the columnar cell variant demonstrate cohesive cell fragments with a prominent papillary architecture. The tumour cells appear columnar in shape, with pale cytoplasm that tapers at one end. Nuclear palisading and stratification are prominent at the periphery of papillary fragments. Intranuclear grooves and pseudoinclusions are rare, as are psammoma bodies and multinucleated tumour giant cells. Due to the scarcity or absence of

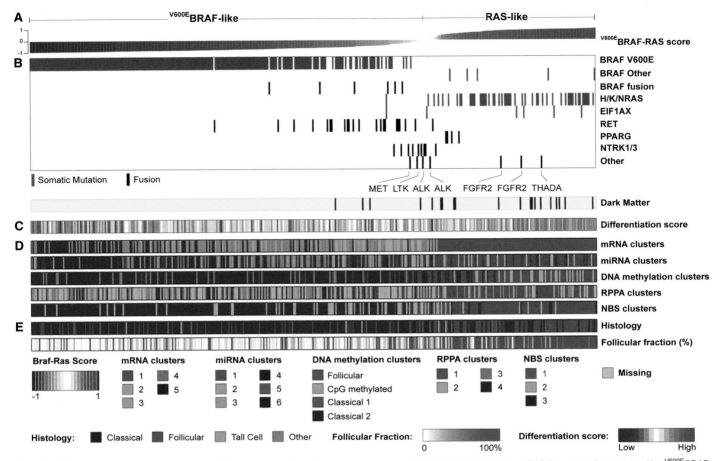

Fig. 2.49 Integrated genomic characterization of 402 papillary thyroid carcinomas along a spectrum from *BRAF* V600E–like to RAS-like expression patterns (the [V600E]*BRAF*-RAS score; BRS) with associated mutations and other correlative studies. **A** Thyroid samples (n = 391) were ranked by BRS, with *BRAF* V600E–like and RAS-like samples having negative scores (−1 to 0) and positive scores (0 to 1), respectively. **B–E** BRS is strongly associated with driver mutation status (**B**), thyroid differentiation score (**C**), single datatype clusters (**D**), and histology and follicular fraction (**E**). The RAS-like samples (normalized score > 0, in red on the top bar) consistently emerged as a distinct subgroup, characterized by a higher thyroid differentiation score. Abbreviations: miRNA, microRNA; NBS, network-based stratification; RPPA, reverse phase protein array. Reprinted from The Cancer Genome Atlas (TCGA) Research Network {375}.

diagnostic nuclear features, aspirates of the columnar cell variant of PTC can be mistaken for medullary carcinoma or metastasis (especially from colon) to the thyroid gland.

Genetic profile

The most relevant genetic alterations in PTC are summarized in Table 2.06 (p. 88). These alterations are generally mutually exclusive and in the large majority of cases cause activation of the MAPK pathway {1992,3024}. The molecular mechanisms are point mutations (e. g. *BRAF* V600E and *NRAS* mutations) in approximately 75% of cases, and gene fusions in approximately 15% of cases; copy-number variations are believed to play a tumorigenic role in approximately 7% of cases {375} (see Fig. 2.48). Overall, papillary carcinoma has a more stable genome and contains a lower number of

mutations (~0.4 non-synonymous somatic mutations per Mb of DNA) compared with carcinomas arising in other organs {375}. *BRAF* V600E mutation is the most common driver mutation in PTC, typically found in conventional PTC and the tall cell variant {6,534,1371,2593}. Other, less frequent types of *BRAF* alterations include K601E point mutation and small insertions or deletions surrounding codon 600 {170,1172,2816}, as well as chromosomal rearrangements such as *AKAP9-BRAF* fusion {375,521}. Mutations in the RAS genes (*NRAS*, *HRAS*, and *KRAS*) are also common in PTC {375}. Most PTCs carrying RAS mutations are of the follicular variant {3123}. Many RAS-like tumours are now reclassified as non-invasive follicular thyroid neoplasm with papillary-like nuclear features or well-differentiated tumour of uncertain malignant potential. *EIF1AX* mutation is another likely driver

mutation found predominantly in FVPTC {375}. Chromosomal rearrangements leading to fusions involving the *RET* gene, called *RET*/PTC rearrangements, are the most common rearrangements in PTC, followed by rearrangements leading to fusions involving *NTRK3*, *NTRK1*, *ALK*, and other genes {375}. Rearrangements typically predominate in radiation-related papillary carcinomas and in younger patients {845,1073,1993,2280}. Progression of PTC is associated with accumulation of mutations in other genes, such as *TP53*, *PIK3CA*, and *AKT1* {1998,2281}. *TERT* mutations (C228T and C250T) are also found in more-advanced-stage PTC and are associated with higher risk of recurrence, distant metastasis, and tumour-related mortality {344,922,1806,3026}. The mutation profile of PTC is changing. Over recent decades, the proportion of tumours carrying *BRAF* V600E mutations has remained stable or has even increased (particularly in conventional PTC), and the prevalence of RAS mutations has sharply increased, whereas the prevalence of *RET*/PTC rearrangements has been steadily decreasing {1281, 2322}.

The Cancer Genome Atlas (TCGA) Research Network {375} has identified two major groups of PTC based on their gene expression profiles: one with a *BRAF* V600E–like signature and one with a RAS-like signature (see Fig. 2.48). *BRAF* V600E–like tumours have conventional papillary morphology (conventional or tall-cell papillary carcinoma), a high prevalence of *BRAF* V600E mutation (or rearrangements such as *RET*/PTC and *NTRK1/3* fusions), high levels of MAPK pathway signalling, a low thyroid differentiation score (based on the expression of 16 genes involved with follicular cell function and metabolism), and a relatively heterogeneous molecular profile. RAS-like tumours have a follicular growth pattern and are encapsulated in > 80% of cases. They have a high prevalence of RAS mutations (or *EIF1AX* mutations and *BRAF* mutations other than V600E), low levels of MAPK pathway signalling, a high thyroid differentiation score, and a relatively homogeneous molecular profile.

Papillary carcinoma typically has euploid DNA content and few chromosomal alterations {1139}. Aneuploidy has been associated with the tall cell variant, high-grade features, and aggressive disease {1396,3010}. The microRNA expression pattern of papillary carcinoma is distinctive, with specific profiles seen in the various tumour subtypes {987}. miR-146b, miR-221, and miR-222 are often upregulated {1115}, and the analysis of microRNAs may provide useful prognostic information {3068}. miR-21 is epigenetically regulated and overexpressed in the tall cell variant of PTC, likely contributing to the clinically more aggressive behaviour of these tumours {375}.

Genetic susceptibility

Approximately 5% of PTCs occur on a familial basis as a component of the hereditary cancer syndrome called familial adenomatous polyposis, an autosomal dominant disease caused by germline mutation in the *APC* gene located on 5q21. About 1–2% of the patients develop thyroid carcinoma (primarily PTC and in particular of the cribriform-morular variant). Other hereditary cancer syndromes associated with PTC include Carney complex and Werner syndrome.

Non-syndromic familial thyroid cancer (familial non-medullary thyroid cancer) develops in individuals belonging to families with a history of thyroid cancer but no known hereditary cancer syndrome. This cancer tends to be multifocal and arises in association with benign lesions (nodules). One study identified *HABP2* as a possible susceptibility gene {927}, but other studies do not support this possibility {2377,2795}.

Prognosis and predictive factors
Prognosis

As a group, PTCs tend to be biologically indolent and have an excellent prognosis; survival rates of 96% at 5 years, 93% at 10 years, and > 90% at 20 years have been reported {1194}. In large series, the overall mortality rates for PTC are 1–6.5% {393,1783,2399}. The prognosis is influenced by the clinical extent of disease: the 10-year reported survival rate for stage I disease is 99.8%; for stage IV, approximately 41% {1459}. Independent risk factors associated with PTC include patient age at diagnosis, with increased mortality among patients aged > 40–45 years {643,2511}; tumour size, with an increased risk of death associated with tumours measuring > 3–4 cm {643,2511}; staging, with extrathyroidal extension constituting an adverse prognostic indicator {643,2511}, although it may be that only extensive extension (pT4), and not minimal extension (pT3), portends a poor outcome {1233,2309}; and distant metastasis {643,2511}. The site of distant metastasis has an impact on prognosis, with osseous and visceral (other than pulmonary) metastases constituting ominous prognostic findings. Non-independent adverse prognostic factors include male sex, nodal metastasis, incomplete surgical excision, tumour cell type, and/or tumour growth patterns (e.g. columnar cell, tall cell, hobnail cell, solid growth, or insular growth). Adverse molecular prognostic factors reported in PTC include *TERT* promoter mutations {344,1806,3026} and multiple concurrent mutations {2281,2612}. *BRAF* V600E mutation is controversial as an independent prognostic factor {2828,3025}. Several prognostic scoring systems for PTC have been proposed to assess risk, including the AMES (patient age, distant metastasis, extent and size of primary tumour) {356}, AGES (patient age, histological grade, extent and size of primary tumour) {1108}, and MACIS (metastases, patient age, completeness of resection, local invasion, tumour size) {1106} systems.

Predictive factors

Complete excision of PTC, including involved cervical lymph nodes, is an important determinant of outcome. Incomplete surgical resection is associated with increased risk of recurrence {1107, 1663}. After initial therapy, recurrence is most common within the first decade and may be associated with increased mortality {984,1041}. Recurrence may be delayed for decades (> 20 years) after initial diagnosis {1041}. The reported overall recurrence rate is 15–35%, with recurrence occurring in the tumour bed, cervical neck lymph nodes, or (less commonly) at distant sites {1105,1109,1778}. Metastasis to lymph nodes is significantly associated with increased risk of disease recurrence but not with survival {1035, 1052,1663,1777}. Extranodal extension of lymph node metastases is associated with a significantly increased risk of recurrence and cancer-specific mortality {477,2869}, and extrathyroidal extension is associated with a higher incidence of extranodal extension {528}. Measurement of serum thyroglobulin provides the highest sensitivity (95–100%) for the detection of persistent or recurrent disease {178}.

Follicular thyroid carcinoma

LiVolsi V.
Abdulkader Nallib I.
Baloch Z. W.
Bartolazzi A.
Chan J. K. C.
DeLellis R. A.
El-Naggar A. K.
Eloy C.
Eng C.
Fagin J. A.
Ghossein R. A.
Giordano T. J.
Kondo T.
Lloyd R. V.
Mete O.
Nikiforov Y. E.
Nonaka D.
Paschke R.
Perren A.
Rosai J.
Sadow P.
Schneider A. B.
Sobrinho Simões M.
Tallini G.
Williams M. D.

Definition
Follicular thyroid carcinoma (FTC) is a thyroid malignancy arising from follicular cells in which the diagnostic nuclear features of papillary thyroid carcinoma (PTC) are absent. The lesions are usually encapsulated and show invasive growth. Oncocytic tumours are discussed in a separate section (see *Hürthle (oncocytic) cell tumours*, p. 96).

ICD-O codes
Follicular thyroid carcinoma, NOS 8330/3
  Minimally invasive   8335/3
  Encapsulated angioinvasive   8339/3
  Widely invasive   8330/3

Synonyms
Follicular thyroid adenocarcinoma, follicular carcinoma

Epidemiology
In 1980–2009, the annual incidence rate of FTC in the USA was 1.19 cases per 100 000 women and 0.55 cases per 100 000 men {524}. The highest annual incidence rate of FTC was among patients aged 70–79, at 2.16 cases per 100 000 population. Over the same time period, the ratio of papillary to follicular carcinoma multiplied by about 3.5 times. Unlike the rate of PTC, the worldwide incidence rate of FTC has remained relatively constant, but in some countries,

such as Italy, it decreased between 1960 and 2007 {1516}. Most studies indicate that FTC accounts for 6–10% of thyroid carcinomas {50,1295,1648}.

Etiology
Insufficient dietary iodine is considered an important risk factor for nodular goitre and follicular carcinoma. When iodine supplementation is introduced into iodine-insufficient areas, the ratio of FTC to PTC decreases {695,2860}. However, it is unclear whether iodine supplementation affects the overall rate of thyroid carcinoma {695}. Exposure to ionizing radiation is associated with an increased risk of follicular carcinoma, although the risk is much lower than that of papillary carcinoma {2554}.

Localization
FTC can occur anywhere in the thyroid. It has also been reported to arise in ectopic

locations, including mediastinal thyroid and struma ovarii {549,2240,2958}.

Clinical features
Follicular carcinoma presents in adults and is very rare in children {2036,2347}. A painless neck mass is usually the presenting symptom; its size can vary from < 1 cm to several centimetres. Large tumours can lead to dysphagia or dyspnoea. Regional lymph node enlargement at presentation is extremely uncommon compared with PTC.

In some cases, the initial symptom is metastasis, such as a bone fracture or a lung nodule. Following the pathological diagnosis of the metastasis as being of thyroid origin, examination of the neck usually reveals a thyroid mass. Occasionally, the finding of metastatic disease (usually in bone) is a cause to re-examine a previously resected thyroid mass thought to be an adenoma, which may

Table 2.07 Classification of follicular thyroid carcinoma

Traditional {2596}	Armed Forces Institute of Pathology (AFIP) 2014 {2340}		WHO 2017
Minimally invasive	Minimally invasive	With capsular invasion	Minimally invasive
		With limited vascular invasion (< 4 vessels)	Encapsulated angioinvasive
		With extensive vascular invasion (≥ 4 vessels)	
Widely invasive	Widely invasive		Widely invasive

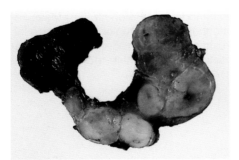

Fig. 2.50 Widely invasive follicular thyroid carcinoma. Gross photograph of a multinodular tumour involving most of the thyroid gland.

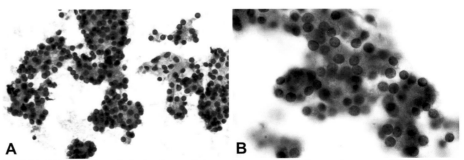

Fig. 2.51 A Fine-needle aspirate showing a cellular specimen consisting of a monotonous population of follicular cells arranged in microfollicles (ThinPrep preparation). **B** A high-power view of the same case shows that the follicular cells are enlarged and round, with uniform nuclear chromatin distribution and barely visible small nucleoli (Papanicolaou-stained, alcohol-fixed smear preparation).

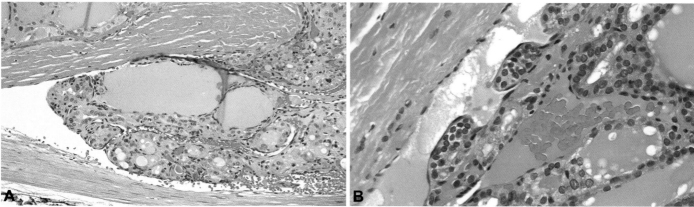

Fig. 2.52 Follicular thyroid carcinoma with vascular invasion. **A** Low magnification. **B** Higher magnification.

reveal underdiagnosis or inadequate sectioning of the capsule.

Rare examples of so-called functioning FTC with associated hyperthyroidism have been documented {362,1867}.

Macroscopy

FTCs vary in appearance from completely encapsulated solid lesions with thick capsules (sometimes demonstrating calcification) to tumours mimicking follicular adenomas, although the capsules are usually more prominent in carcinoma. Rarely, foci of invasion into the tumour capsule can be noted. In lesions that have been biopsied, areas of haemorrhage may be noted. In widely invasive tumours, obvious extension into surrounding thyroid or extrathyroidal tissue is present. Tumour thrombi may be noted in large veins in the neck.

Microscopy

The diagnosis of FTC requires demonstration of capsular and/or vascular invasion. FTC is subclassified into three groups: (1) minimally invasive (capsular invasion only), (2) encapsulated angioinvasive, and (3) widely invasive {145,543}. The cytoarchitectural features of FTC are similar to those of follicular adenoma. Trabecular/solid, microfollicular, normofollicular, macrofollicular, and other patterns (e.g. cribriform) can be observed. Mixed architectural types also occur. FTC lacks the nuclear features of PTC.

FTC is generally surrounded by a thick and irregular capsule, which may be calcified. Most authors require that neoplastic cells penetrate the entire thickness of the tumour capsule; irregular contour of the inner capsular border, capsular pushing by the tumour cells, or tumour cell nests embedded within the capsule

are considered by many authors to be insufficient for the diagnosis. Searching for capsular and vascular invasion in additional sections may be useful. Capsule rupture due to surgical manipulation, changes (pseudoinvasion) secondary to biopsy trauma, and curling of tumour at tissue edges (due to block handling) are not equated with invasion.

When neoplastic cells/follicles penetrate the adjacent normal thyroid parenchyma, a stromal reaction forming a secondary limiting fibrous band is a common finding. Tumour invasive buds may have a mushroom-like appearance.

Vascular invasion is invasion into veins, no matter the vessel size. Although this definition seems straightforward, this aspect of pathology has been controversial in practice {1819}. Intravascular tumour cells should be adherent to the vessel walls, either covered by endothelium or in a context of thrombus or fibrin. Invasion must occur in vessels within or beyond the tumour capsule; the finding of something resembling vascular invasion within the substance of the tumour is not diagnostic of carcinoma, because this finding alone is not associated with malignant behaviour. The extent of vascular invasion is prognostically relevant. Lymphatic invasion by FTC is virtually unknown, as is nodal metastases; the finding of lymphatic involvement should redirect the pathologist to a diagnosis of the follicular variant of PTC (see *Papillary thyroid carcinoma*, p. 81). Tumours with limited invasion of vessels (< 4) have a better prognosis than do those with extensive vascular invasion {925,1230, 3029}. Immunohistochemistry has been used, primarily by using CD31, CD34, factor VIII–related antigen, and TTF1 to highlight endothelium and therefore

vascular channels {1626}. Alternatively, some researchers have used special histochemical stains (trichrome and elastin stains) to highlight vascular invasion by tumour {1A}. However, some authors question the diagnostic utility of these methods.

Widely invasive FTCs show extensive invasion of the thyroid and extra-thyroidal soft tissues. Vascular invasion is often prominent, but alone, does not categorize an FTC as "widely-invasive". More important than the extent of thyroid or soft tissue invasion is the identification of extensive angioinvasion, which is associated with a worse prognosis {2596}. Widely invasive FTCs are usually large tumours {621}.

Widely invasive FTC with a solid or trabecular growth pattern must be distinguished from poorly differentiated thyroid carcinoma {2891}. Distinction from the solid/trabecular variant of PTC and the diffuse/multinodular follicular variant of PTC is difficult, and is ultimately supported by the distinctive nuclear features of these entities {2596}.

Cytology

Benign and malignant follicular-patterned lesions cannot be distinguished using thyroid fine-needle aspiration {141,411, 1746,2274,3017}. The cytological diagnosis of "follicular neoplasm" reflects the limitations of thyroid cytology, because the diagnosis of follicular carcinoma is based on the demonstration of capsular and/or vascular invasion.

Immunophenotype

Like other thyroid conditions (both benign and malignant) arising from follicular cells, FTC expresses the lineage-specific antigens thyroglobulin and TTF1. PAX8 is

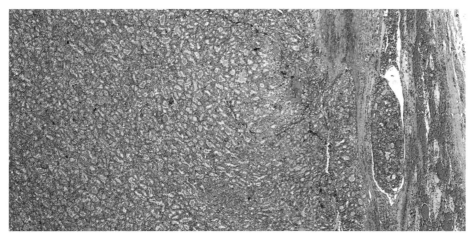
Fig. 2.53 Angioinvasive follicular thyroid carcinoma. Intracapsular blood vessel with tumour thrombus.

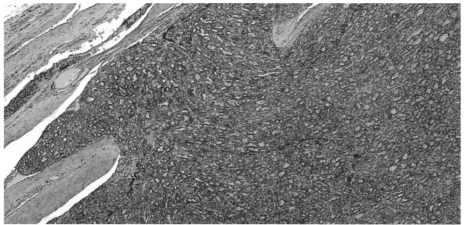
Fig. 2.54 Minimally invasive follicular thyroid carcinoma. Capsular invasion in follicular thyroid carcinoma (FTC). This is an example of the so called mushroom configuration of capsular invasion in this minimally invasive FTC.

usually positive. The value of a variety of markers in the distinction between benign and malignant follicular nodules is questionable. An isolated marker is usually not of much use; some studies have recommended combinations of markers, including CK19, galectin 3, and HBME1. HBME1 may be positive in some follicular carcinomas {2198}. Some authors have had success with immunohistochemistry using these markers on either tissue or cytological samples {163}, but this has not been uniformly noted by other investigators.

Variants

Clear cell variant
Clear-cell changes have been described in various thyroid conditions, including adenomatous hyperplasia, papillary and medullary carcinoma, and FTC, particularly in oncocytic neoplasms {392,527, 2475}. Although focal clear-cell change is not uncommon in many thyroid nodules,

clear cell FTC (defined by > 50% clear cells in the tumour) accounts for < 1% of thyroid malignancies {1429,2158}. Clear-cell cytoplasm predominates, but the co-existence of oncocytic neoplastic cells is not uncommon. Generally, neoplastic cells show uniform round or oval nuclei with small nucleoli. Substantial nuclear pleomorphism, clearing, or groves are not detected. The cytohistological features of PTC are absent.

Cytoplasmic clearing results from accumulation of glycogen, lipid, mucin, and thyroglobulin, or can occur due to dilatation and hypertrophy of mitochondria and Golgi complexes {392,527,2439}. Therefore, overstimulation by TSH may also play a role in generating this phenotype {78,677}.

The diagnosis of clear cell FTC requires exclusion of metastatic clear cell carcinoma arising from the kidney, medullary thyroid carcinoma, and parathyroid tumours. For the very rare cases of

less-differentiated clear cell FTC, which could potentially be thyroglobulin-negative, the combined use of antibodies to TTF1 and PAX8 could be diagnostically useful.

Some authors have suggested that clear cell thyroid carcinomas are more aggressive than conventional types {2475}, whereas others believe that the clear-cell phenotype is prognostically irrelevant and clinical outcome is determined only by the extent of vascular invasion {392,527}.

Other variants
The other variants of FTC reflect relatively minor differences in histopathology. Many of these lesions are extremely unusual and rarely encountered. Such variants include the signet-ring cell type {392,2474}, in which (usually focally) there are intracellular vacuoles filled with mucin. The cells may be bland, with cystic spaces in the stroma filled with extracellular mucin. The vacuoles contain thyroglobulin. Because these lesions are so rare, their biology is not well understood {2326}. Accumulation of extracellular mucinous material is often associated with a microcystic growth pattern of the tumour cells. These tumours must be distinguished from metastatic mucinous adenocarcinoma from other sites {1873,2214,2626, 2940}, as well as from follicular carcinoma with fat cells, in which there are nests of mature adipose cells admixed with the follicular carcinoma elements {998}. Other extremely rare lesions are FTC with a glomeruloid pattern, which has a peculiar architectural growth pattern in which the follicles contain round to oval epithelial tufts growing within them, mimicking a renal glomerulus {291,370}, as well as spindle cell FTC, in which some or nearly all of the tumour cells are spindle-shaped and produce intersecting fascicles. The cells are positive for cytokeratin and TTF1 {990,1869}. Distinction from anaplastic carcinoma is dependent on the bland cytology of the cells and the absence of pleomorphism, mitotic activity, and necrosis. Distinction from postbiopsy spindle cell artefact is facilitated by the presence in such artefact of haemosiderin-laden macrophages, inflammatory cells, and fresh haemorrhage.

Genetic profile

Follicular carcinomas have a significantly higher rate of numerical chromosomal abnormalities and loses and gains of specific chromosomal regions than do papillary carcinomas. Cytogenetic changes are found in about 65% of FTC {1127,2335,2336}. Loss of heterozygosity is present at a rate of 20% per chromosome arm in FTC, 6% in follicular adenoma, and only 2.5% in papillary carcinoma {2947}.

The most common somatic mutations in follicular carcinomas are RAS point mutations and *PPARG* gene fusions. RAS family mutations are found in 30–50% of tumours {792,1257,1997,2911}. The most frequently affected hotspot is *NRAS* codon 61, followed by *HRAS* codon 61. *PPARG* rearrangements, either *PAX8-PPARG* or *CREB3L2-PPARG*, occur in 20–30% of FTCs {492,1481,1688}. *PAX8-PPARG*–positive tumours tend to present in younger patients and more often have vascular invasion {893,1997}. RAS mutations and *PPARG* fusions are also found in some follicular adenomas, supporting a link between these two tumour types. Mutations involving the PI3K/PTEN/AKT pathway genes also occur in FTCs. *PIK3CA* mutations are found in up to 10% of tumours {1171,2597,2943}, and *PIK3CA* copy-number gains may also be seen {3013}. Inactivating *PTEN* mutations are identified in up to 10% of FTCs {1065, 1171,2943}. Activating *TSHR* mutations may be seen, particularly in hyperfunctioning FTCs {1998}.

TERT promoter mutations are found in about 20% of FTCs {1634,1806}. *TERT* mutations have been shown to be associated with more-aggressive clinical behaviour in thyroid carcinomas, including a more-advanced stage at presentation and higher rates of tumour recurrence and tumour-related mortality {1634,1806}. Recent data have shown that *TERT* promoter mutation occurs as an early genetic event in follicular thyroid tumours that have not developed capsular or vascular invasion, raising the possibility that such lesions are preinvasive tumours {2935}.

Genetic susceptibility

As noted in the chapter on inherited tumour syndromes (see *Cowden syndrome and* PTEN-*related lesions*, p. 275), *PTEN* hamartoma tumour syndrome (which includes Cowden syndrome) and other syndromes are associated with tumours of follicular origin, including malignancies; and these cancers are often follicular carcinoma. Cowden syndrome is an autosomal dominant inherited cancer syndrome associated with FTC and the follicular variant of PTC. It is caused by germline mutations in several genes, most importantly the tumour suppressor gene *PTEN*. Thyroid lesions are found in two thirds of patients with Cowden syndrome {1087,1563,1984A,2631,2712}. Younger patient age and multiple well-defined and frequently encapsulated thyroid nodules are characteristic {1087, 1563,1984A,2026,2712}. Follicular carcinoma may also arise in patients with Werner syndrome, an autosomal recessive disease caused by *WRN* gene mutation. Thyroid cancer, typically FTC, occurs in about 3% of affected patients {1223}. Follicular carcinoma is a rare manifestation of Carney complex, an autosomal dominant disorder caused by germline mutations in *PRKAR1A* and other genes {2033,2656}.

A family history of thyroid carcinoma is identified in 3.7% of patients diagnosed with FTC in the USA {1193}.

Prognosis and predictive factors

Follicular carcinomas that show only capsular invasion without vascular invasion have an excellent prognosis {2848}; tumours with any vascular (venous) invasion may show evidence of haematogenous metastasis even if only 1–2 vessels are invaded. However, the larger the number of vessels involved, the worse the prognosis {2037}. The most common sites of distant metastases are bone, lung, brain, and liver {3112}. There have been rare reports of dermal metastases {2012,2222}. *TERT* mutation is an independent marker of a higher risk of disease recurrence and cancer-related mortality {1634,1806}. Because many FTCs are well differentiated, responsiveness to radioactive iodine treatment is expected, and may be associated with prolonged survival.

Hürthle (oncocytic) cell tumours

LiVolsi V.
Baloch Z.W.
Sobrinho Simões M.
Tallini G.

Definition

Hürthle (oncocytic) cell tumours are neoplasms (usually encapsulated) composed of oncocytic cells. Non-invasive cases are called Hürthle cell adenoma and cases with capsular and/or vascular invasion are called Hürthle cell carcinoma (HCC).

Follicular neoplasms that are only in part composed of Hürthle cells are also considered by some authors to be included within the group of Hürthle cell tumours. Most pathologists prefer to diagnose a lesion as a Hürthle cell tumour only if the majority (greater than 75%) of the tumour is composed of Hürthle (oncocytic) cells. Lesions with fewer Hürthle cells are then designated thyroid neoplasms with Hürthle (oncocytic) cell features.

Less common oncocytic tumours, including variants of papillary carcinoma, medullary carcinoma, and poorly differentiated carcinoma are discussed separately (see *Papillary thyroid carcinoma*, p.81; *Medullary thyroid carcinoma*, p.108; and *Poorly differentiated thyroid carcinoma*, p.100).

Unfortunately, it is often unclear whether a given published study about the clinical and prognostic features of Hürthle cell tumours has taken the definitions above into account. The variation in survival statistics and reported metastatic potential suggests that the definitions of these lesions used in many reported series are not consistent.

ICD-O codes

Hürthle cell adenoma	8290/0
Hürthle cell carcinoma	8290/3

Synonyms

Hürthle cell adenoma
Oncocytic adenoma; oxyphilic adenoma; follicular adenoma, Hürthle cell type; follicular adenoma, oncocytic variant
Hürthle cell carcinoma
Oncocytic carcinoma; oxyphilic carcinoma; follicular carcinoma, Hürthle cell type; follicular carcinoma, oncocytic variant

Epidemiology

The frequency of Hürthle cell tumours in the population is unknown, due to the comingling of these lesions with non-Hürthle follicular tumours and the inclusion of hyperplastic Hürthle cell nodules as occur in lymphocytic thyroiditis.

Most series of HCC show that these lesions are more common in men and tend to affect older patients compared with papillary thyroid carcinoma or follicular thyroid carcinoma. The average patient age is 57 years. An analysis of large numbers of cases with long-term follow-up showed that patients with HCC had larger tumours, higher-stage disease, and lower survival rates than did patients with non-Hürthle thyroid carcinomas {1003}.

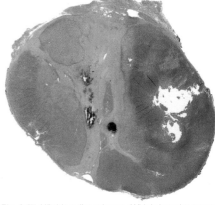

Fig. 2.57 Hürthle cell carcinoma. Widely invasive tumour with wide fibrous bands simulating multinodular goitre.

Etiology

There are no known exogenous factors that predispose an individual to the development of Hürthle cell tumours.

Localization

Hürthle cell tumours can arise in any part of the thyroid gland, including in ectopic thyroid tissue in the mediastinum. HCC has no site predilection.

Clinical features

Hürthle cell tumours usually present as painless masses. The size is variable; a few are < 1 cm, but most are ≥ 2 cm. Occasional examples that have spontaneously infarcted may present with neck pain. Spontaneous haemorrhage may lead to rapid enlargement of the tumour resulting in respiratory compromise.

Macroscopy

Grossly, Hürthle cell tumours have a brown coloration ranging from tan to mahogany. A capsule of variable thickness is usually present; adenomas tend to have thinner capsules than do carcinomas. Calcification of the capsule or of parts of the tumour may be identified; some examples show ossification. These lesions have a propensity to undergo infarction following minor trauma (e.g. fine-needle aspiration or core biopsy) {1275,1386}; in such cases, the tumour may grossly

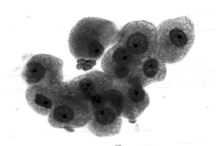

Fig. 2.55 Hürthle cell tumour. Cluster of monotonous large cells with granular cytoplasm and round nuclei. Note the prominent central nucleoli. The uniform cytology defines this as a neoplasm (Papanicolaou stain).

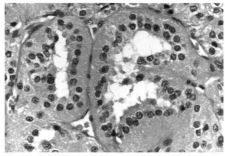

Fig. 2.56 Hürthle cell adenoma. Neoplastic cells with granular eosinophilic cytoplasm. The accumulation of mitochondria displaces nuclei towards the luminal side of the neoplastic follicles.

appear partly or totally necrotic. Some HCCs show gross invasion of the tumour through the tumour capsule into nearby thyroid or perithyroidal soft tissues.

Microscopy

Hürthle cells are large cells with voluminous granular cytoplasm and large centrally located nuclei, which often have prominent nucleoli. The granular cytoplasm, which resembles that of normal hepatocytes, is occupied at the ultrastructural level by numerous abnormally large mitochondria {1769,2597}. Technically, the name "Hürthle cell" is incorrect, because the cells described by Hürthle were not what we now term Hürthle cells; however, the name is now too engrained in the literature to be changed.

The related terms "oncocytes" and "oxyphil cells" have been used interchangeably to describe Hürthle cells. The cytoplasm of these cells is filled with mitochondria, with complete loss of cell polarity {2807A}. To avoid confusion (which could have diagnostic and prognostic implications) these cells should be distinguished from "mitochondria-rich" cells that do not have complete loss of cell polarity and at the ultrastructural level have fewer mitochondria compared with Hürthle (oncocytic) cells. Tumours with mitochondria-rich cells can be papillary (tall cell variant, Warthin-like variant, hobnail variant) or medullary and not be composed of Hürthle (oncocytic) cells {2827}.

Hürthle cell adenoma is usually encapsulated and is composed of follicles or trabeculae of oncocytic cells with the characteristic nuclei of Hürthle cells. Most adenomas show a follicular growth pattern (which is less common in HCC). No invasion is seen. The tumours may arise in a background of normal or goitrous thyroid; many occur in the setting of chronic lymphocytic thyroiditis.

HCCs may show intersecting fibrous bands between nests and clusters of tumour cells. Patterns of growth include solid, trabecular, and follicular. Because the tumours contain little stroma, the lesions may show a pseudopapillary histological pattern {2339}. Rare examples of true papillary growth in HCC have been reported; nuclear features are helpful in distinguishing these tumours from the oncocytic variant of papillary carcinoma. Invasion (capsular and/or vascular) defines the tumour as malignant.

Hürthle cell tumours of all types can show calcifications, usually within the colloid in tumour follicles. Such structures are usually not lamellated and should not be considered psammoma bodies. In Hürthle cell tumours these calcifications may be the result of a physicochemical reaction to altered thyroglobulin within the colloid of the tumour follicles. They are more frequent in benign than malignant tumours. Hürthle cell tumours have a propensity to undergo infarction due to minor trauma such as fine-needle aspiration or core biopsy {1275,1386}. The resulting inflammatory changes may cause irregularities in the capsule and mimic invasion. Association of inflammatory cells and granulation tissue in these areas should warn the pathologist that this is probably not true invasion and instead constitutes a postinflammatory state.

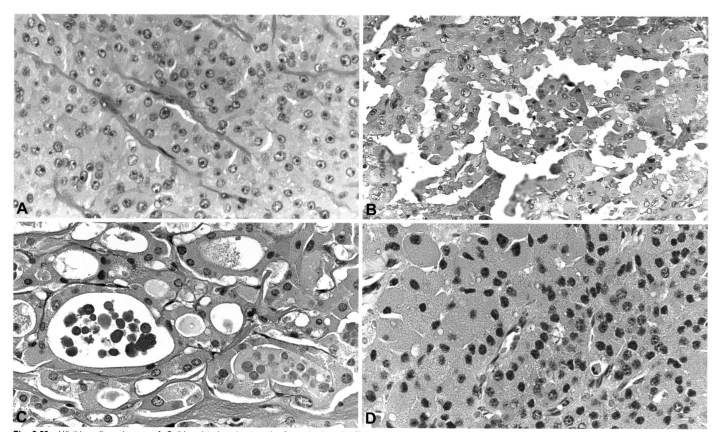

Fig. 2.58 Hürthle cell carcinoma. **A** Solid and trabecular growth of neoplastic cells. This pattern is more common in Hürthle cell carcinoma than in adenoma, where follicular structures tend to predominate. **B** Discohesive growth of neoplastic cells can simulate papillary structures. **C** Colloid concretions inside follicles are often basophilic and may simulate psammoma bodies. **D** Some tumour cells have higher N:C ratios (at right); this feature is more common in Hürthle cell carcinoma than in adenoma.

Five decades ago {1051,2770}, it was believed that all Hürthle cell tumours were malignant; the histopathological features of these lesions were not considered. But pathologically well-controlled studies of Hürthle cell tumours published in the latter half of the 20th century showed that adenomas could be histologically distinguished from carcinomas in this subgroup of tumours using criteria similar to those used for non-Hürthle follicular tumours {333,391,784,864}. It became clear that larger Hürthle cell tumours were more likely to show invasive characteristics {469}, which was not true for usual follicular neoplasms. In one study, Hürthle cell tumours that measured ≥ 3.5 cm harboured a 67% risk of malignancy {469}. However, as with non-Hürthle cell tumours, small lesions can show invasive growth and be associated with malignant clinical behaviour {2405}.

HCCs have some unusual features compared with non-Hürthle or follicular carcinomas. Although follicular carcinomas virtually never metastasize embolically to regional lymph nodes and do not invade lymphatic channels, HCC can spread to cervical nodes {258}. However, many HCCs also invade veins and metastasize haematogenously to liver, lungs, and other distant organs, especially bone {1083, 2776}. Metastases can present several years after the original lesion has been removed; examples of large solitary liver metastases may be misinterpreted clinically and even pathologically as primary hepatocellular carcinoma.

An interesting pattern of metastatic spread involves intravascular (venous) tumour thrombi presenting as multiple nodules in the neck, mimicking nodal metastases {258}.

Although the grading of Hürthle cell tumours is not common practice, certain features are more commonly seen in HCCs than in adenomas: a trabecular/solid growth pattern, rare follicular formation, and foci of small cells. In large HCCs (> 4 cm), foci of tumour necrosis, numerous mitoses (including abnormal forms), and foci of small tumour cells are prominent; these tumours have recently been identified as a subcategory of HCC: poorly differentiated HCC {130,1143}. Such tumours have a worse prognosis than usual HCCs and are more likely to be radioiodine-resistant {2306}. Pathologists should be aware that the poorly differentiated/small-cell component may be

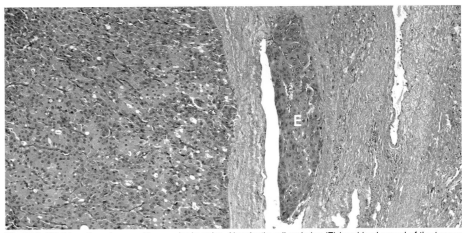

Fig. 2.59 Hürthle cell carcinoma with vascular invasion. Neoplastic cell embolus (E) in a blood vessel of the tumour capsule.

the dominant pattern in metastases, and immunostaining may give problematic results: both thyroglobulin and TTF1 stains may be negative. Therefore, these lesions may be misdiagnosed as primary tumours of non-thyroid origin {130}.

Immunophenotype
Hürthle (oncocytic) cells stain for thyroid transcription factor-1 (TTF-1) and thyroglobulin. Some of these tumours have a perinuclear punctate positivity for thyroglobulin {2339}.

Cytology
Fine-needle aspirates of Hürthle cell tumours show a monotonous population of Hürthle cells. The cells show voluminous granular cytoplasm and large, usually centrally located nuclei with prominent round nucleoli. When Hürthle cells grow in sheets or clusters without other intervening cell types, the lesion is a neoplasm. However, distinction between benign and malignant lesions is not possible on fine-needle aspiration alone. It has been reported that cytological features such as nucleolation, multinucleation, and nucleolar size and shape may be suggestive of carcinoma {1956}.

Genetic profile
Several studies have shown that Hürthle (oncocytic) cell tumours have a higher frequency of mitochondrial DNA mutations than do non-Hürthle tumours, with the mutations ranging from point substitutions, to small insertions and deletions that can lead to frameshifts or premature stop codons, to large-scale deletions (i.e. the 4977 bp deletion) {940,1768,

1770,1771,2708}. It is now recognized that the biochemical and metabolic alterations, as well as the phenotypic alterations (i.e. accumulation of mitochondria) of oncocytic lesions are caused by defects in genes coding for subunits of the five multimeric complexes of the inner mitochondrial membrane that constitute the oxidative phosphorylation system. If these subunits are missing or defective due to a mutation, the multimeric complex does not assemble properly, oxidative phosphorylation is impaired, and there is a compensatory accumulation of mitochondria {938,1767}. In the thyroid gland and other organs, > 50% of the mutations occur at homoplasmic levels in coding mitochondrial DNA regions, which usually (in > 70% of cases) affect the mitochondrial ND genes for complex I (NADH coenzyme Q reductase) subunits {284,940,1775}. Mutations of the complex I subunit encoded by the *NDUFA13* nuclear gene (also called *GRIM19*) are the only nuclear gene mutations specific to oncocytic tumours reported to date. They have been found in 1 of 11 oncocytic follicular carcinomas, in 2 of 20 oncocytic papillary carcinomas, and as a germline mutation in one patient who developed an oncocytic variant of papillary carcinoma and multiple benign oncocytic thyroid nodules {1766}. Although these mutations in mitochondrial and nuclear genes affecting oxidative phosphorylation function are responsible for the oncocytic phenotype, their relationship with tumour development is complex, and there is no proof that they have a direct tumorigenic role {938,939, 1767}. A comprehensive analysis of tumorigenic mutations, DNA copy-number changes, and expression profiling of 27 oncocytic tumours (8 adenomas and 19 carcinomas) has shown that oncocytic tumours have a genetic profile different from that of the other common types of thyroid cancer, with transcriptome signatures consistent with activation of the WNT/beta-catenin and PI3K/AKT/mTOR pathways {924}. Oncocytic follicular tumours (Hürthle cell tumours) have a lower prevalence of RAS gene mutations and PAX8/PPARG rearrangement compared with their counterparts lacking oncocytic change {924,1997,2379}. TP53 mutations have been identified in 10–20% of oncocytic follicular carcinomas lacking high-grade or poorly differentiated features {803,1998}, sometimes in association with PTEN mutations {2959}. Aneuploidy, which is common in oncocytic tumours, more frequently results from chromosomal DNA gains than losses, and usually involves whole chromosomes or large chromosome sections. Gains on chromosomes 5, 7, 12, and 17 are typical; losses are often detected at 2q, 9q, and 22 {674, 783,924,2707,2913}. Gains at chromosomes 12q, 19q, and 20p have been as-

sociated with tumour recurrence {2913}. One study identified chromosome 22 loss in 3 of 11 oncocytic follicular carcinomas from patients who died of disease {783}. Several studies have associated aneuploidy detected by cytometric DNA measurements with aggressive behaviour and poor prognosis {333,753,2234}.

Genetic susceptibility

Certain genetically defined syndromes are associated with a significantly increased risk of Hürthle cell tumours. The most prominent of these is Cowden syndrome, which is part of the spectrum of PTEN hamartoma tumour syndrome (see Familial non-medullary thyroid cancer, p. 275). Hyperplastic nodules, Hürthle cell adenomas, and HCCs are found in affected patients.

Prognosis and predictive factors

Hürthle cell adenoma is benign; it will not recur. The prognosis of HCC is believed to be related to the extent of vascular invasion: the more veins invaded by tumour, the less favourable the prognosis. However, encapsulated HCC may show focal vascular invasion, and such tumours may

be underdiagnosed; after several years, metastases may occur {967}. Widely invasive HCC with extensive vascular invasion is associated with a high mortality rate (> 90% at 10 years) {495}. One study has shown that there are molecular changes that correlate with extensive vascular invasion (> 4 vessels); these changes are associated with a more aggressive clinical phenotype {924}.

Because Hürthle cell tumours are radio-iodine-resistant {495}, treatment options are more limited than for papillary thyroid carcinoma and non-oncocytic follicular thyroid carcinoma.

The overall survival rate for HCC ranges from 85% for minimally invasive lesions to about 10% for widely invasive cases {495,924}. Tumours with poorly differentiated histology have a worse prognosis.

A small proportion of HCCs undergo transformation to anaplastic carcinoma; this may occur after a history of HCC with recurrences or may be noted at the initial diagnostic biopsy, with anaplastic carcinoma as the main lesion and HCC found in the background {2666}.

Poorly differentiated thyroid carcinoma

Tallini G.
Asioli S.
Aubert S.
Carcangiu M.L.
Chernock R.D.
Fellegara G.
Ghossein R.A.
Kakudo K.

LiVolsi V.
Lloyd R.V.
Matias-Guiu X.
Nikiforov Y.E.
Papotti M.
Perren A.
Rosai J.
Sobrinho Simões M.

Definition
Poorly differentiated thyroid carcinoma (PDTC) is a follicular cell neoplasm that shows limited evidence of follicular cell differentiation and is morphologically and behaviourally intermediate between differentiated (follicular and papillary) carcinomas and anaplastic carcinoma. The histopathological diagnostic criteria for PDTC are listed in the Turin consensus proposal {2891}.

ICD-O code   8337/3

Synonyms and related terms
Poorly differentiated follicular carcinoma; insular carcinoma {394}; solid-type follicular carcinoma {2385}; trabecular carcinoma {355}; poorly differentiated carcinoma with a primordial cell component {2099}; high-risk thyroid carcinoma of follicular cell origin {1299}; poorly differentiated papillary carcinoma; grade III papillary carcinoma

Epidemiology
PDTC accounts for a small proportion of all thyroid cancers: 0.3% in Japan and 1.8% in the USA {106}; the proportion is somewhat higher in some geographical regions of Latin America and Europe, with reported prevalence rates of 4% {394, 997} to 6.7% {106}. The mean patient age at diagnosis is 55–63 years {997,2891}, with rare cases diagnosed in young patients {106,1099,1647}. There is a slight female preponderance, with a female-to-male ratio of 1.1–2.1:1 {394,1335,2891}.

Etiology
Iodine deficiency may be a contributing environmental factor, given the association of poorly differentiated carcinoma with longstanding goitre {2099,2893}. There is no association with radiation exposure {1647}. Some tumours arise as a result of loss of differentiation (synchronous or metachronous) of follicular or papillary carcinomas (often of the follicular variant) {106,139,394}; others appear de novo.

Localization
PDTC can arise at any site where thyroid parenchyma may be present, including the mediastinum {693} and struma ovarii {1352}.

Clinical features
The most common presentation is that of a large solitary thyroid mass {394}. In some cases there is a history of recent growth in a longstanding uninodular or multinodular thyroid. Distant metastases are reported at presentation in about 15% of cases {394,1143}. Ultrasonography shows inhomogeneous hypoechoic tumours. They typically appear cold on scintigraphy and positive on FDG-PET {1143,1205,1284}. PDTCs account for about 50% of thyroid tumours that are FDG-PET–positive and radioiodine-resistant {2306}. In the context of a PDTC diagnosis, clinicians should rely on FDG-PET rather than only serum thyroglobulin measurements and radioiodine scans for staging and follow-up {1205,2306}.

Tumour spread and staging
The tumours are widely invasive, extending to perithyroidal soft tissues in 60–70% of cases. Vascular invasion is found in 60–90% of cases, regional lymph node metastases in 15–65%, and distant metastases (most commonly to the lung, followed by bone and other sites, such as brain, liver, skin, spleen, and kidney) in 40–70% {106,394,997,1143,1205,2891}. The staging criteria are the same as those used for well-differentiated follicular and papillary carcinomas. PDTCs have a higher pTNM stage than do well-differentiated carcinomas {670,997,2893}.

Macroscopy
The tumours are large (median size: 5 cm {997}), solid, and light-brown to grey. Some show soft, pale areas of necrosis. The growth margins are often pushing, and the tumour may be partially encapsulated. Frequently, there are satellite nodules within the thyroid parenchyma; in some cases, multinodular tumour growth can simulate thyroid goitre. Extension beyond the thyroid capsule is common and resection margins are often positive, but extrathyroidal infiltration is less pervasive than in anaplastic carcinoma.

Microscopy
The prototypical example of this entity, originally described as poorly differentiated (insular) carcinoma, is characterized by high-grade microscopic features and poor prognosis {394}. Insular carcinoma consists of well-defined solid nests (or 'insulae'), which may contain microfollicles. The tumour cells are small and uniform, with round hyperchromatic nuclei, or may have convoluted nuclei reminiscent of those seen in papillary carcinoma. Mitoses are common. Extensive necrosis can result in a peritheliomatous appearance {394}.
Other tumours share the high-grade microscopic features (mitoses and

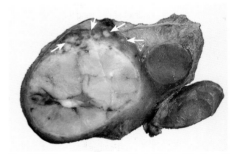

Fig. 2.60 The tumour replaces the left lobe of the thyroid gland, with infiltrative satellite nodules (arrows).

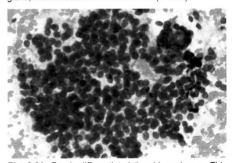

Fig. 2.61 Poorly differentiated thyroid carcinoma. This preoperative fine-needle aspiration specimen shows an insular cluster of small cells with fragile, poorly defined cytoplasm, round, hyperchromatic nuclei with little pleomorphism and a 3D microfollicle (top right).

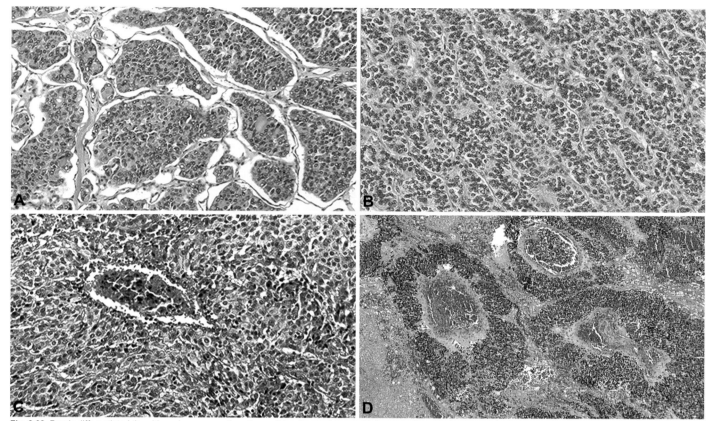

Fig. 2.62 Poorly differentiated thyroid carcinoma: growth patterns. **A** Insular carcinoma with tumour cell nests showing artefactual separation from the surrounding fibrovascular stroma. **B** Trabecular growth pattern. **C** Solid growth pattern with a focus of necrosis. **D** Peritheliomatous pattern due to large areas of tumour necrosis, the surviving neoplastic cells are grouped around blood vessels.

Table 2.08 Immunohistochemical expression of common markers of thyroid follicular cell differentiation (cytokeratins, thyroglobulin, TTF1, TTF2, and PAX8), proliferation (Ki-67 proliferation index as determined using the MIB1 antibody), survival (BCL2), and cell-cycle regulation (p53, Cyclin D1, p21, and p27).

	Cytokeratins	Thyroglobulin	TTF1 [a]	TTF2 [a]	PAX8 [a]	Ki-67 index	BCL2	p53	Cyclin D1	p21 and p27
Normal thyroid follicular cells	Positive	Positive	Positive	Positive	Positive	< 3%	Positive	Negative	Negative	Positive
Well-differentiated thyroid carcinoma	Positive	Positive	Positive	Positive	Positive	< 10%	Positive	Negative	Variably positive	Variably positive
Poorly differentiated thyroid carcinoma	Positive [b]	Decreased (microfollicular and perinuclear staining only)	Positive	Positive	Positive	10–30%	Usually positive	Focally positive [c]	Positive	Focally positive
Anaplastic thyroid carcinoma	Positive, focal/weak, heterogeneous staining	Negative, may be focal/weak, equivocal	Usually negative	Usually negative	Usually positive	> 30%	Negative	Positive	Positive	Negative

[a] Lineage-specific transcription factors are not expressed only by thyroid follicular cells (e.g. clear cell carcinoma of the kidney is PAX8-positive); a panel of immunostains may be useful for diagnosing difficult cases.
[b] Poorly differentiated thyroid carcinomas are immunoreactive for high-molecular-weight cytokeratins. They are typically CK7-positive and CK20-negative, although some cases lack CK7 expression.
[c] p53 expression (partially correlating with *TP53* mutation) is not as diffuse as in anaplastic carcinoma, and may be limited to areas of infiltrative growth.
   Data estimated from the pertinent literature {202,257,1299,1538,2022,2099,2174,2706,2937}.

necrosis) seen in prototypical insular carcinoma, but are composed of larger, more-pleomorphic cells. They usually exhibit a solid and/or trabecular growth pattern {355,2099,2385,2598}. As in insular carcinoma, colloid formation is minimal or absent. Some cases are predominantly composed of oncocytic cells {2105}; others have foci of clear cells, mucinous differentiation {1434}, signet-ring cells {840}, or rhabdoid cells {46}. PDTC can coexist with other thyroid cancer histotypes, including the tall cell {2306, 2895}, hobnail {66}, and cribriform-morular {1947} variants of papillary thyroid carcinoma. Marked nuclear pleomorphism and cellular anaplasia indicate progression to anaplastic carcinoma {1758}.

The Turin proposal, which was developed in 2006 during a consensus meeting held in Turin, Italy, recommends an algorithmic approach to the histopathological diagnosis of this tumour using the following criteria: (1) diagnosis of carcinoma of follicular cell derivation by conventional criteria; (2) a solid, trabecular, or insular growth pattern; (3) absence of the conventional nuclear features of papillary thyroid carcinoma; and (4) at least one of the following three features: convoluted nuclei (i.e. dedifferentiated nuclear features of papillary carcinoma), ≥ 3 mitoses per 10 high-power fields, and tumour necrosis {2891}. The algorithm has also been applied to Hürthle cell (oncocytic) carcinomas, which when poorly differentiated often show a small-cell component {110, 130,671}.

When the Turin consensus criteria are met in only a part of the entire tumour this should be noted and the proportion involved reported. Some studies have shown that the focal presence of PDTC (even accounting for as little as 10% {670} of an otherwise well-differentiated tumour) may be associated with aggressive features and/or may unfavourably affect prognosis {641,670,2000,2423}.

PDTC in metastatic lymph nodes should be reported, because it has been associated with a fatal outcome even in patients in whom papillary microcarcinoma was the only primary tumour {965,2166}.

It has been reported that completely encapsulated tumours with mitotic activity or necrosis and with high-grade cytoarchitectural features that meet the

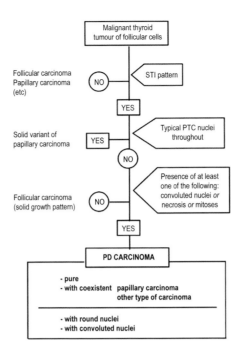

Fig. 2.63 Algorithm for the diagnosis of poorly differentiated (PD) thyroid carcinoma using the Turin consensus criteria. PTC, papillary thyroid carcinoma; STI, solid, trabecular, or insular. Reprinted from Volante M, Collini P, Nikiforov YE, et al. (2007) {2891}.

consensus criteria, except for invasion, of PDTC did not recur or metastasize after a median follow-up of > 10 years {2308}. The Turin consensus criteria define a group of poorly differentiated tumours with a poor prognosis intermediate between that of well-differentiated and undifferentiated (anaplastic) carcinomas {997,1229,2891}. These tumours are not the only thyroid cancers with such a prognosis {2705}. The finding of necrosis or increased mitotic activity {1143} also identifies thyroid carcinomas (other than anaplastic carcinoma) with a poor outcome, with considerable overlap with the Turin criteria {997}. Aggressive forms of

papillary or follicular carcinomas {1860, 1861,2012,2306} should not be included in the poorly differentiated category if their distinctive features of differentiation (papillary carcinoma nuclei, papillae or follicles) are retained throughout the tumour {2891}.

The differential diagnosis includes primarily medullary thyroid carcinoma, followed by parathyroid carcinoma and carcinoma metastatic to the thyroid gland.

Immunophenotype
The immunohistochemical profile of PDTC is summarized in Table 2.08 (p. 101). These tumours show general features intermediate between those of well-differentiated and anaplastic carcinomas.

Cytology
The cytological features most predictive of poorly differentiated carcinoma are severe crowding; clusters with solid, trabecular, or insular morphology; single cells; and a high N:C ratio {280}.

Genetic profile
The genetic alterations found in PDTC are summarized (and compared with those found in well-differentiated and anaplastic carcinomas) in Table 2.09. They include alterations that are early driver events in thyroid carcinogenesis (i.e. RAS family {933} and *BRAF* {1996} mutations, *ALK* {1000,1342} fusions) and others that typically occur as late events associated with tumour dedifferentiation (i.e. mutations of *TP53* {687,696,2180, 2701}, *TERT* {1541,1638,1806}, *CTNNB1* {931,2180}, and *AKT1* {2281}).

PDTCs have a mutation load intermediate between that of anaplastic and well-differentiated papillary carcinomas {1542}. They carry multiple genetic alterations

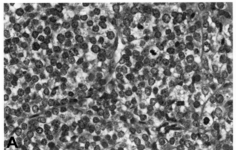 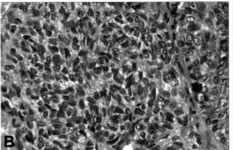 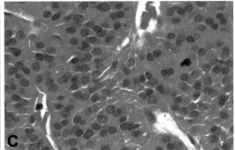

Fig. 2.64 Poorly differentiated thyroid carcinoma. Mitoses are evident in all 3 cases shown. **A** Insular carcinoma with solid nests of small, uniform cells with round hyperchromatic nuclei and minimal pleomorphism. **B** Insular carcinoma with cells showing irregular, convoluted, so-called raisin-like nuclear membranes, corresponding to dedifferentiated nuclear features of papillary carcinoma; compared with that of conventional papillary carcinoma, the chromatin is darker and there are no nuclear pseudoinclusions. **C** Poorly differentiated oncocytic cell carcinoma.

Table 2.09 Genetic alterations in poorly differentiated thyroid carcinoma (PDTC) compared with those in anaplastic (undifferentiated) thyroid carcinoma (ATC) and well-differentiated thyroid carcinoma (WDTC) – follicular thyroid carcinoma (FTC) and conventional papillary thyroid carcinoma (PTC) – with published estimated mutation prevalence rates.

Tumour type		TP53	TERT[a]	RAS[b]	BRAF V600E[c]	PIK3CA	PTEN	CTNNB1[d]	EIF1AX[e]	ALK[f]	Chromosomal DNA[g]
ATC		40–80%	30–75%	10–50%	10–50%	5–25%	10–15%	0–5%	5–15%	0–10%	Unstable and highly aneuploid, complex karyotypic alterations
PDTC		10–35%	20–50%	20–50%	5–15%	0–15%	5–20%	0–5%	5–15%	0–10%	Unstable, complex karyotypic alterations
WDTC	FTC	0%	10–35%	30–50%	0%	0–10%	0–10%	0%	0%	0%	Unstable, ~65% of cases have karyotypic alterations
	PTC	0%	5–15%	0–5%	40–80%	0–5%	0–5%	0%	0–5%	0–5%	Stable

[a] Activating mutation (C228T or C250T) in the promoter region of the TERT gene. In well-differentiated carcinomas, these mutations are associated with unfavourable clinicopathological features.
[b] The most frequently affected RAS gene hotspot is codon 61 of NRAS, followed by codon 61 of HRAS.
[c] The prevalence of BRAF V600E mutation is ~40% in aggressive, radioiodine-refractory and FDG-PET–positive thyroid cancers {2281}.
[d] Some studies have reported a higher prevalence of CTNNB1 mutation in poorly differentiated and anaplastic carcinomas {931}. Mutations in other WNT pathway genes (AXIN1 and APC) have been reported in < 5% of poorly differentiated and anaplastic carcinomas {1542}.
[e] In poorly differentiated and anaplastic carcinomas, EIF1AX mutations are associated with RAS gene mutations {1542}.
[f] In most cases, ALK is fused with STRN. Tumours with ALK rearrangement typically develop from pre-existing papillary carcinomas with follicular architecture. The rearrangement can be identified with the same FISH probes and antibodies used to detect ALK rearrangement in lung carcinomas. Tumours with ALK rearrangement may respond to molecular treatment with ALK inhibitors {1000,1342}.
[g] Assessed by cytogenetics, nuclear DNA content, loss of heterozygosity, comparative genomic hybridization, and DNA copy-number alteration.

more frequently than do well-differentiated tumours: usually one of the early changes in combination with late alterations {563,1542,1998,2281}. Activating AKT1 mutations have been reported in 19% of aggressive, radioiodine-refractory PDTCs, nearly always in combination with BRAF V600E mutation {2281}. In composite tumours, in which a well-differentiated component is associated with poorly differentiated or undifferentiated areas, early alterations are typically found in both components, whereas late changes appear to be restricted to the less-differentiated areas {696,1996,2174, 2224,2701}. TERT mutations are clonal in poorly differentiated and anaplastic carcinomas, whereas they are typically subclonal in well-differentiated papillary carcinoma {1542}. Disruption of the SWI/SNF chromatin remodelling complex, mutation of histone methyltransferases, and inactivation of the DNA mismatch repair system each occurs in as many as 5–10% of PDTCs, and in a higher proportion of anaplastic carcinomas {1542}.

These data support a multiple genetic hits model, which is seen in many types of aggressive cancer, indicating a multistep progression from well-differentiated to poorly differentiated or anaplastic carcinoma {1542}.

Some rearrangements frequently found in well-differentiated tumours are uncommon: RET/PTC and PAX8/PPARG are detected in about 10% and 5% of cases,

Table 2.10 Prognostic factors independently associated with survival in poorly differentiated carcinomas by multivariate analysis.

Poor prognosis		
Clinicopathological factors – Patient age ≥ 45 years {106} – Tumour size ≥ 5 cm {997} – Macroscopically evident extrathyroidal extension (pT4a) at surgery {1205} – Distant metastases (M1) at presentation {1205}	**Histological and immunohistochemical factors** – Tumour necrosis {106} – IMP3 immunoreactivity {106} – Oncocytic features[a] {671}	**Molecular genetic factors** – RAS gene mutation {2895} – Downregulation of miR-150[b] {672}

Good prognosis
Histological factor – Convoluted (papillary carcinoma–like) neoplastic cell nuclei {106}

[a] This association is controversial; poorly differentiated oncocytic carcinomas were not statistically associated with poor survival in other series {106,1143}.
[b] Downregulation of miR-23b was independently associated with tumour recurrence in the same study {672}.

respectively, suggesting that they do not promote dedifferentiation to poorly differentiated or anaplastic carcinoma {285, 1542,2281,2419,2895}.

The microRNA profile of PDTC is different from those of well-differentiated and undifferentiated tumours {672,2883}.

The gene expression pattern of poorly differentiated and anaplastic carcinomas is consistent with marked dysregulation of cell-cycle control mechanisms, and may contribute important prognostic information {1894,2180}.

Prognosis and predictive factors

In most series, the overall 5-year survival rate is 60–70% {106,933,1205,2891}. Recurrences usually develop within the first 3 years {394,997,1143}. The mean disease-specific survival time is approximately 5 years after diagnosis {2891}. Response to radioiodine treatment is generally poor {394,1205,2306}. The prognostic factors that have been associated with survival by multivariate analysis are summarized in Table 2.10. The most robust prognostic factors are stage and patient age. The presence of a tumour capsule is associated with favourable prognosis {2308}.

Anaplastic thyroid carcinoma

El-Naggar A. K.
Baloch Z. W.
Eng C.
Evans H. L.
Fagin J. A.
Faquin W. C.
Fellegara G.
Franssila K. O.

Giuffrida D.
Katoh R.
Kebebew E.
Kondo T.
Matias-Guiu X.
Nikiforov Y. E.
Papotti M.
Smallridge R.

Sugitani I.
Tallini G.
Wakely P. E.
Westra W. H.
Wick M. R.
Williams M. D.

Definition

Anaplastic thyroid carcinoma (ATC) is a highly aggressive thyroid malignancy composed of undifferentiated follicular thyroid cells.

ICD-O code   8020/3

Synonyms

Undifferentiated thyroid carcinoma; sarcomatoid carcinoma; metaplastic carcinoma; spindle cell carcinoma; giant cell carcinoma; carcinosarcoma; pleomorphic carcinoma

Epidemiology

ATC is the most aggressive form of primary thyroid malignancies, with a median 1-year survival rate of only 10–20% {325, 558,1253,1336,2585}. Patients are typically elderly and present with advanced-stage tumours; the female-to-male ratio is 2:1 {234}.

Etiology

The causative factors of ATC remain unknown. However, areas of differentiated thyroid carcinomas are not uncommon, suggesting high-grade/anaplastic evolution from these entities.

Localization

In addition to considerable local invasion, ATC often presents with metastatic spread to regional lymph nodes and distant sites. All ATCs are considered high–stage (IV) tumours {234,275,325,1336}.

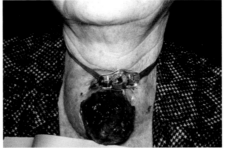

Fig. 2.66 Anaplastic thyroid carcinoma. An 81-year-old woman with a large protruding tumour at presentation.

Clinical features

Patients typically present with a rapidly enlarging, firm, fixed, and widely infiltrative neck mass. The most common symptoms are pain, hoarseness, breathing difficulty, and dysphagia {2905}. Other symptoms include vocal cord paralysis, cervical pain, and dyspnoea. Approximately 30–40% of patients present with distant metastasis, most frequently to the lung, bone, and brain.

Macroscopy

Tumours are commonly bulky and infiltrative, with a homogeneous and/or variegated appearance. On cut section, ATCs are typically light tan and fleshy, with zones of haemorrhage and necrosis.

Microscopy

The highly variable microscopic appearances of ATC are broadly categorized into three patterns, which can occur singly or in any combination: sarcomatoid, giant cell, and epithelial. The sarcomatoid form is composed of malignant spindle cells with features commonly seen in high-grade pleomorphic sarcoma. The giant cell form is composed of highly pleomorphic malignant cells, some of which contain multiple nuclei. The epithelial form manifests squamoid or squamous cohesive tumour nests with abundant eosinophilic cytoplasm; occasional keratinization can be noted. Common to all three forms are necrosis, an elevated mitotic rate, and an infiltrative pattern of growth. Vascular invasion is often present, defined as permeation of the vessel wall by neoplastic spindle cells that protrude into the vascular lumen. Secondary features of ATCs include an acute inflammatory infiltrate and tumour-infiltrating macrophages {357,2365}, heterologous differentiation (e.g. neoplastic bone and cartilage), and osteoclast-like multinucleated giant cells {915,1014,1493}.

Additional rare variants of ATC have also been described, including the paucicellular variant (characterized by abundant fibrous tissue with few atypical spindle cells), which may be mistaken for Riedel thyroiditis {2925}, and angiomatoid {1847, 2013}, rhabdoid {396,1526}, lymphoepithelioma-like, and small cell variants.

The currently available evidence supports the assumption that both de novo and dedifferentiated forms arise from either uncommitted or follicular epithelial cells. Differentiated carcinoma (most

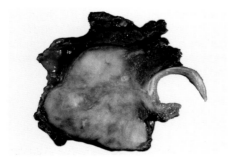

Fig. 2.65 Anaplastic thyroid carcinoma. Gross photograph of a tumour with extension to soft tissue and trachea.

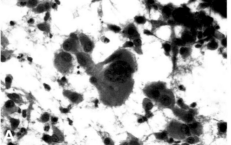
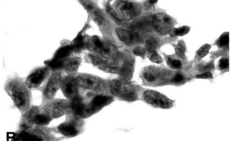

Fig. 2.67 Anaplastic thyroid carcinoma. **A** Markedly pleomorphic tumour cells and occasional multinucleated cells in a background of cell debris (Papanicolaou stain). **B** Fine-needle aspiration specimen demonstrating markedly pleomorphic spindle cells (Papanicolaou stain).

commonly of the papillary phenotype) is a well-recognized precursor.

Immunophenotype
Common thyroid-lineage markers such as TTF1 and thyroglobulin are usually absent, whereas PAX8, also a thyroid-lineage marker, is retained in approximately half of all cases {257,2022}. Positive cytokeratin expression supports the epithelial nature of ATC, but negative immunostaining for cytokeratin does not exclude the diagnosis. A major role of immunohistochemistry is to help distinguish this entity from other undifferentiated malignancies using CD45 and other lymphoid markers along with melanocytic markers to exclude lymphoma and melanoma, respectively {1061,1694,2260}.

Cytology
Fine-needle aspirates of ATC can show either markedly sparse or abundant cellularity, depending on the part of the mass sampled. Fine-needle aspirates can readily be recognized as high-grade malignancy due to malignant cellular features and overt nuclear pleomorphism {1263}. The cellular elements typically include both epithelioid and spindle cells, as well as osteoclast-like tumour giant cells, in a background of tumour diathesis. Tumour cell clusters are commonly infiltrated by neutrophils. In ATC arising in association with a differentiated carcinoma, smears may show cells

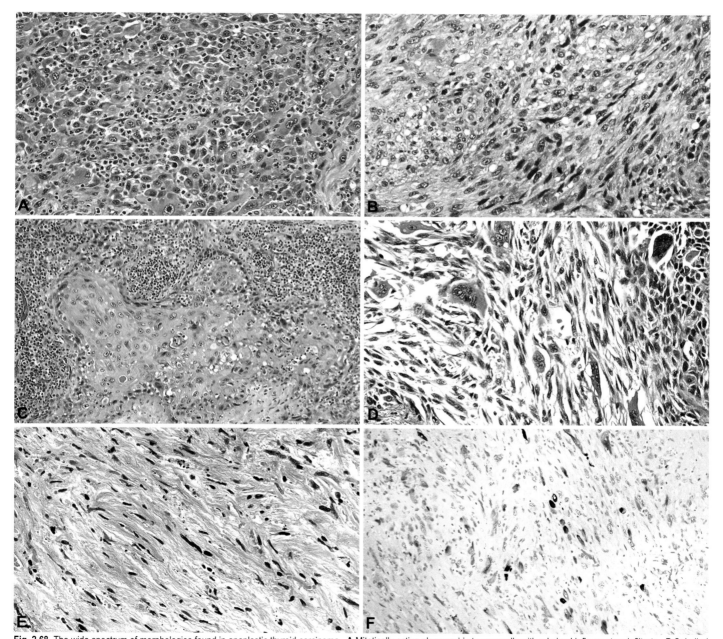

Fig. 2.68 The wide spectrum of morphologies found in anaplastic thyroid carcinoma. **A** Mitotically active pleomorphic tumour cells with admixed inflammatory infiltrate. **B** Spindled sarcoma-like fascicles of tumour cells. **C** Squamous morphology with surrounding dense inflammation. **D** Spindle and epithelioid malignant cells with multinucleated (osteoclast-like) giant cells may be prominent. **E** Paucicellular variant. **F** Cytokeratin highlights scattered spindle cells, which support an epithelial lineage (cytokeratin immunostain).

from a papillary carcinoma or follicular neoplasm. Occasionally, aspirates of ATC consist almost entirely of necrotic debris and inflammatory cells, which can result in a non-diagnostic sample; in such cases, core biopsy can be used in conjunction with fine-needle aspiration. In elderly patients with a rapidly growing neck mass, a thyroid aspirate that shows a necrotic and inflammatory background with rare pleomorphic cells is suggestive of ATC {870,1061,1694,2260}.

Genetic profile

A wide variety of genetic alterations are found in ATC. The most frequently mutated gene is *TP53* (mutated in 30–70% of cases) {275,819,1722}. Other recurring alterations include *BRAF* V600E mutation (present in 20% of cases) and alterations involving RAS genes (*NRAS*, *KRAS*, or *HRAS*; mutated in 20% of cases), *PIK3CA* (in 10–20%), *PTEN* (in 10–15%) {898, 1498,1642,2415}, and *ALK* {1935,2996}. Recent evidence also suggests that alterations in p73, beta-catenin genes {932}, RAF genes {1420,2032,2224}, and a gene named "overexpressed in anaplastic thyroid carcinoma-1" (*OEATC1*) {1871} may be associated with both de novo ATC and cases that arise in differentiated thyroid carcinomas {870,1788,2697, 2995}. Copy-number gains have been found in ATCs, in genes such as *EGFR* (with copy-number gains found in 46% of cases), *FLT1* (also called *VEGFR1*; in 45%), *PDGFRB* (in 38%), and *PIK3CA/B* (in 38%). Epigenetic and microRNA changes have also been reported to be associated with ATC {912,2883}. Evidence that ATC can evolve through pro-

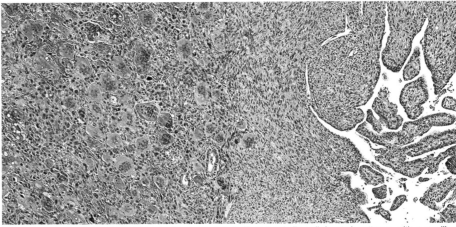

Fig. 2.69 Anaplastic thyroid carcinoma. Giant cell–rich (left) and spindle cell (centre) patterns, with a papillary component (right).

gressive acquisition of genetic alterations in pre-existing differentiated carcinoma is mounting {1046,2398,2997,3023}.

Genetic susceptibility

There are no known genetic susceptibility findings specifically associated with the development of non-syndromic ATC. However, this tumour can occur in patients with inherited cancer syndromes, including Cowden syndrome, Werner syndrome, Carney complex, and familial adenomatous polyposis, all of which are associated with differentiated epithelial thyroid cancer risk (see the respective sections in Chapter 7: *Inherited tumour syndromes*, p. 241).

Prognosis and predictive factors

The prognosis of ATC is grave, with a mortality rate of > 90%. Generally, a primary presentation with bulky infiltrative disease is a poor prognostic sign. Older patient age, acute symptoms, and leukocytosis have also been identified as clinical risk factors associated with a lower survival rate {1336,2674}. Although most ATCs are unresectable at presentation, carefully selected patients can undergo extensive surgery with curative intent, often with adjuvant radiation and chemotherapy {1336,2673}. ATC found incidentally in a resected differentiated thyroid carcinoma may have a better clinical course; the percentage of ATC should be indicated within the report {234,325, 558,3072}. There are no known biological predictors of the clinical behaviour or response to therapy of ATC.

EGFR is expressed in ATC and has been used to guide targeted treatment in selected patients {179,760,1049,1569}. VEGFR and *ALK* gene alterations may also be considered for targeted therapeutic stratification of certain patients {1935,2996}.

Squamous cell carcinoma

Carcangiu M. L.
Lam A. K. Y.
Montone K. T.

Definition
Squamous cell carcinoma is a malignant epithelial tumour composed entirely of cells with squamous differentiation.

ICD-O code   8070/3

Synonym
Epidermoid carcinoma

Epidemiology
This extremely rare tumour occurs in elderly individuals and is more common in women, with a female-to-male ratio of 2:1 {809,1008,1536}.

Clinical features
The clinical features are the same as those of anaplastic thyroid carcinoma. The tumour grows rapidly and often presents with pressure symptoms resulting from tracheal or oesophageal compression {1536}. A longstanding history of thyroid disease, such as Hashimoto thyroiditis, is noted in some cases {462, 551}. Rarely, patients with squamous cell carcinoma develop a paraneoplastic syndrome, with hypercalcaemia and leukocytosis {2288,2381}.

Imaging studies (e.g. laryngoscopy, bronchoscopy, oesophagoscopy, and chest X-ray) are important for the exclusion of primaries from other sites and the determination of extent of disease.

Tumour spread and staging
The most common route of spread is local extension into adjacent structures. Nodal metastases are common and distant metastases develop in approximately 20% of cases {551,1536,2212}. The staging is identical to that of anaplastic (undifferentiated) carcinoma.

Macroscopy
Squamous cell carcinoma is typically a large tumour involving one or both lobes of the thyroid gland {2569}. Satellite tumour nodules are often present. The tumour frequently has a firm consistency and a greyish-white colour, with areas of necrosis.

Microscopy
By definition, squamous cell carcinoma of the thyroid should consist predominantly or entirely of tumour cells with squamous differentiation. Anaplastic and papillary carcinomas can show areas of squamous differentiation {1535,3121}, but there should be no evidence of these or other types of thyroid carcinoma in squamous cell carcinomas. The tumours are graded similarly to squamous carcinomas in other locations. Approximately half of the cases are poorly differentiated or undifferentiated {551,1536}. Squamous cell carcinoma of the thyroid often shows extensive infiltration of perithyroidal soft tissue, as well as prominent vascular and perineural invasion.

The differential diagnosis includes extension or metastasis from a squamous cell carcinoma of other sites, squamous differentiation in papillary carcinoma, squamous metaplasia associated with nodular goitre and lymphocytic thyroiditis, and carcinoma showing thymus-like differentiation. Some squamous cell carcinomas may have arisen in remnants of the branchial arches.

Immunophenotype
Squamous cell carcinoma of the thyroid is strongly positive for CK19, but negative for CK1, CK4, CK10/13, and CK20 {1536, 1538}. Focal positivity for CK7 and CK18 may be present in some tumours. Occasional cases have been reported to be positive for thyroglobulin, but this most likely reflects non-specific absorption from adjacent follicular cells. EMA has also been reported to be positive {3121}. The tumours often have a high proliferation index {2961}.

Genetic profile
Expression of abnormal p53 has been noted in approximately 50% of squamous cell carcinomas of the thyroid. Loss of p21 expression is seen in all cases.

Prognosis and predictive factors
The prognosis is similar to that of anaplastic thyroid carcinoma {551,1536}.

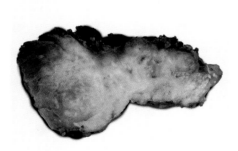
Fig. 2.70 Squamous cell carcinoma. This tumour has replaced an entire lobe of the thyroid.

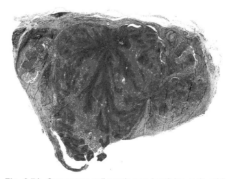
Fig. 2.71 Squamous cell carcinoma involving a thyroid lobe.

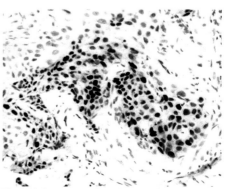
Fig. 2.72 Squamous cell carcinoma. p53 staining.

Medullary thyroid carcinoma

DeLellis R. A.
Al Ghuzlan A.
Albores Saavedra J.
Baloch Z. W.
Basolo F.
Elisei R.
Kaserer K.

LiVolsi V.
Matias-Guiu X.
Mete O.
Moley J. F.
Nikiforov Y. E.
Nosé V.
Pinto A. E.

Definition
Medullary thyroid carcinoma (MTC) is a malignant tumour of the thyroid gland composed of cells with evidence of C-cell differentiation.

ICD-O code   8345/3

Synonyms
Solid carcinoma with amyloid stroma; C-cell carcinoma; parafollicular cell carcinoma

Epidemiology
MTC accounts for < 2–3% of all thyroid malignancies, a lower range than is frequently cited, due to the marked increase in the relative incidence of papillary thyroid carcinoma over the past two decades {2252,2976}. Sporadic forms of the tumour, which account for approximately 70% of cases, occur with similar frequencies in different parts of the world, with a slight female predominance. The peak incidence of sporadic tumours occurs among patients in their fifth or sixth decade of life, with younger patient ages in hereditary cases {1337}. About 30% of MTCs are heritable, with an autosomal dominant pattern of inheritance caused by gain-of-function germline mutations in the *RET* proto-oncogene. Multiple endocrine neoplasia type 2 (MEN2) includes the phenotypes MEN2A, MEN2B, and familial MTC (FMTC) {771,1473,2976,2977}. Currently, FMTC is considered a variant along the spectrum of disease expression in MEN2A {2976} (see *Multiple endocrine neoplasia type 2*, p. 248).

Etiology
The etiology of sporadic MTC is unknown. There is no apparent relationship between external ionizing irradiation of the head and neck and the development of these tumours. The tumours may arise in the setting of Hashimoto thyroiditis, but this association is probably coincidental {2968}. There are very limited data suggesting that chronic hypercalcaemia may be associated with an increased risk of MTC {1649}. In the familial form, germline

mutations in the *RET* proto-oncogene are present (see *Multiple endocrine neoplasia type 2*, p. 248).

Localization
MTCs are usually located at the junctions of the upper and mid portions of the thyroid lobes, corresponding to areas in which C cells are normally concentrated.

Clinical features
Most patients with sporadic tumours present with a painless thyroid mass, which typically appears cold on scanning {2252}. As many as 70% of patients who present with a palpable thyroid nodule have cervical nodal metastases, and 10% have distant metastases {1337, 2976}. Upper airway obstruction and dysphagia may develop due to extensive local tumour growth. Serum levels of calcitonin correlate with tumour burden {880}; however, the tumours can be non-secretory (in < 1% of cases) {1700}. Patients with metastatic disease may have severe diarrhoea and flushing related to high circulating levels of calcitonin and other tumour-related products {1337}. Carcinoembryonic antigen (CEA) is one of the most important markers for the follow up of MTC patients and it is particularly useful for those patients whose tumours produce low levels of calcitonin {2976}. Some tumours produce ACTH or CRH, which are responsible for the development of Cushing syndrome {2991}. The development of calcitonin screening studies in the 1970s and *RET* mutation analysis in the 1990s has altered the

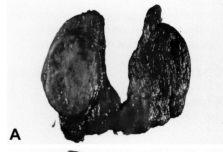
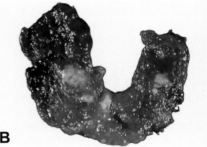

Fig. 2.73 Medullary thyroid carcinoma. **A** This sporadic tumour is unilateral and sharply circumscribed. **B** This multiple endocrine neoplasia type 2A–associated tumour is bilateral and multicentric.

clinical landscape of the heritable forms of these tumours, resulting in younger patient ages at diagnosis and the identification of precursor lesions or early invasive tumours in appropriately screened individuals {2977}.

Macroscopy
The tumours vary in size from < 0.1 cm in diameter to those that replace the entire thyroid lobe. Sporadic MTC typically presents as a single, sharply circumscribed but unencapsulated, greyish-tan to yellow

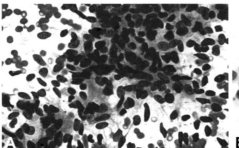
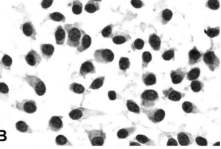

Fig. 2.74 Medullary thyroid carcinoma. Fine-needle aspirate **A** Tumour cells are spindle-shaped (Romanowsky stain). **B** The cells have a plasmacytoid appearance (Papanicolaou stain).

mass of variable consistency, measuring 2–3 cm in diameter. In contrast, heritable tumours are typically bilateral and multicentric {2342}. Prophylactic thyroidectomies in patients with familial syndromes require complete examination of the thyroid, because gross tumours may not be seen. Tumours measuring < 1 cm in diameter have been called medullary thyroid microcarcinomas {47,608,1059, 1864}. Microcarcinomas have been identified as incidental findings in thyroid glands removed for other reasons and in patients with nodular thyroid disease who were screened for calcitonin abnormalities. One study has suggested that the term "microcarcinoma" should be applied only to MTCs measuring < 0.5 cm, since none of the patients with tumours of that size had evidence of metastatic disease {2173}.

Microscopy

MTCs exhibit a wide variety of histological appearances that can mimic the entire spectrum of thyroid malignancies. The prototypical tumour has a solid, lobular, trabecular, or insular growth pattern {1114,2990}. Individual tumour cells are variably sized and can be round, polygonal, plasmacytoid, or spindle-shaped, with frequent admixtures of these cell types. Nuclei are generally round with coarsely clumped chromatin and small nucleoli; occasional nuclear pseudoinclusions may be present. There is a low to moderate degree of nuclear pleomorphism, although scattered markedly pleomorphic nuclei are present in some cases. In most primary tumours, mitotic activity is relatively low {2786}. The cytoplasm varies from eosinophilic to

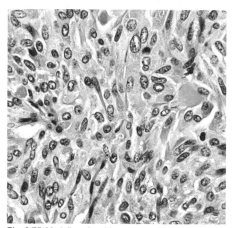

Fig. 2.75 Medullary thyroid carcinoma. The tumour has a diffuse growth pattern and is composed focally of spindle-shaped cells.

amphophilic and appears finely granular in well-fixed samples. Electron microscopy reveals two types of secretory granules, with mean diameters of 280 nm and 130 nm, respectively; both granule types contain calcitonin {651,652}. Occasional mucin-positive vacuoles may be present {3084}, and psammoma-like bodies occur in occasional cases. Stromal amyloid deposits are present in as many as 90% of cases, and spectrometric analysis has shown that full-length calcitonin is their major constituent {1353}. Katacalcin, which flanks calcitonin in the precursor molecule, has also been identified in the amyloid deposits {787}.

Individual tumours from patients with heritable forms of MTC are virtually indistinguishable from those occurring sporadically, except for their bilaterality, multicentricity, and association with primary C-cell hyperplasia {405,678,1319,2157}. Primary C-cell hyperplasia has also been

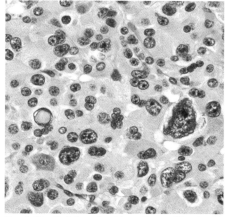

Fig. 2.76 Medullary thyroid carcinoma. The tumour contains scattered cells with enlarged hyperchromatic nuclei. A nuclear pseudoinclusion is present in this field.

referred to as "neoplastic" C-cell hyperplasia and thyroid intraepithelial neoplasia of C-cells (THINC) {405,678,1319,2157}. In addition to the presence of primary C-cell hyperplasia in patients with MEN2, similar changes have been reported adjacent to the tumours in a subset of patients with sporadic micro-MTC, in the absence of germline *RET* mutations {1319,1320,1321}. The C-cell hyperplasia-MTC sequence is discussed in detail in the section on *Multiple endocrine neoplasia type 2* (p. 248).

Immunophenotype

The tumour cells are usually positive for calcitonin and calcitonin gene–related peptide {2636}, but occasional cases express only calcitonin gene–related peptide {1946}. Tumours that are negative for both proteins may give positive signals for their corresponding mRNAs {1652}. A variety of other peptide products, including

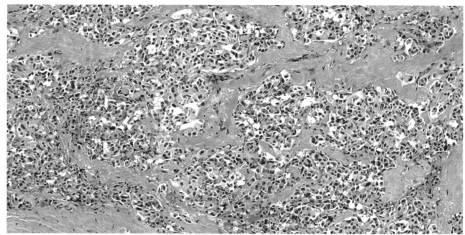

Fig. 2.77 Medullary thyroid carcinoma. The tumour is transected by dense bands of fibrous tissue.

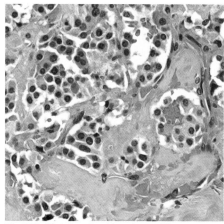

Fig. 2.78 Medullary thyroid carcinoma. The component cells have a distinctive plasmacytoid appearance.

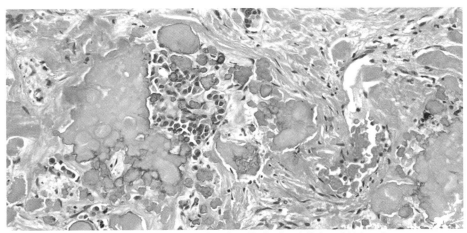

Fig. 2.79 Medullary thyroid carcinoma. The tumour is replaced by focally calcified amyloid deposits.

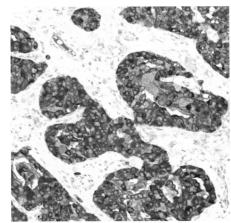

Fig. 2.80 Medullary thyroid carcinoma. Intense immunoperoxidase staining of tumour cells for calcitonin.

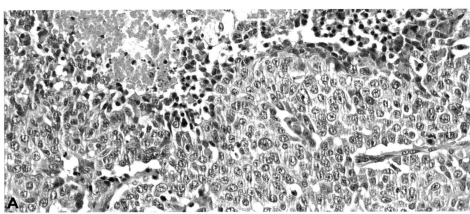
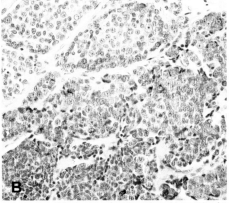

Fig. 2.81 Medullary thyroid carcinoma. A The tumour is focally necrotic and is composed of pleomorphic cells. B The tumour cells in this case are focally and weakly positive for calcitonin.

ACTH, somatostatin, gastrin-releasing peptide, and neurotensin, can also be present in some cases {153,384,2342}. The tumour cells are also positive for generic neuroendocrine markers, including chromogranin and synaptophysin. TTF1 is positive in most cases, although the intensity of staining is less than that seen in follicular cell neoplasms {1328}. PAX8 staining is variable and weak {2022}. The tumour cells are negative for thyroglobulin, but entrapped thyroid follicles are positive. CEA is present in the vast majority of tumours {653}; in some cases, the cells lose their ability to produce calcitonin but retain CEA positivity {1809}.

Variants
There are numerous, although infrequent, cytoarchitectural variants of MTC. Most of these variants have no significant impact on prognosis, but their identification is important to avoid confusion with other tumour types {1755}. The quantitative criteria used to define these subtypes in heterogeneous tumours have yet to be established. Rarely, MTCs may exhibit a true papillary pattern, in which the component cells are aligned on fibrovascular stalks {1297,2401}. More commonly, there is a pseudopapillary pattern, in which there is artefactual separation of groups of tumour cells from the adjacent stroma {1334}. The follicular (tubular/glandular) variant is composed predominantly of neoplastic follicle formations, which are calcitonin-positive and thyroglobulin-negative {1088,2401}. The spindle cell variant consists of elongated cells present singly and in loose clusters {2215}. The giant cell variant is characterized by cells with multiple nuclei and/or enlarged hyperchromatic nuclei {1296}. The clear cell variant is composed of cells with optically clear cytoplasm {1545}, whereas the oncocytic variant is composed of cells with abundant granular eosinophilic cytoplasm {692,1085}. The melanotic variant is composed of cells with variable amounts of melanin pigment {199,2574}. The squamous variant is composed of cells with evidence of squamous differentiation {692}. The amphicrine variant is composed of cells containing both mucin and calcitonin {1010}. The paraganglioma-like variant is composed of cells with a broad trabecular pattern reminiscent of hyalinizing trabecular tumour {1199}. The angiosarcoma-like variant has pseudo-sarcomatous features resembling those of angiosarcomas {1522}. Tumours of the encapsulated variant are surrounded by a complete fibrous capsule {235,1426}. In some series, these tumours have been referred to as C-cell adenomas; however, until more is known about their natural history, it is best to classify them as encapsulated MTCs {1199}. The small cell variant is characterized by cells with round to ovoid nuclei and scant cytoplasm, with growth in compact, trabecular, or diffuse patterns; foci of necrosis may be evident in some of these cases {44,1808}. The small cell variant tends to be more aggressive than conventional MTC and must be distinguished from metastasis to the thyroid. Two cases of calcitonin-negative small cell thyroid car-

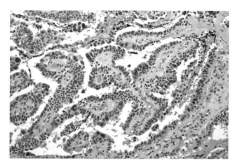
Fig. 2.82 Papillary variant of medullary thyroid carcinoma.

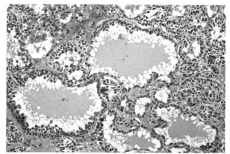
Fig. 2.83 Follicular (tubular/glandular) variant of medullary thyroid carcinoma. The component follicles are large and irregularly shaped.

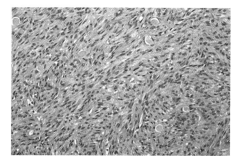
Fig. 2.84 Spindle cell variant of medullary thyroid carcinoma. The tumour is composed of interweaving fascicles of spindle cells.

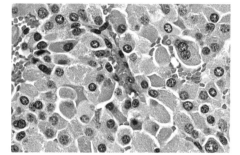
Fig. 2.85 Oncocytic variant of medullary thyroid carcinoma. Tumour cells are large, with abundant granular eosinophilic cytoplasm.

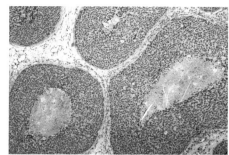
Fig. 2.86 Small cell variant of medullary thyroid carcinoma. The tumour is made up of centrally necrotic cellular nests composed of small tumour cells.

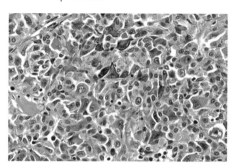
Fig. 2.87 Melanotic variant of medullary thyroid carcinoma. The tumour contains scattered groups of melanin-containing cells.

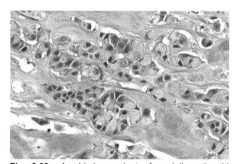
Fig. 2.88 Amphicrine variant of medullary thyroid carcinoma. The tumour is composed of vacuolated cells containing mucin and calcitonin.

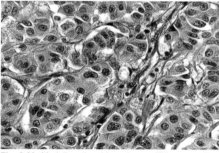
Fig. 2.89 Medullary thyroid carcinoma. This tumour has a predominant trabecular pattern.

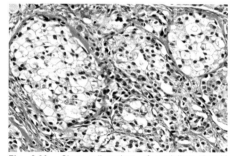
Fig. 2.90 Clear cell variant of medullary thyroid carcinoma.

cinoma have been classified as apparent primary thyroid oat cell carcinomas {802}. It has been suggested that some small cell thyroid carcinomas may be related to the Ewing tumour family, on the basis of *EWSR1-FLI1* rearrangements {761}.

Cytology
Fine-needle aspiration biopsy specimens from MTCs display a spectrum of morphological features similar to those noted on histopathological examination. Most aspirates consist of round, ovoid, or spindle-shaped cells arranged singly or in loosely cohesive groups {1387,2089}. The tumour cells have ample granular cytoplasm with eccentric nuclei, imparting a plasmacytoid appearance to the

tumour cells. The chromatin is similar to that of other neuroendocrine tumours and frequently has a salt-and-pepper appearance. Nuclear pseudoinclusions and multinucleated tumour cells may also be present. Amyloid is present in a smaller proportion of aspirates (50–70%) than of histological sections (~90%) because of the more limited sample sizes. The amyloid appears as acellular material that can be distinguished from the thick colloid of papillary carcinomas on the basis of its congophilia. Immunostains may be helpful in identifying this entity. Despite these well-known cytological features, a recent multicentric study involving 12 institutions found that the cytological diagnosis of MTC was obtained in only 46.1%

of cases, highlighting the difficulty of making this diagnosis in clinical practice; measurement of serum calcitonin can be of great help {796}.

Genetic profile
Germline gain-of-function mutations in the *RET* proto-oncogene are the major molecular drivers in the pathogenesis of hereditary forms of MTC (see *Multiple endocrine neoplasia type 2*, p. 248). Somatic *RET* mutations have been reported in 40–60% of sporadic MTCs {726, 776,1917,2323}. The M918T mutation in exon 16, which is present as a germline mutation in 98% of patients with MEN2B, is the most common somatic mutation in sporadic tumours {2323}. The distribution

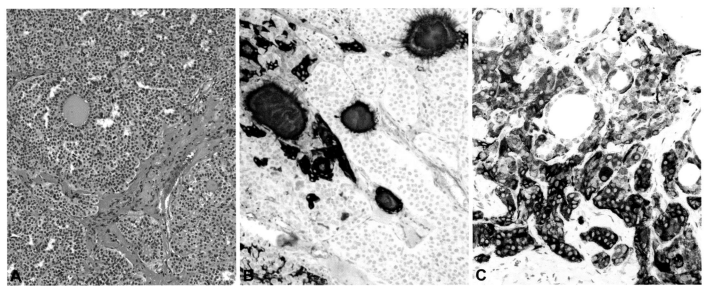

Fig. 2.91 Medullary thyroid carcinoma. **A** Tumour-induced stromal fibrosis is an early sign of invasion in medullary microcarcinoma. **B** Basement membrane, highlighted by collagen IV immunostaining, is lost in areas of stromal invasion. **C** Synaptophysin immunostaining helps to identify infiltrating medullary carcinoma cells.

of this mutation in sporadic MTCs is inhomogeneous, occurring only in subpopulations of most primary tumours and among various subsets of multiple metastases {776}. The prevalence of the M918T mutation is substantially lower in medullary thyroid microcarcinomas than in larger tumours {2323}, which suggests that *RET* mutations might be secondary events driving tumorigenesis rather than initiators of tumour development {1186}. Few non-*RET* molecular alterations have been reported in MTC. RAS family mutations occur in variable proportions of sporadic MTCs {522,1916}. In one study, *HRAS* and *KRAS* mutations were found in 56% and 12%, respectively, of *RET* mutation-negative sporadic MTCs, whereas only 2.5% of *RET* mutation-positive cases had a RAS family gene mutation {1918}. In a larger case series, the overall prevalence of RAS mutations was 10.1%, and 17.6% of *RET*-negative tumours harboured RAS mutations {522}; none of the *RET* mutation-positive tumours in the series was RAS-positive {522}. The mutual exclusivity of *RET* and RAS family mutations suggests that RAS activation may constitute an alternative molecular pathway for the development of the malignancy. A *RET* fusion, *MYH13-RET*, has been proposed as a novel driver mutation of sporadic MTC, because it was present in the absence of point mutations of *RET* and RAS genes {1042}. *ALK* fusions (*GFPT1-ALK* and *EML4-ALK*) have also been reported in these tumours {1259}.

Genetic susceptibility
See *Multiple endocrine neoplasia type 2,* Chapter 7 (p. 248).

Prognosis and predictive factors
Among patients with MTC presenting with a palpable thyroid nodule, the rate of clinical cervical lymph node involvement is as high as 75% in some series {2354}. Nodal metastases most commonly involve central compartment nodes (affected in 50–75% of cases), the ipsilateral jugulocarotid chain (in 50–60%), and the contralateral jugulocarotid chain (in 25–50%) {1899,2489}. Haematogenous metastases occur most commonly in lung, liver, and bone, but have also been reported to occur in a variety of other sites, including the adrenal glands, pituitary gland, and breast {2976}.

Reported 5-year and 10-year survival rates are 65–90% and 45–85%, respectively, depending primarily on disease stage {221,324,1874,2253,2492}. Patient age (≤ 50 years vs > 50 years) and TNM stage were the only independent prognostic factors identified in a series of > 100 cases of sporadic and heritable MTCs; the 5-year and 10-year cause-specific mortality rates were 10.7% and 13.5%, respectively {1337}. In the series, one third of the patients with heritable tumours were diagnosed by biochemical or genetic screening studies, and they had a lower incidence of nodal metastases than did patients with sporadic tumours. In contrast, patients with sporadic or heritable tumours who presented with systemic symptoms of diarrhoea, bone pain, and flushing generally had widespread metastatic disease {1337}. Extrathyroidal extension {2492} and substantial postsurgical calcitonin elevations {2492} have been considered as poor prognostic features. Therefore, early diagnosis of MTC, while it is still intrathyroid, is a fundamental aspect of maximizing the possibility of cure. Early diagnosis of the hereditary forms can be achieved with genetic screening, but for sporadic cases the only possibility is through routine screening of thyroid nodules for serum calcitonin {756A}.

Multiple histological and immunohistochemical parameters, including cellular composition (spindle cell vs round cell), pleomorphism, extent of amyloid deposition, and extent of calcitonin staining, have also been investigated as potential prognostic parameters, but none has proven to be significant in multivariate analyses. Higher proliferation rates, as assessed by Ki-67 staining, have been associated with aggressive biological behaviour {880,2786}. Vascular invasion has been reported as an adverse predictor of disease-free status {3,2299}, and stromal desmoplasia has been suggested as an important parameter to predict metastatic potential {1450}.

RET mutations play an important prognostic role in MTC. MTCs in patients with MEN2B are commonly more aggressive than those in patients with MEN2A

{2024,2354,2976}, but as noted above, the most important *RET* mutation in MEN2B is M918T, whereas in MEN2A it is C634R. It has been demonstrated that the *RET* M918T mutation is the most aggressive and most transforming *RET* mutation {757}. Given these findings, it is not surprising that somatic M918T mutation in sporadic MTC has been associated with poor clinical outcome {757,1832, 1917}. Patients with RAS-mutated sporadic MTCs may have a less aggressive clinical course than those without RAS gene mutations {522,1916}. In one study, tumours with RAS mutations were associated with an intermediate risk of aggressive disease, whereas tumours with *RET* mutations in exons 15 and 16 had the highest risk and those with other *RET* mutations had the most indolent course {1916,1917}.

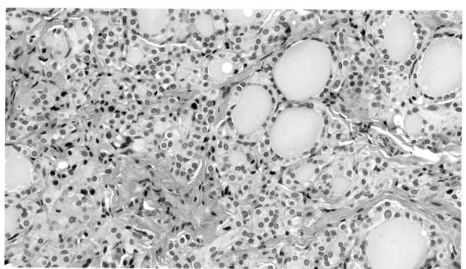

Fig. 2.92 Primary C-cell hyperplasia in a patient with multifocal medullary thyroid carcinoma associated with multiple endocrine neoplasia type 2A.

Mixed medullary and follicular thyroid carcinoma

Volante M.
Hunt J. L.
Komminoth P.
Lax S. F.
Matias-Guiu X.
Papotti M.
Shimizu M.

Definition

Mixed medullary and follicular thyroid carcinoma (MMFTC) is a primary malignant epithelial neoplasm of the thyroid showing morphological and immunophenotypical evidence of the coexistence of follicular and parafollicular cell–derived tumour populations within the same lesion.

ICD-O code   8346/3

Synonyms

Mixed follicular and C-cell carcinoma; mixed medullary and papillary carcinoma; composite carcinoma; biphasic carcinoma; simultaneous carcinoma; compound medullary–follicular carcinoma; concurrent medullary–follicular carcinoma; stem cell carcinoma; differentiated carcinoma, intermediate type (all obsolete)

Epidemiology

MMFTC is extremely rare, with < 60 cases reported, generally as single case reports. Data from the SEER database and small series indicate that about 8% of patients with medullary carcinoma have simultaneous differentiated thyroid carcinoma {3003}. However, among patients affected by medullary thyroid carcinoma (MTC), the prevalence of cases fulfilling the criteria of MMFTC is expected not to exceed 5% {2101}. Among 1420 consecutive differentiated thyroid carcinomas, only 4 cases had a simultaneous MTC, with only one of these showing MMFTC features {780}. There is a slight female predominance, with a female-to-male ratio of 1.2:1, and the mean patient age is 53 years (range: 7–78 years).

Localization

MMFTC can occur anywhere in the thyroid, with no lobe predilection.

Clinical features

MMFTC usually presents as an incidentally discovered, solitary, scintigraphically cold nodule, or as plurimetastatic disease. A considerable number of reported cases have had preoperative serum calcitonin (and CEA) levels within the normal range or only slightly elevated. Thyroglobulin serum levels may be elevated, with increased 131I uptake, especially in patients with disseminated disease {244}.

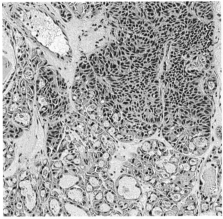

Fig. 2.93 Mixed medullary and follicular thyroid carcinoma. The medullary carcinoma component, with predominant spindle cell features, is closely admixed with a follicular carcinoma of the oncocytic type.

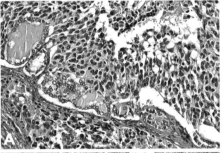
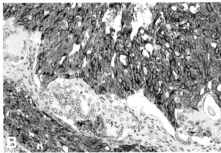

Fig. 2.95 Mixed medullary and follicular thyroid carcinoma. **A** Follicular structures of a papillary carcinoma (at right) merge with the medullary carcinoma component. **B** The papillary carcinoma component is calcitonin-negative, the medullary carcinoma calcitonin-positive.

Ultrasonographic features are unspecific but suggestive of malignancy, including hypoechoic, solid nodules with irregular borders and intranodular vascularization. Preoperative fine-needle aspirates may suggest MMFTC, but in most cases,

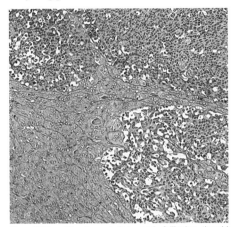

Fig. 2.94 Mixed medullary and follicular thyroid carcinoma. The medullary carcinoma component (at top right) is closely admixed with a papillary carcinoma of the solid variant.

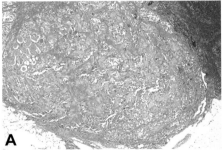
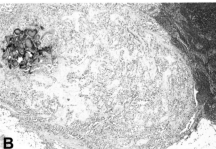

Fig. 2.96 Lymph node metastasis of mixed medullary and follicular thyroid carcinoma. **A** There is a mixed pattern, with a predominant medullary carcinoma component and a minor follicular-variant papillary carcinoma component (at right). **B** The papillary carcinoma component is thyroglobulin-positive.

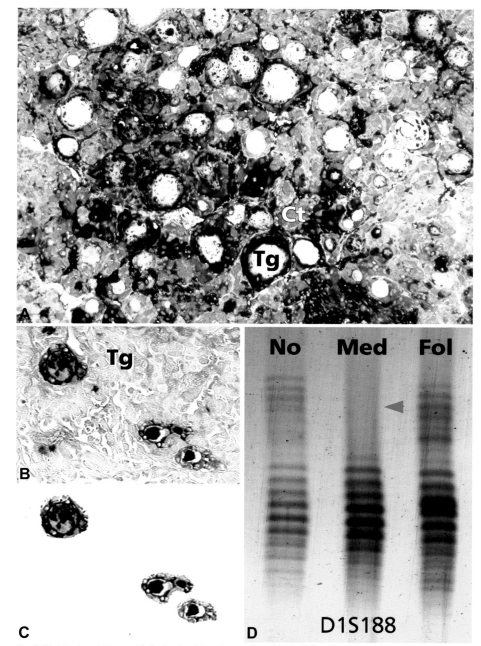

Fig. 2.97 Mixed medullary and follicular thyroid carcinoma. **A–C** The medullary thyroid carcinoma component stains positively (red) for calcitonin (Ct), and the intermingled follicular structures stain positively (black) for thyroglobulin (Tg). **D** Clonality analysis of the microdissected components compared with normal control tissue (No) shows a monoclonal pattern in the medullary carcinoma component (Med) and a polyclonal/oligoclonal pattern in the follicular carcinoma component (Fol).

Microscopy

The histopathological hallmark is coexistent tumour cell populations of MTC and a follicular cell–derived neoplasm {2368} within a thyroid nodule. The relative proportions of the two components are variable, and there is no recommendation on a specific cut-off point supporting the diagnosis of MMFTC. Synchronous medullary and follicular cell–derived carcinomas growing in close proximity but not intermingled constitute collision tumours and should not be classified as MMFTC. The MTC component is similar to the conventional type. The follicular cell–derived component includes conventional or follicular-variant papillary thyroid carcinoma (by far the most common), or follicular, poorly differentiated, or (rarely) anaplastic carcinoma {2108,2118}. Lymph node metastases may have the same morphology as the primary tumour or may contain only one neoplastic component. Immunohistochemistry is mandatory to prove the dual parafollicular (positive for calcitonin and CEA) and follicular (positive for thyroglobulin) cell differentiation, either in separate cell clusters or within individual cells (as confirmed by mRNA and ultrastructural studies). TTF1 is expressed by both components. The differential diagnosis includes the follicular variant of MTC (thyroglobulin-negative throughout), MTC with entrapped non-neoplastic follicles (lacking signs of malignancy), and follicular carcinoma with neuroendocrine differentiation (chromogranin A–positive but calcitonin-negative). In the absence of the appropriate morphological background, thyroglobulin staining should be interpreted with caution, due to potential protein adsorption by MTC cells.

Genetic profile

No genetic data are available on the follicular counterpart. Somatic *RET* mutations have been detected in some cases, mostly affecting codon 918 in exon 16. In a molecular study based on laser capture microdissection of 11 cases, somatic *RET* mutations were detected exclusively in the MTC component. Clonality analysis demonstrated that in all cases, the two tumour components were unrelated, and that in at least some cases, the follicular component was polyclonal/oligoclonal, indicating its sequestration within the MTC component (the so-called hostage histogenetic theory) {2894}.

MTC, a follicular neoplasm, or papillary carcinoma is suspected, depending on the associated component {1079,1680, 1953}. The clinical behaviour of MMFTC is more similar to that of conventional MTC than to that of differentiated thyroid carcinoma. Disease-related fatal outcome is documented in approximately one fifth of reported cases, even 10 years after initial diagnosis {1460}. Lymph node involvement and distant metastases occur in as many as 25% of cases.

Macroscopy

The gross features are not specific, and depend on the predominant tumour cell component. MMFTC frequently presents as a solid, firm, whitish unencapsulated nodule, with a mean size of 29 mm (range: 4–55 mm).

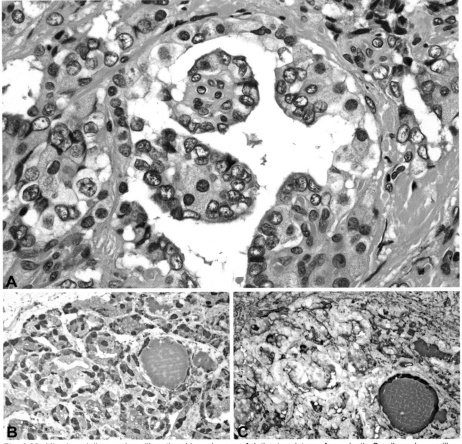

Fig. 2.98 Mixed medullary and papillary thyroid carcinoma. **A** Intimate mixture of neoplastic C cells and a papillary thyroid carcinoma component with classic cleared nuclei. **B** Calcitonin staining highlights the neoplastic C cells, with negative staining in the papillary thyroid carcinoma component. **C** Thyroglobulin staining highlights the neoplastic papillary thyroid carcinoma component.

Genetic susceptibility

Most reported cases are sporadic. However, MMFTC has also been described in the setting of multiple endocrine neoplasia type 2 {878,1865,2894}, with no specific link to any particular germline *RET* mutation.

Prognosis and predictive factors

As is the case with MTC and differentiated thyroid carcinoma, radical surgery is the most important prognostic factor. Response to radioactive iodine treatment has also been documented in metastatic cases {244}.

Mucoepidermoid carcinoma

Cameselle Teijeiro J. M.
Albores Saavedra J.
Baloch Z. W.
Sobrinho Simões M.
Wenig B. M.

Definition
Mucoepidermoid carcinoma is a malignant epithelial neoplasm characterized by the combination of epidermoid cells and mucin-producing cells.

ICD-O code   8430/3

Epidemiology
Mucoepidermoid carcinoma is a rare thyroid tumour {887} that can affect a wide range of age groups, with a median patient age of 47 years (range: 10–91 years). The female-to-male ratio is about 2:1. The epidemiology is similar to that of papillary thyroid carcinoma (PTC) {2311}. Previous radiation exposure of the neck during childhood has been documented in occasional cases {278,826,1892,2980}. Chronic lymphocytic thyroiditis (Hashimoto thyroiditis) occurs in 40% of cases {243,826,2635,2980}.

Etiology
The etiology is unknown. Origins from a solid cell nest, ectopic salivary gland, and thyroglossal duct remnant have been proposed; however, a metaplastic follicular cell derivation is favoured {371, 2202,2203,2873}.

Localization
It occurs in the thyroid gland. It rarely occurs within the thyroglossal duct {2950}.

Clinical features
Patients are usually euthyroid and present with a hypofunctioning mass in the thyroid gland; extrathyroidal extension is observed in 25% of cases at presentation {147,887,2278,2980}. Oesophageal, tracheal, or recurrent laryngeal nerve involvement occurs in about 20% of cases {147,887,2402,2980}. Regional lymph node metastases are seen in 40%, and distant metastases, mainly to lung and bone, have been reported in < 10% of cases {147,887,2551,2980}.

Macroscopy
The tumours range from incidental microscopic foci to 10 cm in size. The

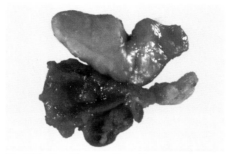

Fig. 2.99 Thyroid mucoepidermoid carcinoma appearing as a circumscribed solid mass (top) separated from adjacent thyroid gland (bottom).

cut surface reveals a tannish-brown to yellowish-white, well-demarcated but rarely encapsulated tumour, occasionally displaying mucoid and/or cystic areas {2980}. Foci of necrosis and infiltration of the thyroid capsule and surrounding tissues are observed occasionally {88, 366}.

Microscopy
Mucoepidermoid carcinoma consists of solid sheets or large confluent epithelial nests showing epidermoid and mucous cells surrounded by a fibrotic stroma. The epidermoid component is arranged in sheets with or without keratin

pearl formation; mucous (goblet) cells are cuboidal epithelial cells lining ducts or glandular spaces. Mucin-producing cells may contain intracytoplasmic droplets (hyaline bodies) that give a positive periodic acid–Schiff (PAS) reaction and resemble colloid {366,1086}. A cribriform-like pattern with elongated lumina containing colloid-like material and papillary infoldings can occur. Ciliated cells are sometimes present {77,1282, 2980}. Extracellular mucin {1554,1957, 2980} and/or cysts with mucin or keratinized debris may be found; psammoma bodies occasionally occur. The tumour cells have medium-sized nuclei with pale chromatin, resembling PTC nuclei; nuclear grooves and pseudoinclusions can be seen {278,887,1252}. Mitotic figures and necrosis are rare. About 50% of mucoepidermoid carcinoma cases are associated with PTC (conventional, follicular variant, or tall cell variant) {147, 906,1854,1957}. Some mucoepidermoid carcinomas (with or without PTC) transform to anaplastic (undifferentiated) carcinoma or display a poorly differentiated (insular) pattern of growth {366,887,2551, 2980}. Continuity with follicular carcinoma or Hürthle cell carcinoma is much

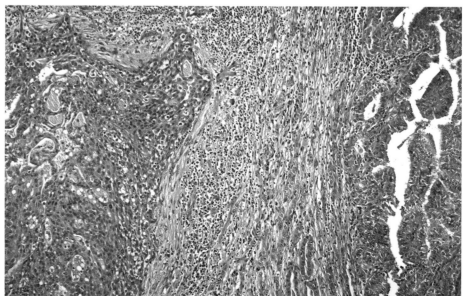

Fig. 2.100 Mucoepidermoid carcinoma (at left) is associated with papillary thyroid carcinoma (at right).

less common {2203}. Chronic lymphocytic thyroiditis (Hashimoto thyroiditis) is frequently seen in the background thyroid parenchyma {1325,1849,2278}.

Immunophenotype
Mucoepidermoid carcinomas are positive for keratins, and most express thyroglobulin, PAX8, and TTF1 {147,2682, 2720,2980}. Epidermoid cells and ductal basal cells are p63-positive {826,2314}. P-cadherin expression and E-cadherin abnormalities can also be observed in epidermoid areas {2311}. Polyclonal CEA positivity is mainly seen in mucocytes and duct-like elements {906,2203}. Calcitonin and neuroendocrine markers are absent {2203,2402,2858,2980}.

Cytology
Aspirates are cellular, containing mucin-producing and epidermoid cells. Mucin-producing cells show vacuolated cytoplasm containing mucin and/or signet-ring cell features {278,372,1957, 2858}. Cellular sheets with a microcystic-like pattern containing hyaline bodies and/or amorphous material can also be seen {367}. Anaplastic change occurs rarely {367}.

Genetic profile
mRNA expression of the *TTF1*, *TTF2*, *PAX8*, *SLC5A5* (also known as *NIS*), and *TPO* genes has been reported in mucoepidermoid carcinoma {1849}. The translocation t(11;19), associated with the *CRTC1-MAML2* fusion transcript identified in salivary and bronchial gland mucoepidermoid carcinomas, was detected in 1 of 3 thyroid mucoepidermoid carcinomas examined {2779}. Absence of this translocation with a slightly increased chromosomal copy number was observed in another thyroid mucoepidermoid carcinoma {2950}. *RET*/PTC1 and *RET*/PTC3 rearrangements were detected in a combined PTC and mucoepidermoid carcinoma {906}, whereas no mutations in *BRAF*, *HRAS*, *KRAS*, or *NRAS* were detected in mucoepidermoid carcinoma {906,2816}.

Prognosis and predictive factors
Mucoepidermoid carcinoma is a low-grade malignant tumour with an indolent biological behaviour. Cervical lymph node metastases are common and distant metastases are rare. Transformation to anaplastic carcinoma has been reported in about 10% of cases {366, 2858}. Death due to tumour progression has occurred in 18% of patients, usually associated with older age and coexistence of poorly differentiated or anaplastic carcinoma {147,366,887,2858}.

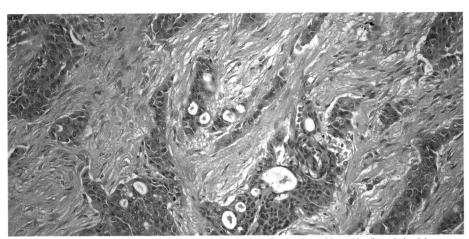

Fig. 2.101 Mucoepidermoid carcinoma. Solid sheets of epithelial cells showing epidermoid cells and glandular spaces in a fibrotic stroma.

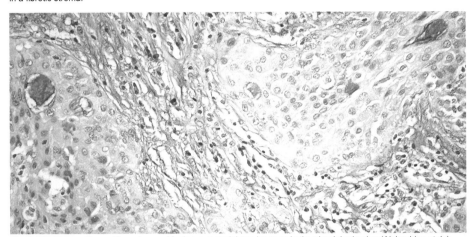

Fig. 2.102 Mucoepidermoid carcinoma. Mucinous material can be seen in the glandular lumina (Alcian blue stain).

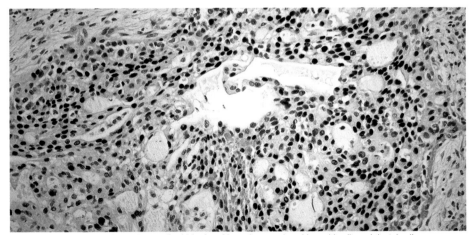

Fig. 2.103 Mucoepidermoid carcinoma. Positivity for p63 can be seen in epidermoid cells and ductal cells.

Sclerosing mucoepidermoid carcinoma with eosinophilia

Sobrinho Simões M.
Albores Saavedra J.
Chan J.K.C.
El-Naggar A.K.
Geisinger K.R.
LiVolsi V.

Definition

Sclerosing mucoepidermoid carcinoma with eosinophilia is a malignant epithelial neoplasm showing epidermoid and glandular differentiation and displaying a sclerotic stroma with eosinophilic and lymphocytic infiltration.

ICD-O code   8430/3

Epidemiology

This rare thyroid tumour occurs in adults and shows a female predilection, with a female-to-male ratio about 7:1 {519,1195, 1524,1672}. Sclerosing mucoepidermoid carcinoma with eosinophilia is consistently associated with fibrosing Hashimoto thyroiditis {42,147,446,2223}.

Clinical features

The tumour typically presents as a slow-growing, painless neck mass and/or a so-called cold thyroid nodule. Occasional cases can show rapid growth, causing dysphagia, airway compression, and recurrent laryngeal nerve involvement {613, 890}. Cervical lymph node metastases are detected in about 35% of patients at presentation {948,2223,2524,2565}.

Macroscopy

The tumours measure 1–13 cm {446,519, 2223}. They usually show poorly defined borders but can be well circumscribed. The cut surface is usually firm and solid.

Table 2.11 Clinical and pathological features of mucoepidermoid carcinoma (MEC) and sclerosing mucoepidermoid carcinoma with eosinophilia (SMECE)

	MEC	SMECE
Median patient age (range)	47 years (10–91 years)	55 years (32–89 years)
Female-to-male ratio	2:1	7:1
Extrathyroidal extension	~25%	~40%
Cervical lymph node metastasis	~40%	~35%
Distant metastasis	< 10%	~22%
Perineural invasion	Rare	Common
Chronic lymphocytic thyroiditis (Hashimoto thyroiditis)	~40%	Common
Association with papillary thyroid carcinoma	~50%	Rare
Thyroglobulin	Usually positive	Usually negative
TTF1	Usually positive	~50%

Microscopy

Sclerosing mucoepidermoid carcinoma with eosinophilia is characterized by small nests and/or short strands of epithelial cells infiltrating a sclerotic stroma richly infiltrated by eosinophils, lymphocytes, and plasma cells {446}. Lymphocytes and plasma cells frequently outnumber eosinophils. The tumour cells are polygonal, with mild to moderate nuclear pleomorphism and distinct nucleoli. Interspersed with the epidermoid nests are mucous-secreting cells with squashed nuclei and small pools of mucin. In some cases, glycogen-rich clear epidermoid cells can predominate {42}. A pseudoangiomatous pattern may be present due to cellular dyscohesion. Perineural invasion and vascular invasion are common. The non-neoplastic thyroid tissue always shows chronic lymphocytic thyroiditis (Hashimoto thyroiditis), often with prominent fibrosis and squamous metaplasia. Rarely, a coincidental separate papillary carcinoma can be seen {360,2223}.

The differential diagnosis includes conventional mucoepidermoid carcinoma, anaplastic carcinoma, primary and secondary squamous carcinoma, intrathyroid thymic carcinoma and florid squamous metaplasia. Lymph node metastases from sclerosing

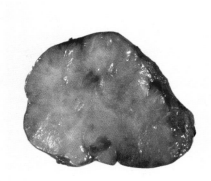

Fig. 2.104 Sclerosing mucoepidermoid carcinoma with eosinophilia. Predominantly solid and focally cystic tumour with poorly defined borders.

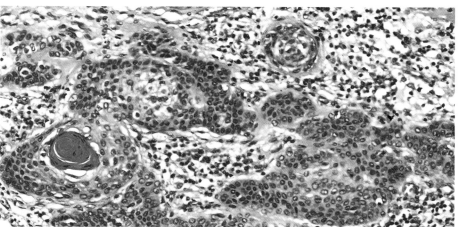

Fig. 2.105 Sclerosing mucoepidermoid carcinoma with eosinophilia. The tumour contains a squamous pearl.

mucoepidermoid carcinoma with eosinophilia can mimic Hodgkin lymphoma (see Table 2.11, p. 119) {147}.

Immunophenotype
The tumour cells express cytokeratins (including CK19), p63, CD10, and galectin 3, but are negative or only focally positive for thyroglobulin {1195,1524, 1672,2223}. Approximately 50% of cases are positive for TTF1 {42,2054,2223}. Calcitonin and S100 protein are negative {1524,2223,2519}.

Cytology
These tumours have a polymorphic appearance due to the presence of several distinct cell lines. The background typically contains a population of lymphocytes with a predominance of small mature cells. The major inflammatory cell type is the eosinophil. Neoplastic glandular and squamous epithelial cells are present. The epithelial cells have polygonal to spindled contours, opaque cytoplasm, and centrally located nuclei, which are large and hyperchromatic, often with coarse chromatin; keratinization may be evident. The malignant glandular cells have cuboidal or columnar shapes, polarized round nuclei, and cytoplasmic vacuoles; they may be present in small cohesive aggregates {277,947,948,1957}.

Prognosis and predictive factors
Sclerosing mucoepidermoid carcinoma with eosinophilia was initially considered to be a low-grade tumour {446}; however, recent studies have highlighted its potentially aggressive behaviour, with extrathyroidal extension in as many as 40% of patients at presentation {360,446,1672, 2223} and distant metastases (to lung, liver, or bone) in approximately 20% {277, 948,2223,2524,2565}. Isolated cases of death due to tumour progression have been reported {1672,2223}. The predictive factors are unclear.

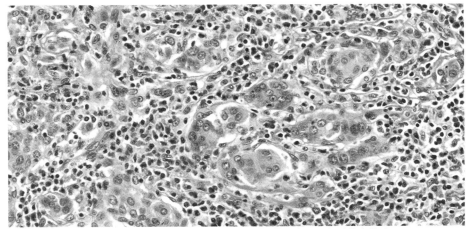
Fig. 2.106 Sclerosing mucoepidermoid carcinoma with eosinophilia. Abundant eosinophilic infiltrate.

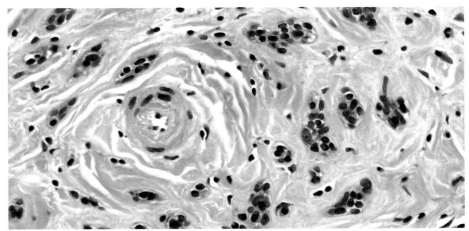
Fig. 2.107 Sclerosing mucoepidermoid carcinoma with eosinophilia. Short strands of epithelial cells in a sclerotic stroma.

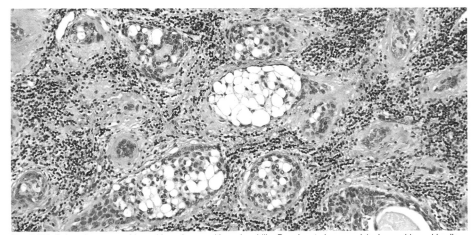
Fig. 2.108 Sclerosing mucoepidermoid carcinoma with eosinophilia. Prominent glycogen-rich clear epidermoid cells.

Mucinous carcinoma

Sobrinho Simões M.
Cameselle Teijeiro J. M.
Kondo T.

Definition
Mucinous carcinoma is a malignant epithelial neoplasm characterized by clusters of neoplastic cells surrounded by extensive extracellular mucin deposition.

ICD-O code   8480/3

Epidemiology
Mucinous carcinoma is rare, with only 9 cases reported in the English-language literature. The patients were aged 32–86 years, and there is no sex predominance {598,1434,1873,3051}.

Etiology
The etiology is unknown. Although derivation from both thyroglossal duct remnant and ectopic salivary gland have been proposed, an origin from ultimobranchial body remnant is more likely, specifically, via acid mucin–containing follicles {1084,2202}.

Clinical features
Mucinous carcinoma presents as either a rapidly or a slow-growing, so-called cold thyroid nodule, often accompanied by regional lymph node metastases {598,1434, 2599}. Distant metastases to skin, lung, and/or bone have been documented in 3 of 9 cases evaluated {583,1434,2599}.

Macroscopy
The tumour presents as either a well-circumscribed or (more often) a poorly circumscribed gelatinous nodule, 2.8–8 cm in diameter {2599,2600}.

Microscopy
Mucinous carcinoma is characterized by abundant mucoid lakes around trabeculae or clusters of tumour cells that usually show large nuclei and prominent nucleoli. The histology of mucinous carcinoma of the thyroid is identical to that of mucinous (colloid) carcinoma of other sites. By definition, features typical of other types of thyroid carcinoma should not be present. Focal squamous differentiation may occur {2600}. Mitotic figures are present but usually not numerous. Capsular and/or vascular invasion is frequently observed. Foci of necrosis were observed in one case, which are thought to constitute an anaplastic transformation of the mucinous carcinoma {868}. The mucosubstance is of the sulfated type, as evidenced by the iron diamine method; it stains positively with mucicarmine and Alcian blue, and gives a diastase-resistant positive periodic acid–Schiff (PAS) reaction {679,2599, 3051}. Mucinous carcinoma of the thyroid should be distinguished from other thyroid primaries that can produce mucins (mostly intracellular and occasionally extracellular). These include follicular adenoma; papillary, follicular, medullary, and mucoepidermoid carcinomas; and sclerosing mucoepidermoid carcinoma with eosinophilia {2339}. Metastatic carcinoma from lung, gastrointestinal tract, breast, or other organs must always be considered in the differential diagnosis when dealing with a thyroid tumour with a large mucinous component.

Immunophenotype
Mucinous carcinomas show focal immunoreactivity for thyroglobulin, TTF1, and PAX8, and are negative for calcitonin and calcitonin gene–related peptide {598,1434,1873,3051}. Thyroglobulin and TTF1 may be negative in areas of anaplastic transformation {868,3051}. The Ki-67 proliferation index (as determined using the MIB1 antibody) is usually high (> 10%) {1434}. The cells are positive for low-molecular-weight cytokeratins {598}. Nuclear immunoreactivity for p53 is often observed {1434}. Several mucins (MUC1, MUC2, MUC3, and MUC4) have been inconsistently detected in mucinous carcinoma of the thyroid, as well as in other types of thyroid carcinoma (papillary, follicular, and medullary) with focal mucin production {63}.

Cytology
Aspirates contain isolated or small aggregates of malignant cells with large nuclei and prominent nucleoli {1434,2599, 3051}. Signet-ring cells can occasionally be seen {598}. Variable amounts of mucous material may also be identified {598,1434,3051}.

Prognosis and predictive factors
Of the 8 patients with follow-up, 6 died of metastatic disease at 6 months to 4 years after diagnosis {583,598,868,1434,1873, 2599}.

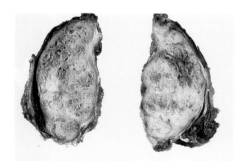
Fig. 2.109 Mucinous carcinoma. Prominent gelatinous appearance on cross-section.

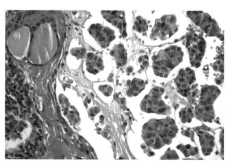
Fig. 2.110 Mucinous carcinoma. Clusters of neoplastic cells within pools of mucin.

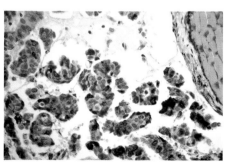
Fig. 2.111 Mucinous carcinoma. Some neoplastic cells stain strongly for thyroglobulin.

Ectopic thymoma

Chan J.K.C.
Cheuk W.
Dorfman D.M.
Giordano T.J.
Kakudo K.
Rosai J.

Definition
Ectopic thymoma is an organotypic thymic epithelial tumour occurring within or attached to the thyroid.

ICD-O code   8580/3

Epidemiology
Ectopic thymoma of the thyroid gland is very rare {448,533,1509,1582,2017, 2045,2731,2748}. Most patients are middle-aged, and there is a strong female predominance.

Localization
Ectopic thymoma of the thyroid gland is predominantly a localized tumour.

Clinical features
Patients present with a neck mass noticed for a few months to several years, with or without compression symptoms. Paraneoplastic syndromes are most uncommon. Thyroid scan reveals a so-called cold nodule, and thyroid function tests are normal.

Microscopy
Ectopic thymoma displays the same histological subtypes seen in mediastinal thymoma. The tumour typically forms jigsaw puzzle–like lobules separated by sclerotic septa. There is an intimate admixture of ovoid or spindled epithelial cells with variable numbers of small lymphocytes. Almost all reported cases are non-invasive. Residual ectopic thymus tissue is identified in the periphery in some cases. The epithelial component can be highlighted by immunostaining for cytokeratins, and the accompanying lymphocytes are characteristically immature T cells, which express TdT.

The differential diagnosis includes ectopic hamartomatous thymoma, which is not a genuine thymoma but rather a benign tumour that occurs in the soft tissues of the lower neck without involvement of the thyroid gland {448,2970}. Histologically, it is a circumscribed tumour lacking a lobulated growth pattern. It shows haphazard blending of the following features: (1) fascicular or lattice-like bland-looking spindle cells; (2) epithelial units in the form of squamous islands, syringoma-like tubules, anastomosing networks, simple glands, and cysts; and (3) adipocytes, which are present in highly variable proportions. There are few lymphocytes. The spindle cells are immunoreactive for cytokeratins, particularly high-molecular-weight cytokeratin.

Prognosis and predictive factors
Ectopic thymoma of the thyroid gland does not usually recur after surgical excision {448,2017}. To date, only one reported case has been complicated by cervical lymph node metastasis, which occurred 1 year after diagnosis {1509}.

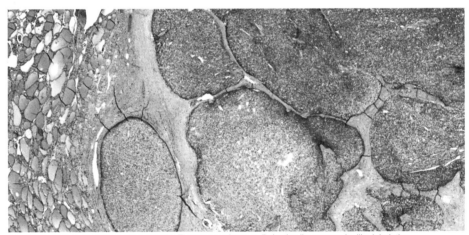

Fig. 2.112 Ectopic thymoma of the thyroid. The tumour shows a distinctive jigsaw puzzle–like lobulation.

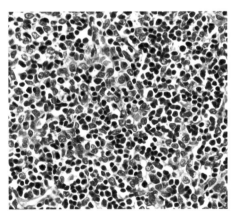

Fig. 2.113 Ectopic thymoma of the thyroid. There is an intimate admixture of neoplastic epithelial cells and small lymphocytes.

Spindle epithelial tumour with thymus-like differentiation

Chan J.K.C.
Dorfman D.M.
Giordano T.J.

Definition

Spindle epithelial tumour with thymus-like differentiation is a rare malignant tumour of the thyroid characterized by a lobulated architecture and a biphasic cellular composition featuring spindled epithelial cells that merge into glandular structures {448}.

ICD-O code   8588/3

Synonyms

Spindle cell tumour with thymus-like differentiation; spindle epithelial tumour with thymus-like element (SETTLE)

Epidemiology

Spindle epithelial tumour with thymus-like differentiation predominantly affects children and young adults, with a mean patient age of 19 years (range: 2–59 years). There is a male predilection, with a male-to-female ratio of 1.5 : 1 {1221,2262}.

Localization

Primary location is the thyroid. The tumour shows a tendency for late metastasis to lung, lymph node, and other visceral sites {865}.

Clinical features

The most common presentation is a painless thyroid mass, present for variable durations. Less common presentations include a rapidly enlarging neck mass, local tenderness, and diffuse thyroid enlargement. The tumour appears cold on thyroid scan and shows heterogeneous solid and cystic density on CT. Approximately 10% of patients have cervical lymph node metastasis at presentation {1221,2262}.

Macroscopy

The tumour is grossly encapsulated, partially circumscribed, or infiltrative, with an average size of 4.2 cm (range: 1.1–12 cm) {1221}. The cut surface is firm, greyish-white to tan, and vaguely lobulated.

Microscopy

Spindle epithelial tumour with thymus-like differentiation is a highly cellular tumour with a vaguely lobulated pattern imparted by fibrous septa. Most cases are biphasic, but occasional cases (the so-called monophasic variant) consist almost exclusively of spindled cells or glandular structures {483}. Compact interlacing to reticulated fascicles of spindled cells merge imperceptibly with tubulopapillary glands, with areas of stromal hyalinization. The spindled cells have elongated nuclei, with fine chromatin and inconspicuous nucleoli, and scant cytoplasm. Mitotic figures are typically rare, although high mitotic activity and necrosis may be present in rare cases {1389}. The glandular component usually takes the form of glomeruloid glands, tubules, papillae, cords, small pale-staining islands, and epithelium-lined cystic spaces. The epithelial cells are cuboidal to columnar and are sometimes mucinous or ciliated. Their nuclei are similar to those of the spindled cells except for an oval or round contour. Exceptionally, there is focal squamous differentiation. Lymphocytes are typically scant. Vascular invasion may be present.

Immunophenotype

Both spindled and glandular cells extensively express high-molecular-weight cytokeratin and CK7, but express low-molecular-weight cytokeratin only focally {865}. Rarely, the spindled cells may demonstrate myoepithelial differentiation {2669,3028}. The tumour cells are negative for thyroglobulin, calcitonin, CEA, TTF1, S100 protein, and CD5. Ultrastructurally, the epithelial nature of the spindle cells is evidenced by the presence of tonofilaments, desmosomes, and basal lamina {448}.

Spindle epithelial tumour with thymus-like differentiation can be distinguished from its histological mimic, synovial sarcoma, by the lower overall nuclear grade, glomeruloid glandular structures, absence of intraglandular necrotic debris, stromal hyalinization, paucity of mast cells, and diffuse expression of high-molecular-weight cytokeratin {865}.

Genetic profile

The tumour lacks the *SS18* gene translocation that characterizes synovial sarcoma {865,2262}. *KRAS* mutation has been reported in one case {3028}.

Prognosis and predictive factors

Spindle epithelial tumour with thymus-like differentiation is a slow-growing tumour with an overall survival of 86% at a median follow-up of 6.3 years {2262}. The metastatic rate is 26%, which increases to 41% with follow-up > 5 years {2262}. The latency period to develop metastasis is usually long (mean: 10 years) {2262}. Cervical lymph node metastasis is associated with a high risk of subsequent development of distant metastasis {2262}; however, metastatic disease can be compatible with long survival after treatment {485}.

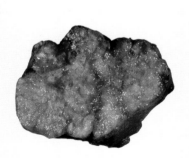

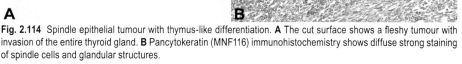

Fig. 2.114 Spindle epithelial tumour with thymus-like differentiation. **A** The cut surface shows a fleshy tumour with invasion of the entire thyroid gland. **B** Pancytokeratin (MNF116) immunohistochemistry shows diffuse strong staining of spindle cells and glandular structures.

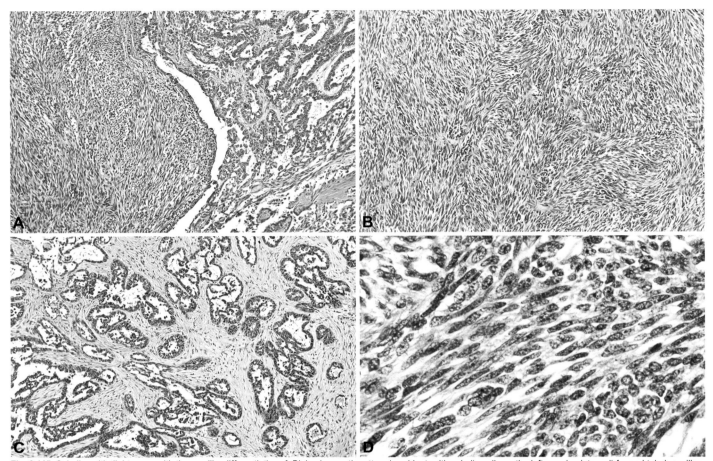

Fig. 2.115 Spindle epithelial tumour with thymus-like differentiation. **A** Biphasic growth pattern is evident, with spindle cells on the left merging into well-formed tubulopapillary structures on the right. **B** This tumour is composed of interlacing bundles of spindle cells. **C** Tumour with a predominantly monophasic appearance dominated by epithelial cells forming glomeruloid glandular structures. **D** The spindle tumour cells have relatively uniform nuclei, but are not as densely packed as in synovial sarcoma.

Intrathyroid thymic carcinoma

Kakudo K.
Chan J.K.C.
Cheuk W.
Dorfman D.M.
Giordano T.J.
Nosé V.

Definition

Intrathyroid thymic carcinoma {2696} is a malignant epithelial tumour of the thyroid gland with thymic epithelial differentiation. It is the malignant counterpart of ectopic thymoma of the thyroid gland.

ICD-O code   8589/3

Synonyms

Intrathyroidal epithelial thymoma {1862}; carcinoma showing thymus-like differentiation {448}; primary thyroid thymoma {96}; carcinoma showing thymus-like features {606}; carcinoma showing thymus-like element (CASTLE) {1974}; lymphoepithelioma-like carcinoma of the thyroid {1266,2018}; CD5-positive thyroid carcinoma {1294}

Epidemiology

Intrathyroidal thymic carcinoma showing thymus-like differentiation is a very rare thyroid carcinoma that affects middle-aged adults. The female-to-male ratio is nearly equal, with only a slight female predominance. This entity has been estimated to account for 0.083% of primary malignant tumours of the thyroid gland (8 of 9582 cases) in Japanese patients and 0.15% (3 of 2033 cases) in Chinese patients {510,1294}.

Etiology

The etiology of intrathyroidal thymic carcinoma showing thymus-like differentiation is unknown. Most reported cases have occurred in Asia, specifically China {510,1188,1643,2945} and Japan {1232, 1294,1862}. The fact that intrathyroidal thymic carcinoma showing thymus-like differentiation is more prevalent in Asian populations may suggest that genetic, ethnic, and/or environmental factors could contribute to tumorigenesis. There is no known association with EBV {1294}.

Localization

The great majority of cases occur within the thyroid gland, most commonly in the lower poles of the lateral lobes {1232, 1862}.

Clinical features

The reported subjective symptoms are neck tumour and hoarseness due to recurrent nerve paralysis {1232}. Lymph node metastasis was found in 9 of 18 patients (50%) who underwent lymph node dissection. Neither leukocytosis nor elevated granulocyte colony-stimulating factor has been reported. On ultrasound, the tumour appears as a hypoechoic solid mass without calcification {20,3045}. Thyroid scan normally reveals a cold nodule, and thyroid function tests are generally normal. Paraneoplastic syndrome, such as myasthenia gravis, has not been reported to date {1294}.

Macroscopy

Grossly, the tumour is solid, and neither calcification nor cystic change is found. The cut surface is ivory-white after fixation. The tumour is usually well demarcated but not encapsulated. A sharp border between the tumour and thyroid parenchyma is a characteristic feature in the early stage.

Microscopy

The histopathological characteristics of intrathyroidal thymic carcinoma showing thymus-like differentiation are identical to those of thymic carcinoma of the mediastinum. The tumour is basically a squamous cell carcinoma with lymphocyte-rich stroma without follicular or papillary structures. Occasional single-cell keratinization or stratification of keratinizing tumour cells is observed. The tumour is usually well demarcated at an early stage, and it invades into surrounding structures beyond the thyroid capsule at the advanced stages. The histological grade of intrathyroidal thymic carcinoma showing thymus-like differentiation is low compared with that of primary squamous cell carcinoma; nuclear atypia is mild

Fig. 2.116 Intrathyroidal thymic carcinoma showing thymus-like differentiation. A well-demarcated but unencapsulated tumour mass occupies the lower pole of the lateral lobe of the thyroid. The cut surface shows an ivory-white solid tumour without calcification or cystic change.

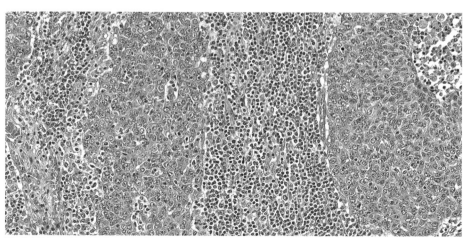

Fig. 2.117 Lymphoepithelioma-type intrathyroidal thymic carcinoma showing thymus-like differentiation. There is dense lymphocytic infiltration in the stroma separating tumour nests.

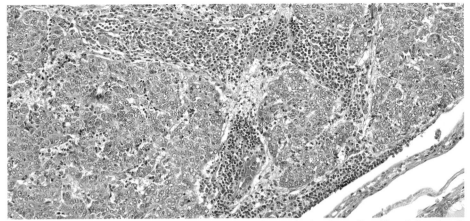

Fig. 2.118 Lymphoepithelioma-type intrathyroidal thymic carcinoma showing thymus-like differentiation. A well-circumscribed but unencapsulated tumour interfaces with the thyroid parenchyma.

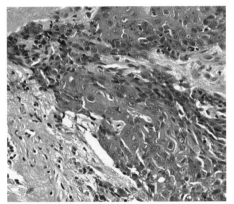

Fig. 2.119 Squamous cell carcinoma–type intrathyroidal thymic carcinoma showing thymus-like differentiation. Stratification of keratinizing tumour cells is seen in the tumour nest.

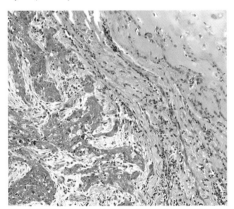

Fig. 2.120 Intrathyroidal thymic carcinoma showing thymus-like differentiation. This tumour has locally invaded the tracheal cartilage in the upper right field.

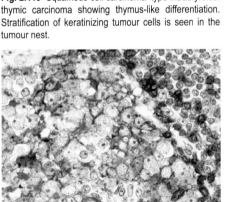

Fig. 2.121 Intrathyroidal thymic carcinoma showing thymus-like differentiation. Immunoperoxidase staining for CD5 reveals membrane positivity in the tumour cells and in the cytoplasm of T cells (upper right).

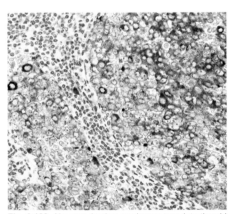

Fig. 2.122 Neuroendocrine carcinoma type intrathyroid thymic carcinoma. Immunohistochemical stain for synaptophysin demonstrated neuroendocrine nature with cytoplasmic positivity.

itive markers {1147,1643,2945} for the differential diagnosis of primary squamous cell carcinoma (CD5-negative and Ki-67 proliferation index > 50%), anaplastic (undifferentiated) carcinoma (CD5-negative and Ki-67 proliferation index > 50%), C-cell (medullary) carcinoma (CD5 and p63-negative and C-cell markers–positive), malignant lymphoma (CD5 and p63-negative and lymphocyte markers–positive), and solid-type follicular cell carcinoma (CD5-negative and follicular cell markers–positive). Neuroendocrine nature has been confirmed with chromogranin A, synaptophysin, and neuron-specific enolase in some cases, which were confirmed to be positive for CD5 and negative for calcitonin {1294,3047}. Three histological subtypes have been reported: (1) squamous cell carcinoma type, (2) lymphoepithelioma or basaloid type, and (3) neuroendocrine carcinoma type similar to mediastinal thymic carcinoma {1294}.

Prognosis and predictive factors

Patients with intrathyroidal thymic carcinoma showing thymus-like differentiation have excellent outcomes after curative resection; the reported 5-year and 10-year disease-specific survival rates are 90% and 82%, respectively {1232}. Intrathyroidal thymic carcinoma showing thymus-like differentiation is locally invasive, with regional lymph node metastasis at presentation; haematogenous metastases (to lung, liver, bone, and pleura) have been reported at advanced stages {389, 1232,1298,1505}. The absence of nodal metastasis and tumour extension to adjacent organs has been reported to be an indicator of a favourable prognosis {1232, 2319}. Postoperative external radiation has been reported to be effective {510, 1232,2677,2826}. Accepted prognostic and predictive factors have not been established.

and mitoses are rare. The Ki-67 proliferation index is approximately 10–30%, whereas it is often > 50% in anaplastic carcinoma and primary squamous cell carcinoma {1294}.

Immunophenotype

The immunohistochemical profile of intrathyroidal thymic carcinoma showing thymus-like differentiation is summarized in Table 2.12. CD5 {218,699,2269}, KIT (also known as c-KIT and CD117), and p63 have been reported to be useful pos-

Paraganglioma and mesenchymal/stromal tumours

Paraganglioma

Matias-Guiu X.
Costinean S.
DeLellis R. A.
Wakely P. E.

Definition
Intrathyroidal paraganglioma is an intrathyroidal neuroendocrine tumour of paraganglionic origin.

ICD-O code   8693/3

Epidemiology
Thyroid paragangliomas are uncommon, accounting for approximately 0.5% of head and neck paragangliomas {2899}. There is a strong female predominance, and the mean patient age at presentation is 48 years.

Localization
Paraganglioma occurs adjacent to or inside the thyroid gland, probably arising from inferior laryngeal paraganglia.

Clinical features
Most patients present with an asymptomatic neck mass.

Macroscopy
Intrathyroidal paraganglioma is typically a circumscribed or encapsulated solitary nodule, grey to tan or brown in colour. The mean tumour size is 3 cm {1523}.

Microscopy
Microscopically, intrathyroid paragangliomas are similar to head and neck parasympathetic paragangliomas. There is a thin, fibrous capsule. Occasionally, thyroid follicles may be entrapped within the periphery of the nodule. Tumour cells are arranged in nesting (Zellballen) or trabecular architectural patterns, although a solid pattern of growth can be identified focally {424,2899,3078}. Lobules and nests are separated by fibrovascular connective tissue. The tumour cells are round, polyhedral, or spindle-shaped, with a moderate amount of granular, eosinophilic, and amphophilic cytoplasm. The nuclei are round to ovoid, with finely granular nuclear chromatin. Hyperchromatic nuclei and binucleated cells (so-called endocrine atypia) are occasionally seen, but do not correlate with malignant behaviour. Mitoses are uncommon. Sustentacular cells are present at the periphery of the nests or intermingled with chief cells.

The main differential diagnoses are medullary thyroid carcinoma, hyalinizing trabecular tumour, and metastatic neuroendocrine tumours. Medullary thyroid carcinoma is usually positive for cytokeratins, calcitonin, calcitonin gene–related peptide, TTF1, and CEA, and negative for enzymes involved in mitochondrial respiratory functions. Hyalinizing trabecular tumours are positive for thyroglobulin. Metastatic neuroendocrine tumours are usually positive for cytokeratins and show a prominent interstitial growth pattern, multiple tumour foci, and folliculotropism {1757}.

Immunophenotype
The tumour cells are positive for chromogranin A and synaptophysin, whereas staining for cytokeratin, calcitonin, calcitonin gene–related peptide, and TTF1 is usually negative. Sustentacular cells are positive for S100 {424}.

Cytology
Cytological aspirates contain single cells and loose clusters of large epithelioid, plasmacytoid to spindle-shaped cells, with ovoid to elongated nuclei, fine chromatin, focally discrete nucleoli, moderate anisocytosis, and anisonucleosis {568, 2730,2885,3103}. There is an occasional acinar pattern with nuclear overlapping, crush artefact, and naked nuclei.

Genetic profile
The genetic profile is similar to that of head and neck paragangliomas.

Genetic susceptibility
SDHA, *SDHB*, *SDHC*, and *SDHD* germline variants have been detected in some cases {568,2899,3091}. Heterozygous SNP and extragenic mutation in the nicotinamide *NNMT* gene at the *SDHD* (also known as *PGL1*) locus were identified in one case {568}.

Prognosis and predictive factors
The vast majority of thyroid paragangliomas have been cured by surgery, but a few tumours have been reported to metastasize {1030,1880}.

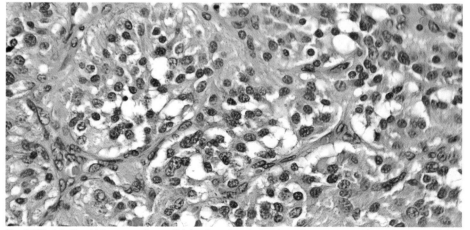

Fig. 2.123 Intrathyroidal paraganglioma. Chief cells and sustentacular cells are arranged in nests, surrounded by fibrovascular septa.

Peripheral nerve sheath tumours

Thompson L.D.R.
Chan J.K.C.
Volante M.

Definition
Thyroid gland peripheral nerve sheath tumours are benign or malignant neoplasms showing Schwann cell or perineurial differentiation, arising from peripheral nerves within the thyroid gland. The benign neoplasms are called schwannomas and the malignant neoplasms malignant peripheral nerve sheath tumours (MPNSTs).

ICD-O codes
Schwannoma   9560/0
Malignant peripheral nerve
  sheath tumour   9540/3

Synonyms
Neurilemmoma; malignant schwannoma; neurofibrosarcoma

Epidemiology
Primary thyroid gland peripheral nerve sheath tumours are rare, accounting for < 0.01% of all primary thyroid gland tumours {32,1308,2094,2765}. They can affect individuals of any age and show no sex predilection.

Etiology
There is no known etiology for thyroid gland peripheral nerve sheath tumours {2765}.

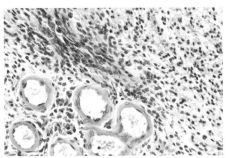

Fig. 2.125 Thyroid schwannoma. Perivascular hyalinization is noted in this schwannoma. There is a palisaded spindled cell population.

Localization
The tumours tend to develop from the medium to large nerves (sympathetic, parasympathetic, and sensory nerves) at the thyroid gland periphery {713,1009, 2765,2859}.

Clinical features
The presenting symptoms include a mass increasing in size (rapidly in MPNST), dyspnoea, and difficulty breathing, as well as weight loss in patients with MPNST. Symptoms are usually present for several months. Imaging studies show an inhomogeneous, low-density mass. Airway compression, destructive growth, and necrosis suggest malignancy {32,2672,2765}. Direct extension from neoplasms in the neck and metastatic MPNSTs to the thyroid gland must be excluded {92,126,468,3001}. Staging is not performed.

Macroscopy
The tumours can reach 7 cm in size; MPNSTs are usually larger than

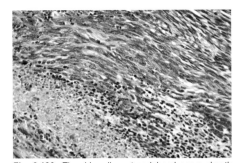

Fig. 2.126 Thyroid malignant peripheral nerve sheath tumour. Highly cellular spindle cell proliferation associated with necrosis.

schwannomas. Schwannomas are encapsulated, and the cut surface may show cystic foci. MPNSTs show infiltrative growth with effacement of thyroid parenchyma; the tumours are firm and tan, and may show necrosis {73,1308, 2082,2094,2765}.

Microscopy
Schwannomas show variable cellularity, with densely packed spindle-cell areas (Antoni A regions) and loosely arranged hypocellular myxoid-degenerated areas (Antoni B regions). The slender, fusiform cells have wavy, elongated cytoplasmic extensions and are arranged in interlacing fascicles within a variably hyalinized matrix. Nuclear palisading (Verocay bodies) may be present. The cells contain an elongated nucleus with dense chromatin. Mitoses are inconspicuous. Small to medium-sized blood vessels may show ectasia, hyalinization, or fibrinoid deposition {1308,2765}.
MPNSTs show infiltrative growth, often with tumour necrosis and haemorrhage.

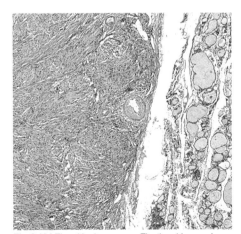

Fig. 2.124 Thyroid schwannoma. The thyroid parenchyma is noted at the periphery of this schwannoma. There is an interlacing spindled cell proliferation.

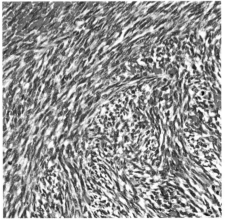

Fig. 2.127 Thyroid malignant peripheral nerve sheath tumour. The highly cellular interlacing fascicles create a herringbone pattern. Three mitoses are visible in this high-power field.

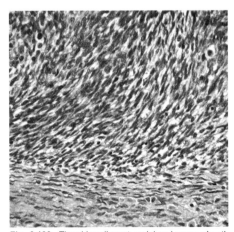

Fig. 2.128 Thyroid malignant peripheral nerve sheath tumour. A highly cellular spindled cell population is directly apposed to an area of lower cellularity.

The tumours are highly cellular, with the neoplastic cells arranged in tightly packed fascicles, often imparting a marbled appearance. Wavy cells with fibrillar cytoplasmic extensions are more common in areas that have a loose background. Cellular pleomorphism and mitotic figures, including atypical forms, are easily identified {32,713,2082,2765}. Rarely, malignant triton tumours (MPNSTs with rhabdomyoblastic differentiation) have been reported {286,1954}. A specific grading system for MPNSTs of the thyroid gland has not been proposed, but the general grading criteria include nuclear anaplasia, increased mitoses, and tumour necrosis {713,2765}.

The neoplastic cells are typically diffusely and strongly immunoreactive for S100 protein and SOX10, but negative for thyroglobulin, pancytokeratin, HMB45, and melan-A {32,79,1385,1839,2765}. S100 protein staining is often more patchy and less intense in MPNSTs. TTF1 staining may be seen in MPNSTs.

Genetic susceptibility
Peripheral nerve sheath tumours are increased in frequency in neurofibromatosis type 1, although neurofibromin gene mutations have not been documented in thyroid gland primary tumours.

Prognosis and predictive factors
Schwannomas have a benign course, whereas thyroid gland MPNSTs show a poor clinical outcome irrespective of clinical features or tumour size, grade, or stage {32,2765}; all patients with available follow-up have died from their disease {32,2765}.

Benign vascular tumours

Papotti M.
Rosai J.
Tsang W.Y.W.
Volante M.

Definition
Benign vascular tumours of the thyroid include haemangioma and lymphangioma.

ICD-O codes
Haemangioma	9120/0
Cavernous haemangioma	9121/0
Lymphangioma	9170/0

Synonyms
Angioma; cavernous haemangioma

Epidemiology
Haemangiomas are very rare, with only 19 cases, generally of the cavernous type, reported in the English-language literature. Lymphangiomas are exceedingly rare.

Etiology
It is uncertain whether haemangiomas are genuine neoplasms or congenital/acquired vascular malformations, because rare cases are preceded by fine-needle aspiration {2115,2300,2821}.

Localization
The localization is usually intrathyroidal.

Clinical features
Haemangiomas of the thyroid are usually incidental findings, although they may be suspected on ultrasonography, appearing as well-circumscribed, hypoechoic heterogeneous and hypovascular nodules with linear echogenic septal lines {1058,2115}. There is no sex predilection. The median patient age is 53 years (range: 0.2–84 years). Hemithyroidectomy appears to be the treatment of choice {614}.

Macroscopy
Haemangiomas are well-demarcated, haemorrhagic nodules with variable solid areas, especially in larger or longstanding tumours, due to fibrosis. The mean size is 6.1 cm, but so-called giant tumours, as large as 17 cm, have been reported {1572,1703}.

Microscopy
Fine-needle aspiration cytology is generally non-diagnostic. Histologically, thyroid haemangioma resembles its soft

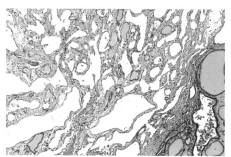

Fig. 2.129 Thyroid haemangioma. Ectatic vascular spaces are lined by flat endothelium and are well demarcated from the surrounding thyroid follicles.

tissue counterpart of the cavernous type: a circumscribed collection of blood-filled ectatic vascular spaces lined by flat or plump endothelial cells, with occasional atypia and papillary endothelial projections {2097,2115}. Variable degrees of fibrosis and calcification can be observed. The differential diagnoses include the extremely rare thyroid lymphangioma {1580}, papillary endothelial hyperplasia (also known as Masson tumour), and angiosarcoma (see the next section). Papillary endothelial hyperplasia, a mimic of various benign and malignant vascular neoplasms on imaging and microscopy, is a hyperplastic intravascular proliferation of endothelial cells arranged in papillae with fibrin cores. Rarely, it occurs in longstanding nodular goitre as part of the post-haemorrhagic reparative process {2097,2420}.

Angiosarcoma

Wick M.R.
Eusebi V.
Lamovec J.
Ryška A.

Definition
Thyroid angiosarcoma is a malignant primary thyroid tumour showing evidence of endothelial cell differentiation.

ICD-O code   9120/3

Synonyms
Malignant haemangioendothelioma; haemangiosarcoma

Epidemiology
Angiosarcomas of the thyroid were originally reported in patients who lived in the alpine countries of central Europe. Iodine

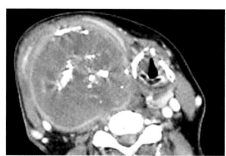

Fig. 2.130 Thyroid angiosarcoma. CT showing angiosarcoma in the right thyroid lobe, markedly displacing the trachea and other cervical structures.

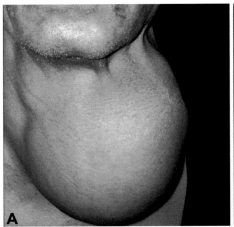

Fig. 2.131 Thyroid angiosarcoma. **A** This patient has marked thyromegaly. **B** The excision specimen shows effacement of the thyroid parenchyma by tumour tissue, which is haemorrhagic.

deficiency was identified as a potential cause. In Switzerland, they accounted for 4.3% of all thyroid neoplasms during the time period of 1962–1973 {1122}. This geographical restriction of thyroid angiosarcomas has since been challenged by reports of such tumours in flatlands and seaside regions. They have also been reported in Hong Kong SAR, China {453}; Singapore {1006}; the Republic of Korea {1365}; Spain {2059}; northern France {2213}; Portugal {1025}; Germany {1097}; Tunisia {2013}; the UK {198}, and the USA {801,1330}. In a review of thyroid lesions of patients living in non-mountainous areas of Italy between 1990 and 1994, angiosarcoma was found to account for 2.3% of all malignant neoplasms, excluding lymphomas {1718}. Thyroid angiosarcomas manifest as so-called cold nodules in elderly patients. The mean patient age is in the seventh decade of life

{1718,2097} and the female-to-male ratio is 4.5:1 {2097}. These lesions appear to develop most often in longstanding multinodular goitres. When the lesions are cystic, they can easily be misdiagnosed by fine-needle aspiration biopsy {1718}.

Etiology
Iodine deficiency has been suggested as a possible etiological factor {1066}.

Localization
Either thyroid lobe can be affected by the tumour.

Clinical features
With the exception of occasional cases that initially manifest with signs of metastasis, these tumours present with neck pain, pressure symptoms relating to encroachment on the trachea {1539}, or a rapidly growing but painless mass {2721}.

Macroscopy
Grossly, thyroid angiosarcomas often appear to be circumscribed, but they are nonetheless invariably invasive. The cut surface is variegated, with cystic and solid areas. Haemorrhage is usually present and the solid areas are often necrotic. The lesions are 3–10 cm in size {1718, 2721}. Occasional cases are extensively infiltrative, with growth into the trachea and surrounding soft tissues {801}.

Microscopy
Thyroid angiosarcomas are microscopically similar to angiosarcomas of deep soft tissues {861}. The solid areas of the lesions show extensive necrosis admixed with fibrosis and dense inflammation. Those changes may obscure the remaining viable neoplastic tissue, which tends to be present only peripherally. Anastomosing channels containing papillary fronds lined by endothelial cells are regularly found. Sheet-like cellular growth is also frequent, producing a histological appearance that overlaps with that of anaplastic (undifferentiated) carcinomas. Thyroid angiosarcomas frequently demonstrate epithelioid cytological features {801,2097}. The neoplastic cells have abundant eosinophilic cytoplasm, with round hyperchromatic or vesicular nuclei, well-defined nuclear membranes, and prominent eosinophilic nucleoli {801, 2366}. Occasional binucleated and multinucleated forms may be present. Numerous mitoses are usually seen.

Immunophenotype
Thyroid angiosarcomas have been reported to be immunoreactive for factor VIII–related antigen, Ulex europaeus lectin receptors, CD34, and CD31 {735, 1718,2162,2721}, and often for pankeratin {801,1034,1718}. Thyroglobulin was not detected by mRNA expression in situ hybridization in one assessment {2109}, nor has it been seen immunohistochemically. There is little information about possible immunoreactivity in thyroid angiosarcomas for adjunctive epithelial markers such as EMA, E-cadherin, p40, and p63 {595}. Similarly, there have been no systematic assessments of ERG or FLI1 proteins {1631,1830} as additional endothelial-selective determinants; of those, ERG appears to be the most reliable marker.

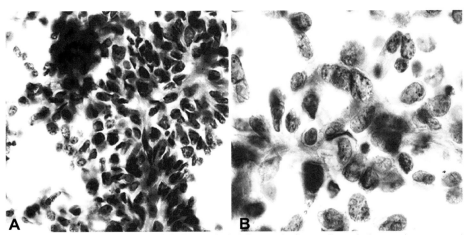

Fig. 2.132 Thyroid angiosarcoma. **A,B** The cytological features in fine-needle aspiration specimens are not diagnostically definitive. They include variable cohesion of the tumour cells, with moderate nuclear pleomorphism. Similar findings can be seen in other differential diagnostic entities.

Ultrastructure

Ultrastructurally, single, membrane-bound, internally striated, rod-shaped cytoplasmic structures, compatible with Weibel–Palade bodies, have been identified {801,1718,2721} in thyroid angiosarcomas. Intercellular or intracytoplasmic lumina may also be seen, together with numerous cytoplasmic intermediate filaments and intercellular junctional complexes {61,1704,2366}.

Cytology

Fine-needle aspiration biopsy preparations of thyroid angiosarcoma usually demonstrate abundant necrotic material and haemorrhage. In that background, variably cohesive large neoplastic cells can be seen that have abundant amphophilic cytoplasm, round central nuclei with coarse chromatin, and nucleoli {1222, 1625,1694}. The cytological appearance is not diagnostically definitive {1300}; it can be imitated by primary anaplastic thyroid carcinoma, metastases of other carcinomas, and metastatic melanoma.

Differential diagnosis

The differential diagnosis of angiosarcoma in this location includes primary angiomatoid anaplastic carcinoma {1540, 1847,2013,2097,2305} and angiomatoid medullary carcinoma {2104} of the thyroid, metastatic melanoma with angiomatoid features {151,3097}, and metastatic angiomatoid carcinoma of the lung and other locations {150}. Other considerations are intrathyroidal haemangiomas (which are typically cytologically bland and evolve slowly {1494,2300}) and endothelial hyperplasia, which may appear in nodular goitres that have undergone degenerative changes {2420}. A peculiar angioproliferative lesion may appear in the thyroid after fine-needle aspiration biopsy; this lesion has been termed "worrisome alterations following fine-needle aspiration of the thyroid" {1651}. It features intraglandular fibrosis and nuclear atypia in regenerating thyroid epithelial cells.

Histogenesis

For more than three decades, there has been debate over the lineage(s) of differentiation pertaining to thyroid angiosarcoma {1066}, and two main postulates have emerged. The first is that angiosarcoma of the thyroid is a singular and distinct entity that is basically pathologically

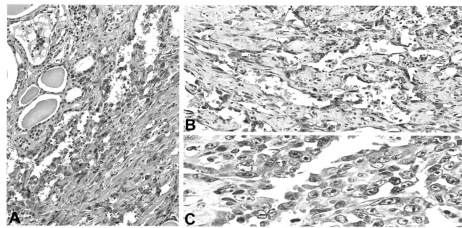

Fig. 2.133 Thyroid angiosarcoma. This composite image shows (**A**) the relationship of the neoplasm to remaining thyroid tissue, as well as (**B,C**) the formation of interanastomosing vascular channels that are lined by epithelioid tumour cells.

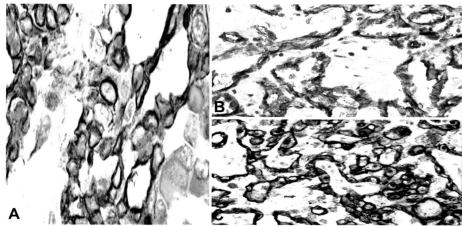

Fig. 2.134 Thyroid angiosarcoma. There is immunoreactivity for pankeratin (**A**); CD31 (**B**); and CD34 (**C**).

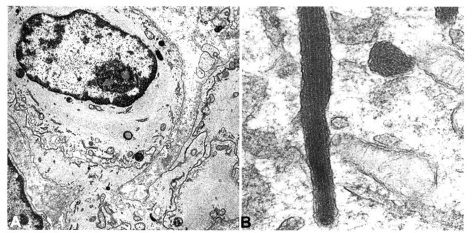

Fig. 2.135 Thyroid angiosarcoma. These electron micrographs show numerous cytoplasmic intermediate filaments and intercellular junctional complexes (**A**), as well as Weibel–Palade bodies (**B**).

comparable to angiosarcoma of the deep soft tissues, and that it has no relationship whatsoever to anaplastic thyroid carcinomas {801,2059,2366,2805}. Reports of cases that support this hypothesis have

described tumours that lack all epithelial markers on immunohistochemistry and molecular analysis, and instead demonstrate reactivity for endothelial determinants or show the ultrastructural phenotype of a pure endothelial proliferation {2097,2109}. Alternatively, other authors have suggested that thyroid angiosarcoma is in fact merely a variant of anaplastic carcinoma in that gland {1847, 1848,2097,2897}. Currently, there seems to be no concrete means of resolving this conceptual issue.

Prognosis and predictive factors

Most patients with thyroid angiosarcoma die from their tumours in < 6 months {740, 1521}, regardless of treatment modality, with very few surviving as long as 5 years {801,1521,1539,1718}. Lesions that are confined by the thyroid capsule may have a somewhat better prognosis than those with extraglandular extension.

Smooth muscle tumours

Thompson L. D. R.
Kim N. R.

Definition

Thyroid leiomyoma (benign) and leiomyosarcoma (malignant) are tumours showing smooth muscle differentiation arising from thyroid gland vascular smooth muscle.

ICD-O codes

Leiomyoma	8890/0
Leiomyosarcoma	8890/3

Epidemiology

Leiomyosarcoma, which is more common than leiomyoma {247,789,2766}, accounts for < 0.01% of all primary thyroid gland tumours {67,550,2766}. Leiomyosarcoma is the second most common primary thyroid sarcoma (after angiosarcoma), accounting for about 11% of cases {2681}. Leiomyoma develops in young to middle-aged patients; leiomyosarcoma develops primarily in older patients, with a female predominance.

Etiology

An association with EBV was reported in a patient with congenital immunodeficiency disease {2829}.

Localization

There is a peripheral predilection, where larger smooth muscle–walled vessels are identified {1331,2766}.

Clinical features

Non-specific symptoms, including a mass (usually increasing in size in leiomyosarcoma), may be associated with dyspnoea and/or stridor. Imaging studies reveal the location, size, and extent of the

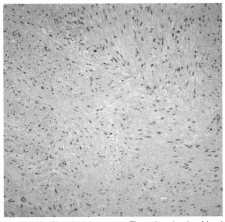

Fig. 2.136 Thyroid leiomyoma. There is a benign bland spindle cell proliferation showing a fascicular arrangement.

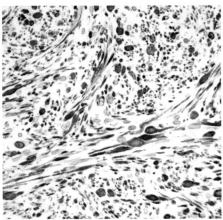

Fig. 2.137 Thyroid leiomyoma. There is a strong and diffuse cytoplasmic reaction with desmin in this example.

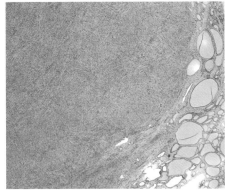

Fig. 2.138 Thyroid leiomyosarcoma. A highly cellular, malignant spindle cell tumour has destroyed much of the thyroid parenchyma. This fascicular-patterned tumour represents a primary leiomyosarcoma.

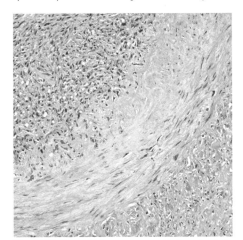

Fig. 2.139 Thyroid leiomyosarcoma. Malignant spindle cell neoplasm arising from the vessel wall. It is common to see a vascular origin for smooth muscle tumours.

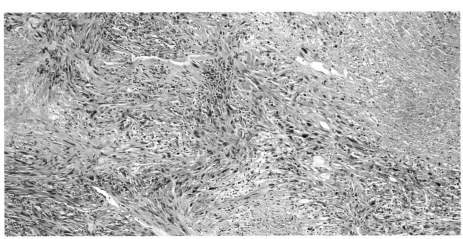

Fig. 2.140 Thyroid leiomyosarcoma. Atypical spindle cell proliferation arranged in irregular fascicles with easily identified tumour necrosis and pleomorphism.

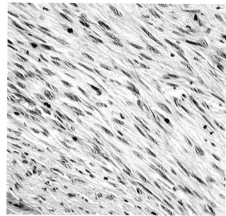

Fig. 2.141 Thyroid leiomyosarcoma. There are many mitoses in the atypical spindle cell population of this example.

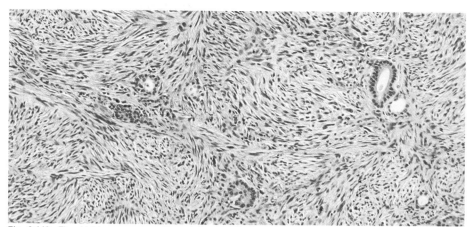

Fig. 2.142 Thyroid leiomyosarcoma. Several thyroid follicular epithelial cells are entrapped within this atypical, fascicular spindled cell tumour.

tumour. Tracheal compression, infiltrative extension beyond the thyroid, and necrosis suggest malignancy {2681,2698, 2766}. Staging is not performed.

Macroscopy
Leiomyosarcomas are typically larger than leiomyomas, with average sizes of 6 cm and 2 cm, respectively {67,247, 550,2766}, but these tumours can reach 12 cm in size. Leiomyomas have a well-defined border, whereas leiomyosarcomas tend to be widely infiltrative.

Microscopy
The tumour cells are arranged in bundles or fascicles of smooth muscle fibres, often intersecting. The tumour cells are spindled, with centrally located, blunt-ended, cigar-shaped, slightly hyperchromatic nuclei adjacent to perinuclear cytoplasmic vacuoles. Entrapped thyroid follicles, capsular and/or vascular invasion, and necrosis are commonly seen in leiomyosarcoma. Leiomyosarcomas show high cellularity, pleomorphism, and increased mitotic activity (> 5 mitoses per 10 high-power fields), including atypical forms {550,739,1283,2719,2766}. Direct extension from neoplasms in the neck and metastatic leiomyosarcoma (uterine, gastrointestinal, or soft tissue) must be excluded {664,763,1566,3004}.

Immunophenotype
The neoplastic cells are immunoreactive for alpha-SMA, MSA, SMA, caldesmon, calponin, desmin, and vimentin. MYOD1 and myogenin may be focally reactive. Thyroglobulin, pancytokeratin, S100 protein, SOX10, and calcitonin are negative {480,1331,2766}. Undifferentiated

carcinoma (more common) and rare malignant glomus tumour {518} should be excluded. Grading of leiomyosarcoma of the thyroid gland is not performed, but general grading criteria would include nuclear anaplasia, increased mitoses, and necrosis.

Prognosis and predictive factors
Leiomyomas are benign, whereas leiomyosarcomas are associated with a poor outcome {67,550,2719,2766}.

Solitary fibrous tumour

Sobrinho Simões M.
Cameselle Teijeiro J. M.
Matias-Guiu X.
Rosai J.

Definition
Solitary fibrous tumour of the thyroid is a mesenchymal neoplasm indistinguishable from pleural or other extrapleural solitary fibrous tumours.

ICD-O code   8815/1

Synonyms
Fibroma; fibrosarcoma (neither is recommended)
Cases reported in the past as haemangiopericytoma of the thyroid are probably in fact solitary fibrous tumours.

Epidemiology
Solitary fibrous tumour of the thyroid is a rare neoplasm observed in middle-aged men and women; the median patient age is 56 years (range: 28–88 years) {62,

1872,2316,2690}. Solitary fibrous tumour is probably the most frequent spindle cell mesenchymal tumour of the thyroid.

Etiology
The etiology is unknown. Solitary fibrous tumour is not associated with a long-standing pre-existing goitre or thyroid tumour. It has been speculated that the solitary fibrous tumour precursor cell may be a vimentin-positive, CD34-positive primitive mesenchymal cell capable of fibroblastic, myofibroblastic, adipose, and/or haemangiopericytic differentiation {2690}.

Clinical features
Most patients are clinically euthyroid and present with a slow-growing mass that is scintigraphically cold, solid, and usually well circumscribed on ultrasonography {373,1872,2316,2690}. Compressive symptoms and (rarely) respiratory failure can occur {1553,1624,2857}.

Macroscopy
Most tumours present as a well-circumscribed, usually unencapsulated mass measuring 1.5–13.8 cm (median: 5 cm)

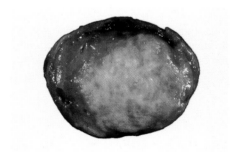

Fig. 2.143 Thyroid solitary fibrous tumour. A fairly well-demarcated, unencapsulated tumour.

{62,123,340,2095}. On cut section, they have a firm, solid appearance; cystic changes are rarely observed {1354,1872, 2716}.

Microscopy

Solitary fibrous tumours display a variegated, wavy, storiform, haemangiopericytic, or desmoid-like arrangement of spindle cells. The neoplastic cells may infiltrate the thyroid parenchyma. Solitary fibrous tumours characteristically have alternation of hypocellular areas (keloid-like collagen) and hypercellular areas, as well as branching haemangiopericytoma-like vessels {373,668,2316,2614}. Myxoid change and interstitial chronic inflammatory cells (mainly mast cells) can be seen. The tumour cells have scant cytoplasm with indistinct borders. Nuclear atypia is rare {1999}. Only very few cases show mitotic figures {62,1999}. Some thyroid solitary fibrous tumours, usually those with a prominent haemangiopericytic growth pattern, contain scattered lipomatous areas with a lobular or cord-like pattern, poorly delimited from the surrounding proliferative spindle cells {368,2690}.

The differential diagnosis includes all spindle cell mesenchymal tumours, post–fine-needle aspiration spindle cell nodules, follicular adenoma and adenomatous goitre with spindle cell features, Riedel thyroiditis, medullary carcinoma, spindle epithelial tumour with thymus-like differentiation, and anaplastic carcinoma of the paucicellular variant.

Immunophenotype

Solitary fibrous tumours are characteristically immunoreactive for CD34, CD99, BCL2, vimentin, and STAT6. They are negative for thyroid markers (TTF1, thyroglobulin, and calcitonin), cytokeratins, desmin, CD31, KIT (also known as CD117), and S100 protein {662,2416, 2716,2863}. Positivity for factor XIIIa, progesterone receptors, and estrogen receptors has been detected in solitary fibrous tumours with a haemangiopericytoma-like pattern and adipocytes {368};

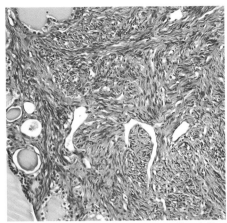

Fig. 2.144 Thyroid solitary fibrous tumour with an infiltrative growth pattern.

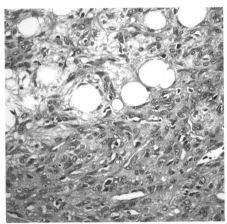

Fig. 2.146 Thyroid solitary fibrous tumour with scattered adipocytes.

there is immunoreactivity for S100 protein in the lipomatous foci {368}.

Cytology

In most cases on record, the correct diagnosis could not be achieved on fine-needle aspiration biopsy, probably due to the frequent occurrence of non-diagnostic samples and features of atypia of undetermined significance or follicular lesions of undetermined significance {829, 1999,2095,2123}.

Genetic profile

The recurring chromosomal abnormalities detected in solitary fibrous tumours of other sites have not been studied in

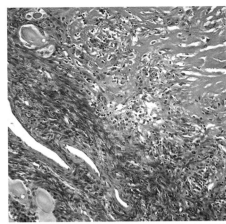

Fig. 2.145 Thyroid solitary fibrous tumour with a hypocellular area displaying keloid-like collagen.

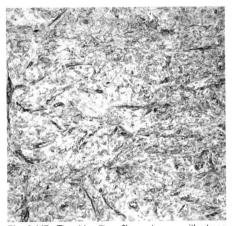

Fig. 2.147 Thyroid solitary fibrous tumour with strong immunoreactivity for CD34.

thyroid solitary fibrous tumours {1160}. This is likely a reflection of the limited number of cases on record, and apparently has no clinical relevance.

Prognosis and predictive factors

Almost all thyroid solitary fibrous tumours display benign clinical behaviour, despite the frequent neoplastic cell infiltration of the adjacent thyroid tissue {273}. The single case on record that manifested unequivocal signs of malignant behaviour had prominent histopathological features of malignancy (numerous mitoses and marked cellular atypia) {1999}.

Haematolymphoid tumours

Langerhans cell histiocytosis

Chan J. K. C.   Thompson L. D. R.
Burke J. S.   Weiss L. M.
Ferry J. A.   Wotherspoon A.
Rosai J.

Definition
Langerhans cell histiocytosis is a clonal proliferation of Langerhans dendritic cells.

ICD-O code   9751/3

Epidemiology
Cases limited to the thyroid are exceedingly rare {759,1664,2767,3032}. Most cases occur in patients with multifocal disease, who tend to be younger. Both sexes are affected.

Etiology
The discovery of frequent *BRAF* and *MAP2K1* mutations in Langerhans cell histiocytosis suggests that it is a neoplastic process of myeloid origin {125,336, 443,661}. Moreover, a subset of cases show antigen receptor gene rearrangements {472}, and cases of synchronous Langerhans cell histiocytosis and acute leukaemias of ambiguous or myeloid lineage have been reported, indicating a possible clonal relationship {3069}. However, the disorder shares features with

other IL17A-related inflammatory diseases {661}, and elevated levels of Merkel cell polyomavirus DNA sequences have been discovered in the peripheral blood and tissues of patients with Langerhans cell histiocytosis, suggesting an inflammatory process in which the Merkel cell polyomavirus infection triggers an IL1 activation loop {1929,1930}. Therefore, despite the neoplastic characteristics, inflammation probably supplements the pathogenesis, and Langerhans cell histiocytosis could be interpreted as a form of inflammatory myeloid neoplasia {57, 228}.

Localization
Thyroid gland involvement can be diffuse or focal, and is accompanied by other sites of involvement in patients with multifocal disease.

Clinical features
Patients typically present with diffuse or localized goitre or an isolated thyroid nodule {2767}, but some are incidentally found to have Langerhans cell histiocytosis in surgical specimens of the thyroid {2823}. Thyroid hormone status is variable: 41% of patients are euthyroid and as many as 20% are hypothyroid. Some cases are associated with Hashimoto thyroiditis, with antithyroglobulin or antimicrosomal antibodies detected in some {2127}.

Microscopy
Microscopic examination reveals a nodular or diffuse proliferation of sheets and groups of round to oval pale cells with deeply grooved or contorted nuclei, delicate chromatin, and moderate amounts of lightly eosinophilic cytoplasm. There are often admixed eosinophils, lymphocytes, and occasional multinucleated giant cells. Infiltration of thyroid follicular epithelium and destruction of thyroid follicles are common. The background commonly shows chronic lymphocytic thyroiditis {661,1745,2127,2767}.

The lesional cells are positive for S100 protein, CD1a, CD207 (also called langerin), and CD68 {661,949,1745,2127}. A subset of cases are immunopositive for V600E-mutated BRAF {2313}.

There have been rare reports of papillary thyroid carcinoma and Langerhans cell histiocytosis synchronously or metachronously affecting the thyroid {1908,2767, 2866,3021}. Both neoplasms may be associated with *BRAF* mutations {1908}, suggesting a common underlying genetic defect.

Genetic profile
Recurrent *BRAF* V600E mutations occur in about half of all cases of Langerhans cell histiocytosis {125}. Mutations in *MAP2K1* are identified in one third to half of the *BRAF*-negative cases {336,443}.

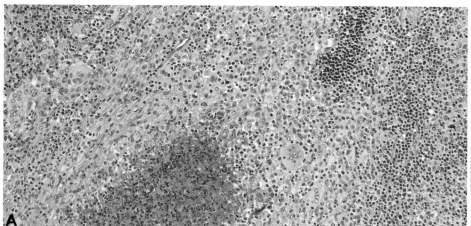
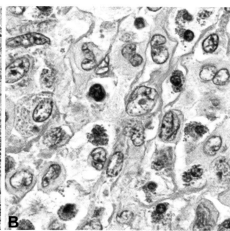

Fig. 2.148 Langerhans cell histiocytosis involving the thyroid. **A** The thyroid shows infiltration by sheets of Langerhans cells. There are many admixed eosinophils, with formation of an eosinophil abscess. **B** The Langerhans cells have deeply grooved nuclei and a moderate amount of pale cytoplasm. Eosinophils are admixed.

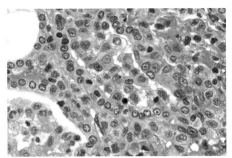

Fig. 2.149 Langerhans cell histiocytosis involving the thyroid. The Langerhans cells infiltrate between and into the thyroid follicles.

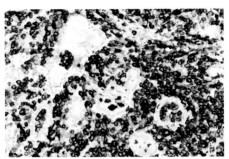

Fig. 2.150 Langerhans cell histiocytosis involving the thyroid. Typical positive immunostaining for CD207 (also called langerin).

Mutations in other genes in the MAPK pathway (*ARAF* and *MAP3K1*) or other signalling pathways (*PIK3CA*) have also been rarely described {1134,1965,1966}.

Prognosis and predictive factors

Cases with thyroid involvement associated with systemic disease have an aggressive course, whereas those with isolated thyroid involvement do not show progression after surgery {2767}.

Rosai–Dorfman disease

Chan J. K. C.
Facchetti F
Rosai J.
Thompson L. D. R.

Definition

Rosai–Dorfman disease is a reactive condition characterized by the proliferation of distinctive histiocytes commonly exhibiting emperipolesis.

Synonym

Sinus histiocytosis with massive lymphadenopathy

Epidemiology

Involvement of the thyroid by Rosai–Dorfman disease is very rare, and is usually accompanied by involvement of cervical lymph nodes {1571,1921,2191, 2908}. In the cases reported to date, the patients were females with a mean age of 48 years; this is in contrast to typical Rosai–Dorfman disease, which is usually seen in young males. The background thyroid often shows chronic lymphocytic thyroiditis.

Clinical features

Patients present with a thyroid mass, which may be rapidly enlarging, clinically mimicking malignancy.

Microscopy

The thyroid shows infiltration by loose aggregates of very large histiocytes with round vesicular nuclei, distinct nucleoli, and voluminous pale-staining cytoplasm. Some histiocytes exhibit emperipolesis of lymphocytes and plasma cells. There are always many admixed plasma cells. The histiocytes are immunoreactive for S100 protein and negative for CD1a.

Prognosis and predictive factors

All patients have remained well after treatment.

Follicular dendritic cell sarcoma

Chan J. K. C.
Rosai J.
Thompson L. D. R.

Definition

Follicular dendritic cell sarcoma is a neoplasm showing morphological and immunophenotypical features of follicular dendritic cells.

ICD-O code　　　　　　　9758/3

Epidemiology

Few cases of primary thyroid follicular dendritic cell sarcoma have been reported, all in adult women {918,2633,3080}. The background thyroid often shows chronic lymphocytic thyroiditis.

Clinical features

Patients present with a painless thyroid mass, often with cervical lymph node metastasis.

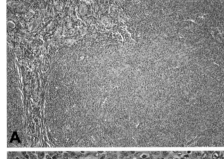

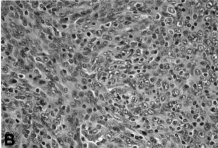

Fig. 2.152 Follicular dendritic cell sarcoma of the thyroid. A The thyroid gland is infiltrated by a tumour consisting of plump spindled cells, with a storiform to whorled growth pattern. B The spindled tumour cells show indistinct cell borders, vesicular nuclei, and distinct nucleoli. There are typically admixed small lymphocytes.

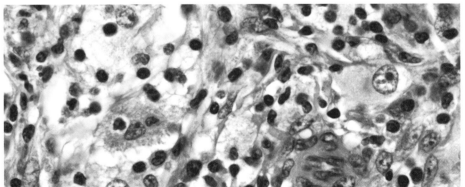

Fig. 2.151 Rosai–Dorfman disease involving the thyroid. The distinctive histiocytes are very large; they have vesicular round nuclei with distinct nucleoli and abundant pale-staining cytoplasm. Some contain lymphocytes or plasma cells in the cytoplasm.

Microscopy

The tumour consists of syncytial-appearing spindled to oval cells, exhibiting storiform, fascicular, or whorled patterns. The nuclei are often vesicular, with distinct nucleoli. There are variable numbers of admixed small lymphocytes. The lesional cells are immunoreactive for follicular dendritic cell markers (i.e. CD21, CD35, CD23, and CXCL13) and negative for cytokeratin.

Genetic profile

Clonal immunoglobulin gene rearrangements {3080} and mutations in *PTEN*, *RET*, and *TP53* {2633} have been reported.

Prognosis and predictive factors

A pooled analysis of the literature shows local recurrence and distant metastasis rates of 28% and 27%, respectively {2439A}.

Primary thyroid lymphoma

Chan J.K.C.
Burke J.S.
Ferry J.A.
Wotherspoon A.

Definition

Primary thyroid lymphoma is a malignant lymphoma originating in the thyroid gland.

Epidemiology

Primary lymphomas of the thyroid are rare. They account for as many as 5% of all thyroid malignancies and approximately 2% of extranodal lymphomas {86, 2135}. The female-to-male ratio is 3–4:1, and the mean patient age is 65 years {65, 2747,2954}.

Etiology

Thyroid lymphomas are almost always associated with chronic lymphocytic (Hashimoto) thyroiditis {500,619,666, 1202,2135}. Patients with chronic lymphocytic thyroiditis have a significantly increased risk of developing thyroid lymphoma; for example, the risk among Japanese patients with chronic lymphocytic thyroiditis is 80 times the risk in the general Japanese population {1158,1323, 2954}. Sequence similarity is reported in the clonal bands of chronic lymphocytic

thyroiditis and the ensuing thyroid lymphoma {1910}. Thyroid lymphomas often exhibit common homologous germline VH genes used by antithyroid antibodies, further implicating derivation from chronic lymphocytic thyroiditis {2345,2433}.

Localization

Lymphoma involves the thyroid, sometimes the cervical lymph nodes, and infrequently more-distant sites {65,666, 1094,2581,2954}.

Clinical features

Patients nearly always present with a mass in the thyroid, with or without cervical lymphadenopathy. Rapid enlargement of the mass, hoarseness, dyspnoea, and increased serum lactate dehydrogenase are more common with aggressive lymphomas than with low-grade cases. Constitutional symptoms are rare {65, 500,666,1094,2581,2954}.

Microscopy

Diffuse large B-cell lymphoma (DLBCL) is most common, followed by extranodal marginal zone B-cell lymphoma of mucosa-associated lymphoid tissue (MALT lymphoma) and follicular lymphoma {124}. Some DLBCLs constitute large cell transformation of MALT lymphoma {65,666,2581,2954}. Other rare types include T-cell lymphomas {65,466,1110, 2954}, Burkitt lymphoma {39}, gamma heavy chain disease {2711}, and classic Hodgkin lymphoma {2938}.

DLBCL shows obliteration of thyroid tissue by large cells, with distinct nucleoli and amphophilic cytoplasm. Most show a germinal-centre B-cell immunophenotype {1986,2954}.

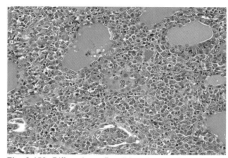

Fig. 2.153 Diffuse large B-cell lymphoma of the thyroid. The thyroid gland shows destructive infiltration by large lymphoma cells. There is also infiltration into the thyroid follicular epithelium and lumen.

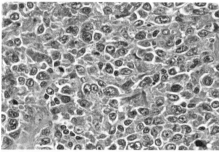

Fig. 2.154 Diffuse large B-cell lymphoma of the thyroid. The large lymphoma cells show vesicular nuclei and prominent nucleoli.

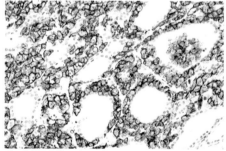

Fig. 2.155 Diffuse large B-cell lymphoma of the thyroid. The lymphoma cells show positive immunostaining for CD20. Infiltration of the thyroid follicular epithelium by the large lymphoma cells is also obvious.

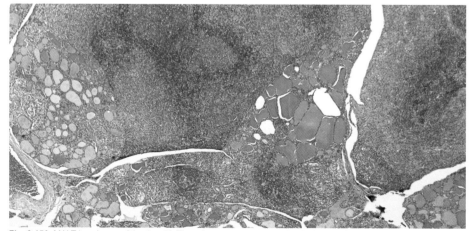

Fig. 2.156 MALT lymphoma of the thyroid. There is a monotonous lymphoid infiltrate effacing the thyroid parenchyma, interspersed with reactive lymphoid follicles.

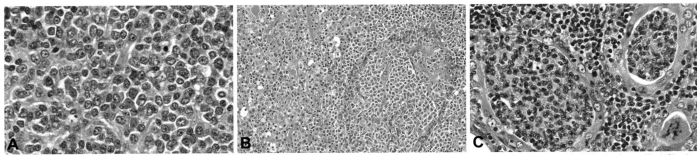

Fig. 2.157 MALT lymphoma of the thyroid. **A** The lymphoma cells are small to medium-sized, and some have plasmacytic features. **B** A lymphoepithelial lesion formed by infiltration and expansion of the thyroid follicle by lymphoma cells. **C** A distinctive so-called MALT-ball lymphoepithelial lesion, characterized by an expansile ball-like aggregate of lymphoma cells plugging the thyroid follicular lumen.

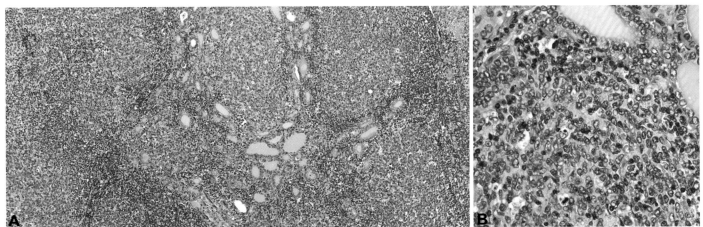

Fig. 2.158 Follicular lymphoma of the thyroid. **A** Abnormal (neoplastic) follicles are present among thyroid follicles. **B** The neoplastic follicles lack mantles and tingible body macrophages. In this example, they show predominance of centrocytes.

MALT lymphoma is characterized by a diffuse infiltrate of small lymphoid cells, centrocyte-like cells, monocytoid cells, and plasma cells, often with interspersed reactive lymphoid follicles. Neoplastic cells tend to invade and expand thyroid follicles, forming lymphoepithelial lesions or occupying their lumina {666,2014, 2954}. This form of lymphoma is positive for CD20; variably positive for cytoplasmic immunoglobulin; and negative for CD5, CD10, and BCL6.

Follicular lymphoma is characterized by extensive lymphoid infiltration and formation of neoplastic follicles, often with a prominent interfollicular component. Lymphoepithelial lesions are common {124}. One group is similar to classic nodal follicular lymphoma, usually with high-stage (stage II–IV) disease, histological grade 1 or 2, CD10 and BCL2 immunopositivity, and BCL2 rearrangement. The other group is similar to extranodal BCL2-negative follicular lymphoma, usually with early-stage (stage I) disease, histological grade 3, variable CD10 staining, BCL2 negativity, and germline BCL2.

Genetic profile

Translocation t(3;14)(p14;q32) with FOXP1-IGH fusion is found in about half of all cases of thyroid MALT lymphoma, whereas other chromosomal translocations characteristic of MALT lymphoma are rarely found {2661,2662}. DLBCLs show genetic features similar to those of their nodal and other extranodal counterparts, with some cases exhibiting translocation involving BCL6 or MYC, or 17p11 alterations {1986}.

Prognosis and predictive factors

Patients with localized thyroid lymphoma have a favourable prognosis, with a median overall survival of 9.3 years and a 5-year disease-specific survival rate of 79%. The lymphoma type also influences survival, with a 5-year disease-specific survival rate of 89–100% for MALT lymphoma, compared with 75% for DLBCL {1028,2755}.

Poor prognostic indicators include poor performance status, high stage, bulky tumour, advanced patient age, extracapsular extension, and vascular invasion {666,1833}.

Germer cell tumours

Furtado L. V.
Thompson L. D. R.

Definition
Germ cell tumours of the thyroid gland are tumours composed of mature or immature tissues derived from all three germ cell layers (i.e. the ectoderm, mesoderm, and endoderm) involving the thyroid gland {1369,2763}.

ICD-O codes
Benign teratoma
    (grade 0 or 1)   9080/0
Immature teratoma (grade 2)   9080/1
Malignant teratoma (grade 3)   9080/3

Epidemiology
Teratomas account for < 0.1% of all thyroid gland primary neoplasms, with about 340 teratoma cases reported in the literature. The patients range from newborn to 85 years of age at initial presentation, but most cases present in newborns, and the mean patient age is < 10 years. The sex distribution is equal overall, but malignant teratomas show a slight male predilection.

Localization
By definition, primary thyroid teratoma involves, is in direct continuity with, or completely replaces the thyroid gland. Thyroid gland tissue may be seen in a teratoma, but a thyroid teratoma has thyroid follicular epithelial cells at the periphery of the tumour {2763,2973}.

Clinical features
Patients present with a neck mass, often of considerable size. Radiographical images usually reveal a multicystic mass, often containing fat and sometimes compressing the upper airway or resulting in neck distortion. Enlarged, peripherally enhancing lymph nodes in the neck suggest malignant teratoma {465,1355,2763, 2837}. Benign (mature or immature) teratoma may cause compression atrophy or maldevelopment of neck organs. Local recurrence with metastatic disease to the regional lymph nodes, followed by metastatic disease to the lungs, is frequently seen in malignant cases {52,298,686, 2763}.

Macroscopy
The tumours can reach 13 cm in greatest dimension, but on average are about 6 cm {52,2763}. The tumour surface is smooth to bosselated or lobulated, firm to soft and cystic, and greyish-tan or yellowish-white to translucent. The cut surface is usually multiloculated, with the cystic spaces containing whitish-tan creamy material, mucoid glairy material, or haemorrhagic fluid with necrotic debris. Material resembling brain tissue is frequently noted. Islands of gritty material consistent with bone and cartilage may be seen.

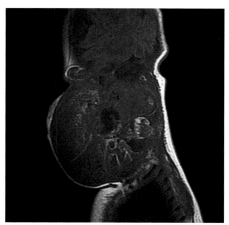

Fig. 2.159 Thyroid teratoma. Sagittal T1-weighted MRI shows a large neoplasm with a lobulated surface in the anterior neck, replacing the thyroid.

Microscopy
All germ cell tumours contain mature or immature tissues from all three embryonic germ cell layers: the ectoderm, mesoderm, and endoderm {2763}. On the basis of the interrelationship of these constituents and the proportions of each element, the tumours are categorized into mature, immature, and malignant types. For a mass to qualify as a thyroid teratoma, thyroid parenchyma should be identified within it, although residual thyroid follicles may be scarce or absent in malignant teratoma. A variety of epithelium types may be seen, including

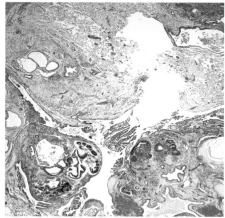

Fig. 2.160 Thyroid teratoma. All germ cell layers are represented in this benign immature teratoma showing primitive neuroepithelium and retinal anlage.

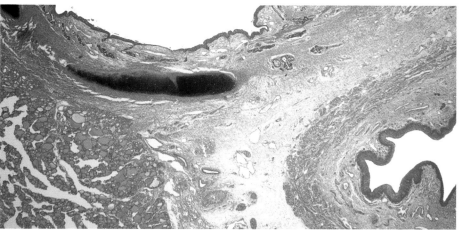

Fig. 2.161 Thyroid teratoma. In this benign teratoma, thyroid follicles are identified at the periphery of the tumour (lower-left corner) alongside a recapitulation of trachea and oesophagus.

squamous, pseudostratified ciliated columnar, cuboidal (with and without goblet cells), glandular, and transitional. Pilosebaceous and adnexal structures may be seen in association with squamous epithelium. True organ (pancreas, liver, or lung) differentiation is uncommon. Nearly all cases contain neural tissue (ectodermal derivation), consisting of mature glial elements, choroid plexus, pigmented retinal anlage, or immature neuroblastemal elements. The neuroblastemal elements are composed of small to medium-sized cells with dense hyperchromatic nuclei accompanied by mitoses, arranged in sheets or rosette-like structures (Flexner–Wintersteiner rosettes). The maturation of the neural-type tissue determines the grade: completely mature tissue defines grade 0; predominantly mature tissue, grades 1 and 2; and exclusively immature tissue, grade 3 or malignant tumour. Cartilage, bone, striated skeletal muscle, smooth muscle, adipose tissue, and loose myxoid to fibrous embryonic mesenchymal connective tissue are seen

intermixed with the neural and epithelial elements {52,578,686,2763}.

Immunoreactivity for epithelial, mesenchymal, and neural markers is seen in the corresponding tissue types, but may be helpful in immature or malignant cases. Reactivity for S100 protein,

GFAP, neuron-specific enolase, and NFP helps identify immature glial constituents. MYOD1 and myogenin reactivity highlights early skeletal muscle differentiation {1251,1567,2763,2906}.

Table 2.13 Partial literature summary (> 3 cases reported per article) {52,136,176,230,586,2763,2906}

	Histology			
	All	**Mature**	**Immature**	**Malignant**
Cases analysed[a] (n)	109	62	29	18
Sex (n)				
Female	58	30	17	12
Male	44	27	11	6
Average patient age at presentation; range	9.8 years; (newborn to 85.0 years)	6.3 years; (newborn to 72.0 years)	Newborn; (newborn to 6.0 years)	31.2 years; (newborn to 85.0 years)
Patient age groups (n)				
Neonates and infants	80	47	28	5
Children and adults	29	15	1	13
Average tumour size	6.5 cm	5.9 cm	6.2 cm	8.7 cm

[a] The number of cases analysed was not stated in all reports; therefore, the numbers in this row do not necessarily equal the sum of the values in the corresponding columns.

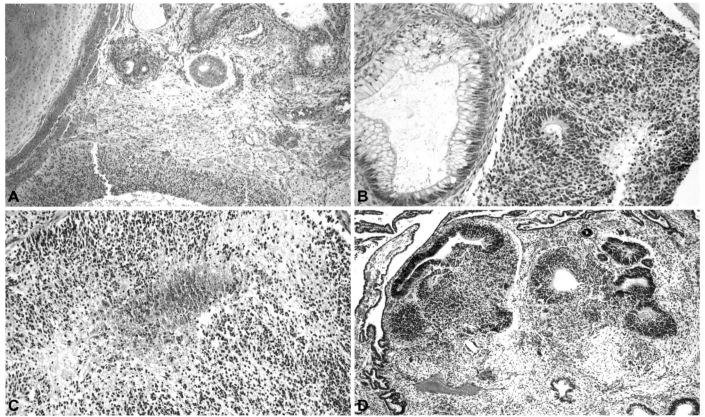

Fig. 2.162 Thyroid teratoma. **A** Benign teratoma with mature cartilage, smooth muscle, and glands interspersed in myxoid connective tissue. **B** Benign immature teratoma (grade 2) with immature neuroepithelium arranged in Flexner–Wintersteiner rosettes. **C** Malignant teratoma (grade 3) showing immature neuroectodermal tissue with areas of central comedonecrosis. **D** This immature teratoma shows foci of immature, embryonic-type neuroepithelial tubules adjacent to glands and loose myxoid stroma.

Grading

Benign, immature, and malignant teratomas are recognized based on the presence of immature neuroectodermal tissues. Grade 0 is defined as a benign tumour with only mature elements. Grade 1 identifies a benign tumour with limited immaturity, defined as embryonal-type tissue in only one low-power (40× magnification) microscopic field. Grade 2 identifies a benign tumour with 2–4 low-power fields of immature foci. Grade 3 (malignant tumours) contain > 4 low-power fields of immature tissue, along with mitoses and cellular atypia. By definition, the presence of embryonal carcinoma or yolk sac tumour places a teratoma in the malignant category (grade 3) {910}.

Prognosis and predictive factors

The outcome is dependent on patient age, tumour size, and degree of tissue immaturity. Neonates and infants show a preponderance of benign teratomas (grade 0–2); whereas children and adults show a preponderance of malignant teratomas (grade 3). Grade 0–2 tumours can cause death due to tracheal compression or a lack of development of vital structures in the neck during fetal growth. Consequently, surgery should be performed promptly, including in utero when necessary, due to considerable preoperative mortality rates. About 30% of patients with grade 3 tumours die due to tumour recurrence or metastasis {1448, 2558,2763}. Tumours > 5 cm in size are associated with a shorter median survival irrespective of the histology {1344,2763, 2822,2837}.

Secondary tumours

Fadda G.
DeLellis R. A.
Sadow P.

Definition
Secondary tumours of the thyroid gland are tumours that arise in the thyroid gland by direct extension from adjacent structures or by vascular spread from non-thyroidal sites.

Epidemiology
Likely due to advanced stage, the thyroid is identified as a site for metastasis in as many as 24% of autopsies {2563}. In current routine practice, the frequency of metastasis is < 0.2% of thyroid malignancies {361,1615,2096,2214}. Thyroid metastases are more common in females, with a female-to-male ratio of 1.2:1, and tend to occur with advancing age (average patient age: > 60 years) {516,2096,2214, 2324,2382}. They may be identified after the diagnosis of the primary tumour; for renal cell carcinoma, the median latency period is 21 years {2881}.

Etiology
The thyroid is relatively vascular and may harbour metastases at a higher frequency than other organs {1948}. Metastases to the thyroid may be favoured by goitre or thyroiditis {1124}, and they may localize within a primary thyroid neoplasm (tumour-to-tumour metastasis {10,143}).

Localization
Clear cell renal cell carcinoma is the most common primary, followed by adenocarcinoma of the lung, breast, or colon {361,516,1124,2324}. Squamous cell carcinoma of the larynx is the most common primary to spread by direct extension {2214}. Less common are metastases from the prostate, uterus, stomach, and pancreas, as well as melanomas and secondary lymphomas {10,361,658, 2214}.

Clinical features
Patients present with a variably symptomatic neck mass, and rarely with pain, hoarseness, or cough {361,2324}. Most nodules are either asymptomatic or detected incidentally on ultrasound {2382}.

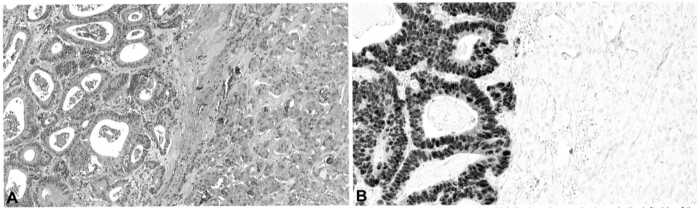

Fig. 2.163 Thyroid metastasis from colonic adenocarcinoma. **A** Metastasis from a colonic adenocarcinoma arising in a thyroid follicular adenoma is shown in the left side of the field. **B** The adenocarcinomatous cells of the metastasis show marked nuclear expression of CDX2, in contrast with the surrounding thyroid tissue.

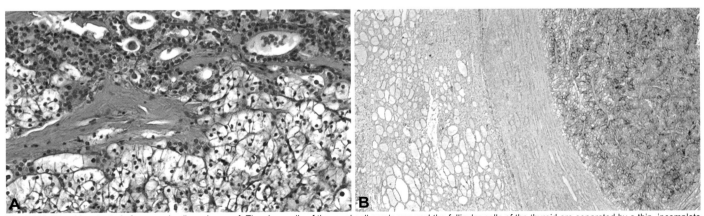

Fig. 2.164 Thyroid metastasis from renal cell carcinoma. **A** The clear cells of the renal cell carcinoma and the follicular cells of the thyroid are separated by a thin, incomplete capsule. **B** The cells of the renal cell carcinoma show strong positivity for CD10.

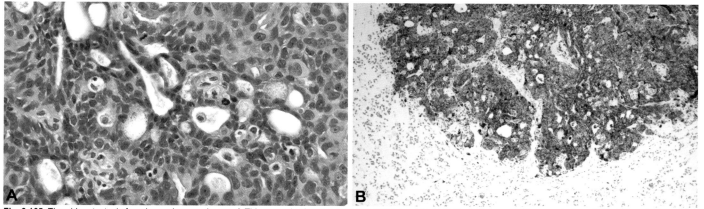

Fig. 2.165 Thyroid metastasis from lung adenocarcinoma. **A** This example shows a solid and glandular pattern. **B** The tumour cells show marked positivity for napsin-A, proving their metastatic origin.

Thyroid enlargement or symptoms of hyperthyroidism caused by parenchymal destruction by the metastasis have been described {2324,2382}. Metastases can be single, multiple, or bilateral {2096, 2324}.

Macroscopy

Multinodular metastasis may be indistinguishable from a nodular goitre {2324}. Clues favouring metastasis are gross features consistent with the primary tumour, such as the yellow, haemorrhagic appearance of a renal cell primary or the mucin pools of a gastrointestinal primary. If metastasis arises from an adjacent structure, gross extension from the primary site is generally clear.

Microscopy

It can be difficult to distinguish between a primary thyroid tumour and metastasis when a metastasis mimics the microfollicular or alveolar structure seen in many thyroid neoplasms. Tumours with clear-cell changes (e.g. renal cell carcinoma and some breast carcinomas) are the most challenging to recognize as metastases, because clear cells are frequently encountered in primary thyroid tumours. Clinical history and immunohistochemistry enable the correct diagnosis in most cases.

Cytology
Haemorrhage and necrosis can distort cytological details, leading to possible misdiagnosis by fine-needle aspiration biopsy unless a secondary tumour is suspected {2214,2346}.

In difficult cases, the immunohistochemistry of secondary tumours can be useful; however, additional specific non-thyroidal markers (e.g. napsin-A for lung or renal cell carcinoma antigen for kidney) must be used in conjunction with non-specific thyroid antibodies (TTF1 and PAX8) {523,752}. Another primary tumour that should be distinguished from metastasis is anaplastic carcinoma: the expression of PAX8 may rule out malignancies from lung or larynx {257,2214}.

Genetic profile

Secondary tumours often have genetic profiles similar to those of their counterparts at primary sites, and testing may be useful in rare cases {156,2606}.

Prognosis and predictive factors

The reported overall 5-year survival rate after the detection of a secondary tumour or after thyroidectomy for removing metastatic disease is 20–30% {361,2324}. The identification of primary tumour site by fine-needle aspiration biopsy of thyroid nodules has provided opportunities to assess for molecular parameters useful in the administration of adjuvant therapy {37,208,459,575}.

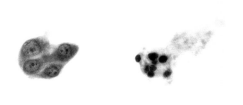

Fig. 2.166 Fine-needle aspiration of a lung adenocarcinoma metastatic to the thyroid. Liquid-based cytology shows a cluster of carcinomatous cells (at left) mixed with a group of typical thyroid follicular cells (Papanicolaou stain).

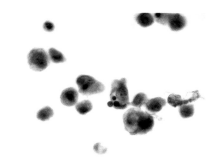

Fig. 2.167 Fine-needle aspiration of a lung adenocarcinoma metastatic to the thyroid. On liquid-based cytology, the neoplastic cells show prominent cytoplasmic vacuolization (Papanicolaou stain).

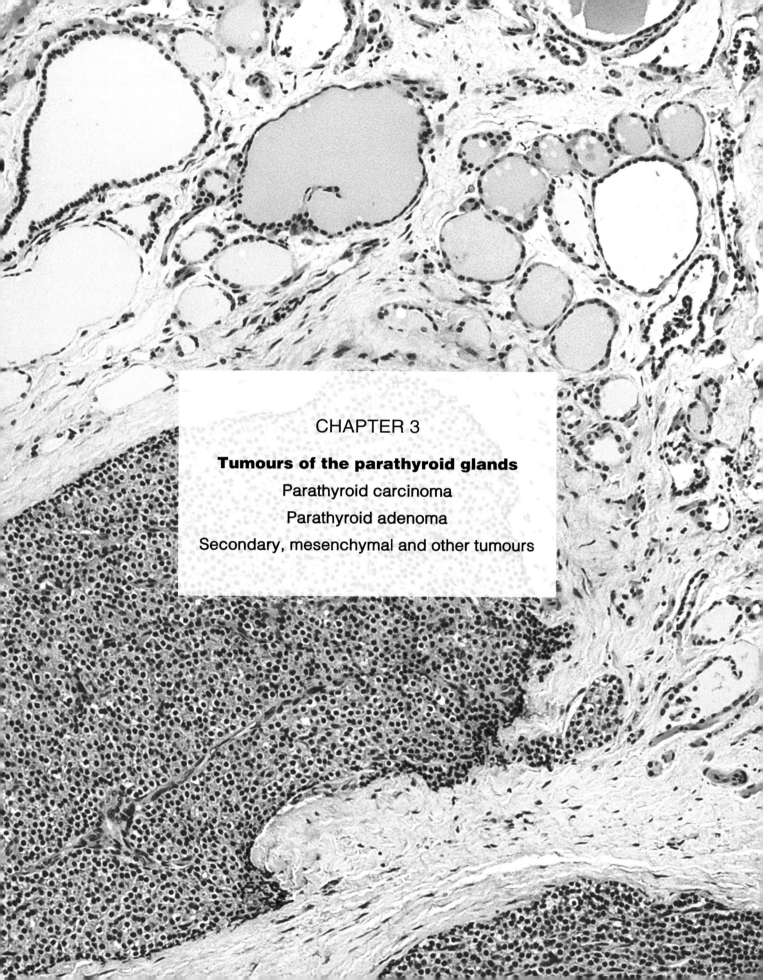

CHAPTER 3

Tumours of the parathyroid glands

Parathyroid carcinoma

Parathyroid adenoma

Secondary, mesenchymal and other tumours

WHO classification of tumours of the parathyroid glands

Parathyroid carcinoma	8140/3
Parathyroid adenoma	8140/0
Secondary, mesenchymal and other tumours	

The morphology codes are from the International Classification of Diseases for Oncology (ICD-O) {898A}. Behaviour is coded /0 for benign tumours; /1 for unspecified, borderline, or uncertain behaviour; /2 for carcinoma in situ and grade III intraepithelial neoplasia; and /3 for malignant tumours. The classification is modified from the previous WHO classification, taking into account changes in our understanding of these lesions.

TNM staging of tumours of the parathyroid glands

T – Primary Tumour

TX	Primary tumour cannot be assessed
T0	No evidence of primary tumour
Tis	Atypical parathyroid neoplasm (neoplasm of uncertain malignant potential)
T1	Localized to the parathyroid gland with extension limited to soft tissue
T2	Direct invasion into the thyroid gland
T3	Direct invasion into recurrent laryngeal nerve, oesophagus, trachea, skeletal muscle, adjacent lymph nodes, or thymus
T4	Direct invasion into major blood vessels or spine

N – Regional Lymph Nodes

NX	Regional lymph nodes cannot be assessed
N0	No regional lymph node metastasis
N1	Regional lymph node metastasis
N1a	Metastasis to Level VI (pretracheal, paratracheal, and prelaryngeal/Delphian lymph nodes) or upper/superior mediastinal lymph nodes
N1b	Metastasis to unilateral, bilateral or contralateral cervical (Levels I, II, III, IV, or V) or retropharyngeal nodes

M – Distant Metastasis

M0	No distant metastasis
M1	Distant metastasis

Stage

There are not enough data to propose a formal staging system at this time.

Adapted from: AJCC Cancer Staging Manual, 8th Edition, 2017. {1545A}

Parathyroid carcinoma

DeLellis R. A.
Arnold A.
Bilezikian J. P.
Eng C.
Larsson C.
Lloyd R. V.
Mete O.

Definition
Parathyroid carcinoma is a malignant neoplasm derived from parathyroid parenchymal cells.

ICD-O code   8140/3

Epidemiology
Parathyroid carcinoma is a rare neoplasm accounting for <1% of cases of primary hyperparathyroidism and 0.005% of all malignancies in North America and most of western Europe {837,1577}. Studies from Japan {2041} and Italy {837} have shown that 5–6% of cases of primary hyperparathyroidism are due to parathyroid carcinomas. Although some of this variation may be due to differences in the diagnostic criteria used, it may also reflect true geographical differences. SEER data indicate that the annual incidence of parathyroid carcinoma in the USA is considerably less than 1 case per million population. However, the incidence increased from 3.58 cases (1988–91) to 5.73 cases (2000–03) per 10 million population {1577}. A similar trend has been noted in other countries {339}. Possible reasons for this increase in incidence include increased screening, evolving diagnostic criteria, and a true increase in the incidence of the disease. The mean patient age at diagnosis is 56 years (range: 15–89 years). Parathyroid carcinoma has a female-to-male ratio of

approximately 1:1 {104}, in contrast to its much more common benign counterpart, whose female-to-male ratio is 3–4:1.

Etiology
There have been few studies on the etiology of sporadic parathyroid carcinoma, but a genetic background has been established for familial forms as well as subsets of sporadic cases {2523}. Parathyroid carcinoma occurs in 10–15% of patients with hyperparathyroidism–jaw tumour syndrome (HPT-JT) {2523} and has also been reported in the setting of familial isolated hyperparathyroidism (FIHP) {2953}. A few case reports have documented parathyroid carcinomas in the settings of multiple endocrine neoplasia type 1 (MEN1) {17,2572} and multiple endocrine neoplasia type 2 (MEN2) {1254}, but these associations are exceptionally uncommon. Parathyroid carcinoma has rarely been reported following radiation exposure {514}, whereas the association between parathyroid adenoma and external radiation of the head and neck (although an unusual cause) is well known. Rare cases of parathyroid carcinoma associated with prolonged chief cell hyperplasia have been documented in patients with renal failure {1843} and coeliac disease {305}.

Localization
Parathyroid carcinoma can arise in any of the normally located parathyroid glands or in a variety of other sites within the neck, retro-oesophageal space, mediastinum, thymus, and thyroid gland, wherever parathyroid tissue is present.

Clinical features
The presenting features of parathyroid carcinoma are dominated by the effects of excess secretion of parathyroid hormone {2515,2521}, with calcium levels often > 14 mg/dL. At presentation, many patients show evidence of renal disease, with the majority having nephrolithiasis. A similar proportion of patients show evidence of bone disease, with osteitis fibrosa cystica, subperiosteal bone resorption, diffuse osteoporosis, and fractures. Many patients show evidence of both renal and bone disease. Additional signs and symptoms include those of hypercalcaemia per se, such as fatigue, weakness, weight loss, anorexia, nausea, vomiting, polyuria, and polydipsia. Rarely, parathyroid carcinomas can be non-functioning, mimicking thyroid carcinomas both clinically and pathologically {849}. A palpable neck mass is present in 30–75% of patients, whereas it is rare in patients with parathyroid adenomas. Recurrent laryngeal nerve paralysis may indicate the presence of parathyroid carcinomas.

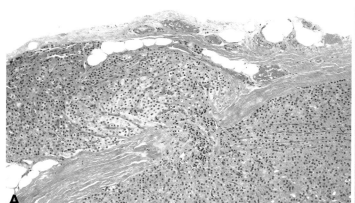
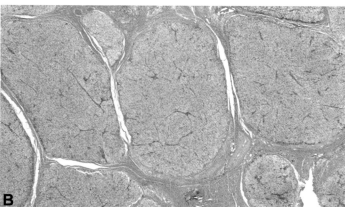

Fig. 3.01 Parathyroid carcinoma. **A** Early capsular invasion. The tumour has extended through the fibrous capsule into the surrounding soft tissues. **B** This invasive tumour has a nodular growth pattern, with individual nodules separated by fibrous bands.

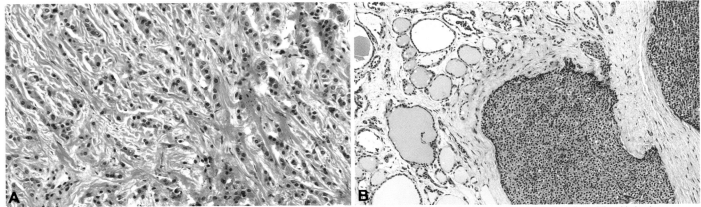

Fig. 3.02 Parathyroid carcinoma. **A** This invasive tumour is associated with a prominent fibrous stroma. **B** This invasive tumour extends into the adjacent thyroid gland.

Macroscopy

Parathyroid carcinomas show considerable variation in their macroscopic features. They are typically large and variably encapsulated tumours, weighing from 1.5 to > 50 g {263,2341}. They often appear as poorly circumscribed masses, which may be densely adherent to the surrounding soft tissues and thyroid gland. On cross-section, they are usually firm and pinkish-tan, with a lobular appearance due to the presence of thick fibrous bands {2444}. However, some of the tumours may be grossly indistinguishable from parathyroid adenomas.

Microscopy

The diagnosis of malignancy should be restricted to tumours with evidence of invasive growth involving adjacent structures such as the thyroid and soft tissues, capsular and/or extracapsular blood vessels or perineural spaces and/or to those with documented metastases {2341}. To qualify as vascular invasion,

a tumour should be located in capsular vessels or vessels in the surrounding soft tissues. The tumour should be attached to the vessel wall at least partially, and fibrin should be present in association with it. An endothelial lining may or may not be present. As with follicular thyroid neoplasms, the presence of intratumoural vascular invasion is not considered a criterion of malignancy {2341}.

The tumours are variably cellular and are often subdivided by broad bands of fibrous connective tissue extending from the peritumoural capsule. Fibrous bands are present in as many as 90% of carcinomas {2444}, but their presence is not specific for malignancy {279}. Occasional carcinomas show evidence of follicle formation, and rarely the tumours can have a carcinosarcomatous growth pattern {2692}. Most carcinomas are composed of chief cells that are intermediate in size, with round to ovoid nuclei containing dense chromatin and inconspicuous nucleoli; carcinomas with these

features can be indistinguishable from adenomas at the cytological level. Variable numbers of oncocytes, transitional oncocytes, clear cells, and spindle cells may be present {425}. Many tumours exhibit some degree of pleomorphism, manifested by intermediate-sized nuclei and small nucleoli; some tumours exhibit marked pleomorphism, with coarsely clumped chromatin and macronucleoli. Occasional carcinomas are composed exclusively of oncocytic (oxyphilic) cells {785}. The diagnostic criteria for oncocytic carcinoma are identical to those for chief cell carcinoma. Ultrastructurally, chief cell carcinomas contain variable numbers of dense-core secretory granules; oncocytic carcinomas also contain numerous mitochondria {60}.

Mitotic figures are present in as many as 80% of carcinomas, and they also occur in substantial numbers of parathyroid adenomas {2444,2589}. However, the presence of atypical mitoses strongly favours the diagnosis of malignancy. The Ki-67

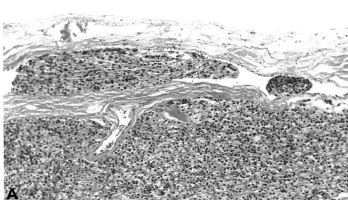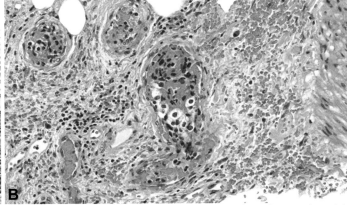

Fig. 3.03 Parathyroid carcinoma. **A** Tumour cells are present within a capsular vessel. **B** Intravascular tumour cells with associated fibrin are present in small venous channels in the surrounding soft tissues.

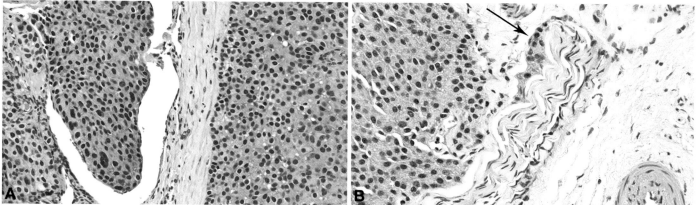

Fig. 3.04 Parathyroid carcinoma. **A** An intravascular tumour embolus surrounded by endothelial cells is present in a large vascular channel in the surrounding soft tissues. **B** The tumour has invaded a perineural space (arrow) in the surrounding soft tissues.

proliferation index (as determined using the MIB1 antibody) is higher in carcinomas (6–8.4%) than in adenomas (≤ 4%), but the overlap between these groups has limited the utility of this approach in equivocal cases. Additionally, expression of CDKN1B (also called p27) is lower in carcinomas than in adenomas {786}. Foci of coagulative necrosis may be present in parathyroid carcinomas, and it has been suggested that the triad of macronucleoli, > 5 mitoses per 50 high-power fields, and necrosis appears to be predictive of aggressive growth in these tumours {279}.

Parathyroid carcinomas are usually positive for parathyroid hormone, although the staining may be less extensive than in parathyroid adenomas. The tumours are also positive for the transcription factors GCM2 (a master regulatory gene of parathyroid development {2019}) and GATA3 {2056}. In addition, tumour cells are positive for cytokeratins (CAM5.2), synaptophysin, and chromogranins. In contrast

to oncocytic adenomas, which are positive for CK14, oncocytic carcinomas are negative for this marker {785}. Staining for RB protein is often negative in parathyroid carcinomas {436,584}, but variable results have been noted in some studies {828}. Many parathyroid carcinomas, with the exception of those occurring in some patients with chronic renal failure, are negative for CDC73 (also called parafibromin), the product of the *CDC73* gene (also called *HRPT2*) {791,974,977,2713}. To ensure reproducibility, the CDC73 staining procedure must be rigorously controlled; variations have been noted across laboratories. Additional ancillary markers that have been reported to be positive in parathyroid carcinomas include galectin 3 {220,851} and PGP9.5 {1176}, whereas APC, CDKN1B, and BCL2 are negative or only weakly expressed in these tumours {1277,2649}. However, most studies of these markers have been limited to relatively small case series, and additional studies are required for validation.

It is often challenging to distinguish parathyroid carcinoma from parathyromatosis {850}, which can result from the inadvertent implantation of hyperplastic or adenomatous parathyroid tissue during surgery for hyperparathyroidism or from persistent embryological remnants of parathyroid tissue {860,876,2263}. Parathyromatosis often has an infiltrative growth pattern similar to that of parathyroid carcinoma. Features favouring carcinoma over parathyromatosis include markedly increased serum levels of calcium and parathyroid hormone, a palpable neck mass, and vascular or perineural invasion {850,2028}.

Genetic profile

Conclusions from the literature on the genetic profile of parathyroid carcinoma require cautious interpretation, because studies can differ in the criteria used for diagnosing and selecting cases. However, among cases selected with rigorous criteria, inactivation of the tumour

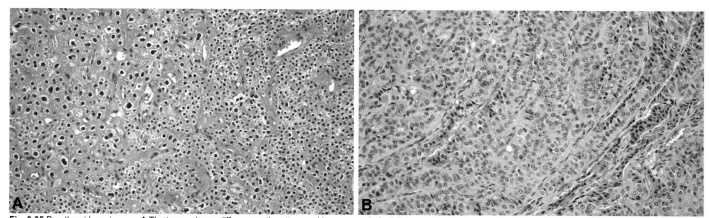

Fig. 3.05 Parathyroid carcinoma. **A** The tumour has a diffuse growth pattern and is composed of mildly to moderately pleomorphic chief cells. **B** The tumour has a trabecular growth pattern.

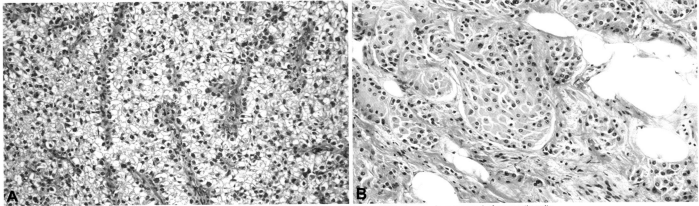

Fig. 3.06 Parathyroid carcinoma. **A** The tumour is composed of chief cells with clear cytoplasm. **B** The tumour is composed of oncocytic cells.

suppressor gene *CDC73* is overwhelmingly the major known molecular driver in the pathogenesis of parathyroid carcinoma (both sporadic and familial forms) {564,1238,1972}. The role of germline *CDC73* mutation in familial predisposition to parathyroid carcinoma, in particular HPT-JT, is discussed in the *Genetic susceptibility* section. The normal CDC73 protein regulates gene expression and inhibits cell proliferation, but exactly how its loss of function drives tumorigenesis in the vulnerable cell types requires further study.

Sporadic parathyroid carcinomas frequently have clonal, somatic inactivating mutations in *CDC73* {564,2523}. Often, biallelic mutation is detected, consistent with a classic tumour suppressor model {435,1177,2523}. Because mutations capable of inactivating *CDC73* would escape detection if located outside the coding region (to which sequencing has been limited in most clinical testing and research studies), it is plausible that even the high (> 75%) reported incidence of *CDC73* inactivation understates the true frequency as a driver of the disease. Importantly, germline *CDC73* mutations are

present in a substantial minority of cases that present clinically as sporadic parathyroid carcinoma, with no familial clustering or syndromic features, indicating that some of these patients may nonetheless have HPT-JT or a phenotypic variant {564,1238,2523}. The recognition that family members of some patients with apparently sporadic disease are also at risk for parathyroid malignancy has broadened the indication for DNA testing in this setting {1238,2521,2523}.

The acquisition of mutations in additional collaborating genes may be necessary for the expression of malignant behaviour in parathyroid neoplasia, even in tumours exhibiting biallelic inactivation of *CDC73*. Genetic studies of parathyroid carcinomas have uncovered recurrent clonal alterations that suggest the involvement or chromosomal location of other candidate contributors. *CCND1*, a parathyroid adenoma oncogene, is overexpressed in many parathyroid cancers (although sample sizes are limited) {2854,3110}; one cause of such overexpression may be clonal *CCND1* DNA amplification {3110}. Recurrent loss of chromosome 13q in parathyroid carcinomas

has been found using both comparative genomic hybridization {1510} and molecular allelotyping {436,584}, and a tumour suppressor gene on chromosome 13 in the vicinity of (but probably distinct from) *RB1* may play a role in some cases {2522}. Somatic inactivation or loss of heterozygosity of *MEN1* (11q13), despite its frequent role in familial MEN1-related hyperparathyroidism and typical sporadic adenomas, has not been a major finding in parathyroid carcinoma, although it has been reported {565,1102,1510}; case ascertainment may have contributed to the inconsistency of results. Notably, parathyroid carcinoma has been documented only as an exceedingly rare event in patients with MEN1.

Unbiased next-generation sequencing of parathyroid carcinomas with whole-genome {1316} or whole-exome {2085, 3082} approaches has confirmed the importance of *CDC73* mutation in this disease, and has also identified several interesting candidate oncogenes with lower levels of potential involvement, including *PRUNE2*, *PIK3CA*, *KMT2D* (previously called *MLL2*), *MTOR*, *ADCK1*, and members of a kinase family with

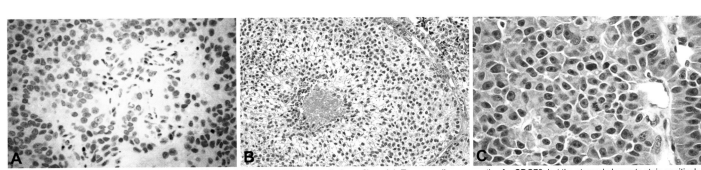

Fig. 3.07 Parathyroid carcinoma. **A** Immunoperoxidase staining for CDC73 (also called parafibromin). Tumour cells are negative for CDC73, but the stromal elements stain positively. **B** This tumour has a nodular growth pattern with central areas of necrosis (comedonecrosis). **C** The tumour cells have macronucleoli.

functions related to cell migration and invasion. These candidates, and others of potential importance to the development of parathyroid carcinoma that are likely to be identified as more tumours are analysed with modern technologies, will need to be carefully validated using genetic and functional–experimental approaches, in order to establish their involvement as pathogenetic drivers. But it is already clear from these early studies that the driver landscape of parathyroid carcinoma is quite distinct from those found in commonly sequenced types of human cancers.

With the exception of patients with germline CDC73 mutations, in whom parathyroid carcinoma development is consistent with a progression model, allelic loss patterns suggest that most sporadic parathyroid carcinomas arise de novo, rather than evolving from clinically recognizable benign adenomas {564,565,1510}.

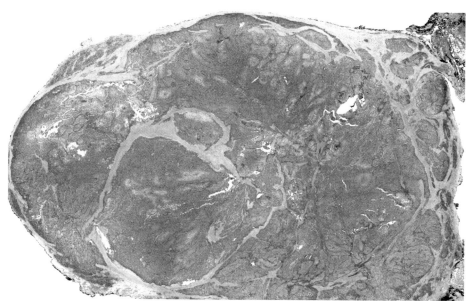

Fig. 3.08 Parathyroid carcinoma. Nodular growth pattern with bands of fibrosis and extension into the surrounding soft tissues.

Genetic susceptibility

The genetic differential diagnoses to consider for parathyroid carcinoma include CDC73-related disorders such as HPT-JT, FIHP, and apparently sporadic parathyroid carcinoma with germline CDC73 mutations {1238}.

HPT-JT is an autosomal dominant tumour disorder characterized by parathyroid adenoma or carcinoma; ossifying fibroma of the mandible and maxilla; and renal cysts, adenomas, and carcinomas (see *Hyperparathyroidism–jaw tumour syndrome*, p. 255). Germline mutations in CDC73 (previously called HRPT2), which encodes the CDC73 protein, are associated with HPT-JT {412,1972}. Diagnosis is based on the biochemical finding of primary hyperparathyroidism, the identification of ossifying fibroma(s) of the maxilla and/or mandible on imaging studies, family history, and detection of a heterozygous germline CDC73 pathogenic variant on molecular genetic testing. Parathyroid carcinoma, manifesting as primary hyperparathyroidism, occurs in approximately 10–15% of affected individuals. A unique pathological feature of parathyroid lesions in HPT-JT is the high frequency of cystic change. About 30% of patients with HPT-JT develop fibro-osseous lesions, primarily in the mandible and/or maxilla. Kidney lesions have also been reported, including bilateral cysts, renal adenoma, hamartomas,

and papillary or chromophobe renal cell carcinoma.

Typically, patients with HPT-JT present with solitary parathyroid adenomas or carcinomas. Rarely, they present with double neoplasms. Parathyroid carcinomas are extremely rare and are not components of any other heritable syndrome, with the exception of single case reports in the settings of MEN1 and MEN2A {17, 1254,2572}. Therefore, these tumours should raise suspicion for the genetic diagnosis of HPT-JT. Approximately 80% of patients with HPT-JT present with hyperparathyroidism, but it is important to be aware that in some families, only parathyroid lesions are present (FIHP). HPT-JT (with CDC73 mutation present in > 50–80% of cases), parathyroid carcinoma (with CDC73 mutation present in 20% of all apparently sporadic cases), and FIHP associated with germline mutations in CDC73 (accounting for 15% of all FIHP cases) are collectively referred to as CDC73-related disorders {1238,1972}. CDC73 has 17 exons, spanning 18.5 kb of genomic distance. HPT-JT–associated mutations are truncating: mainly (in > 80% of cases) frameshift and nonsense mutations, with most occurring in exon 1 {412,1972}. A large germline deletion in CDC73 has been reported {417}, but it remains unknown whether there is a genotype–phenotype association. The penetrance of hyperparathyroidism (which typically develops by late adolescence) is 80%. The CDC73 transcript,

which spans 2.7 kb, is predicted to encode a protein with a length of 531 amino acids. Although the gene is ubiquitously expressed, its function remained unknown for some time. Eventually, CDC73 was shown to bind RNA polymerase II as part of the PAF1 transcriptional regulatory complex {3061}, and importantly, was found to mediate H3K9 methylation, which silences cyclin D1 expression {3056}.

Prognosis and predictive factors

Most parathyroid carcinomas tend to recur locally, with spread to contiguous structures in the neck. Recurrent disease is often accompanied by profound hypercalcaemia and other metabolic complications {1092}. The most common sites of local involvement are the ipsilateral thyroid gland, strap muscles, ipsilateral recurrent laryngeal nerve, oesophagus, and trachea {1427}. Metastatic spread tends to occur late in the course of the disease, with involvement of cervical lymph nodes, lung, liver, and a variety of other sites.

For patients with parathyroid carcinoma, the estimated 5-year and 10-year overall survival rates are 78–85% and 49–70%, respectively {104}. A study of > 700 cases collected in the United States National Cancer Database (NCDB) showed that negative prognostic factors in multivariate analyses included older patient age at the time of diagnosis, larger tumour size, and male sex {104}. When the data

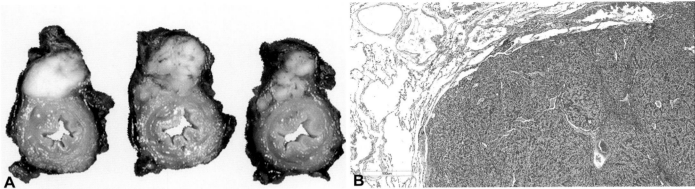

Fig. 3.09 A Recurrent parathyroid carcinoma 1 year after excision of the primary tumour. At laryngo-oesophagectomy with small bowel transplant, the tumour had recurred in the perioesophageal soft tissues with vascular invasion and multiple regional nodal metastases. B Parathyroid carcinoma. The tumour in this pulmonary metastasis has a diffuse growth pattern and is composed of relatively bland chief cells that are indistinguishable from those of chief cell adenoma.

were adjusted for nodal status, patient age and sex, and extent of surgical excision, each centimetre of increase in tumour size was associated with a 2% increase in risk of death. Positive nodal status was not found to be associated with an increased risk of death in that study, but has been reported to be a risk factor for decreased survival in other series {1092}. In general, the extent of local invasion correlates positively with the development of recurrent or metastatic disease {1304,2510,2704}.

As noted by the authors of the 8th edition of the AJCC Cancer Staging Manual, there is no generally accepted staging system for these tumours. They note that proposing a formal staging system at this time would be premature because of the wide variation among existing studies with respect to significant prognostic factors. They propose a working TNM classification with recommendations for recording specific variables to develop a formal staging system to be used in future AJCC manuals (see the proposed TNM classification table on p. 146) {1545A}.

Parathyroid adenoma

DeLellis R. A.
Arnold A.
Eng C.
Erickson L.A.

Franssila K. O.
Haigh P. I.
Hendy G. N.
Hunt J. L.

Definition
Parathyroid adenoma is a benign parathyroid neoplasm composed of chief cells, oncocytes, or transitional oncocytes, or an admixture of these cell types.

ICD-O code   8140/0

Epidemiology
Over the past half-century, primary hyperparathyroidism has gone from being a relatively obscure disorder to being one of the most commonly diagnosed of all endocrine diseases, in particular among postmenopausal women. This dramatic change is in large part a result of the use of multichannel biochemical analysers that include serum calcium determinations, introduced in the mid-1970s {23}. In a recent population-based study, 90% of individuals with hypercalcaemia had primary hyperparathyroidism {3063}. Parathyroid adenoma involving a single gland accounts for 85% of cases of primary hyperparathyroidism worldwide {1735}. Incidence and prevalence rates vary across populations and depend on the detection methods used {888}. The prevalence established by biochemical screening ranges from 1 case (USA) to 21 cases (Finland) per 1000 population. Estimation of the true incidence is difficult, but overall figures in the UK, USA, and Sweden are relatively consistent at 27–30 cases per 100000 person-years {888}. The peak incidence is found among individuals aged 50–60 years, with a female-to-male ratio of 2–3:1; however, the female-to-male ratio varies from close to 1:1 among individuals aged < 40 years to more than 5:1 among individuals older than 75 years {888}. In a study of a racially mixed population of > 13 000 patients with primary hyperparathyroidism who were enrollees within Kaiser Permanente Southern California in the USA, substantial differences were found in the incidence and prevalence of this disorder, with the highest incidence found among Blacks, followed by Whites, and with lower rates among Asians, Hispanics, and other ethnic groups {3063}. Incidence rates fluctuated over the years,

and did not correlate with the frequency of calcium testing, which increased steadily over the study period {3063}. Interestingly, the prevalence of primary hyperparathyroidism tripled during the study period (1995–2010): from 76 cases to 233 cases per 100 000 person-years in females and from 30 cases to 85 cases per 100 000 person-years in males {3063}.

Etiology
The etiology of most parathyroid adenomas is unknown. A relatively small subset of cases is heritable, associated with multiple endocrine neoplasia type 1 (MEN1), multiple endocrine neoplasia type 2A (MEN2A), and the *CDC73*-related disorders, including hyperparathyroidism–jaw tumour syndrome and familial isolated hyperparathyroidism (see *Genetic susceptibility*). More commonly, MEN1 and MEN2A are associated with multiglandular hyperplasia; *CDC73*-related disorders are associated with multiple adenomas and less commonly with carcinomas. External ionizing irradiation of the head and neck, particularly in childhood, has been implicated in the development of these tumours {532}. Primary hyperparathyroidism and thyroid cancer occur together in radiation-exposed individuals more often than would be expected by chance {1650}. Survivors of the atomic bombing of Hiroshima had a 4-fold increase

in parathyroid adenomas, which appeared to be dose-dependent {902}. An increased risk of primary hyperparathyroidism has been noted among cleanup workers following the Chernobyl accident {272}; in this group, the cause of primary hyperparathyroidism may be exposure to strontium-90, a ligand for calcium-sensing receptor molecules. Exposure to diagnostic or therapeutic doses of radioactive iodine does not appear to be a significant risk factor {2244}. Long-term lithium therapy has been implicated in the development of both parathyroid adenomas and primary chief cell hyperplasia {119,1735}.

Localization
Parathyroid adenomas can arise in any of the normally located glands, with the inferior glands involved slightly more often than the superior. They can also occur in other sites, including other areas of the neck, the retro-oesophageal space, the mediastinum, the thymus, and the thyroid gland {410,535,737,2085}. They can also arise from ectopic or supernumerary parathyroid tissue within the pericardium, vagus and hypoglossal nerves, carotid sheath, or soft tissues adjacent to the angle of the jaw {1315,1519}. As many as 15% of patients have double adenomas, which show a predilection for both superior parathyroid glands (so-called fourth pouch disease) {1844}.

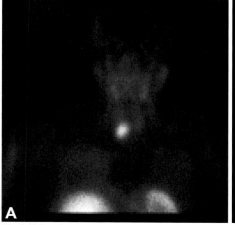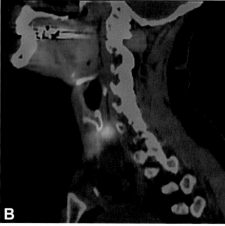

Fig. 3.10 Parathyroid adenoma. **A** Planar technetium sestamibi scan of a large right superior parathyroid adenoma in a descended position. **B** Fused SPECT/CT showing high signal in the left superior adenoma.

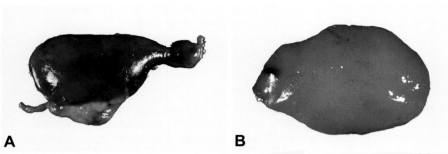

Fig. 3.11 Parathyroid adenoma. **A** External surface of chief cell adenoma. Residual normal parathyroid tissue is present in the adjacent adipose tissue inferiorly. **B** Cross-section of chief cell adenoma.

Clinical features

Prior to the introduction of routine serum calcium screening, most patients with parathyroid adenomas presented with classic symptoms of primary hyperparathyroidism, including severe metabolic bone disease (e.g. osteitis fibrosa cystica, also called von Recklinghausen disease of bone) and renal disease {1735}. In current clinical practice in the developed world, most patients are relatively asymptomatic and are identified by abnormal calcium levels. Common symptoms include weakness, fatigue, anxiety, and some degree of cognitive impairment. The risk of bone fractures is increased in patients with primary hyperparathyroidism {2871}, and 4–15% of patients present with nephrolithiasis {2272}. The diagnostic laboratory finding is an abnormally elevated intact parathyroid hormone (PTH) level concurrent with an elevated albumin adjusted calcium

level {1735}. However, some patients have normocalcaemic primary hyperparathyroidism {2564}.

Preoperative localization studies for focused parathyroidectomy include ultrasonography, sestamibi-technetium-99m scintigraphy usually with single photon emission computed tomography (SPECT), fused SPECT/CT, 4-dimensional parathyroid computed tomography (4DCT), and magnetic resonance imaging {359A,2729A}. The most commonly used approaches include: (1) ultrasonography and sestamibi-SPECT or SPECT/CT and (2) ultrasonography and 4DCT {359A}.

Macroscopy

Parathyroid adenomas vary in size, ranging from < 1 cm to > 10 cm {2342}. The term "microadenoma" has been used to describe tumours measuring < 0.6 cm and weighing < 100 mg {999,2241}. Parathyroid adenomas are generally ovoid in shape and are surrounded by a thin capsule, but some are bilobulated or multilobulated. On cross-section, adenomas are soft and pinkish-tan. A rim of normal gland, recognizable by its pale tan or yellow colour, may be present at the periphery of the tumour {2085}. Foci of cystic change may be present, particularly in larger tumours. The cysts are filled with straw-coloured or brown fluid. Cystic change may be accompanied by prominent areas of fibrosis and foci of calcification {2085}. The walls of cystic adenomas may be markedly thickened, with adherence to the adjacent thyroid gland or soft tissues, raising suspicion for malignancy at surgery. Spontaneous infarction of parathyroid adenomas can occur {1470,1681}. There is some correlation between tumour size, symptomatology, and levels of serum calcium and PTH. In a series from the Massachusetts General Hospital in the United States, adenomas associated with severe bone disease had

an average weight of 10 g, whereas in patients without bone disease, the average tumour weight was 1.3 g, with many examples weighing < 0.5 g {425}.

Microscopy

Most parathyroid adenomas are encapsulated neoplasms composed of chief cells at various stages of their secretory cycles {59}. Microadenomas are usually not encapsulated and can be difficult to distinguish from glands with focal (nodular) hyperplasia. The component cells often have a palisaded arrangement around blood vessels. Neoplastic chief cells are generally round to polyhedral and are slightly larger than those in the adjacent rim of normal parathyroid tissue. Occasional spindle-shaped cells may also be present. The cytoplasm is faintly eosinophilic but may appear clear. In some instances, well-developed perinuclear haloes may be prominent {650}. Nuclei are generally round and centrally located, with dense lymphocyte-like chromatin and inconspicuous nucleoli. Multinucleated cells may be present, in addition to cells with enlarged hyperchromatic nuclei measuring as large as 50 µm (so-called endocrine atypia). As many as 80% of adenomas exhibit some degree of mitotic activity, typically with < 1 mitosis per 10 high-power fields {2589}, which underscores the fact that mitotic activity alone is an unreliable predictor of malignancy in these neoplasms. Follicle formation is not uncommon, and some adenomas have a predominant follicular architecture. Very rarely, the tumours can have a papillary architecture {2378}. Although the capsule surrounding adenomas is usually thin, in some instances it is markedly thickened, with entrapped tumour cells.

In contrast to adenomas, which commonly involve a single gland, chief cell hyperplasia is a multiglandular process, but the hyperplasia may be asymmetrical (pseudoadenomatous), with marked variation in gland size {264}. Cases of asymmetrical hyperplasia can be difficult to differentiate from single or multiple adenomas.

Non-adenomatous glands from patients with parathyroid adenomas are indistinguishable from those of normocalcaemic individuals using standard histopathological criteria {750}. However, parenchymal cells in non-adenomatous glands contain prominent neutral lipid droplets that are

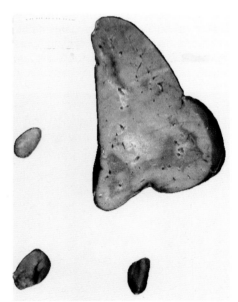

Fig. 3.12 Parathyroid adenoma. Cross-section of formalin-fixed parathyroid adenoma. The other three parathyroid glands are of normal size.

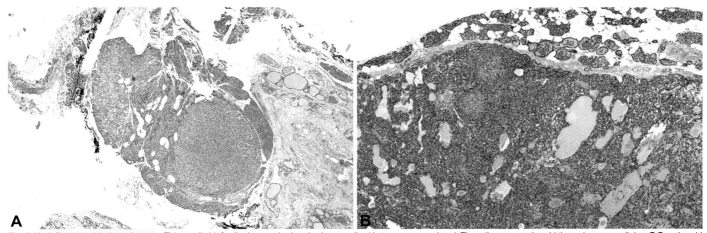

Fig. 3.13 A Parathyroid microadenoma. This small chief cell adenoma is sharply circumscribed but non-encapsulated. The adjacent parathyroid tissue is normocellular. **B** Parathyroid adenoma separated by thin fibrous capsule from a well defined rim of adjacent residual normal parathyroid.

independent of the stromal fat content {2350}. Lipid in the adenoma cells is either absent or finely dispersed throughout the cytoplasm. The secretory setpoint of cells derived from non-adenomatous glands is decreased below normal levels, and the proliferation rate of the cells is also decreased {2111}.

Cytology

Aspirates of parathyroid adenomas are variably cellular and often contain dissociated epithelial cells, in addition to small-cell aggregates with round to ovoid hyperchromatic nuclei. The cytoplasm is pale, amphophilic, and occasionally vacuolated.

Immunophenotype

Parathyroid adenomas are typically positive for PTH, GCM2, GATA3, synaptophysin, and chromogranin {2019, 2056}. CDC73 (also called parafibromin) is usually positive, except in adenomas

occurring in the setting of hyperparathyroidism–jaw tumour syndrome {1176}. Parathyroid adenomas are usually positive for RB {851}; APC {1278}; and the combination of CDKN1B (also called p27), BCL2, and MDM2 {2649}. They are generally negative for galectin 3 {851, 2819} and PGP9.5 {1176}.

Variants

Oncocytic (oxyphilic) adenomas are relatively uncommon, accounting for 3–6% of parathyroid adenomas. They tend to be somewhat larger than chief cell adenomas, although there is considerable overlap in tumour weights {1181}. Grossly, the tumours are soft and reddish-brown on section. Tumour cells may be arranged in sheets, nests, acini, or trabeculae. They are composed exclusively or predominantly (> 75%) of cells with abundant granular eosinophilic cytoplasm and round to ovoid nuclei with coarse chromatin and distinct nucleoli.

Occasional nuclei may be enlarged, irregularly shaped, and hyperchromatic. Early studies suggested that these tumours were either non-functioning or hypofunctioning, but more recent analyses indicate that they are frequently symptomatic, with higher serum calcium and PTH levels than chief cell adenomas {1181}.

Parathyroid lipoadenomas (hamartomas) are rare benign neoplasms characterized by the proliferation of stromal and parenchymal elements. Occasional cases have been associated with hyperparathyroidism {508}. Some lipoadenomas attain a very large size, with weights in excess of 400 g; they can occur in normally positioned parathyroid glands or in a variety of ectopic sites {3070}. Rare examples of double lipoadenomas have been documented {2044}. Grossly, the tumours are encapsulated and yellow. They are composed of mature adipose tissue with

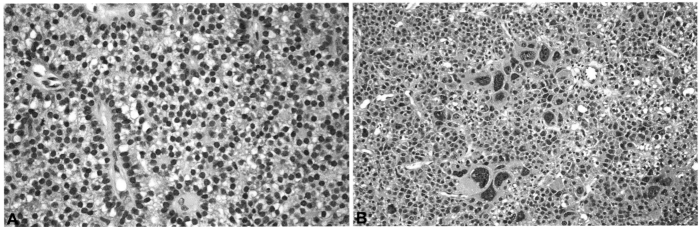

Fig. 3.14 Parathyroid adenoma. **A** The tumour cells form palisaded arrangements around blood vessels. **B** Groups of cells with enlarged hyperchromatic nuclei.

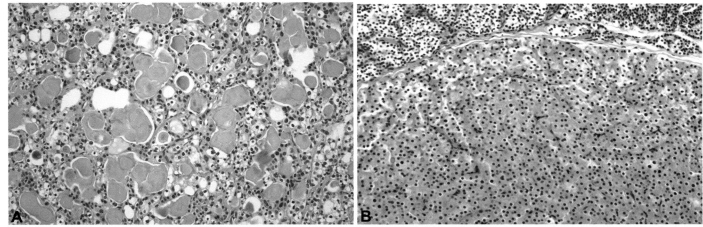

Fig. 3.15 Parathyroid adenoma. **A** Predominant follicular pattern. Individual follicles contain eosinophilic colloid. **B** The tumour is composed exclusively of oncocytic cells. A rim of adjacent normal parathyroid tissue is present.

myxoid change, fibrosis, and chronic inflammation. The parenchymal elements include chief cells and varying numbers of oncocytes arranged in thin, branching, cord-like patterns. Foci of lipoadenomatous change can occur in otherwise typical chief cell adenomas.

Water-clear cell adenomas are exceptionally rare {131}. The tumours are yellowish-tan on section, and are composed of cells with clear cytoplasm containing multiple small vacuoles. The nuclei are relatively small and hyperchromatic, and are located either in the centre of the cell or towards its periphery. Water-clear cell adenoma involving two glands has been documented {1484}.

Atypical parathyroid adenomas are a group of neoplasms composed of chief cells with variable numbers of oncocytes and transitional oncocytes that exhibit some of the features of parathyroid carcinoma but lack unequivocal invasive growth {649,650,850,1048,1220,1596, 2649}. As a group, they may be considered tumours of uncertain malignant potential. Gross and microscopic features can include banding fibrosis (with or without associated haemosiderin deposition), adherence to (but not invasion of) contiguous structures, presence of tumour within the surrounding capsule, solid or trabecular growth patterns, nuclear atypia and prominent nucleoli, and mitotic activity. However, none of these features alone or in combination is diagnostic of malignancy (see *Parathyroid carcinoma*, p. 147). Most patients with atypical adenomas have a benign clinical course; however, close follow-up is mandatory. Studies of CDC73 immunoreactivity have proven useful to predict the potential for recurrence in atypical adenomas as defined by the 2004 WHO criteria {650,

1483}. Recurrence was not documented in any CDC73-positive cases, whereas 10% of CDC73-negative tumours recurred {1483}. In contrast, among carcinomas that satisfied the 2004 WHO criteria for malignancy, recurrence was documented in 36% of CDC73-positive and 38% of CDC73-negative cases. Molecular studies showed that allelic loss of RB, p53, CDC73, and CDKN1A (also called p21) was more frequent in carcinoma cases but also occurred in atypical adenomas; loss of NME1 (also called NM23), the von Hippel–Lindau protein, and APC was found only in the carcinoma group {1785}. In that study, none of the patients with atypical adenomas had evidence of recurrence after a mean follow-up of 5 years.

Genetic profile

Recurrent mutations of a variety of established and candidate oncogenes and

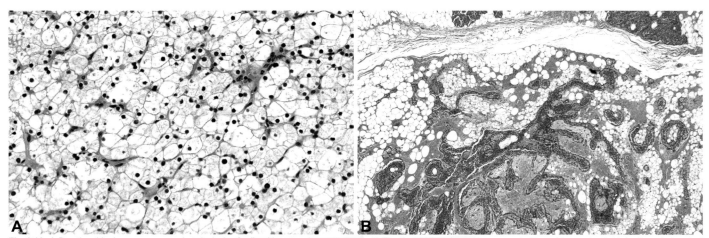

Fig. 3.16 A Parathyroid adenoma composed exclusively of cells with water-clear cytoplasm. **B** Parathyroid lipoadenoma composed of branching cords of chief cells and abundant fat, with areas of myxoid change.

tumour suppressor genes play patho-genetic roles in the development of sporadic parathyroid adenomas {1129}. *CCND1* (previously called *PRAD1*) has been identified as an oncogene activated by clonal DNA rearrangement in parathyroid adenomas {564,1914} and is overexpressed by rearrangement or alternative mechanisms in as many as 40% of cases {564}. Overexpression of cyclin D1, a central regulator of the cell cycle, causes parathyroid neoplasia and biochemical hyperparathyroidism, including an altered PTH–calcium setpoint, in transgenic mice {1215,1725}, establishing its role as a driver oncogene. The tumour suppressor gene *MEN1*, germline mutations of which cause MEN1 {455}, undergoes biallelic somatic inactivation by mutation and/or deletion in 12–35% of sporadic adenomas {564}. A mouse model of *MEN1* deficiency demonstrates a phenotype that includes parathyroid hypercellularity {576,1612}. Germline and somatic mutations in several genes of the CDKN family have been identified in sporadic parathyroid adenomas, and similar germline variants occur in familial MEN1-like settings {15,2141}, but in this different context the findings suggest that rare CDKN gene variants contribute to typical sporadic hyperparathyroidism as reduced-penetrance predisposition alleles {566,567}. Recurrent somatic mutations in *ZFX* and *EZH2* have been discovered in 1–5% of sporadic adenomas {579, 2617}; the intragenic specificity of these mutations suggests that both candidates will be confirmed by functional testing to be direct-acting parathyroid oncogenes. Somatic mutations in *CDC73* (also called *HRPT2*) occur almost exclusively in adenomas from patients with hyperparathyroidism–jaw tumour syndrome or associated predispositions, rather than in truly sporadic cases. With these adenomas, as well as with atypical adenomas, little is known about their somatic genetics apart from driver *CDC73* mutations {564}. Several notable candidate genes, including *CASR*, *VDR*, and *RET*, are not somatically mutated in typical sporadic parathyroid adenomas {1170,2129,2400}, but some (e.g. *CASR* and *VDR*), may play an important secondary role in the hyperparathyroid phenotype.

Genetic susceptibility

The genetic differential diagnoses to consider for parathyroid adenoma

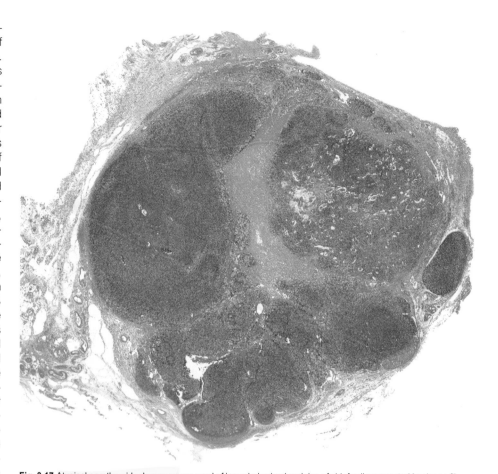

Fig. 3.17 Atypical parathyroid adenoma composed of irregularly sized nodules of chief cells separated by dense fibrous tissue. There is no evidence of extracapsular invasion.

include *CDC73*-related disorders such as familial isolated hyperparathyroidism and apparently sporadic parathyroid carcinoma with germline *CDC73* mutations {1238} (see *Parathyroid carcinoma*, p. 147), MEN1 {991} (see *Multiple endocrine neoplasia type 1*, p. 243), and MEN2A (see *Medullary thyroid carcinoma*, p. 108, and *Multiple endocrine neoplasia type 2*, p. 248).

Multiple endocrine neoplasia type 1 is an autosomal dominant cancer syndrome occurring in 1–2 in 100 000 live births. It is characterized by the classic triad of pituitary tumours, parathyroid hyperplasia, and neoplasia and pancreatic neuroendocrine neoplasia {991}. Multiglandular parathyroid chief cell hyperplasia of nodular type is the major manifestation of MEN1; parathyroid adenomas also occur but are considerably less common. Most, if not all, parathyroid hyperplastic lesions in patients with MEN1 are clonal processes and can even consist of more than one clone {896,1676}. Approximately 90% of individuals affected by MEN1 have hypercalcaemia (the most prevalent manifestation of this disorder) before the age of 25 years.

Germline loss-of-function mutations in the tumour suppressor gene *MEN1* (11q13), encoding menin, have been found in 80–90% of MEN1 familial probands and approximately 65% of non-familial probands {455,991,1555}. Exonic and whole-gene deletions are found in another 1–4% {991}. More than 1400 *MEN1* mutations have been reported to date; like most tumour suppressor gene–associated loss-of-function mutations, they are nonsense, frameshift, and missense mutations, and are scattered throughout the gene, without specific genotypic or phenotypic associations. Many of the menin missense mutants are targeted to the proteasome and are poorly expressed {374}. Rare germline mutations in *CDKN1B* (also called *P27*) and other CDKN genes may be associated with a MEN1-like syndrome {1882,1883,1884}.

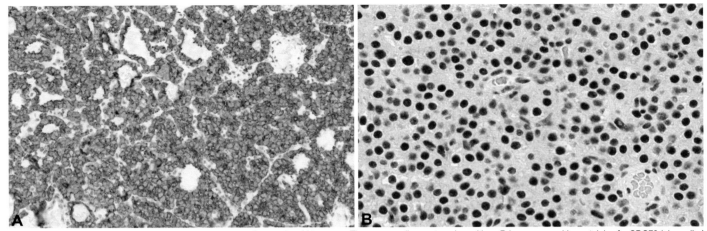

Fig. 3.18 Parathyroid adenoma. **A** Immunoperoxidase staining for parathyroid hormone. The tumour cells are strongly positive. **B** Immunoperoxidase staining for CDC73 (also called parafibromin). Tumour cell nuclei are strongly and uniformly positive.

Multiple endocrine neoplasia type 2 is an autosomal dominant inherited cancer syndrome occurring in 1 in 300 000 live births and comprising three subtypes based on specific combinations of clinical features {774,2459,3095} (see *Medullary thyroid carcinoma*, p. 108, and *Multiple endocrine neoplasia type 2*, p. 248). MEN2A, the most common clinical subtype, is characterized by medullary thyroid carcinoma (MTC), phaeochromocytoma, and hyperparathyroidism. The discovery that *RET* is the susceptibility gene for MEN2 also led to the realization that there exist genotype-related variable penetrance patterns and that the highest threshold exists in the parathyroid glands and the lowest in the C cells {882}. The incidence of hyperparathyroidism, which occurs in 15–30% of patients with MEN2A, is genotype-dependent and is associated with the codon C634R mutation. Parathyroid proliferative lesions are almost always characterized by multiglandular chief cell hyperplasia

of diffuse or nodular types, but occasional examples of adenoma have also been reported. MEN2B, the least common subtype, is similar to MEN2A, except that the component neoplasias of MEN2B occur an average of 10 years earlier than those of MEN2A; clinically apparent hyperparathyroidism is rarely, if ever, seen; and other syndromic features are variably present {1018}. Familial MTC is characterized by MTC only in any given family {827}. Given our current knowledge of the genetics of MEN2, it is thought that familial MTC and MEN2A are artificially divided subtypes, and may in fact lie along a continuum, with the different phenotypes resulting from different penetrance {3094}. The mutation profiles of the MEN2 syndromes are summarized in the section on *Medullary thyroid carcinoma* (p. 108).

Prognosis and predictive factors
The optimal approach for the treatment of parathyroid adenoma includes excision

of the abnormal gland(s), as identified by preoperative localization studies, with intraoperative visualization of the other glands, biopsy of an additional normal gland, or confirmation of an appropriate decrease in PTH levels following excision of the abnormal gland(s) {1037}. Overall cure rates are excellent; however, recurrent or persistent hyperparathyroidism occurs in a subset of patients {410}. The causes of persistent or recurrent disease include initial treatment failure due to the inability to locate a normally positioned gland, anatomical factors such as ectopic or supernumerary glands, the biology of the underlying disease (hyperplasia vs adenoma), and implantation and regrowth of parathyroid tissue (parathyromatosis) resulting from incomplete excision of a lobulated adenoma or capsular rupture with spillage of adenoma cells {2250}. Rarely, recurrent or persistent disease can result from incomplete excision of an unrecognized carcinoma at initial surgery.

Secondary, mesenchymal and other tumours

DeLellis R. A.
Erickson L. A.
Thompson L. D. R.

Secondary tumours

Definition
Secondary tumours of the parathyroid glands are tumours involving the parathyroid glands as a result of direct extension from contiguous structures or lymphovascular spread from a distant primary site.

Epidemiology
Secondary involvement of normal or adenomatous parathyroid glands can occur as a result of direct extension from primary tumours of the larynx, oesophagus, thyroid gland, or adjacent soft tissues, or as a result of lymphovascular metastases from distant tumours. The most common primary sites include the breast, haemolymphatic system, skin (melanoma), lung, and kidney {159,511,630,2540}. Approximately 4% of thyroidectomies performed for cancer reveal direct extension of tumour into the parathyroid glands {1231, 2540}. When multiple parathyroid glands are sampled at autopsy of patients with disseminated malignancies of various types, as many as 12% contain metastatic deposits {1168,2540}. The specific epidemiological features are characteristic of the primary tumour types.

Localization
Secondary tumours can involve normal or hyperplastic parathyroid glands {2541}, in addition to parathyroid adenomas.

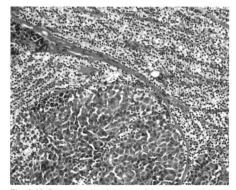

Fig. 3.19 Secondary involvement of the parathyroid gland by direct extension of a medullary thyroid carcinoma. The tumour cells form large nests, which are surrounded by chief cells with clear cytoplasm.

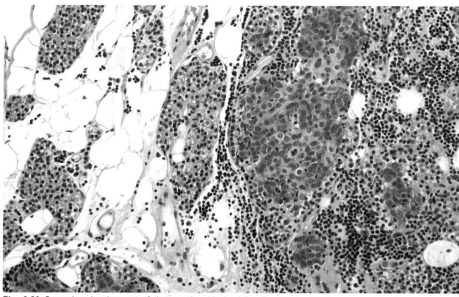

Fig. 3.20 Secondary involvement of the parathyroid gland by direct extension from an adjacent squamous cell carcinoma. Tumour cells form nests characterized by large nuclei and eosinophilic cytoplasm. Lymphocytes are present around the tumour cells and within the adjacent parathyroid tissue.

Clinical features
Many patients with secondary tumours of the parathyroid glands are asymptomatic, but some present with evidence of a neck mass. Depending on the extent of the tumour, there may be hoarseness, dysphagia, and neck pain. Hypoparathyroidism as a result of tumour replacement of the glands is exceptionally rare {1168}. Hypercalcaemia has been reported in a subset of patients with parathyroid metastases, but virtually all of the cases occurred in patients with concurrent osseous metastases {1168}.

Macroscopy
Metastases can be inapparent on gross examination or can cause enlargement of one or more glands {630}. In cases with direct local extension from an adjacent site, the tumours tend to be large and involve one or more glands.

Microscopy
Most tumours that involve the glands by direct extension are thyroid carcinomas (of various types), squamous cell carcinomas, lymphomas, or soft tissue tumours. Metastatic tumours arising from distant primary sites can involve normal or adenomatous glands, and they generally retain the cytohistological features of the primary tumour.

Prognosis and predictive factors
Prognosis depends on the nature of the primary malignancy, but is usually poor.

Mesenchymal and other tumours

Primary parathyroid mesenchymal and stromal tumours are exceptionally rare. There have been 3 reported cases of haemangiomas occurring in adenomatous or hyperplastic glands {1815, 2683} and a single case occurring in a normal parathyroid gland {1977}. It has been suggested that some of these lesions may in fact be exuberant tumour-associated vascular proliferations rather than true vascular neoplasms {2683}. Paraganglioma may arise rarely within the parathyroid {1598}.

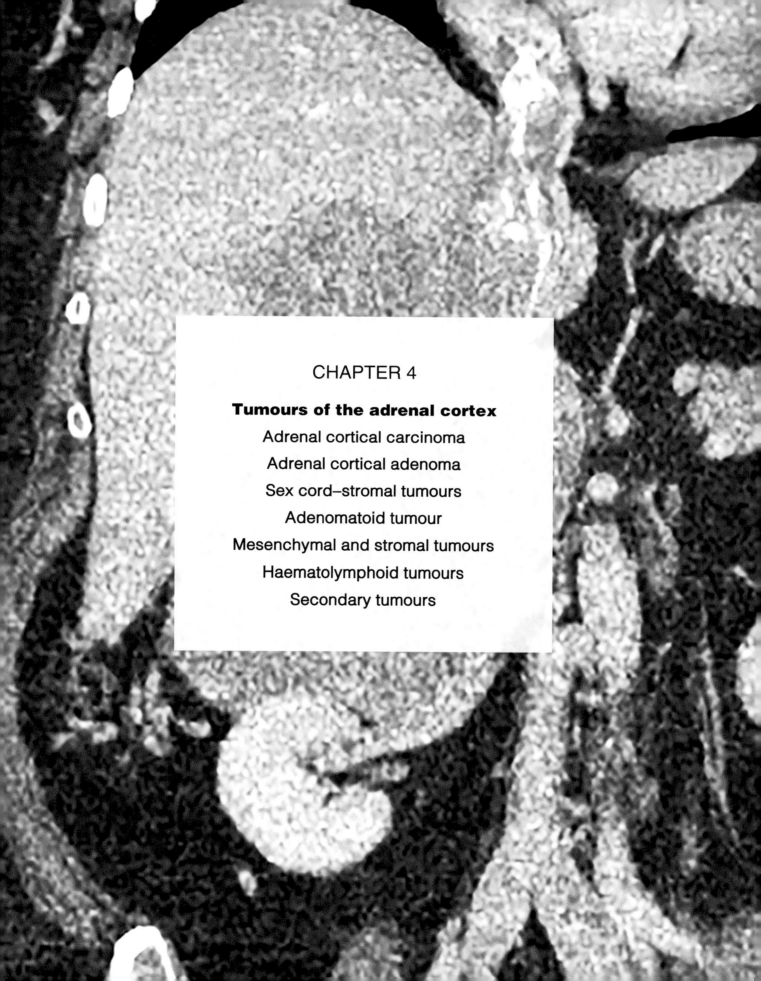

CHAPTER 4

Tumours of the adrenal cortex

Adrenal cortical carcinoma

Adrenal cortical adenoma

Sex cord–stromal tumours

Adenomatoid tumour

Mesenchymal and stromal tumours

Haematolymphoid tumours

Secondary tumours

WHO classification of tumours of the adrenal cortex

Adrenal cortical carcinoma	8370/3	**Haematolymphoid tumours**
Adrenal cortical adenoma	8370/0	**Secondary tumours**
Sex cord–stromal tumours	8590/1	
Adenomatoid tumour	9054/0	
Mesenchymal and stromal tumours		
Myelolipoma	8870/0	
Schwannoma	9560/0	

The morphology codes are from the International Classification of Diseases for Oncology (ICD-O) {898A}. Behaviour is coded /0 for benign tumours; /1 for unspecified, borderline, or uncertain behaviour; /2 for carcinoma in situ and grade III intraepithelial neoplasia; and /3 for malignant tumours. The classification is modified from the previous WHO classification, taking into account changes in our understanding of these lesions.

TNM classification of tumours of the adrenal cortex

T – Primary Tumour

TX Primary tumour cannot be assessed
T0 No evidence of primary tumour
T1 Tumour 5 cm or less in greatest dimension, no extra-adrenal invasion
T2 Tumour greater than 5 cm, no extra-adrenal invasion
T3 Tumour of any size with local invasion, but not invading adjacent organs*
T4 Tumour of any size with invasion of adjacent organs*

N – Regional Lymph Nodes

NX Regional lymph nodes cannot be assessed
N0 No regional lymph node metastasis
N1 Metastasis in regional lymph node(s)

M – Distant Metastasis

M0 No distant metastasis
M1 Distant metastasis

Stage

Stage I	T1	N0	M0
Stage II	T2	N0	M0
Stage III	T1, T2	N1	M0
	T3, T4	N0, N1	M0
Stage IV	Any T	Any N	M1

*Adjacent organs include kidney, diaphragm, great vessels (renal vein or vena cava), pancreas, and liver.

Adapted from: TNM Classification of Malignant Tumours, 8th Edition (2016). {323}

Adrenal cortical carcinoma

Giordano T. J.
Chrousos G. P.
de Krijger R. R.
Gill A.
Kawashima A.
Koch C. A.

Medeiros L. J.
Merino M. J.
Papathomas T. G.
Papotti M.
Sasano H. R.
Weiss L. M.

Definition
Adrenal cortical carcinoma is a malignant epithelial tumour of adrenal cortical cells.

ICD-O code   8370/3

Synonym
Adrenocortical carcinoma

Epidemiology
The annual incidence of adrenal cortical carcinoma is stable, at 0.5–2 cases per 1 million population {764,1338}. The incidence in southern Brazil is higher, due to a founder germline *TP53* R337H mutation {969}. The median patient age at diagnosis is in the fifth to sixth decade of life, but cases also occur in children; some series demonstrate a bimodal distribution with peaks in the first and fifth decades {3008}. There is a predilection for females, with a female-to-male ratio as high as 2.5:1 {1693,1834}.

Etiology
Adrenal cortical carcinomas, like all neoplastic processes, are thought to arise through acquired genetic mutations (see *Genetic profile*) in driver genes, with activation of key cellular signalling pathways {2887}. Many such mutations are believed to be random, arising during DNA replication {2792}. Adrenal cortical carcinomas can also be part of several hereditary syndromes (see *Genetic susceptibility*). Aside from hereditary syndromes, there are no established risk factors, although an equivocal association with smoking has been observed {1500}. Mutation signatures, including those typical of smoking and mismatch repair deficiency, have been reported in a subset of cases {3113}.

Localization
Most cases of adrenal cortical carcinoma involve a single adrenal gland; bilateral adrenal enlargement suggests other entities. For unknown reasons, the left adrenal gland is more commonly involved {835}. Rarely, carcinomas arising in ectopic adrenal tissue have been reported {27}.

Clinical features
Clinical symptoms and signs
Patients with adrenal cortical carcinoma can present in three distinct ways. About half of the patients present with the signs and symptoms of steroid hormone excess {58,1693}. About a third of the patients present with non-specific symptoms related to tumour growth, such as pain and abdominal fullness {833,1693}. The remaining cases are discovered incidentally during unrelated imaging procedures {764}.

The signs and symptoms of hormone excess reflect the particular endocrinopathy, which can be mixed. Hypercortisolism is the most common presentation, occurring in as many as 80% of patients

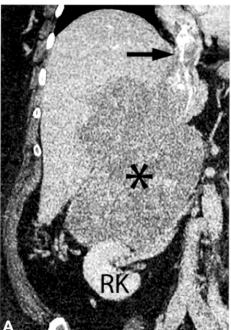 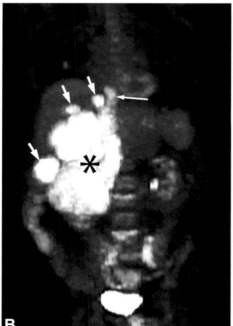 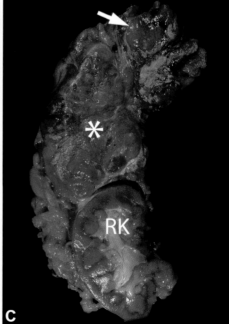

Fig. 4.01 Adrenal cortical carcinoma in a 50-year-old woman who presented with progressive lower extremity oedema. **A** Coronal CT shows a 15 cm soft tissue mass (asterisk) above the right kidney (RK), with an occlusive, partially calcified thrombus in the inferior vena cava extending into the right atrium (arrow). **B** Maximum-intensity projection of FDG-PET/CT demonstrates intense FDG avidity of the tumour (asterisk), with caval thrombus (long arrow) and hepatic metastases (short arrows). **C** Primary adrenal cortical carcinoma (asterisk) with a metastatic lesion in the liver (arrow). The kidney is not involved. RK, right kidney.

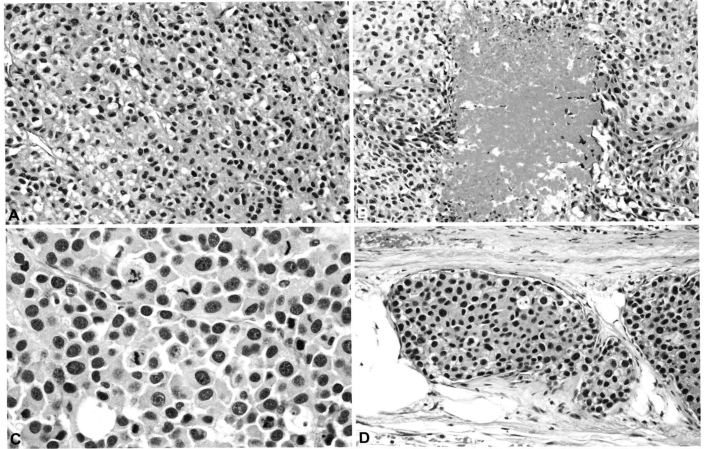

Fig. 4.02 Histological hallmarks and variants of adrenal cortical carcinoma. **A** Diffuse growth pattern. **B** Tumour necrosis. **C** Frequent mitotic figures. **D** Lymphovascular invasion is present.

with hormone excess. The classic signs and symptoms of Cushing syndrome include central obesity, muscle weakness, diabetes, osteoporosis, skin thinning and striae, impaired immune defence, hypertension, psychiatric disturbances, and gonadal dysfunction. Rapid-onset Cushing syndrome is usually indicative of adrenal cortical carcinoma {615}, with relatively little weight gain, marked muscle atrophy, and severe hypertension and diabetes {835}.

In females, androgen excess can be associated with hirsutism, virilization, and menstrual irregularities. In males, androgen excess often goes unrecognized due to a paucity of symptoms. Rare mineralocorticoid excess can lead to hypertension and hypokalaemia. Estrogen secretion, which is also rare in adrenal cortical carcinoma {1902}, results in gynaecomastia and testicular atrophy in males. Both androgen and estrogen production in the setting of an adrenal tumour raises suspicion for adrenal cortical carcinoma.

In general, adrenal cortical carcinomas are relatively large; the median size is > 10 cm and they can grow as large as 25 cm in diameter, particularly if nonfunctioning. Large tumours can cause local compressive symptoms and pain.

Imaging
Adrenal imaging can usually distinguish adenomas from carcinomas with reasonable accuracy {1269,1270}. Benign tumours with haemorrhage and revascularization can mimic carcinomas on

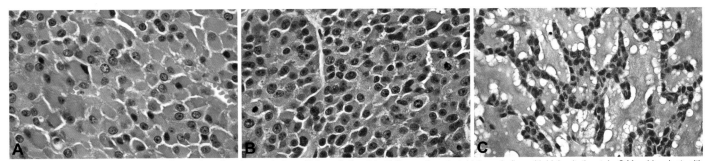

Fig. 4.03 Adrenal cortical carcinoma. **A** Oncocytic variant, low grade (i.e. with low mitotic rate). **B** Oncocytic variant, high grade (i.e. with high mitotic rate). **C** Myxoid variant, with abundant extracellular connective tissue–type mucin.

Table 4.01 Weiss criteria for malignancy in adrenal cortical tumours {2966,2967}; the presence of ≥ 3 of these criteria correlates with malignant behaviour

High nuclear grade (based on Fuhrman criteria)

Mitotic rate of > 5 mitoses per 50 high-power fields

Atypical mitotic figures

< 25% Clear cells

Diffuse architecture

Tumour necrosis

Venous invasion

Sinusoidal invasion

Capsular invasion

imaging {682}. Adrenal cortical carcinomas commonly display the following characteristics on imaging: size > 4 cm, necrosis, haemorrhage, heterogeneous CT density (> 10 Hounsfield units), heterogeneity on CT contrast washout, and heterogeneous signal drop on chemical-shift MRI. Functional imaging with FDG-PET can improve the diagnostic evaluation of adrenal cortical carcinoma {526}.

Tumour spread
Adrenal cortical carcinomas often displace and invade adjacent organs, including the kidneys, liver, pancreas, and inferior vena cava. Advanced disease is characterized by intrahepatic and regional lymph node metastases; local infiltration of the vena cava; and metastases to the liver, lungs, bone, and brain {764}.

Staging
The European Network for the Study of Adrenal Tumours (ENSAT) staging system is recommended {834,1685}. Stage I tumours are confined to the adrenal gland and are < 5 cm in diameter,

whereas stage II tumours are organ-confined and > 5 cm. Stage III tumours are characterized by involvement of surrounding tissue, positive regional lymph nodes, or involvement of regional veins. Stage IV disease is characterized by distant metastasis {835}.

Macroscopy
Most adrenal cortical carcinomas are large, solitary, circumscribed tumours. Some reach massive size and weight (exceeding 25 cm and 2 kg) before being discovered. The cut surface shows a yellowish-tan variegated appearance, with many intratumoural nodules that may reflect histological heterogeneity. Areas of necrosis and haemorrhage are frequent. Extensive sampling of all distinct areas and judicious assessment of the capsule are required. Gross extension into regional veins, extra-adrenal adipose tissue, and adjacent organs (kidney, pancreas, and liver) is usually apparent in stage III and IV disease.

Microscopy
In general, the tightly nested and corded growth patterns typical of adrenal cortical adenomas are replaced by one of several growth patterns in adrenal cortical carcinomas: solid, broad trabecular, or large nested. Other architectural hallmarks, such as true gland formation, are generally absent. Fibrous bands can be present, whereas intratumoural inflammatory cells are usually absent. Tumour encapsulation is the rule, with thick fibrous capsules particularly associated with carcinoma. Tumour necrosis is common, especially in high-grade tumours. Degenerative changes following haemorrhage, an increasingly recognized

Table 4.02 Lin–Weiss–Bisceglia criteria for diagnostic categorization of oncocytic adrenal cortical neoplasms {256}. The presence of 1 major criterion indicates malignancy; the presence of 1–4 minor criteria indicates uncertain malignant potential.

Major criteria
Mitotic rate of > 5 mitoses per 50 high-power fields
Atypical mitotic figures
Venous invasion

Minor criteria
Size > 10 cm and/or weight > 200 g
Necrosis
Sinusoidal invasion
Capsular invasion

occurrence, are not by themselves a sign of malignancy and should not be confused with bona fide tumour necrosis {682}. Tumour invasion, both capsular and vascular, is often striking and often present at the tumour–capsule interface. Mitoses are strong predictors of adrenal cortical carcinoma, an observation borne out by numerous molecular studies that have demonstrated the dominant role of cell proliferation in these tumours (see *Genetic profile*). Accordingly, all of the various clinicopathological algorithms developed for the diagnostic evaluation of adrenal cortical tumours incorporate mitotic rate {1175,2100,2147A,2850, 2966}. The Weiss criteria indicate that mitotic activity is optimally assessed by evaluating at least 10 random high power fields in the area of highest mitotic activity in each of 5 slides. At least 50 fields should be evaluated. If fewer than 50 fields are available {1560A}, immunostaining for phosphohistone may be helpful in highlighting mitoses in tumours with low mitotic count {720}.

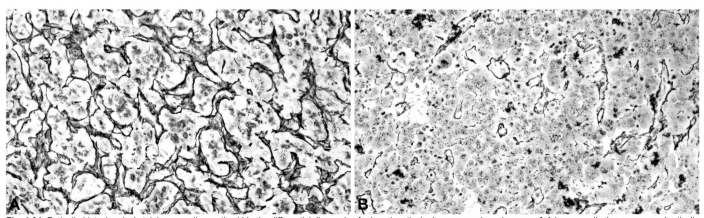

Fig. 4.04 Reticulin histochemical staining as a diagnostic aid in the differential diagnosis of adrenal cortical adenomas and carcinomas. **A** Adenomas display a preserved reticulin network similar to that of normal adrenal cortex. **B** Carcinomas show an altered network.

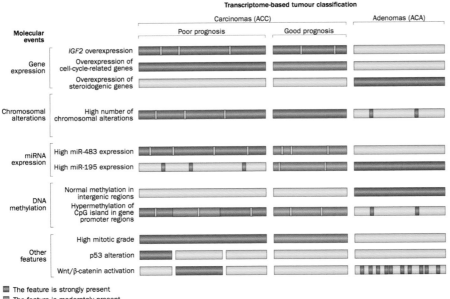

Transcriptome-based tumour classification

Fig. 4.05 Emerging molecular classification of adrenal cortical tumours based on various molecular parameters. Molecular information can distinguish adenomas from carcinomas. Carcinomas can be further divided into good and poor prognostic groups. Mutation of *TP53* and activation of the WNT/beta-catenin pathway are associated with poor prognosis and tend to be mutually exclusive. From Assié G, Jouinot A, Bertherat J {111}. Reprinted by permission from Macmillan Publishers Ltd.

Adrenal cortical carcinomas can be sub-divided on the basis of mitotic frequency into low grade (≤ 20 mitoses per 50 high-power fields) and high grade (> 20 mitoses per 50 high-power fields) {985, 2967}.

Considerable progress has been made in the assessment of adrenal cortical tumours over the past 25 years. Recognizing that individual parameters have low sensitivity for carcinoma diagnosis, several groups have proposed multifactorial diagnostic algorithms, which show a high degree of concordance {1175, 2850,2966}. Of these, the Weiss system (Table 4.01, p. 165) is the most widely accepted, but other systems may be useful in borderline cases and histological variants {2851}.

The recognized histological variants, in decreasing order of frequency, are oncocytic, myxoid, and sarcomatoid carcinomas {629}. Oncocytic tumours are characterized by oncocytes with abundant, densely eosinophilic cytoplasm {256,723, 1621,3002}. The Weiss system cannot be directly applied to oncocytic adrenal cortical neoplasms because of the consistent presence of eosinophilic cytoplasm, diffuse growth pattern, and high-grade nuclei. Therefore, diagnostic schemes specific for oncocytic adrenal cortical neoplasms have been established {256, 629,3002}, such as the Lin–Weiss–Bisceglia system (Table 4.02, p. 165).

Myxoid carcinomas have abundant extracellular connective tissue mucin {1183, 2106}. Sarcomatoid carcinomas show loss of cortical differentiation {540,1740, 3113} and can be biphasic with typical differentiated areas; when monophasic, these tumours can be indistinguishable from true sarcomas of the adrenal gland {1112} and retroperitoneal sarcomas that secondarily involve the adrenal gland {3113}.

The classification of paediatric adrenal cortical tumours is problematic, frequently leading to overdiagnosis of carcinoma {644}. The Weiss system cannot be applied, but a specialized classification system for paediatric tumours has been proposed {2985}.

Differential diagnosis and immunophenotype

The differential diagnosis of adrenal cortical carcinoma includes adrenal cortical adenoma and oncocytoma, phaeochromocytoma, renal cell carcinoma (primary and metastatic), hepatocellular carcinoma (primary and metastatic), sarcoma, metastatic melanoma, and other metastases (lung, colorectal, and bladder). Immunohistochemical evaluation plays an important role in the evaluation of adrenal masses. Adrenal cortical neoplasms express markers specific for steroid-producing cells, such as SF1 {2426,2427, 2440} and inhibin alpha, as well as markers expressed by other tumour types, such as melan-A and calretinin {352,856, 1838,1890,2408}. However, staining for these markers is variable and a panel approach is therefore used. Common epithelial markers, such as cytokeratin, EMA, and CEA are generally negative. Unlike chromogranin A, synaptophysin is frequently expressed and should not be used in the differential diagnosis with phaeochromocytoma.

The differential diagnosis with adrenal cortical adenoma is often straightforward, but cases with intermediate features pose a challenge. Rare cases with equivocal features may sometimes be diagnosed as adrenal cortical neoplasm of uncertain malignant potential. In addition to the accepted diagnostic algorithms, immunostaining for Ki-67 can be useful, with adenomas showing a Ki-67 proliferation index of < 5% and carcinomas of > 5% {91,2615,2912}. Similarly, overexpression of IGF2 supports a diagnosis of carcinoma {2615,2927}. Reticulin staining demonstrates the loss of nested architecture, has diagnostic power, and has been incorporated into a diagnostic algorithm along with necrosis, mitotic rate, and vascular invasion {719}. Despite these advances, the accurate classification of adrenal cortical neoplasms remains a challenge, with major diagnostic discrepancies in as many as 9% of cases {722}.

Genetic profile

Numerous studies have elucidated the molecular pathogenesis of adrenal cortical tumours, leading to a molecular classification of these tumours consistent with histology {111}. There is also emerging molecular evidence for an adenoma-to-carcinoma progression {629,2333}, albeit at an exceptionally low rate, given that most adenomas never progress to carcinoma {167,2072}.

Chromosomal imbalance and copy number alterations

Conventional cytogenetic analysis, comparative genomic hybridization, and high-density SNP arrays have revealed the

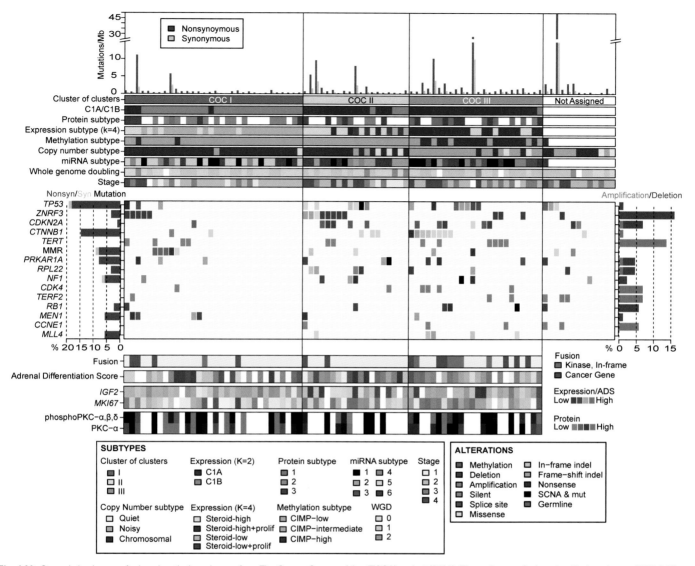

Fig. 4.06 Genomic landscape of adrenal cortical carcinoma, from The Cancer Genome Atlas (TCGA) project {859A}. Three classes of adrenal cortical carcinoma (COC I–III) are shown, along with mutation density, clustering from individual genomic platforms, tumour stage, and other key parameters, such as *MKI67* expression.

important role of chromosomal changes in the pathogenesis of adrenal cortical carcinoma {162,2333,2642,3108}. These findings have been confirmed and expanded by pan-genomic studies {112, 3113}.

Gene expression profiling
Collectively, gene expression profiling studies have defined the transcriptional signatures of adrenal cortical carcinomas and adenomas {986,1562,2583,2793}. *IGF2* is one of the most highly expressed genes in carcinomas {623,988}. The results of one gene expression profiling study have suggested that the expression of two genes, *DLGAP5* (previously called *DLG7*) and *PINK1*, could be used to identify carcinomas, including tumours of uncertain malignant potential (i.e. with a Weiss score of 2–3), and predict recurrence {636}.

MicroRNA expression profiling
MicroRNAs have been investigated as diagnostic and prognostic tools in adrenal cortical tumours {242,2128,2616}. Specific microRNA expression profiles have been associated with adrenal cortical carcinomas, including histological variants {721,2071,2468,2793}. MicroRNAs are also potential serum biomarkers {2125}. The clinical application of microRNAs as diagnostic tools awaits further validation.

DNA methylation profiling
Like gene expression profiling, DNA methylation profiling has been successfully used as a diagnostic tool to distinguish between adrenal cortical adenomas and carcinomas {866,2261}. Methylation profiles have also been used to define classes of adrenal cortical carcinoma with distinct survival rates {161, 3113}.

Integrated genomic characterization
Several integrated genomic characterizations of adult and paediatric adrenal cortical carcinomas have advanced our global understanding of the molecular pathogenesis and classification of these

Table 4.03 Hereditary syndromes associated with adrenal cortical carcinoma (ACC) {764}

Syndrome	Mutated gene(s)	Prevalence among patients with ACC
Li–Fraumeni syndrome	TP53	3–5% in adults 50–80% in children
Lynch syndrome	MSH2, MSH6, MLH1, PMS2	3% in adults
Multiple endocrine neoplasia type 1	MEN1	1–2% in adults
Familial adenomatous polyposis	APC	< 1%
Carney complex	PRKAR1A	< 1%
Beckwith–Wiedemann syndrome	IGF2, H19 at the 11p15 locus	< 1%
Neurofibromatosis type 1	NF1	< 1%

tumours {112,1276,2177,3113}. Collectively, these studies highlight essential molecular aspects of carcinomas, including (1) the highly prevalent role of *IGF2* overexpression; (2) the frequency of *TP53* mutations, their dominance in the paediatric cohort, and their association with aggressive disease; (3) the frequency and diversity of WNT pathway defects (*CTNNB1* point mutations and *ZNRF3* deletions), which are found in as many as 50% of cases; (4) the important role of copy-number alterations and whole-genome doubling as a mechanism for disease progression; (5) the important role of telomeres and telomerase reactivation; and (6) the relative lack of targetable hotspot mutations.

Genetic susceptibility

Most adrenal cortical carcinomas are sporadic. Several hereditary syndromes (Table 4.03) account for rare familial cases, with Li–Fraumeni syndrome accounting for most paediatric cases {2915, 2952}, especially in southern Brazil, where 0.3% of the population carries the founder germline *TP53* R337H mutation {969}. Other hereditary syndromes that can manifest with adrenal cortical carcinoma are Lynch syndrome {1794,2258}, multiple endocrine neoplasia type 1 {346, 941,1548,2582,2918}, familial adenomatous polyposis {942,1734,2587}, Carney complex {231,793,1905}, Beckwith–Wiedemann syndrome {233,1131}, and neurofibromatosis type 1 {1813}. Given

this wide variety of syndromes, it has been recommended that patients with adrenal cortical carcinoma be screened for hereditary diseases associated with *TP53* mutation and mismatch repair deficiency {764,2258}.

Prognosis and predictive factors

The 5-year overall survival rate associated with adrenal cortical carcinoma is 37–47% {764,835}. Several prognostic and predictive factors in adrenal cortical carcinoma have been identified over the past decade. Clinically relevant hypercortisolism has been confirmed to be an adverse prognostic factor in patients with completely resected disease {229}. In patients with advanced disease (stage III–IV), the modified European Network for the Study of Adrenal Tumours (mENSAT) staging system is highly correlated with overall survival, as are patient age > 50 years, symptoms related to tumour or to hormone excess, resection status, and tumour grade {1610}.

Mitotic grading of adrenal cortical carcinoma divides tumours into two prognostically relevant groups: low-grade carcinomas have < 20 mitoses per 50 high-power fields and high-grade carcinomas have ≥ 20 {2967}. This approach has been adopted by many centres {985}. Immunohistochemical assessment of Ki-67 has demonstrated significant prognostic and predictive power in both two-grade and three-grade schemes {241,1904,2093}. However, preanalytical

variability, lack of standardized assessment methods, and interobserver variability pose significant challenges {2093}. Other prognostic factors have also been reported. High expression of SF1, as assessed by immunohistochemistry, is correlated with poorer clinical outcome, an observation validated in an independent tumour set {724,2440}. miR-195 expression and miR-483-5p expression have been proposed as prognostic {2616} and predictive biomarkers {440}. Other emerging biomarkers (e.g. *TOP2A*, *EZH2*, and *BARD1*) might provide additional prognostic information {706,1218}. In two highly concordant studies of transcriptional signatures, adrenal cortical carcinomas were divided into two groups with different survival rates that reflected differences in mitotic rates and expression of cell-cycle genes {636,986}. The expression of two genes, *BUB1B* and *PINK1*, predicted prognosis {636}. The concept of two groups of adrenal cortical carcinoma with different outcomes was further confirmed by consensus clustering analysis of multidimensional genomic data classifying these tumours into two main molecular subgroups (C1A and C1B), which showed distinct genomic alterations {112}. Extending the C1A and C1B distinction, three classes of adrenal cortical carcinomas with significant survival differences were identified in a larger multidimensional genomic study {3113}, a result consistent with the three-grade schemes derived from recent Ki-67 expression studies {241,720}.

The ability to accurately predict treatment response to the adrenolytic agent mitotane would be a major advance, because not all patients respond and the drug is highly toxic. Several candidate biomarkers for mitotane response have been identified. The expression of RRM1 {2896} and CYP2W1 {2334} may be predictive of mitotane response. If validated, these biomarkers could spare many patients from unnecessarily experiencing the adverse effects associated with this drug.

Adrenal cortical adenoma

Giordano T. J.
Chrousos G. P.
Kawashima A.
Koch C. A.
Sasano H. R.
Young W. F.

Definition

Adrenal cortical adenoma is a benign epithelial tumour of adrenal cortical cells.

ICD-O code   8370/0

Synonym

Adrenocortical adenoma

Epidemiology

Adrenal cortical nodules are common, affecting as much as 10% of the population, with incidence increasing with age {1732}. They occur in all age groups and in both sexes. As is true in other endocrine organs, the distinction between hyperplastic nodules and true neoplasms in the adrenal cortex is difficult and arbitrary. Therefore, the true incidence of adrenal cortical adenoma is unknown; however, the incidence seems to have sharply increased recently {1611,3092}, possibly as a consequence of increasing use of CT abdominal imaging and the ageing population {297}. Adrenal cortical adenoma accounts for a large proportion of incidentally discovered adrenal tumours (so-called adrenal incidentalomas) {345,1322,1611,1936}.

Etiology

Adrenal cortical adenomas can be part of several hereditary syndromes (see *Genetic susceptibility*). There are no proven environmental factors that lead to adenoma development. There is emerging evidence that aldosterone-producing adenomas arise from cell clusters within the zona glomerulosa, termed aldosterone-producing cell clusters {294,2002,2003}. The mutations found to be associated with autonomous aldosterone production (see *Genetic profile*) support this model of adenoma formation {846,2004}.

Localization

The vast majority of adrenal cortical adenomas are unilateral masses, almost by definition, because most multinodular processes would more likely be pathologically classified as hyperplasia. Precise localization to the various zones of the adrenal gland is not possible.

Clinical features

Adrenal cortical adenomas can be non-functioning, or they can be associated with several endocrinopathies, depending on the hormonal secretory status of the tumour.

Aldosterone-producing adenoma: Aldosterone production related to an adrenal cortical lesion is called primary aldosteronism (or Conn syndrome) and typically results in hypertension and hypokalaemia/normokalaemia, as well as higher rates of cardiovascular disease. Symptoms are non-specific and include muscle weakness, cramping, headaches, palpitations, polydipsia, polyuria, and nocturia. Physical findings are also non-specific; however, many patients have hypertension. The evaluation of aldosterone production includes measurement of plasma renin activity and plasma aldosterone levels.

Cortisol-producing adenoma: Cortisol hypersecretion typically results in ACTH-independent Cushing syndrome, with weight gain, central obesity, facial rounding, hirsutism, easy bruising, poor wound healing, wide purplish-red skin striae, proximal muscle weakness, hyperglycaemia, hypertension, osteoporosis, and susceptibility to opportunistic infections. Hypercortisolism must be evaluated with baseline morning and evening measurements of serum and saliva free cortisol, and a 24-hour urinary free cortisol test. Autonomy can be confirmed with the dexamethasone suppression test. A suppressed plasma ACTH level classifies the hypercortisolism as ACTH-independent. Subclinical Cushing syndrome is also recognized, in which autonomous glucocorticoid production occurs without the overt specific signs and symptoms of Cushing syndrome {2270}.

Sex-hormone–producing adenoma: Secretion of sex hormones is more commonly observed in adrenal cortical carcinomas; sex-hormone–producing adenomas are rare. Patients with these adenomas have signs and symptoms that reflect the particular sex hormones secreted by the tumours. Androgen excess in females leads to hirsutism, amenorrhoea, and virilization, whereas estrogen excess in males results in gynaecomastia and impotence.

Non-functioning adenomas: The detection of non-functioning adrenal masses incidentally discovered on radiological imaging (adrenal incidentalomas) has increased in parallel with increasing use of computed abdominal imaging. The diagnostic evaluation of adrenal incidentalomas includes physical examination, hormonal evaluation, and dedicated adrenal imaging to assess lipid content. Non-functioning tumours that are lipid-rich on imaging can be followed by observation, whereas tumours that are lipid-poor, tumours with heterogeneity, and tumours with subclinical hormone excess should be considered for surgery. The growth

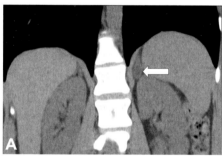

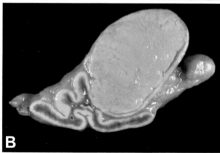

Fig. 4.07 Adrenal cortical adenoma. Aldosterone-producing adenoma in a 34-year-old woman. **A** Coronal CT of the abdomen shows a 1.8 cm left adrenal cortical nodule (arrow). **B** At laparoscopic left adrenalectomy, the adrenal gland contained a 1.6 × 1.6 × 1.1 cm yellow cortical adenoma.

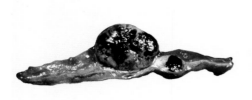

A

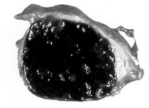

B

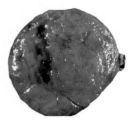

C

Fig. 4.08 Adrenal cortical adenoma. **A** Cushing adenoma. The cut surface of this small tumour has a heterogeneous tan and brown appearance. **B** Pigmented (black) adenoma. **C** Oncocytoma.

rate of adrenal incidentalomas seems to be very low, at 0.02–0.53 cm per year {541}.

Macroscopy

Most adrenal cortical adenomas are well-circumscribed masses confined to the gland. They are typically solitary and tend to be < 5–6 cm and weigh < 50–100 g, although giant adenomas have been reported {665,1496}. Large tumours are often related to acute haemorrhage, followed by central organization and degeneration. They may be encapsulated. Determining hormonal production on the basis of gross appearance is imprecise, but aldosterone-producing adenomas tend to be yellowish-orange and cortisol-producing adenomas are often tan in colour. Black adenomas, usually related to intracellular accumulation of lipofuscin (and rarely, of melanin), have been described {90,1302}. Myelolipomatous foci, which are of no clinical significance, are often found within adenomas. In cortisol-producing adenomas, the adjacent adrenal gland (zona fasciculata and zona reticularis) often shows marked cortical atrophy due to suppression of the hypothalamic–pituitary–adrenal axis secondary to excess cortisol secretion.

Microscopy

Adrenal cortical adenomas consist of lipid-rich cells with abundant intracytoplasmic lipid droplets resembling zona fasciculata and lipid-poor compact cells resembling zona reticularis, in varying proportions. The adenoma growth pattern is characterized by cords, nests, and islands of cortical cells separated by abundant vasculature and sinusoidal structures. Nuclei tend to be small and uniform, although isolated extreme nuclear pleomorphism is common {2424}. Mitotic activity is absent or very low {2648,2966}. In patients treated with spironolactone, adrenal cortical adenomas and non-neoplastic cortex often develop eosinophilic intracytoplasmic inclusions called spironolactone bodies {617}. Lipomatous or myelolipomatous foci can be seen {1898}. Importantly, the histological hallmarks of adrenal cortical carcinoma (see *Adrenal cortical carcinoma*, p. 163), such as tumour cell invasion (capsular and vascular), diffuse growth pattern, necrosis, high nuclear grade, mitoses, and atypical mitoses, are generally absent. Reticulin histochemical staining reveals an intact network, a validated observation with diagnostic power {719, 2889}. Myxoid change is occasionally encountered in adenomas, but is a more frequent finding in carcinoma.

Oncocytoma

Adrenal cortical oncocytomas are composed of large cells with dense eosinophilic cytoplasm {2428}. They often show isolated nuclear pleomorphism and prominent nucleoli {1621}, features shared with oncocytomas found at other sites. Oncocytomas are most often nonfunctioning, but can be associated with androgen excess and virilization {2518}. On CT, oncocytomas are indistinguishable from lipid-poor adenomas {1349}.

Immunophenotype

The cells of adrenal cortical adenomas are immunoreactive for several proteins, including SF1 {778,2409,2425}, inhibin alpha {499,1781}, synaptophysin {1432},

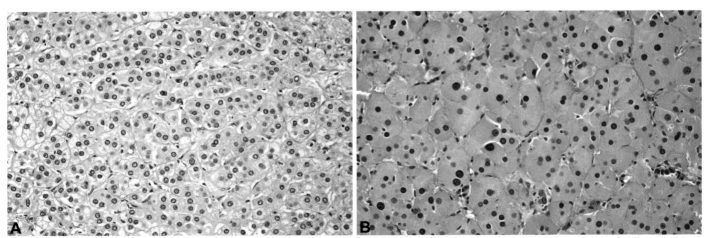

Fig. 4.09 Adrenal cortical adenoma. **A** Cushing adenoma with nested growth pattern and lipid-poor cortical cells with eosinophilic cytoplasm. **B** Adrenal cortical oncocytoma composed of large cells with intensely eosinophilic cytoplasm.

Haematolymphoid tumours

Weiss L.M.
Jaffe E.S.

Definition
Primary haematolymphoid tumours involving the adrenal gland are essentially limited to lymphoma and plasmacytoma.

Synonym
Primary adrenal lymphoma

Epidemiology
Secondary involvement of the adrenal gland by leukaemia and lymphoma occurs in as many as 20% of cases, whereas primary involvement is rare. Most haematolymphoid tumours involving the adrenal gland are lymphomas, although very rare cases of extramedullary plasmacytoma have also been described. Most lymphomas occur in older adults, with a male predominance.

Etiology
Primary haematolymphoid disorders in the adrenal gland may be rare due to the secretion of endogenous steroids, which have a suppressive effect on lymphoid proliferation. An association with EBV has been described for both B-cell and T-cell lymphomas {2242}.

Localization
Both unilateral and bilateral involvement can occur as primary cases. Effacement of both the cortex and medulla is usually seen. Involvement of adjacent para-aortic lymph nodes can be seen in some cases, but should be less prominent than the primary adrenal mass.

Clinical features
Most cases present either as a solitary mass (typically very large) or, even more commonly, as bilateral masses, which are solid or, less commonly, cystic {1039, 1317,2242,2472}. Many patients have B symptoms. About half of all patients, particularly those with bilateral tumours, have concomitant symptoms of adrenal insufficiency.

Microscopy
Both B-cell and T-cell lymphomas have been described, with B-cell lymphomas predominating {1039,1317,1920,2242}. Diffuse large B-cell lymphoma, NOS, is the most common B-cell lymphoma, although plasmablastic lymphoma, Burkitt lymphoma, and even low-grade B-cell lymphomas have also been reported. A variety of T-cell lymphomas have been reported, including peripheral T-cell lymphoma, NOS, and extranodal NK/T-cell lymphoma of nasal type. Rare cases of extranodal plasmacytoma primary in the adrenal gland have been reported, mostly in the older literature {376}.

Genetic profile
Most diffuse large B-cell lymphomas primary to the adrenal gland are of activated B-cell type {1920}. Many of these cases have *BCL6* gene rearrangement.

Prognosis and predictive factors
Prognosis depends on the classification of the haematolymphoid malignancy. Poor prognosis has been reported in some series {1920}.

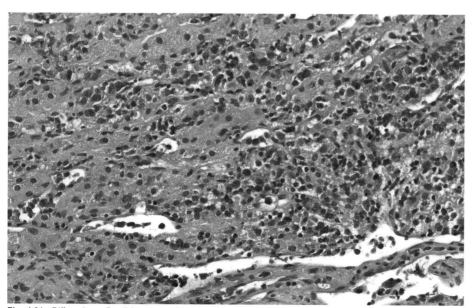

Fig. 4.21 Diffuse large B-cell lymphoma involving the adrenal gland. A diffuse infiltrate of large lymphoid cells is apparent, with sinusoidal infiltration seen in the adjacent adrenal cortex.

Secondary tumours

Sasano H. R.
Cheng L.
DeLellis R. A.
Kawashima A.

Lack E.
Lam A. K. Y.
Lloyd R. V.
Tischler A. S.

Definition
Secondary tumours of the adrenal cortex are tumours that originate in extra-adrenal locations and spread to the adrenal gland by either metastasis or direct infiltration.

Synonym
Metastatic adrenal tumours

Epidemiology
Adrenal metastasis is reported in as many as 27% of cancer cases {310,996, 1534}. The adrenal gland is the fourth most common site of metastasis, after the lungs, liver, and bone. The most common primary sites are the breast, lung, kidney, stomach, pancreas, oesophagus, and liver / bile duct {1534,2035}. Adrenal metastasis is usually detected in the setting of advanced-stage disease. Presentation with a solitary adrenal metastasis is uncommon {2259}.

Localization
Bilateral metastases are detected in more than half of patients {1534,2375}.

Clinical features
Most cases are identified at staging or follow-up of patients with known cancer diagnoses. Adrenal cortical insufficiency may occur due to destruction of adrenal tissues {1534,2265,2497}. Metastasis of ACTH-producing neuroendocrine carcinoma can result in hyperplasia

and more-pronounced cortisol overproduction in the adjacent adrenal cortex {2434}. CT is a valuable imaging procedure for evaluating adrenal tumours {127, 381,1773}. MRI may facilitate differential diagnosis {2825,3005}. FDG-PET/CT is useful {3027}. PET/CT has high sensitivity and specificity for adrenal metastasis in non-small cell lung carcinoma {2651}, but accurate diagnosis requires biopsy confirmation {2163,2651}. Endoscopic ultrasound in conjunction with fine-needle aspiration has been used diagnostically {2836}.

Macroscopy
In contrast to the appearance of primary adrenal cortical tumours, which are commonly yellow, the gross appearance of metastatic tumours depends on the type of tumour.

Microscopy
Carcinoma, primarily adenocarcinoma, constitutes > 90% of metastatic tumours. Some tumours, such as renal cell carcinoma, large cell neuroendocrine carcinoma of the lung, hepatocellular carcinoma, and melanoma, can prove particularly challenging diagnostically at the time of adrenal biopsy. Immunohistochemistry may provide valuable information in this differential diagnosis. Markers used to identify adrenal cortical tumours include inhibin alpha, calretinin, melan-A, and SF1 {352,856,1838,2426}. SF1 may

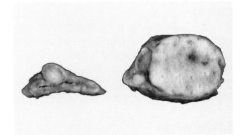

Fig. 4.22 Secondary tumour of the adrenal cortex. Bilateral adrenal metastasis from colon adenocarcinoma. The foci of metastasis appear white to light grey on the cut surface.

be the most valuable marker in this differential diagnosis {2408,2426}. Adrenal cortical tumours are typically negative for cytokeratins, although there are exceptions {1550,1891,2971}. It can be difficult to distinguish between adrenal cortical tumours and metastatic neuroendocrine tumours or phaeochromocytoma. Synaptophysin, but not chromogranin or CD56, is commonly positive in adrenal cortical tumours {2972}.

Prognosis and predictive factors
Patients with metastasis to the adrenal glands are at an advanced stage of disease. Systemic therapy tailored to the type of primary tumour has been the treatment of choice. Adrenalectomy or surgical resection of adrenal metastasis has been performed, with improved survival in some highly selected cases {1044,2259,2325,2429}.

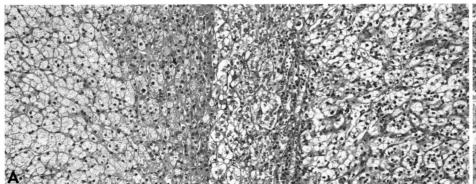
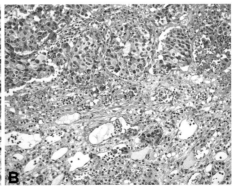

Fig. 4.23 Secondary tumour of the adrenal cortex. **A** Adrenal tissue (left) with metastasis from clear cell renal cell carcinoma (right). Histologically, the tumour cells resemble adrenal cortical parenchymal cells. **B** Metastatic adrenal tumour from large cell neuroendocrine carcinoma of the lung.

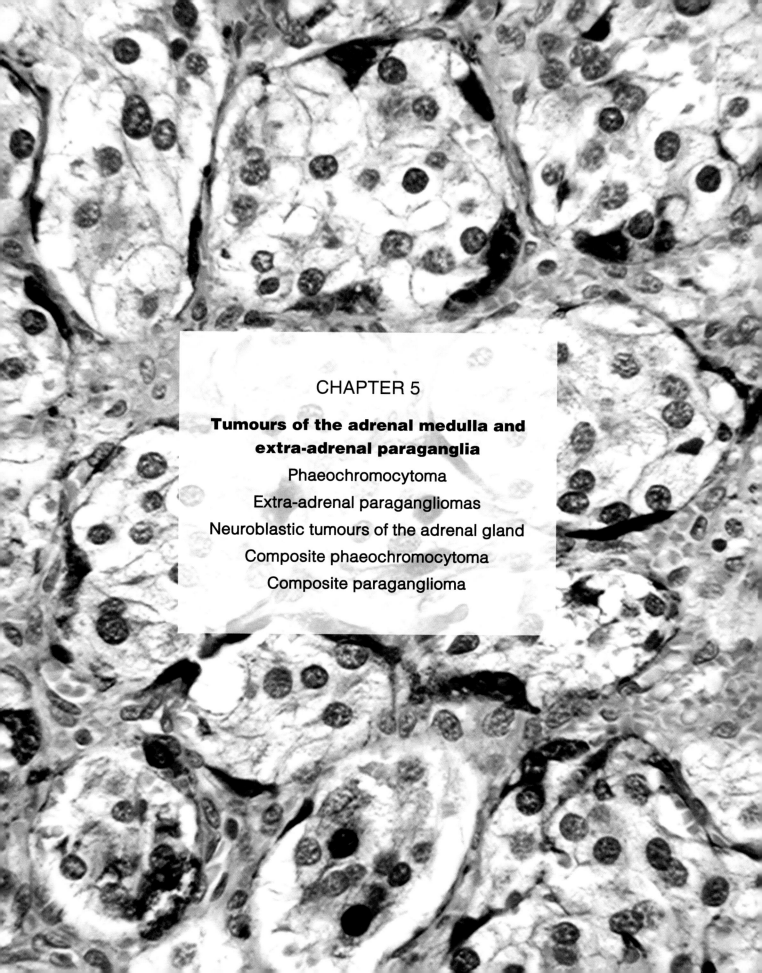

CHAPTER 5

Tumours of the adrenal medulla and extra-adrenal paraganglia

Phaeochromocytoma

Extra-adrenal paragangliomas

Neuroblastic tumours of the adrenal gland

Composite phaeochromocytoma

Composite paraganglioma

WHO classification of tumours of the adrenal medulla and extra-adrenal paraganglia

Phaeochromocytoma	8700/3
Extra-adrenal paragangliomas	
Head and neck paragangliomas	
Carotid body paraganglioma	8692/3*
Jugulotympanic paraganglioma	8690/3*
Vagal paraganglioma	8693/3
Laryngeal paraganglioma	8693/3
Sympathetic paragangliomas	8693/3

Neuroblastic tumours of the adrenal gland	
Neuroblastoma	9500/3
Ganglioneuroblastoma, nodular	9490/3
Ganglioneuroblastoma, intermixed	9490/3
Ganglioneuroma	9490/0
Composite phaeochromocytoma	8700/3
Composite paraganglioma	8693/3

The morphology codes are from the International Classification of Diseases for Oncology (ICD-O) {898A}. Behaviour is coded /0 for benign tumours; /1 for unspecified, borderline, or uncertain behaviour; /2 for carcinoma in situ and grade III intraepithelial neoplasia; and /3 for malignant tumours. The classification is modified from the previous WHO classification, taking into account changes in our understanding of these lesions.

TNM staging of tumours of the adrenal medulla and extra-adrenal paraganglia (phaeochromocytoma and paraganglioma)

T – Primary Tumour

TX — Primary tumour cannot be assessed
T0 — No evidence of primary tumour
T1 — Phaeochromocytoma within adrenal gland less than 5 cm in greatest dimension, no extra-adrenal invasion
T2 — Phaeochromocytoma within adrenal gland 5 cm or more in greatest dimension, or functional paraganglioma of any size, no extra-adrenal invasion
T3 — Tumour of any size with invasion into surrounding tissues (e.g., liver, pancreas, spleen, kidneys)

N – Regional Lymph Nodes

NX — Regional lymph nodes cannot be assessed
N0 — No regional lymph node metastasis
N1 — Metastasis in regional lymph node(s)

M – Distant Metastasis

M0 — No distant metastasis
M1 — Distant metastasis

Stage

Stage I	T1	N0	M0
Stage II	T2	N0	M0
Stage III	T1	N1	M0
	T2	N1	M0
	T3	Any N	M0
Stage IV	Any T	Any N	M1

Adapted from: AJCC Cancer Staging Manual, 8th Edition, 2017. {72A}

Introduction

Tischler A. S.
de Krijger R. R.
Gill A.
Kawashima A.
Kimura N.
Komminoth P.

Papathomas T. G.
Thompson L. D. R.
Tissier F.
Williams M. D.
Young W. F.

Since the publication of the 2004 WHO classification, new genetic discoveries have profoundly altered our understanding of phaeochromocytoma and paraganglioma. At least 30% of these tumours are now known to be hereditary. Germline mutations in at least 19 hereditary susceptibility genes have been reported to date, and somatic mutations of some of the same genes have been identified in sporadic tumours. Genotype–phenotype correlations determine tumour distribution, hormonal function, multiplicity, risk of metastasis, and syndromic associations (Table 5.02). A surprising development has been the identification of the Krebs cycle as a nidus of hereditary tumour susceptibility genes responsible for distinct but overlapping tumour syndromes. Mutations in genes encoding succinate dehydrogenase subunits, collectively known as the SDH gene family, have been identified as the most common cause of hereditary phaeochromocytoma and paraganglioma, surpassing mutations of VHL and RET. Germline mutations in malate dehydrogenase genes and FH have also been reported in a few cases, as have somatic mutations in isocitrate dehydrogenase genes.

Additional new developments have been the discovery of overlap between phenotypes associated with different genes and the expansion of the spectra of syndromic lesions to include new and sometimes common tumours. Syndrome overlap can occur not only with newly recognized syndromes but also with long-established ones. Hereditary gastrointestinal stromal tumour, previously

thought to be associated with neurofibromatosis, is now recognized as a component of the SDH-related syndromes and termed succinate dehydrogenase–deficient gastrointestinal stromal tumour. Common tumours now included in some syndromes include pituitary adenoma and renal cell carcinoma.

The expanded known genetic landscape presents new challenges to both clinicians and pathologists. With patients who present with an apparently sporadic phaeochromocytoma, paraganglioma, or syndromically associated tumour, the challenge is to determine whether there

is occult hereditary susceptibility. Targeted genetic testing based on tumour location, biochemical phenotype, and pathology plays an important role in identifying cases of hereditary disease {593}. Targeted testing has some limitations such as the size of the testing panel, so some hereditary lesions with rare or unknown mutations {421} will not be detected. Therefore targeted gene panels will have to be expanded to include all known susceptibility genes. Alternatively, next-generation sequencing can be done to detect variants of uncertain significance that could otherwise lead to overdiagnosis if they ultimately prove to be inconsequential {1970}. When there is evidence suggesting a hereditary syndrome, the challenges are to exclude the possibility that the suspected syndromic tumours are in fact merely coincidental, to determine to which syndrome the tumours are related, and to devise an appropriate follow-up strategy {663,1244}. Pathologists can contribute to meeting these challenges by recognizing the distinct morphological features sometimes associated with syndromic gastrointestinal stromal tumour {976}, renal cell carcinoma {978}, and pituitary adenoma {663}. Immunohistochemical staining for SDHB and SDHA can be a valuable ancillary tool for assessing the involvement of SDH gene mutations {727,976, 978,2092} and for validating variants of uncertain significance. Above all, pathologists must be aware of the rapidly changing status of this field, in order to effectively communicate new information to clinical colleagues {2784}.

Table 5.01 Somatic mutations in sporadic phaeochromocytoma and paraganglioma

Mutated gene	Frequency	Reference
NF1	21–41%	{599}
ATRX	12.6%	{859}
HRAS	5–10%	{580,1682,2067}
VHL	9.2%	{351}
EPAS1 (also called HIF2A)	5–7.4%	{547,2974}
CDKN2A	7%	{430}
RET	5%	{351}
TP53	2.35–10%	{430,1682}
MET	2.5%	{430}
BRAF	1.2%	{1682}
MAX	1.65–2.5%	{349,351}
IDH1	Very rare	{913}
KIF1B	Very rare	{2461}
SDH gene family	Very rare	{182,593,989,2124}

Table 5.02 Genotype–phenotype correlations of hereditary phaeochromocytoma (PCC) and paraganglioma (PGL) susceptibility genes

Gene (locus) Syndrome	Approximate frequency[a]	Distribution[a]			Approximate risk of metastasis[a]	Syndromic lesions
		PCC	PGL of abdomen or thorax	PGL of head and neck		
VHL (3p25.5) VHL	9%	+++	Rare	Very rare	5%	RCC; HB; pancreatic and other NETs; pancreatic serous cystadenoma; renal, hepatic, and epididymal cysts; endolymphatic sac tumours {507}
RET[b] (10q11.2) MEN2	5%	+++	Rare	Very rare	< 5%	MTC, parathyroid hyperplasia/adenoma, Marfanoid habitus, mucocutaneous neuroma, gastrointestinal ganglioneuromatosis, cutaneous lichen amyloidosis {2251}
NF1 (17q11.2) NF1	2%	++	Rare	Very rare	12%	Neurofibroma, café-au-lait spots, Lisch nodules, GIST, MPNST, duodenal NET (SOM) {807,3033}
SDHD (11q23) PGL1/CSS	5–7%	+	++	++	< 5%	RCCc, SDH-deficient GIST, PA {807,1984}
SDHAF2 (11q12.2) PGL2/CSS	< 1%	–	–	++	Low	None reported {807}
SDHC (1q23.3) PGL3/CSS	1–2%	Rare	Rare	++	Low	SDH-deficient RCC, SDH-deficient GIST {807}
SDHB (1p36.13) PGL4/CSS	6–8%	+	+++	+	30–70%	SDH-deficient RCC, SDH-deficient GIST, PA {807}
SDHA (5p15.33) PGL5/CSS	1–2%	Rare	+	+	Low	SDH-deficient RCC[c], SDH-deficient GIST, PA {807,3033}
TMEM127 (2q11.2)	1%	++	+	+	Low	RCC[c] {1136,2220}
MAX (14q23.3)	1%	+	+	+[c]	10%	None reported {349}
EPAS1[b] (2p21) PZS[d]	Very rare	+[c]	+		29%	Polycythaemia, duodenal NET (SOM), ocular abnormalities {595A,1673,2074}
EGLN2 (19q13.2)	Very rare	+	+		Unknown	Polycythaemia {3050}
EGLN1 (1q42.1)	Very rare	+	+		Unknown	Polycythaemia {1520,3050}
FH (1q42.1)	1%	+	+	+	> 50%	HLRCC-associated RCC, cutaneous and uterine leiomyoma {529,2181}
MDH2 (7q11.23)	Very rare		+		Unknown	None reported {416}
KIF1B (1p36.22)	Very rare				Unknown	Ganglioneuroma, leiomyosarcoma, lung adenocarcinoma, neuroblastoma {3062}
MEN1 (11q13.1)	Very rare	+		+	Unknown	Parathyroid adenoma/hyperplasia; pancreatic NET; enteric, bronchopulmonary, and thymic NET; PA; adrenal cortical adenoma, lipoma, angiofibroma, collagenoma, and meningioma {941,1244}

CSS, Carney–Stratakis syndrome (paraganglioma and gastric stromal sarcoma); GIST, gastrointestinal stromal tumour; HB, haemangioblastoma; HLRCC, hereditary leiomyomatosis and renal cell carcinoma; MEN2, multiple endocrine neoplasia type 2; MPNST, malignant peripheral nerve sheath tumour; MTC, medullary thyroid carcinoma; NET, neuroendocrine tumour; NF1, neurofibromatosis type 1; PA, pituitary adenoma; PGL1–5, paraganglioma syndrome types 1–5; PZS, Pacak–Zhuang syndrome; RCC, renal cell carcinoma; SDH, succinate dehydrogenase; SOM, duodenal somatostatinoma; VHL, von Hippel–Lindau syndrome.

[a] Unless otherwise specified, data for frequency, distribution, and risk of metastasis are approximations based on compilations encompassing several databases {271,342, 599,2077}. Frequency indicates the proportion of all PCCs and PGLs (as combined data) associated with mutations of each gene.
[b] Proto-oncogene/gain-of-function mutations.
[c] Insufficient data available.
[d] PZS is a recently described endocrine tumour syndrome caused by gain-of-function mutations in EPAS1 (also called HIF2A) {595A,1673,2076,2807}. The manifestations include PCCs, multiple PGLs, somatostatin-producing NETs in the duodenum, polycythaemia, and bilateral ocular manifestations including dilated capillaries, retinal neovascularization, and fibrosis overlying the optic disc {2074}. Most cases are caused by somatic mosaicism {3048}. One hereditary case has been reported {1673}.

Phaeochromocytoma

Tischler A. S.
de Krijger R. R.
Gill A.
Kawashima A.
Kimura N.
Komminoth P.
Papathomas T. G.
Thompson L. D. R.
Tissier F.
Williams M. D.
Young W. F.

Definition
A tumour of chromaffin cells that arises in the adrenal medulla.

ICD-O code
8700/3

Synonyms
Benign phaeochromocytoma; malignant phaeochromocytoma; paraganglioma; chromaffinoma

Historical annotation
A phaeochromocytoma is an intra-adrenal sympathetic paraganglioma. The name, meaning "dusky-coloured tumour" in Latin, derives from the brown colour that develops when catecholamines in the tumour tissue react with chromate or other weak oxidizing agents (the chromaffin reaction).

Epidemiology
The annual incidence of phaeochromocytoma is 0.4–9.5 cases per 1 million population, with geographical variations likely attributable both to founder mutations resulting in different prevalence rates of hereditary tumours {75,848,1156, 2641} and to variable reporting of cases to cancer registries. Most historical series included both phaeochromocytomas and extra-adrenal sympathetic paragangliomas, which are approximately one tenth as common as phaeochromocytomas in adults and one third as common in children. Some series were based on combinations of clinical and autopsy diagnoses {186,2983}. Currently, as many as 61% of phaeochromocytomas are discovered as incidentalomas {128,2062}. Most phaeochromocytomas present in the fourth to fifth decades of life, with a roughly equal sex distribution. However, they can occur in patients of any age, including very young children and elderly individuals {2962}. The youngest reported patient was 2.7 years old {2621}. Hereditary disease tends to first manifest before the age of 40 years, but can also present late in life {2962}. As many as 70% of children aged < 10 years with an apparently sporadic phaeochromocytoma are

eventually shown to have hereditary disease {2916}.

Etiology
The only known causative factor for human phaeochromocytoma is hereditary susceptibility.

Localization
By definition, phaeochromocytomas arise exclusively in the adrenal glands. Morphologically and functionally similar tumours arising in extra-adrenal paraganglia are classified as paragangliomas.

Clinical features
Clinical symptoms and signs
All phaeochromocytomas are capable of catecholamine synthesis, and most signs and symptoms are caused by excess catecholamine production and release. The most common sign is hypertension, which can be sustained or paroxysmal. The classic triad of headache, tachycardia/palpitations, and sweating is seen in < 25% of patients. At least one component of the triad occurs in slightly less than 50% of patients {128}. Less frequent findings include orthostatic hypotension, pallor, tremors, anxiety, and panic attacks. So-called spells, defined as recurrent, self-limited, and stereotypical symptoms or groups of symptoms with sudden onset, are a diagnostically useful but non-specific finding {3077}. A lesser-known finding is severe constipation, seen in about 6% of patients and associated with norepinephrine production {2773}. Increasingly, patients whose tumours are discovered as incidentalomas or after positive screening for a hereditary susceptibility gene are asymptomatic {2062}. Factors contributing to the absence of symptoms include small tumour size and O-methylation of catecholamines within tumour cells to produce metanephrines {741,742}.

Phaeochromocytomas occasionally cause paraneoplastic syndromes by producing ectopic regulatory peptides. The most common is Cushing syndrome, caused by ACTH {1987} or (rarely) CRH

{183} secretion. The syndrome of watery diarrhoea, hypokalaemia, and achlorhydria (WDHA syndrome, also called Verner–Morrison syndrome) can be caused by production of VIP {1662}, most often in composite phaeochromocytomas containing areas of ganglioneuroma or ganglioneuroblastoma {1260,2783}. Polycythaemia attributed to tumoural and systemic production of erythropoietin {2076} or increased sensitivity of erythropoietin receptors {3050} is associated with phaeochromocytomas/paragangliomas caused by mutations in *EPAS1* (also called *HIF2A*) or *EGLN1/2* (also called *PHD2/1*), respectively.

In patients with hereditary phaeochromocytomas, signs and symptoms may result from syndromically associated abnormalities in addition to or instead of phaeochromocytoma itself. These often present before phaeochromocytomas and can be the first clue to the presence of genetic disease (see *Genetic profile*).

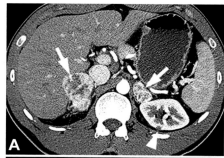
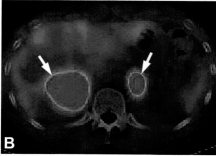

Fig. 5.01 Bilateral phaeochromocytoma in von Hippel–Lindau syndrome. **A** Enhanced CT reveals hyperenhancing bilateral adrenal masses (arrows), with the larger mass on the right. **B** The corresponding ^{123}I-MIBG SPECT image shows intense uptake of tracer in the adrenal masses.

They include gastrointestinal stromal tumour, renal cell carcinoma, medullary thyroid carcinoma, and other neoplasms (Table 5.02, p. 182).

Biochemical testing
Clinical suspicion of phaeochromocytoma must be confirmed by biochemical testing to demonstrate catecholamine production. The specific test used depends on the institution. Current guidelines recommend that initial testing should include measurements of plasma free metanephrines or urinary fractionated metanephrines {1587}, which are the most sensitive analytes because they reflect intratumoural O-methylation of catecholamines leaked from storage vesicles in tumour cells {741,742}. The catecholamine metabolite profile can point to specific genetic disorders (see *Genetic profile*). Phaeochromocytomas associated with multiple endocrine neoplasia type 2 (MEN2) or neurofibromatosis type 1 typically produce epinephrine, resulting in increased concentrations of metanephrine. In contrast, isolated increases in normetanephrine and norepinephrine suggest von Hippel–Lindau syndrome. Additional or isolated production of the dopamine metabolite 3-methoxytyramine points to the presence of *SDHB*, *SDHD*, or *SDHC* mutation and is also associated with potentially metastatic tumours {744,746}.

Imaging
Imaging studies should only be initiated if there is clear biochemical evidence of phaeochromocytoma {1587}. Anatomical imaging, which is usually performed first, can be CT or MRI {1587}. MRI classically shows an enhancing mass with high T2-weighted signal intensity (the so-called lightbulb sign), seen in approximately one third of cases {427}. Other findings

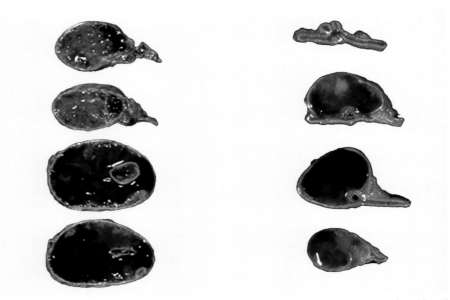

Fig. 5.02 Bilateral phaeochromocytoma in von Hippel–Lindau syndrome. Macroscopic appearance of the bilateral adrenal masses seen in Fig. 5.01 in the right (**A**) and left (**B**) adrenal glands.

may include cystic change, necrosis, haemorrhage, and calcification. Functional imaging by ¹²³I-MIBG scintigraphy has excellent sensitivity and specificity and can be helpful in confirming a diagnosis. MRI and ¹²³I-MIBG scintigraphy are preferable to CT for detecting phaeochromocytoma metastases or additional paragangliomas in patients with hereditary tumour syndromes {1587}. Newer modalities of functional imaging (including ¹⁸F-FDOPA PET/CT and somatostatin receptor imaging, particularly by ⁶⁸Ga-DOTATATE PET/CT) offer greater sensitivity than other functional imaging modalities for these purposes {427,1247}, but are not yet widely available.

Tumour spread and staging
Approximately 10% of phaeochromocytomas metastasize {748}. This contrasts with an almost 40% risk of metastasis from extra-adrenal sympathetic paragangliomas, as estimated by meta-analysis of multiple series {748}. The most common sites of metastases are local lymph nodes, axial skeleton, liver, and lung {2462}. Metastases sometimes develop years or decades after resection of a primary tumour {2491}. Extensive local invasion, which is much less frequent than metastasis, is by itself a poor predictor of metastasis {3122}.
The 2004 WHO classification defined malignant phaeochromocytoma by the development of metastases, but noted that the definition did not account for the potentially lethal behaviour of tumours with extensive local invasion. Confusion due to this incongruity was noted by several authors {2782,3122}, resulting in the use of the more informative and precise terms "metastatic" and "non-metastatic" in recent papers {1376,2773}. Metastatic deposits should only be considered as such at sites where normal chromaffin

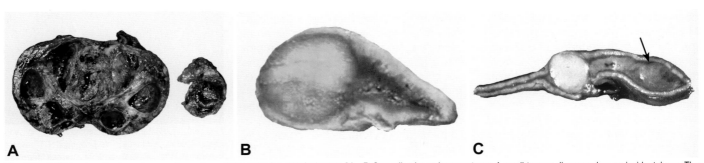

Fig. 5.03 A Bilateral cystic phaeochromocytomas in multiple endocrine neoplasia type 2A. **B** Sporadic phaeochromocytoma. A small tumour discovered as an incidentaloma. The adjacent adrenal medulla is normal. **C** Phaeochromocytoma and adrenal medullary hyperplasia in multiple endocrine neoplasia type 2A. Note the small phaeochromocytoma on the left, the prominent adjacent adrenal medulla, and a poorly circumscribed second phaeochromocytoma on the right (arrow), which has the same colour as the medulla.

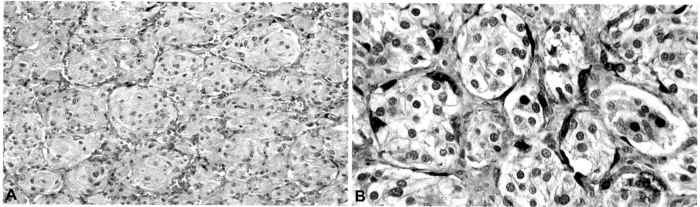

Fig. 5.04 Phaeochromocytoma. **A** Classic histoarchitecture with prominent uniform cell nests (Zellballen). **B** Immunohistochemical stain for S100 showing classic distribution of sustentacular cells, mostly at the periphery of cell nests.

tissue is not present, in order to avoid the misclassification of multicentric primary tumours as metastases. These sites include bone, liver, histologically confirmed lymph node, and lung. Rare primary paragangliomas arising in the lung {117} or in the hilum of the liver should not be confused with metastases. A staging system for phaeochromocytoma was introduced in the 8th edition of the American Joint Committee on Cancer staging manual.

Macroscopy

Phaeochromocytomas are circumscribed but typically unencapsulated tumours that arise in the adrenal medulla. With increasing size, they expand to the capsule of the adrenal gland and compress or obliterate the cortex. The adrenal capsule thereby becomes the apparent capsule of the tumour. Occasionally, a pseudocapsule is present between tumour and adjacent adrenal tissue {1518}. The cut surface is pinkish-grey to tan (in contrast to the bright-yellow colour of adrenal

cortical tumours) but may undergo slight yellowing after exposure to air or during formalin fixation. Haemorrhage, central degenerative changes, fibrosis, and cystic change are variably present. The tumour diameter is usually about 3–5 cm, but can be > 10 cm {1518} or < 1 cm. Molecular analyses suggest that adrenal medullary nodules measuring < 1 cm, which have previously been arbitrarily classified by some authors as hyperplastic nodules, are in fact better considered small phaeochromocytomas {1457}.

During examination of a specimen containing phaeochromocytoma, the adrenal gland should be carefully searched for additional medullary nodules and diffuse medullary hyperplasia, which can indicate hereditary disease (see *Genetic profile* and *Genetic susceptibility*) {406}. In the absence of superimposed nodules, diffuse hyperplasia can be recognized if there is prominent extension of medullary tissue (which is normally confined to the head and body of the adrenal gland) into

the alae and tail {654,1518}. Mild diffuse hyperplasia may only be detectable by morphometric analysis {654}. A careful effort should also be made to confirm the origin of the tumour within (rather than adjacent to) the adrenal gland. This may require careful gross and microscopic examination of the tumour periphery to search for residual adrenal cortex.

Microscopy

Tumour may extend to the adrenal capsule, or a pseudocapsule may be present {1518}. The border with the adjacent cortex may be sharp or irregular, with intermingling of tumour cells and cortical cells. A range of architectural and cytological features can be seen, often within an individual tumour. Most phaeochromocytomas exhibit an alveolar (Zellballen) pattern, consisting of nests of polygonal tumour cells separated by peripheral capillaries. Architectural variations include trabecular and diffuse growth patterns and prominent

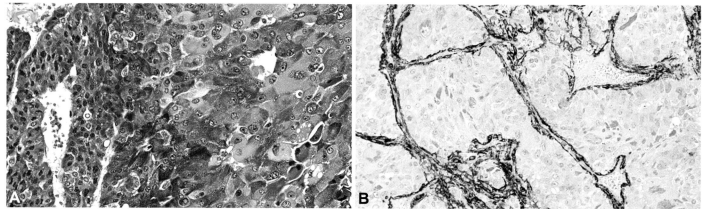

Fig. 5.05 **A** Phaeochromocytoma with irregular histoarchitecture and a gradient of cell size, with varied cytological features. Note the transition from small cells with nondescript nuclei on the left to large cells with vesicular nuclei and prominent nucleoli on the right. **B** Phaeochromocytoma with irregular histoarchitecture highlighted by immunohistochemical staining for CD31 to outline blood vessels.

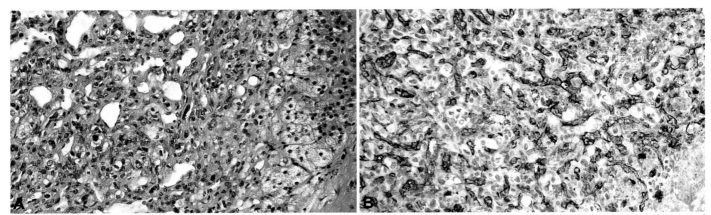

Fig. 5.06 Phaeochromocytoma. **A** Unusual noradrenergic phaeochromocytoma composed of small cells with amphophilic clear or vacuolated cytoplasm and numerous interspersed small branching blood vessels. Adrenal cortex is at the right. **B** The vascular pattern is highlighted by immunohistochemical staining for CD31. Similar features have been associated with von Hippel–Lindau syndrome.

vascularity that may mimic that of an angioma {2550}. Haemorrhage, haemosiderin deposition, and sclerosis are sometimes marked. Cytologically, phaeochromocytoma cells can closely resemble normal chromaffin cells, or may be smaller or larger; larger cells often have vesicular nuclei with prominent nucleoli. Cytoplasmic staining is typically granular and basophilic to amphophilic, and can be markedly affected by fixation conditions. Nuclear pseudoinclusions and intracytoplasmic hyaline globules that give a diastase-resistant positive periodic acid–Schiff (PAS) reaction are often present. Nuclear pleomorphism and cellular pleomorphism are sometimes conspicuous, but mitoses are usually rare {2663}. Less common features include spindle cells (occurring as a typically minor component in a small proportion of cases), clear cells (so-called lipid degeneration) that can mimic neoplastic adrenal cortex, and oncocytic cells that can be focal or diffuse {1318}. Lipofuscin, neuromelanin,

or cutaneous-type melanin pigment is sometimes present {482,1291}. Amyloid is present very rarely and is usually a systemic type {1855}. Some phaeochromocytomas contain scattered ganglion cells; those tumours should not be diagnosed as composite phaeochromocytomas, which show complete histoarchitecture of an additional tumour type {1518} (see *Composite phaeochromocytoma*, p. 204).

Histopathological features in risk stratification
Current thinking is that all phaeochromocytomas have some metastatic potential. Therefore, the previous categories of benign and malignant phaeochromocytoma have been eliminated in favour of an approach based on risk stratification. Putative adverse features have been variably identified in mostly retrospective studies of phaeochromocytomas that metastasized. These features fall into five categories: invasion (vascular, adrenal capsular,

and periadrenal soft tissue), architectural variation (irregular, enlarged, and confluent cell nests; diffuse growth), cytological variation (spindling, small cells, high cell density, cellular monotony, and extreme pleomorphism), necrosis (focal or confluent, comedonecrosis in cell nests), and proliferative activity (increased mitotic count, atypical mitoses, and increased Ki-67 proliferation index) {1376,2761}. Other reported adverse findings include tumour size > 5 cm {748}, coarse nodularity {1628}, absence of hyaline globules {1628}, vascular pattern abnormalities {2068}, and reduced numbers or absence of sustentacular cells {2841}.
Studies assessing adverse features individually have reached conflicting conclusions regarding their predictive value, in particular for tumour size and Ki-67 proliferation index. The reasons for these discrepancies might include differences in the approach to tumour measurement {748}, the use of different scoring protocols {2781}, the generally low mitotic

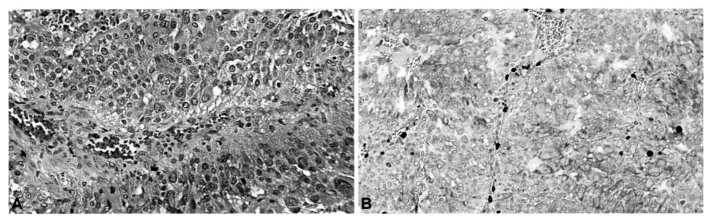

Fig. 5.07 Phaeochromocytoma. **A** Unusual phaeochromocytoma showing diffuse growth and perivascular cuffing around prominent intratumoural blood vessels (so-called pseudorosette pattern). **B** Immunostaining for Ki-67 shows proliferative activity almost exclusively in the blood vessels.

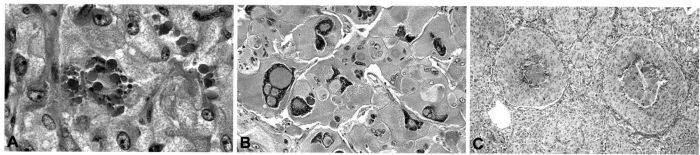

Fig. 5.08 A Phaeochromocytoma in multiple endocrine neoplasia type 2A (MEN2A). Hyaline globules such as those shown here are particularly prevalent in phaeochromocytomas associated with MEN2A. **B** Phaeochromocytoma with pleomorphic nuclei containing prominent pseudoinclusions formed by invagination of cytoplasm. **C** Phaeochromocytoma with irregular Zellballen and comedonecrosis.

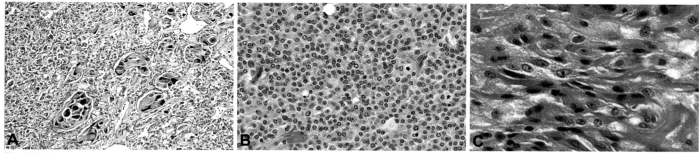

Fig. 5.09 A Phaeochromocytoma with irregular Zellballen and extreme atypia. **B** Phaeochromocytoma with diffuse architecture and a monomorphous population of small cells. Note the two mitoses present at the right. **C** Phaeochromocytoma containing spindle cells.

count even in tumours that do metastasize {2663}, and the subjectivity of some parameters resulting in poor agreement between pathologists {2068}. An overarching consideration is the difficulty in assessing the independent predictive value of some parameters; for example, monotonous architecture typically coexists with increased cellularity and small cell size {2761}, and there may be a subordinate association of the Ki-67 proliferation index to adverse conventional histological features {2663}.

In order to improve the predictive value of histological risk assessment, combinatorial systems that score multiple parameters have been developed {1376, 1628,2761}. However, there is currently no consensus on the use of any scoring system for phaeochromocytoma or paraganglioma. The best-known systems are the Phaeochromocytoma of the Adrenal Gland Scaled Score (PASS), which applies only to phaeochromocytoma {2761}, and the Grading System for Adrenal Phaeochromocytoma and Paraganglioma (GAPP) {1376}. PASS provides a threshold for identifying tumours unlikely to metastasize, and GAPP provides a stepwise, incremental assessment of both risk of metastasis and patient survival. PASS was established in 2002 and has been found to be useful in

some studies {926,2663} but not others {13}, possibly in part due to poor concordance between pathologists {3012}. A modified PASS excluding several of the original parameters has been reported to have higher predictive value {926}. GAPP also omits several PASS parameters, and weights others somewhat differently. Good predictive value was reported in a preliminary GAPP study {1380} and a large follow-up study {1376}. PASS was developed using histological features alone, without knowledge of tumour genotype and without immunohistochemistry for Ki-67, which is a GAPP parameter {1376}. In the GAPP follow-up study, SDHB immunohistochemistry served as a surrogate for genetic testing; 13 immunonegative tumours were reported, all of which were of intermediate or high grade and 10 of which metastasized {1376, 1377}.

Immunophenotype
The diagnosis of phaeochromocytoma can be confirmed by immunohistochemistry if necessary. The major differential diagnosis is adrenal cortical neoplasia, and the major diagnostic pitfall is misdiagnosis of oncocytic tumours {722}. The most reliable marker for distinguishing phaeochromocytoma from adrenal cortical neoplasms, renal cell carcinomas,

and non-endocrine metastatic tumours is expression of chromogranin A {1518}. Staining for chromogranin A should be strong and diffuse. If chromogranin A expression is absent, the diagnosis of phaeochromocytoma should be questioned. Expression of tyrosine hydroxylase and dopamine beta-hydroxylase, which is required for catecholamine synthesis, can help to rule out neuroendocrine tumours metastatic to the adrenal gland {1374, 2781}. Other helpful findings are the usual absence of keratins {484} and the absence of adrenal cortical markers {722}. Oncocytic tumours in any location may show weak non-specific staining with some antibodies {95}. Immunostaining for S100 highlights sustentacular cells, which can be found in varying numbers at the periphery of Zellballen or interspersed between tumour cells {1653}. Neoplastic chromaffin cells are sometimes also positive for S100, but typically stain more weakly than do sustentacular cells in the same area. Immunohistochemistry for regulatory peptides is not usually required but can be helpful in determining whether a phaeochromocytoma is ectopically producing a hormone known to be present in excess (e.g. ectopic ACTH) {138}. A relatively new use of immunohistochemistry is as an adjunct to genetic testing for hereditary tumours

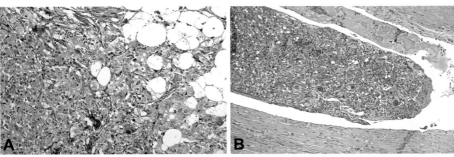

Fig. 5.10 A Phaeochromocytoma invading periadrenal adipose tissue. **B** Phaeochromocytoma invading the adrenal vein. Note the associated thrombus.

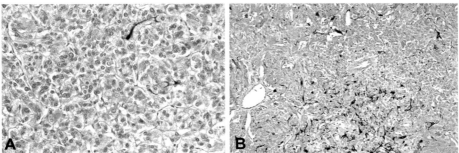

Fig. 5.11 Phaeochromocytoma in multiple endocrine neoplasia type 2A. Immunohistochemical staining for S100 highlights intertumoural and intratumoural heterogeneity in the number and distribution of sustentacular cells in separate tumours from the same adrenal gland. **A** One tumour shows uniform histoarchitecture and contains extremely rare sustentacular cells apparently enveloping individual neoplastic chromaffin cells. **B** A second tumour from the same adrenal gland shows mixed architectural patterns and varied density of sustentacular cells.

caused by SDH mutations, all of which result in loss of SDHB protein {601,975, 2849} (See the *Genetic profile* section and *Familial paraganglioma–phaeochromocytoma syndromes caused by SDHB, SDHC, and SDHD mutations*, p. 262). Many additional immunohistochemical markers have been associated with metastatic tumours in small series but require further validation {748}.

Correlations between histopathology and genotype

A few histological features can provide clues both to the presence of hereditary disease and to specific genotypes {1377,

2784} (see *Genetic profile*). Multicentric phaeochromocytomas and adrenal medullary hyperplasia suggest MEN2 and, less often, non-syndromic germline mutations in *TMEM127* {2790}. Numerous hyaline globules are often seen in epinephrine-producing tumours, including those associated with MEN2. Reported characteristics of phaeochromocytomas in patients with von Hippel–Lindau syndrome include stromal myxoid or oedematous change, a thick vascular capsule, and small to medium-sized tumour cells with clear cytoplasm and many interspersed small blood vessels {1424}. Because these features are variable and are

affected by tissue fixation, they are more reliable for distinguishing MEN2 from von Hippel–Lindau syndrome in patients with multiple tumours than for characterizing an apparently sporadic solitary tumour {2784}.

Genetic profile

Phaeochromocytomas must be considered part of a disease spectrum that also includes sympathetic and parasympathetic paragangliomas in other locations. At least 30% of these tumours develop in patients harbouring germline mutations in hereditary susceptibility genes, making phaeochromocytomas and paragangliomas collectively the most strongly hereditary of all human tumours {213,2077}. Occult germline mutations in susceptibility genes are present in 11–24% of patients presenting with an apparently sporadic phaeochromocytoma or paraganglioma {69, 326,1968}. For this reason, it is recommended that genetic testing for at least the most frequent germline mutations be considered for all patients, regardless of family history {1587}. At least 19 hereditary susceptibility genes have been identified to date {2077} (see *Introduction*, p. 181), with the specific gene determining tumour location, biochemical phenotype, risk of metastasis, and syndromic associations. Most of the genes are tumour suppressor genes characterized by autosomal dominant inheritance and loss or inactivation of the wildtype allele in the tumours. Exceptions are the *RET* proto-oncogene and *EPAS1*, with gain-of-function mutations that do not require a second hit, although allelic imbalance can occur {1423}. Inheritance of three genes (*SDHD*, *SDHAF2*, and *MAX*) involves a parent-of-origin effect: the mutation can be inherited from either parent,

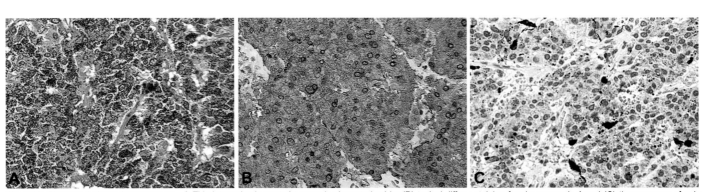

Fig. 5.12 Pigmented phaeochromocytoma. **A** This intensely pigmented tumour is characterized by (**B**) typical diffuse staining for chromogranin A and (**C**) the presence of only scattered S100-positive sustentacular cells, distinguishing it from melanoma.

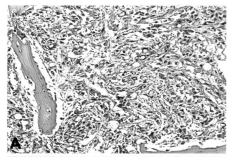

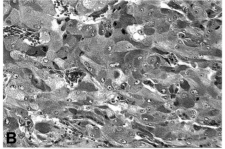

Fig. 5.13 A Phaeochromocytoma metastatic to vertebral bone. There is no discernible histological architecture. **B** Phaeochromocytoma with a mosaic-like pattern of admixed large polygonal cells with basophilic to slightly acidophilic cytoplasm. These so called embracing cells, with cytoplasm moulded by the cytoplasm of adjacent cells, are often associated with this tumour architecture.

but disease usually manifests only following paternal transmission. Several mechanisms have been proposed for this effect {184,1151} (see *Familial paraganglioma–phaeochromocytoma syndromes caused by SDHB, SDHC, and SDHD mutations*, p. 262). Mutations of different hereditary susceptibility genes are usually mutually exclusive. Although double mutations do rarely occur, DNA sequence variants of unknown significance detected by genomic screening often prove to have no effect on protein structure, and therefore no pathogenic effect {790}.

Truly sporadic phaeochromocytomas and paragangliomas in patients without germline mutations are now known to harbour somatic mutations of hereditary susceptibility genes in 14% {351} to > 20% {599} of cases. Interestingly, the most common somatic mutations involve *NF1* {348,599,2975}, which is a relatively

uncommon cause of hereditary phaeochromocytoma and paraganglioma. In contrast, somatic mutations in the SDH genes are extremely rare in the absence of germline mutation {348,2124,2975} (see *Introduction*, p. 181). Somatic mutations of *HRAS* or *BRAF* have been identified in almost 9% of sporadic tumours, and *TP53* mutations in 2.3% {1682}. Mutations in these common cancer genes and hereditary susceptibility genes are almost always mutually exclusive {1682}. Phaeochromocytomas and paragangliomas cluster into two broad groups with distinct transcriptional and functional profiles. The first group (cluster 1) is characterized by pseudohypoxic signalling and consists of tumours with SDH and *VHL* mutations, whereas cluster 2 is associated with abnormalities of tyrosine kinase pathways and mutations of *NF1*, *RET*, RAS genes, and *TMEM127* {980}. *MAX*-related tumours constitute an intermediate cluster {2219}. Cluster 1 can be further subdivided according to molecular profile {351} and tumour location {2517}.

Genetic susceptibility

Driver gene mutations alone are not sufficient for tumorigenesis of either hereditary or sporadic tumours, and the complete requirements remain unknown. Integrated genomic analyses show distinct landscapes of molecular alterations associated with mutations of individual susceptibility genes. These alterations include chromosomal gains and losses, mutations of additional genes, copy-number changes, and epigenetic alterations {430,859A,1682,2733}, with consequent effects on the microRNAome, transcriptome, proteome, signalling pathway activation, and metabolome {2284}. Frequent chromosomal changes include early losses of apparent tumour suppressor genes on chromosomes 1p and 3q; losses of 11p, 11q, 6q, 17p, and 22; and gains of 9q, 17q, 19p13.3, and 20q {1682}. Extensive genome methylation is associated with all SDH mutations {951,1595}.

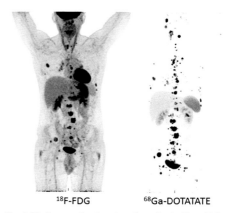

¹⁸F-FDG   ⁶⁸Ga-DOTATATE

Fig. 5.14 Comparative imaging of a patient with multiple paraganglioma metastases by ¹⁸F-FDOPA PET/CT and ⁶⁸Ga-DOTATATE PET/CT. Somatostatin receptor imaging (i.e. with ⁶⁸Ga-DOTATATE or other somatostatin analogues) is the most sensitive modality available for tumours that express somatostatin receptors.

Prognosis and predictive factors

The prognosis is highly dependent on resectability and the genetic profile. Complete resection is the only cure. Hereditary *SDHB* mutations, which are associated with the highest risk of metastasis {69,265}, also predict shorter survival times than do other mutations after metastases occur {68}. Histological parameters {1376,1377} and methylation patterns {622} might provide further prognostic information. The overall 5-year survival rate when metastases are present is 34–60%. Survival times tend to be < 5 years when metastasis involves the liver or lung, and longer when metastasis involves bone {2075}. Local invasion alone is a poor predictor of metastasis and is compatible with long-term survival if excision is complete {1793}. Incomplete excision of a locally invasive tumour can lead to local recurrence without metastasis years after the initial surgery {2570}. Early genetic testing for predisposing germline mutations facilitates risk-reduction strategies that may reduce the risk of metastasis from both phaeochromocytomas and associated tumours {69,2077}. Molecular profiling predicts a number of potential targeted therapies for metastases {838, 1063,1682}.

Extra-adrenal paragangliomas

Kimura N.
Capella C.
DeLellis R. A.
Epstein J. I.
Gill A.
Kawashima A.

Koch C. A.
Komminoth P.
Lam A. K. Y.
Merino M. J.
Mete O.
Papathomas T. G.

Sadow P.
Thompson L. D. R.
Tischler A. S.
Williams M. D.
Young W. F.

Paragangliomas are non-epithelial tumours originating from neural crest–derived paraganglion cells situated in the region of the autonomic nervous system ganglia and accompanying nerves. The paraganglion system can be divided into the adrenal medulla and the extra-adrenal paraganglion system. The latter can be further subdivided into the para-sympathetic and sympathetic paraganglia. The parasympathetic paraganglia are primarily located in the head and neck and are less frequently located in the thorax and pelvis. The sympathetic paraganglia are primarily located along the sympathetic nerve chains bordering the vertebrae in the abdomen and pelvis.

Head and neck paragangliomas

Definition
Head and neck paragangliomas (HNPGLs) are neural crest–derived neuroendocrine neoplasms arising from extra-adrenal paraganglia distributed along the parasympathetic nerves in the head and neck. These paragangliomas are named according to their anatomical sites of origin, which include the carotid body, jugulotympanicum (middle ear), vagus nerve, and larynx. The tumours are generally non-functioning, and only rare cases secrete catecholamines {1403,1938}.

ICD-O codes
Carotid body paraganglioma   8692/3
Jugulotympanic paraganglioma   8690/3
Vagal paraganglioma   8693/3
Laryngeal paraganglioma   8693/3

Synonyms
Parasympathetic paraganglioma; non-chromaffin paraganglioma; chemodectoma; carotid body tumour; glomus caroticum tumour; glomus jugulare tumour; jugular glomus tumour; glomus tympanicum tumour; tympanic glomus tumour

Epidemiology
HNPGLs account for approximately 20% of all paragangliomas in unselected series, for 0.6% of head and neck tumours, and for 0.03% of all tumours {1728,2685}. The overall annual incidence of HNPGLs is 1 case per 30 000–100 000 population. Carotid body paragangliomas are the most common (accounting for 57% of cases), followed by jugular (23%), vagal (13%), and tympanic (6%) paragangliomas. Laryngeal paragangliomas are very rare {781,3115}.
Patients are aged 5–85 years (mean: 41–47 years) {458,781,2757,3115}. There is a female predominance, which is more pronounced in populations at high altitudes, in which the female-to-male ratio is 8:1 {1573,2317}. On average, inherited cases occur about a decade earlier {350}. Bilateral paragangliomas are noted in as many as 10–25% of cases {3115}, with multicentric tumours present in 17–37% of unselected cases and in as many as 80% of patients with a positive family history {383}.
About 4–6% of HNPGLs metastasize {70, 1549,2038,2383}. Metastatic HNPGLs, compared with their primary counterparts, are associated with a younger patient age at presentation (37 vs 45 years), have a higher rate of multifocality (46% vs 20%), and are more likely to be functioning (in 27% vs 5% of cases) {1795}. They are also more likely to occur near the carotid bifurcation.

Etiology
HNPGLs are frequently hereditary {350, 1620,1970,2287}. Chronic hypoxic conditions, such as cyanotic heart disease and a high-altitude environment are additional risk factors {115,2052}.

Localization
Paragangliomas can be derived from the carotid body (carotid body paraganglioma), or they can arise in the vicinity of the jugular bulb or on the medial promontory of the middle ear (jugulotympanic paraganglioma), within or adjacent to the vagus nerve in the vicinity of the ganglion nodosum (vagal paraganglioma), or in the larynx (laryngeal paraganglioma).

Clinical features
HNPGLs are usually non-secreting. They are often diagnosed because of cervical nerve compression or are incidentally detected during imaging of the thyroid gland or neck vessels {2167}. In one series, only 3.6% of these tumours were

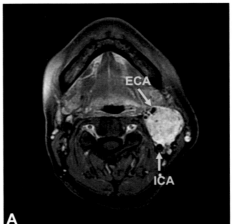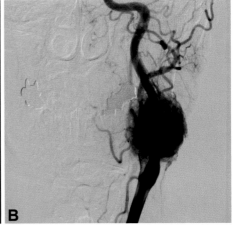

Fig. 5.15 Carotid body paraganglioma. **A** Axial-view gadolinium-enhanced T1-weighed MRI shows a highly enhanced tumour located at the left bifurcation of the carotid artery. The distance between the external carotid artery (ECA) and the internal carotid artery (ICA) is enlarged. The salt-and-pepper sign is evident in the tumour. **B** A left common carotid angiogram in the frontal view shows a tumour at the left bifurcation of the carotid artery that shows high uptake of the iodine-containing contrast medium due to the hypervascular character of the tumour.

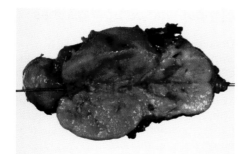

Fig. 5.16 Head and neck paraganglioma. A solitary, tan-coloured tumour grows around the carotid artery (indicated by a probe).

documented to have catecholamine hypersecretion {781}. Metastasis occurs in 3–5% of cases, with a lower risk (2–6%) among carotid body paragangliomas and jugulotympanic paragangliomas, and a higher risk (16%) among vagal paragangliomas {1240,1378,1412,1730}. The most common sites of metastases are the cervical lymph nodes (accounting for 68.6% of metastases); other sites include bone, lung, and liver {1573,1911}. The overall 5-year survival rate for patients with metastatic tumours is generally good (60–84%) {1573,1911}. Hereditary cases can occur in association with sympathetic paragangliomas in the retroperitoneum, adrenal gland, and thorax, and may be associated with other stigmata of syndromic disease {350,1728,1970, 2287}.

Macroscopy

Paragangliomas are firm, rubbery, and well circumscribed, ranging from 2.0–6.0 cm in size. Carotid body paragangliomas can encase and infiltrate the carotid artery, which may have to be sacrificed during surgery.

Microscopy

Typically, the organoid (Zellballen) pattern of the normal paraganglion is seen. The Zellballen pattern is composed of two cell types: chief cells, which have abundant pale cytoplasm and hyperchromatic nuclei, and sustentacular cells, which are slender, spindle-shaped, and peripherally located around the nests. There is a prominent vascular network separating the tumour nests. Mitotic figures are usually rare. The tumour cells of HNPGLs are smaller and show higher cellularity than those of sympathetic paragangliomas. A wide range of variant morphologies may be observed, including trabecular, spindled, angioma-like, and sclerosing

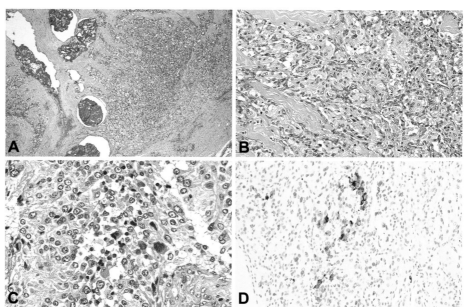

Fig. 5.17 Head and neck paraganglioma (HNPGL). **A** Foreign materials used for embolization can be identified in tumour blood vessels. **B** Tumour cells are arranged in a Zellballen pattern, with abundant collagenous stroma (sclerosing pattern). **C** Embolization prior to surgery results in nuclear pyknosis and focal necrosis; these are not worrisome features. **D** Chromogranin A immunoreactivity is variable in HNPGL, and is often focal and weak.

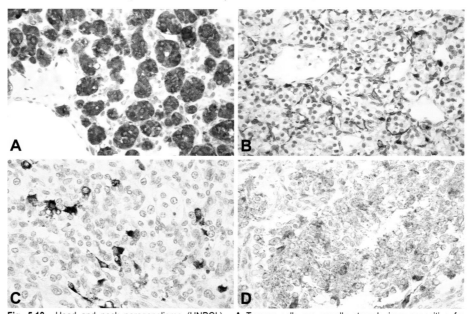

Fig. 5.18 Head and neck paraganglioma (HNPGL). **A** Tumour cells are usually strongly immunopositive for synaptophysin. **B** Sustentacular cells surrounding chief cells are immunopositive for S100 protein. **C** Dopamine beta-hydroxylase–positive cells are occasionally sparsely observed. **D** Granular cytoplasmic staining is characteristic of paragangliomas with wildtype SDH genes.

patterns. Preoperative therapeutic embolization may result in degenerative atypia and focal necrosis, and embolic material is usually present {2781}.

Immunophenotype

The chief cells usually express synaptophysin, chromogranin A, CD56, and SSTR2A {768,1378}, and are usually negative for cytokeratin, CEA, and calcitonin. In contrast to phaeochromocytomas and paragangliomas elsewhere, HNPGLs can sometimes be negative for chromogranin A, or it may be expressed only focally, in a perinuclear dot-like (Golgi) pattern. Tyrosine hydroxylase and dopamine beta-hydroxylase, enzymes for catecholamine synthesis, are focally expressed in approximately 30% and 11% of cases, respectively, consistent with the usual lack of catecholamine-related clinical function {2063,2781}. The sustentacular cells express S100 protein and/or GFAP. The Ki-67 proliferation index (as determined using the MIB1 antibody) is typically < 1%, consistent with the slow growth of most HNPGLs {645}. The loss of immunohistochemical staining for SDHB protein occurs in the vast majority of paragangliomas associated with germline mutation in any of the SDH genes {975,2849}. Paragangliomas associated with *SDHA* mutation also show loss of SDHA expression {1456}.

Genetic profile and susceptibility

The germline mutation rate is as high as 18.8% in HNPGLs that present as apparently sporadic, and much higher in patients with a family history {2167}. The mutations that cause HNPGL occur mostly in genes encoding the subunits of the succinate dehydrogenase component of mitochondrial complex II. Mutations occur most commonly in *SDHD* (in 80% of cases), followed by *SDHB*, then *SDHAF2*, *SDHA*, and *SDHC* {185}. Mutations in *VHL*, and rarely in *TMEM127*, *RET*, and *NF1*, have also been reported in association with HNPGLs {1378,2167}.

Prognosis and predictive factors

Optimal management depends on the tumour location, local involvement of neurovascular structures, estimated metastatic risk, and the patient's age and general health. Surgery has historically been the

treatment of choice, although recurrence can occur (in < 10% of cases). Radiotherapy (fractionated or stereotactic radiosurgery) provides short-term symptomatic relief and tumour growth retardation, but the long-term consequences are unclear {383}. In selected patients, close observation is increasingly preferred to surgery {307,1246,1549}.

Paragangliomas associated with *SDHB* mutations have a high risk of metastasis, which occurs in at least a third of patients by the age of 70 years {271,838,973}. Metastases are confined to regional lymph nodes in the majority (68.6%) of cases, with carotid body paragangliomas found to have the highest rate of regional confinement (93.8%) {1573,2507}. Metastasis does not necessarily signify a poor short-term prognosis, because of the slow disease course {1795}. Distant metastasis and patient age > 50 years are associated with shorter patient survival {2507}. Given the high risk of hereditary disease, even in the absence of a family history, it has been recommended that genetic testing be considered for at least the most common genes in all patients, depending on local resources {973}.

Sympathetic paragangliomas

Definition

Sympathetic paraganglioma is a neural crest–derived neoplasm arising from extra-adrenal paraganglia distributed along the prevertebral and paravertebral sympathetic chains and the sympathetic nerve fibres innervating the retroperitoneum, thorax, and pelvis.

ICD-O code   8693/3

Synonyms

Extra-adrenal paraganglioma;
extra-adrenal phaeochromocytoma

Epidemiology

The prevalence of phaeochromocytoma and paraganglioma is estimated to be about 1 case per 2500–6500 population, with an incidence of 500–1600 cases per year in the USA {470}. Paragangliomas account for 10–15% of all phaeochromocytoma/paraganglioma cases {589, 1376}. Paragangliomas can develop at any age, with the highest incidence among individuals aged 40–50 years and an approximately equal sex distribution {1728}. Compared with adult cases, paediatric phaeochromocytomas and paragangliomas are more frequently familial, bilateral, multifocal, and malignant {935}. The risk of metastasis in phaeochromocytomas and paragangliomas overall is estimated to be 10–20%; the risk in extra-adrenal sympathetic paraganglioma is 2.5–50% depending on genotype {1004,1091,1454}.

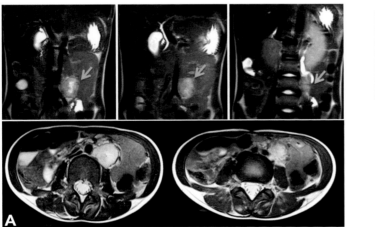
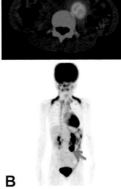
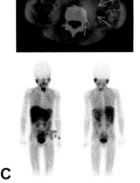

Fig. 5.19 Retroperitoneal paraganglioma. **A** Gadolinium-enhanced MRI shows a tumour (arrows) located at the bifurcation of the descending aorta, lower pole of the left kidney, and left ureter. **B** PET/CT and (**C**) ^{123}I-MIBG scintigraphy highlight a paraganglioma (arrows) in the same location shown in (A); the lack of accumulation in other sites suggests an absence of metastasis.

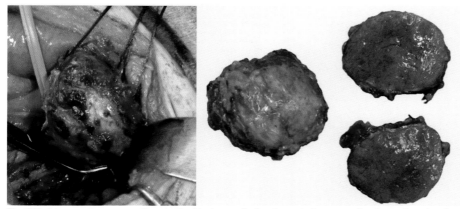

Fig. 5.20 Intraoperative paraganglioma in situ. The tumour firmly adheres to the surrounding tissue. On cut surface, the tumour is solid and tan-coloured.

Etiology

At least 30% of paragangliomas are known to be hereditary, a proportion that has increased with the discovery of new susceptibility genes {980}. Paediatric-onset paragangliomas are almost always hereditary, even in the absence of a family history, and genetic testing should be offered for all paediatric patients with paragangliomas {1076,1214,1584}. A prolonged hypoxic state has also been implicated {209,434,857,2840}.

Localization

Approximately 85% of sympathetic paragangliomas arise below the diaphragm: 42% in or around the adrenal gland and renal hilum or pedicle, 28% around the organ of Zuckerkandl, 10% in the urinary bladder {201,1128,2225}, about 12% within the thorax, and the remainder in other locations. Cardiac paragangliomas constitute less than 2% of all cases {1845,2929}.

Clinical features

Sympathetic paragangliomas are capable of catecholamine synthesis, and most signs and symptoms are caused by excess catecholamine production and release, as is the case with phaeochromocytomas (see the *Clinical symptoms and signs,* subsection of *Phaeochromocytoma,* p. 183). However, patients with sympathetic paragangliomas usually have elevated norepinephrine only, or norepinephrine and dopamine, but not elevated epinephrine; this is because phenylethanolamine N-methyltransferase, the enzyme required for converting norepinephrine to epinephrine, is not expressed in paragangliomas as it is in the adrenal medulla. Non-functioning tumours (clinically silent, with non-elevated catecholamine levels) account for 17–43% of sympathetic paragangliomas {589,1376,2487,2979}.

Invasion and metastasis

Direct invasion into other organs is rare; however, retroperitoneal paragangliomas invading the duodenum (mimicking a submucosal tumour) {1372,2702} and into the vena cava {1729} have been reported. About 40–50% of patients with urinary bladder paragangliomas experience haematuria or micturition-induced signs and symptoms.

The most common sites of metastasis are the local lymph nodes, bone, liver, and lung; rare sites include the peritoneum, pleura, ovary, and testis {1380,2487}. Metastases sometimes develop years or decades after resection of a primary tumour {2491}.

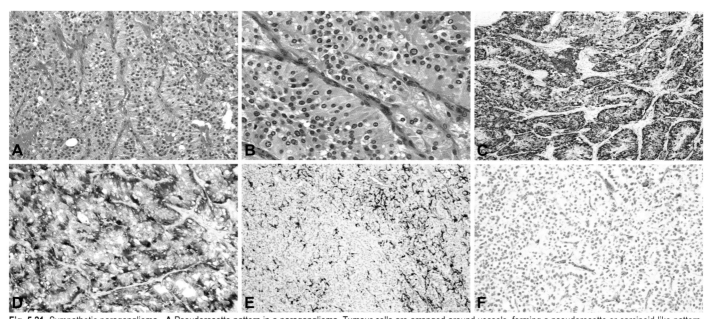

Fig. 5.21 Sympathetic paraganglioma. **A** Pseudorosette pattern in a paraganglioma. Tumour cells are arranged around vessels, forming a pseudorosette or carcinoid-like pattern. **B** Higher magnification shows that the tumour cells have abundant cytoplasm and monomorphic, hyperchromatic nuclei. **C** Chromogranin A immunoreactivity is polarized. **D** The pattern of dopamine beta-hydroxylase immunostaining is identical to that of chromogranin A immunoreactivity, showing polarization like that seen in carcinoid tumours. **E** S100 protein immunostaining shows many sustentacular cells. **F** SDHB immunostaining is negative in the tumour cells of *SDHB*-mutated paraganglioma, with positive endothelial cells serving as internal controls.

Macroscopy

Sympathetic paragangliomas are usually well-circumscribed, solid, soft, tan tumours. Haemorrhagic or cystic degeneration may be seen in larger tumours. The tumours may firmly adhere to and occasionally invade adjacent tissues such as vessels and nerves.

Microscopy

Sympathetic paragangliomas exhibit histology similar to that of phaeochromocytoma. Architectural variations include irregular combined large and small Zellballen and pseudorosette patterns. The pseudorosette pattern is suggestive of *SDHB* mutation–associated tumours {1377}. Urinary bladder paragangliomas may be misdiagnosed as urothelial carcinoma due to their histological similarity {3119}.

Immunophenotype

Neuroendocrine markers (e.g. chromogranin A, synaptophysin, and CD56) are almost always positive in paragangliomas. If chromogranin A is negative, the diagnosis of sympathetic paraganglioma should be questioned. Positive reactions for catecholamine-synthesizing enzymes (dopamine beta-hydroxylase and tyrosine hydroxylase) are helpful for excluding other neuroendocrine tumours in the differential diagnosis. The sensitivity and specificity of dopamine beta-hydroxylase has been reported to be 100%, even in non-functioning paragangliomas {1374}. Combined with diffuse positivity for neuroendocrine markers, a negative keratin reaction helps to rule out neuroendocrine

tumours of the pancreas and gastrointestinal tract, adrenal cortical tumours, renal cell carcinoma, and urothelial carcinoma of the bladder. However, paragangliomas can be focally positive for keratin {484, 1375}. The Ki-67 proliferation index is usually low {755}.

Tumours associated with germline mutations in any of the SDH genes show greatly decreased or absent immunoreactivity for SDHB {975,2849}, and tumours associated with *SDHA* mutation also show loss of SDHA expression {1456}.

Histological grading and risk stratification

Current thinking is that all paragangliomas have some metastatic potential. Therefore the previous categories of benign and malignant paragangliomas have been eliminated for an approach based on risk stratification. The criteria are similar to those used for phaeochromocytomas in the adrenal glands. The Phaeochromocytoma of the Adrenal Gland Scaled Score (PASS) is not intended for use in extra-adrenal paraganglioma and only provides a single threshold for predicting metastatic risk.

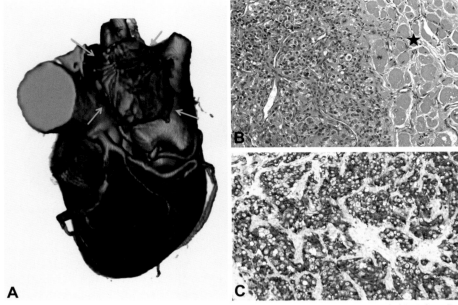

Fig. 5.22 Cardiac paraganglioma. **A** CT angiography shows a tumour (arrows) located on the roof of the left cardiac atrium and truncus of the pulmonary artery. **B** Tumour cells invade the myocardium (star) and (**C**) are strongly positive for dopamine beta-hydroxylase.

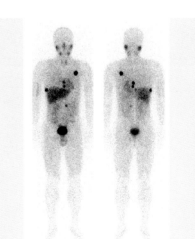
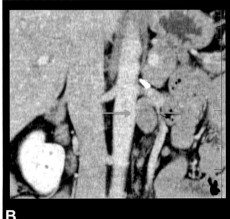
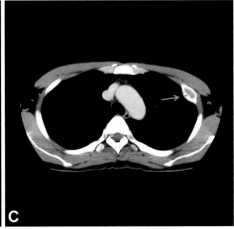

Fig. 5.23 Malignant sympathetic paraganglioma. **A** ^{123}I-MIBG scintigraphy shows multiple metastases of paraganglioma in ribs, paravertebral ganglia, and retroperitoneum. **B** Gadolinium-enhanced MRI shows metastatic paraganglioma (arrows) located between the abdominal aorta and the left renal artery. **C** Enhanced CT shows a metastasis (arrow) in a rib.

The Grading System for Adrenal Phaeochromocytoma and Paraganglioma (GAPP), developed in Japan, classifies phaeochromocytomas and paragangliomas into a three-tiered grading system reflecting a continuum of metastatic risk, on the basis of histological features, Ki-67 immunohistochemistry, and hormone data {1376,2761}. The reported risks of metastasis and 5-year survival rates, respectively, for these three groups are 3.6% and 100% for well-differentiated tumours, 60% and 66.8% for moderately differentiated tumours, and 88.2% and 22.4% for poorly differentiated tumours {1376}. Additional risk factors include tumour size > 5 cm and *SDHB* mutation or loss of immunohistochemical expression of SDHB {1376,1377}.

Genetic profile and susceptibility
See *Phaeochromocytoma* (p. 183).

Prognosis and predictive factors
The prognosis for phaeochromocytoma or paraganglioma is closely linked to the genetic profile, with a higher metastatic potential documented in *SDHB*-mutated and *MAX*-mutated paraganglionic tumours {838}. However, germline *SDHB* mutations explain only 55% of metastatic phaeochromocytomas/paragangliomas; 45% of patients have apparently sporadic tumours {2831}. Other factors that might be related to metastatic potential include larger tumour size {743,2039, 2831}, older patient age at initial diagnosis {505,747}, and a noradrenergic and/ or dopaminergic biochemical phenotype {743,744}.

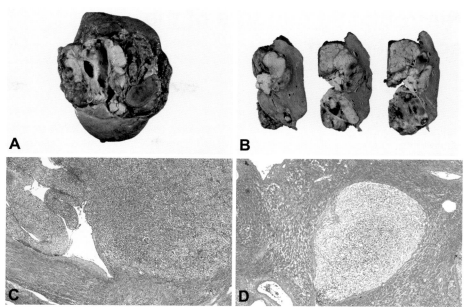

Fig. 5.24 Sympathetic paraganglioma. **A** Macroscopic view of metastases of paraganglioma to the inferior vena cava (IVC) and liver. **B** Cut surface (step sections) of the same metastases. **C** Paraganglioma invades and extends to the IVC wall. **D** Paraganglioma metastasis in the liver.

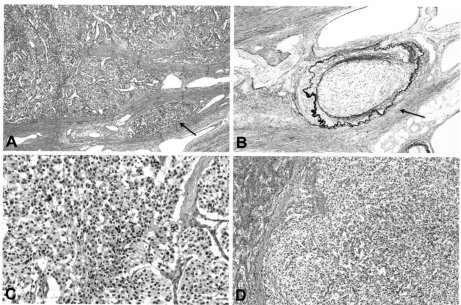

Fig. 5.25 Sympathetic paraganglioma. **A** Primary paraganglioma in retroperitoneum shows vessel invasion (arrow). **B** The same section shown in panel A, with the elastica stained by Masson trichrome. The Zellballen pattern is evident even in an intravenous embolus (arrow). **C** Primary paraganglioma in retroperitoneum shows an irregular Zellballen pattern with central degeneration. **D** Metastatic tumour in the liver showing histology similar to that of the primary retroperitoneal paraganglioma shown in panel C.

Neuroblastic tumours of the adrenal gland

Shimada H.
DeLellis R. A.
Tissier F.

Definition
Neuroblastic tumours of the adrenal gland are a group of tumours arising from the sympathoadrenal lineage of the neural crest during development. They are included within the broader classification of peripheral neuroblastic tumours.

ICD-O codes
Neuroblastoma	9500/3
Ganglioneuroblastoma, nodular	9490/3
Ganglioneuroblastoma, intermixed	9490/3
Ganglioneuroma	9490/0

Terminology
The word "neuroblastoma" is often used as an omnibus term for all types of peripheral neuroblastic tumours of neural crest origin; however, it is recommended that this term instead be used to designate a specific type of tumour within this broader group, characterized by the grade of neuroblastic differentiation and the degree of Schwannian stromal development. The International Neuroblastoma Pathology Classification (INPC) defines four categories of peripheral neuroblastic tumours (Table 5.03, p. 198) {2542}: neuroblastoma (Schwannian stroma–poor); ganglioneuroblastoma, intermixed (Schwannian stroma–rich); ganglioneuroblastoma, nodular (composite, Schwannian stroma–rich/dominant and Schwannian stroma–poor) and ganglioneuroma (Schwannian stroma–dominant). The degree of Schwannian stromal development is noted in parentheses after the tumour category (see *Microscopy*). It is believed that all ganglioneuromas were once neuroblastomas in their early stage of tumour development.

Epidemiology
Peripheral neuroblastic tumours are the third most common childhood neoplasm, after leukaemias and brain tumours. They are the most common neoplasms during the first year of life and the most common extracranial solid tumours during the first 2 years of life. In the USA, the prevalence of this disease is 1 case per 7000 live births, and 650–700 new cases are diagnosed each year. About 40% of patients are aged < 1 year, and nearly 90% are diagnosed before 5 years of age (median patient age at diagnosis: 17.3 months). The disease is slightly more common in boys than in girls, with a male-to-female ratio of 1.2:1 {328,1056,1179}.

Etiology
By definition, this disease is caused by transformation of neural crest cells secondary to genetic or epigenetic events. Although a great deal has been discovered about the genetic and transcriptional regulation of neural crest development, the events leading to tumorigenesis remain poorly understood.

The young patient age at onset of disease suggests a role of preconceptional or gestational factors. Indeed, neuroblastic tumours not infrequently present as congenital tumours {2053}. Numerous parental factors have been speculated to be associated with increased risk {552, 892,1811,2120}. However, to date there

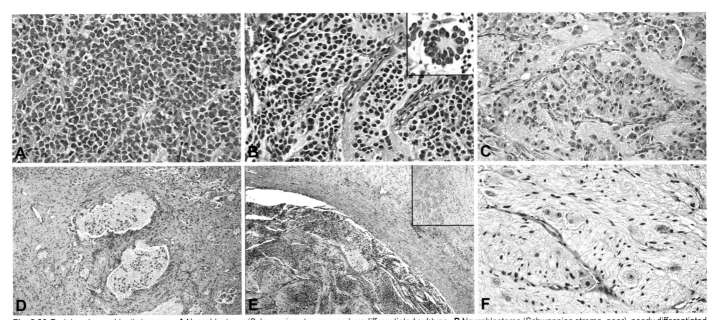

Fig. 5.26 Peripheral neuroblastic tumours. **A** Neuroblastoma (Schwannian stroma–poor), undifferentiated subtype. **B** Neuroblastoma (Schwannian stroma–poor), poorly differentiated subtype (inset: Homer Wright rosette). **C** Neuroblastoma (Schwannian stroma–poor), differentiating subtype. **D** Ganglioneuroblastoma, intermixed (Schwannian stroma–rich). **E** Ganglioneuroblastoma, nodular (composite, Schwannian stroma–rich/dominant and Schwannian stroma–poor). Inset: ganglioneuromatous component in which ganglion cells are distributed in Schwannian stroma. **F** Ganglioneuroma (Schwannian stroma–dominant), maturing subtype. Completely mature ganglion cells are covered with satellite cells.

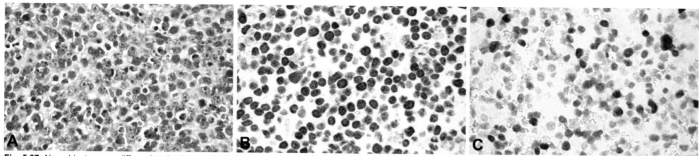

Fig. 5.27 Neuroblastoma, undifferentiated subtype. **A** *MYCN*-amplified neuroblastoma showing an appearance of undifferentiated subtype, with a high mitosis-karyorrhexis index (MKI). Note the presence of one to several prominent nucleoli in the tumour cell nuclei. **B** PHOX2B immunohistochemistry of the same tumour reveals intense nuclear staining. **C** MYCN immunohistochemistry of the same tumour shows nuclear staining of various intensities.

are no definite factors accepted to consistently increase the incidence of this disease.

Localization
The primary sites reflect the migration pattern of neural crest cells during fetal development and include the adrenal glands (involved in 40% of cases) as well as the abdominal ganglia (in 25%), thoracic ganglia (15%), pelvic ganglia (5%), and cervical sympathetic ganglia (3–5%). Rare tumours occur in the paratesticular region, and 1% of patients are reported to have no detectable primary tumour.

Clinical features
Peripheral neuroblastic tumours are well known to demonstrate spontaneous regression, tumour maturation, and aggressive progression refractory to therapy. These specific clinical features are now considered to be closely associated with the molecular properties of individual tumours.

Clinical symptoms caused by the primary tumour include abdominal distension and constipation caused by an abdominal mass, respiratory distress caused by a mediastinal mass, and neurological symptoms caused by paraspinal tumours extending into the spinal canal. Metastases can cause lymphadenopathy, hepatomegaly, bone pain, and raccoon eyes (exophthalmia associated with bruising and swelling around the eyes). Metastatic dissemination to the lung and brain is rare {711,1341}. CNS involvement, when present, often shows a diffuse spreading along the meningeal surfaces.

Several paraneoplastic syndromes have been reported, including (1) the syndrome of watery diarrhoea, hypokalaemia, and achlorhydria (WDHA syndrome, also called Verner–Morrison syndrome), caused by the tumour secreting VIP {295}; (2) Horner syndrome (unilateral ptosis, miosis, and anhidrosis associated with a thoracic or cervical tumour) {1715}; (3) opsoclonus-myoclonus-ataxia syndrome (dancing eyes and acute cerebellar ataxia, possibly via an autoimmune mechanism) {2351}; and (4) hypertension, due to catecholamine secretion or renal artery compression by the tumour {2494,2552}. Rare cases with constitutional mutations of *PHOX2B* have also been documented; patients with such cases present with congenital central hypoventilation and Hirschsprung disease {1125}.

Macroscopy
Neuroblastomas (Schwannian stroma–poor) can reach 1–10 cm in diameter, and form a soft, greyish-tan mass (often haemorrhagic), with or without foci of necrosis and calcification. The tumours can be well encapsulated or can show invasive growth into the surrounding tissue. In the nodular subtype of ganglioneuroblastoma (composite, Schwannian stroma–rich/dominant and Schwannian stroma–poor), there are one or more grossly visible, usually haemorrhagic and/or necrotic nodules of soft consistency (the stroma-poor component) coexisting with tannish-white tumour tissue (the stroma-rich or stroma-dominant component). The intermixed subtype of ganglioneuroblastoma (Schwannian stroma–rich) and ganglioneuroma (Schwannian stroma–dominant) have firmer or elastic consistencies and tannish-white cut surfaces.

Microscopy
Surgically resected primary tumour samples obtained prior to chemotherapy or radiation therapy are optimal for histological examination and prognostic evaluation. A diagnosis of peripheral neuroblastic tumour can be established by incisional or core needle biopsy or fine-needle aspiration biopsy of the primary or metastatic tumour. However, fine-needle aspiration does not allow for histopathological classification, which is required for proper risk assessment, so it should only be performed if incisional or core needle biopsy is not feasible for clinical reasons. At the surgical pathology bench, securing an adequate sample for histological examination should be the first priority. Saving snap-frozen material for molecular tests is critical for determining the biological characteristics of a given tumour. Making touch preparations for *MYCN* and other analyses by FISH is recommended.

Whenever feasible, it is recommended to obtain biopsy or surgical materials before starting chemotherapy. This is critical for patient stratification and appropriate protocol assignment at the time of diagnosis.

Lymph nodes attached to the primary tumour should not be sampled separately; they should be included in the histological section with the main tumour, because involvement of contiguous lymph nodes does not influence clinical staging.

Histopathological classification
The INPC defines four categories of peripheral neuroblastic tumours (Table 5.03, p. 198) and clearly delineates the distinction between neuroblastoma, ganglioneuroblastoma, and ganglioneuroma {2542}. The maturation sequences of the tumours are promoted by the so-called cross-talk between neuroblasts and Schwann cells {1635}, comparable to the embryologically well-defined relationship in neural crest development towards ganglion structures of the autonomic nervous system.

Neuroblastoma
(Schwannian stroma–poor)

This category contains tumours composed of neuroblastic cells forming groups or nests demarcated by thin fibrovascular stromal septa with no to limited Schwannian proliferation. Three subtypes are recognized: undifferentiated, poorly differentiated, and differentiating. The undifferentiated neuroblastoma subtype is rare and requires supplementary diagnostic techniques (e. g. immunohistochemistry and/or molecular tests), because the proliferating cells have a uniformly primitive so-called small round blue cell appearance, without clearly recognizable neuropil formation. The poorly differentiated neuroblastoma subtype is defined as a tumour with a background of readily recognizable neuropil with or without Homer Wright rosettes. Less than 5% of the neuroblastic cells have cytomorphological features of differentiation towards mature neurons. The nuclear morphology of the neuroblasts in both the undifferentiated and poorly differentiated subtypes is often described as salt-and-pepper (with an admixture of heterochromatin and inconspicuous nucleoli). However, careful microscopic examination reveals the presence of one to several prominent nucleoli in about 30% of the tumours {2671,2934}, especially when the MYCN oncogene is amplified {1421}. These two subtypes also include rare tumours, designated large cell neuroblastoma, composed of neuroblastic cells with a slightly enlarged and uniquely open nucleus containing one to several prominent nucleoli {2800} (see the subsection *Augmented expression of MYC family proteins* in the section *Prognosis and predictive factors*, p. 203). Infrequently, tumours of these subtypes show unusual histological features (e. g. large, pleomorphic, fusiform, spindle, and pseudorhabdoid cells) focally or diffusely. The differentiating neuroblastoma subtype is defined as a tumour usually with abundant neuropil, and in which > 5% of the tumour cells have an appearance of differentiating neuroblasts, characterized by synchronous differentiation of the nucleus (i. e. enlarged, eccentrically located, with a vesicular chromatin pattern and usually a single prominent nucleolus) and of the cytoplasm (i. e. eosinophilic or amphophilic with a diameter at least twice that of the nucleus).

Ganglioneuroblastoma, intermixed
(Schwannian stroma–rich)

This category contains tumours composed of well-defined microscopic nests of neuroblastic cells in a background of naked neuropil, which are intermixed or randomly distributed in the ganglioneuromatous tissue (see below). These nests are composed of a mixture of neuroblastic cells in various stages of differentiation, usually dominated by differentiating neuroblasts. By definition, > 50% of tumour tissue shows a ganglioneuromatous appearance, with ganglion cells embedded in abundant Schwannian stroma.

Ganglioneuroblastoma, nodular
(composite, Schwannian stroma–rich/dominant and Schwannian stroma–poor)

Tumours in this category are characterized by the presence of one or more grossly visible, usually haemorrhagic and/or necrotic neuroblastic nodules (a stroma-poor component) coexisting with the intermixed subtype of ganglioneuroblastoma (a stroma-rich component) or with ganglioneuroma (a stroma-dominant component). The term "composite" denotes that the tumour is composed of biologically different clones.

Ganglioneuroma
(Schwannian stroma–dominant)

Tumours in this category are characterized by the presence of ganglion cells individually distributed in Schwannian stroma. Neuritic processes produced by ganglion cells are enveloped by the cytoplasm of Schwann cells, so that there are no microscopic foci of naked neuropil without Schwannian coverage. Two subtypes, maturing and mature, are included in this category. The maturing ganglioneuroma subtype has both maturing and mature ganglion cells, whereas the mature

Table 5.03 Categories and subtypes of peripheral neuroblastic tumours as defined in the International Neuroblastoma Pathology Classification (INPC)

Category	Definition	Subtype	Remarks
Neuroblastoma (Schwannian stroma–poor)	Cellular neuroblastic tumour without prominent Schwannian stroma	Undifferentiated	- No clearly identifiable neuropil formation - Supplementary diagnostic techniques required
		Poorly differentiated	- Diagnosis can be made by pure morphological criteria - Characteristic neuropil is present - Differentiating neuroblasts < 5%
		Differentiating	- Usually with abundant neuropil - Differentiating neuroblasts > 5%
Ganglioneuroblastoma, intermixed (Schwannian stroma–rich)	Intermingled microscopic foci of neuroblastic elements in an expanding Schwannian stroma, constituting > 50% of the tumour volume		- Neuroblastic foci are microscopic, without grossly visible nodular formation - Neuroblastic foci are composed of a mixture of neuroblastic cells in various stages of differentiation, in a background of naked neuropil
Ganglioneuroblastoma, nodular (composite, Schwannian stroma–rich/dominant and Schwannian stroma–poor)	A grossly visible neuroblastic nodular (stroma-poor) component coexisting with an intermixed ganglioneuroblastoma (stroma-rich) or ganglioneuroma (stroma-dominant) component		- The proportion of the components varies - The stroma-poor component is usually haemorrhagic and/or necrotic
Ganglioneuroma (Schwannian stroma–dominant)	Predominantly composed of Schwannian stroma, with individually distributed neuronal elements. No detectable naked neuropil	Maturing	- Contains both maturing and mature ganglion cells
		Mature	- Contains exclusively mature ganglion cells surrounded by satellite cells

ganglioneuroma subtype has exclusively mature ganglion cells in the Schwannian stroma. The mature ganglion cells are surrounded by satellite cells. The stromal tissue is usually well organized and has a fascicular profile of Schwann cells bundled with perineurial cells.

Immunophenotype
The tumour cells are variably positive for neuronal markers. A panel approach is advised, which may include synaptophysin, chromogranin, PGP9.5, CD56, and NFP. The tumour cells are also positive for neural crest markers such as tyrosine hydroxylase and PHOX2B {248, 1100}, and for the neuroblastoma marker NB84 {1836}. It is recommended to have positive staining for a combination of these markers along with negative staining for markers of other small round cell tumours. In most *MYCN*-amplified tumours, neuroblasts express MYCN protein {2934}. Mature Schwann cells are S100-positive in the intermixed subtype of ganglioneuroblastoma and in ganglioneuroma. In some neuroblastomas, S100 can also stain putative Schwann cells (Schwannian blasts) in the fibrovascular septa {2544}.

Genetic profile
DNA content
Tumours presenting with whole-chromosome copy-number gains without structural abnormalities (hyperdiploid tumours) are associated with an excellent prognosis {955,1668}. Hyperdiploidy presumably results from chromosome-segregation failure during mitosis. In contrast, tumours in the diploid range are associated with a poor clinical outcome. Flow cytometric analysis for determination of DNA index has been used as a simple and semiautomated method of measuring total cell DNA.

Segmental chromosomal loss/gain and mutations
Tumours presenting with segmental chromosome copy-number changes (losses or gains) and with somatic mutations are associated with a higher risk of relapse than are tumours without those changes {1013}. Chromosomal instability seems to be a dynamic process that cannot be accurately measured at a single time point in the clinical course of individual cases.

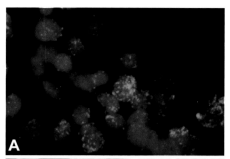
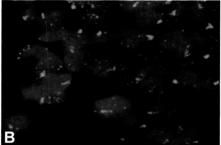

Fig. 5.28 Neuroblastoma cells with *MYCN* amplification. FISH using a *MYCN* probe (green) and a chromosome 2 reference probe (red) reveals amplified *MYCN* organized extrachromosomally in so-called double minutes (**A**) and in double minutes and small homogeneously staining regions (**B**).

Chromosomal loss
Loss of heterozygosity (LOH) of chromosome 1p has been reported in 25–35% of cases {116,397,1737,2460}. Most of the deletions are located distal to 1p36. Distal 1p likely harbours tumour suppressor genes or genes controlling differentiation of neuroblastic cells. A relationship between LOH of 1p and *MYCN* amplification has been described. LOH of chromosome 11q has been identified in 35–45% of cases; 11q23 is the most common site for deletion. Chromosome 11q deletions resulting in LOH are often associated with older patient age, and rarely occur in combination with *MYCN* amplification.

Chromosomal gain
Trisomy 17q may be the most prevalent genetic abnormality in neuroblastomas, and has been detected in about 60% of cases {299,685,2161}. Although the gain can occur independently, it frequently occurs as part of an unbalanced translocation between chromosomes 1 and 17. The 17q breakpoints vary, but a region has been defined at 17q22-qter. Chromosome 1q gain is also reported in neuroblastomas.

MYCN amplification
The *MYCN* oncogene, located on chromosome 2p24.3, is considered a major oncogenic driver of neuroblastoma {71,197,332,2495}. Recently, elevated *LIN28B* expression enhanced by *MYCN* has been reported to contribute to neuroblastoma tumorigenesis. *MYCN* amplification is seen in approximately 20–25% of all neuroblastoma cases. A large region including the *MYCN* locus becomes amplified as extrachromosomal double minutes, and may be linearly integrated into a chromosome as homogeneously staining regions. By FISH, *MYCN* status is determined as amplified (i.e. with ≥ 4 times as many signals vs reference signals of chromosome 2), gain (with increased signals but < 4 times as many vs reference signals of chromosome 2), or unamplified. It is recommended to report the extent of the amplification (i.e. 4–10 times, 10–30 times, or > 30 times) and the type of amplification (i.e. double minutes or homogeneously staining regions).

ALK mutations and amplification
Abnormalities of the *ALK* oncogene seem to account for most cases of hereditary neuroblastoma {473,956,1245,1912, 1913}. About 6–10% of sporadic neuroblastomas carry somatic *ALK*-activating mutations, and an additional 3–4% have *ALK* amplification. ALK is expressed in the developing sympathoadrenal lineage of the neural crest, where it may regulate the balance between cellular proliferation and differentiation through multiple pathways, including the MAPK and RAP1 signal transduction pathways {1913}.

ATRX mutations
ATRX mutations occur in 17% of patients aged 18 months to 12 years with stage 4 disease, and in 44% of patients aged > 12 years, who uniformly have a very poor prognosis {487,488}. *ATRX* mutations have not been reported in tumours with *MYCN* amplification. Little is known about how *ATRX* contributes to the development and differentiation of the sympathoadrenal lineage. Most tumours with *ATRX* mutations show alternative lengthening of telomeres. A high level of telomerase activity is reported to be predictive of reduced patient survival {487, 2138}. However, telomere length does not necessarily correlate with telomerase activity.

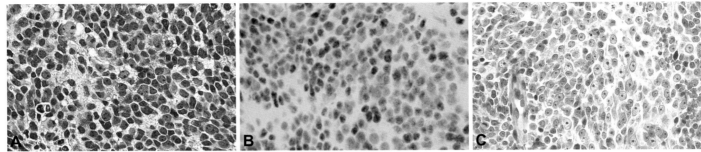

Fig. 5.29 Neuroblastoma. **A** Poorly differentiated subtype with MYC protein overexpression. Note the presence of one to several prominent nucleoli. **B** MYC protein immunostaining of the same tumour. **C** Large cell neuroblastoma with a unique nuclear morphology showing the presence of one to several nucleoli in a clear, so-called euchromatin-rich nucleus.

Expression of neurotrophin receptors

Neurotrophins, a family of growth factor proteins, control survival, differentiation, and growth of neurons. Among the neurotrophin receptors, the expression of three tyrosine kinase receptors (TrkA, TrkB, and TrkC) is important in neuroblastoma biology. Their preferred ligands are nerve growth factor, brain-derived neurotrophic factor, and neurotrophin-3, respectively. Neurotrophin-4/5 appears to function through TrkB. A high level of TrkA expression is inversely correlated with *MYCN* amplification and is associated with a favourable clinical outcome. The nerve growth factor / TrkA pathway may play a critical role in regression or neuroblastic differentiation in selected patients. In contrast, TrkB is more commonly expressed in tumours with *MYCN* amplification. TrkB and its preferred ligand (brain-derived neurotrophic factor), which are both expressed by the same tumour cells, may form an autocrine or paracrine loop providing some tumour survival and growth advantage. TrkC expression is often correlated with TrkA expression {329,1940}.

Genetic susceptibility

About 1–2% of affected individuals have familial neuroblastoma {2553}. This condition has an autosomal dominant inheritance pattern with incomplete penetration. Patients with hereditary predisposition to neuroblastoma are usually diagnosed at an earlier age (mean: 9 months) than are patients with sporadic cases (mean: 17.3 months), and at least 20% of them have bilateral adrenal or multifocal primaries. A genome-wide study identified a linkage of familial neuroblastoma with 16p12-13 {1739}. Germline mutations reported in familial neuroblastoma cases are located in *PHOX2B* (2p12) and *ALK* (2p23).

PHOX2B mutation has been identified in a small number of inherited cases {1125}. *PHOX2B* encodes a homeodomain transcription factor that promotes cell cycle exit and neuronal differentiation; therefore, it plays a crucial role in the development of neural crest–derived autonomic neurons. Non–polyalanine repeat expansion mutations of *PHOX2B* are associated with neuroblastoma, Hirschsprung disease, and congenital central hypoventilation syndrome {72,1125}. Inherited changes in the *ALK* oncogene are observed in most cases of hereditary neuroblastoma {1913}. Several mutations lead to constitutive phosphorylation of ALK, leading to dysregulation of cell signalling and then uncontrolled proliferation of the neuroblastic cells. *ALK* could be an oncogenic driver, and the activating mutations or amplifications are associated with aggressive disease.

Table 5.04 The International Neuroblastoma Pathology Classification (INPC), with favourable and unfavourable histology groups defined on the basis of age, degree of neuroblast differentiation, nodular pattern, degree of Schwannian stromal development, and mitosis-karyorrhexis index (MKI)

Patient age at diagnosis	Favourable histology group	Unfavourable histology group
Any age	- Ganglioneuroblastoma, intermixed (Schwannian stroma–rich) - Ganglioneuroma (Schwannian stroma–dominant) of either subtype (maturing or mature)	- Neuroblastoma (Schwannian stroma–poor) of the undifferentiated subtype - Neuroblastoma (Schwannian stroma–poor), of any subtype, with a high MKI
< 18 Months (< 548 days)	- Neuroblastoma (Schwannian stroma–poor) of the poorly differentiated subtype, with a low or intermediate MKI - Neuroblastoma (Schwannian stroma–poor) of the differentiating subtype, with a low or intermediate MKI	
18–60 Months (548 days to 5 years)	- Neuroblastoma (Schwannian stroma–poor) of the differentiating subtype, with a low MKI	- Neuroblastoma (Schwannian stroma–poor) of the poorly differentiated subtype - Neuroblastoma (Schwannian stroma–poor) of the differentiating subtype, with an intermediate MKI
> 60 Months (> 5 years)		- Neuroblastoma (Schwannian stroma–poor) of any subtype

Ganglioneuroblastoma, nodular (composite, Schwannian stroma–rich/dominant and Schwannian stroma–poor) is classified in either the favourable or unfavourable histology group depending on the characteristics of its neuroblastomatous nodules. For this distinction, the same age-dependent evaluation criteria for grade of neuroblastic differentiation and MKI are applied to the neuroblastomatous components as are used in the neuroblastoma (Schwannian stroma–poor) category.

Genome-wide association studies

Whole-genome sequencing reveals recurrent genetic lesions in the RAC-RHO pathway and in *ARID1A* and *ARID1B*. Several predisposing SNPs have been identified within or adjacent to genes including *CASC15* (also called *LINC00340*), *BARD1*, *LMO1*, *DUSP12*, *HSD17B12*, *DDX4*, *IL31RA*, *HACE1*, and *LIN28B* {292,382,684,1738,1976,2211, 2436,2930}.

Prognosis and predictive factors

Clinical staging

Two systems, the International Neuroblastoma staging system (INSS) {330, 331} and the International Neuroblastoma Risk Group (INRG) staging system {1888}, are widely recognized as significant predictive factors. At diagnosis, > 50% of patients present with metastatic disease. Of those, 7% are so-called special neuroblastoma, evaluated as INSS stage 4S (INRG stage MS). Approximately 20–25% have localized disease and 15% have regional extension.

Age at diagnosis

In neuroblastoma, patient age at diagnosis is a powerful prognostic indicator, and the age of 1 year has historically been used as the cut-off point. Age is considered a surrogate for genetic or biological risk factor markers. The prognostic impact of age on clinical outcome is continuous in nature; survival rates are always better among younger patients than older patients, regardless of the cut-off point used. London et al. {1666} reported the statistical evidence of an age cut-off point > 1 year for risk stratification, and the Children's Oncology Group (COG) is in the process of updating the cut-off point from 1 year (365 days) to 1.5 years (548 days) in their neuroblastoma risk grouping system {2114}.

The International Neuroblastoma Pathology Classification

The INPC was first established in 1999 {2542,2543} (as a slightly modified version of the original Shimada classification {2545}) and then revised in 2003 {2160}. It defines four categories of peripheral neuroblastic tumours (see Table 5.03, p. 198): neuroblastoma (Schwannian stroma–poor); ganglioneuroblastoma, intermixed (Schwannian stroma–rich); ganglioneuroblastoma, nodular (composite, Schwannian stroma–rich/dominant and Schwannian stroma–poor); and ganglioneuroma (Schwannian stroma–dominant), on the basis of the cross-talk between neuroblastic cells and Schwannian stromal cells (see *Microscopy*). The neuroblastoma (Schwannian stroma–poor) category contains three subtypes, defined by the grade of neuroblastic differentiation: undifferentiated, poorly differentiated, and differentiating {2546}. Neuroblastoma (Schwannian stroma–poor) tumours are

Table 5.05 The Children's Oncology Group (COG) neuroblastoma risk grouping system {2114,2963}

INSS stage	Patient age	*MYCN* status	Ploidy (DNA index)	INPC histology group	Other	Risk group[a]
1	Any	Any	Any	Any		Low
2A/2B	Any	Unamplified	Any	Any	Resection ≥ 50%	Low
					Resection < 50%	Intermediate
					Biopsy only	Intermediate
		Amplified	Any	Any	Any degree of resection	High
3	≤ 547 days	Unamplified	Any	Any		Intermediate
	> 547 days	Unamplified	Any	Favourable		Intermediate
				Unfavourable		High
	Any	Amplified	Any	Any		High
4	< 365 days	Unamplified	Any	Any		Intermediate
		Amplified	Any	Any		High
	365–547 days	Unamplified	> 1	Favourable		Intermediate
		Any	1	Any		High
		Any	Any	Unfavourable		High
		Amplified	Any	Any		High
	> 547 days	Any	Any	Any		High
4S	< 365 days	Unamplified	> 1	Favourable	Asymptomatic	Low
			Any	Any	Symptomatic	Intermediate
				Unfavourable	Asymptomatic or symptomatic	Intermediate
			1	Any	Asymptomatic or symptomatic	Intermediate
		Unknown	Unknown	Unknown	Patient too sick for biopsy	Intermediate
		Amplified	Any	Any	Asymptomatic or symptomatic	High

INPC, International Neuroblastoma Pathology Classification; INSS, International Neuroblastoma staging system.

[a] The intermediate-risk group is further divided into three subgroups (not shown) on the basis of patient age, *MYCN* status, ploidy, INPC histology group, and the presence or absence of loss of heterozygosity of 1p/11q.

also evaluated for mitotic activity and karyorrhectic activity (which are significantly associated with *MYCN* oncogene status {1020,2547}); the mitosis-karyorrhexis index (MKI), which is defined as the number of cells undergoing mitosis or karyorrhexis per 5000 cells, is classified as low (< 100), intermediate (100–200), or high (> 200). *MYCN*-amplified tumours typically have a high MKI. The prognostic implications of MKI class are age-dependent {2740}.

The INPC distinguishes between favourable and unfavourable histology groups, with each case classified within the framework of age-appropriate maturation sequence and age-appropriate MKI (See Table 5.04, p. 200). Two age cut-off points, 18 months (548 days) and 60 months (5 years), are used in the INPC. The vast majority of neuroblastomas (Schwannian stroma–poor) are diagnosed in infants and young children. In contrast, ganglioneuroblastoma, intermixed (Schwannian stroma–rich); ganglioneuroblastoma, nodular (composite, Schwannian stroma–rich/dominant and Schwannian stroma–poor); and ganglioneuroma (Schwannian stroma–dominant) are often diagnosed in older children.

Prognostic classification with this system, for either primary or metastatic tumours, should only be performed before starting chemotherapy or radiation therapy. MKI determination is not feasible in bone marrow metastases. For evaluation of histological changes after chemotherapy or radiation therapy, there are currently no reliable guidelines for predicting clinical outcome.

Biochemistry

Elevated levels of serum neuron-specific enolase (> 100 ng/mL) {3099}, ferritin (> 150 ng/mL) {1078}, and lactic dehydrogenase (> 1500 IU/L) {2557}, as well as a VMA-to-HVA ratio < 1.0 {1561} are associated with poor prognosis.

DNA index

As mentioned in the *Genetic profile* section, hyperdiploidy indicates an excellent prognosis {955} and diploidy indicates a poor prognosis {1668}. However, the prognostic significance of ploidy seems to be lost in children aged > 2 years, possibly because hyperdiploid tumours in older children typically have a number of structural abnormalities.

MYCN status

MYCN amplification is associated with tumours of advanced stage and aggressive clinical behaviour {332,1737,2495}. The vast majority of *MYCN*-amplified tumours overexpress MYCN protein. However, there are rare *MYCN*-amplified neuroblastomas without protein overexpression, and also rare *MYCN*-unamplified neuroblastomas with protein overexpression. Recent studies support the supposition that MYCN protein overexpression and MYC-MAX heterodimer formation (rather than *MYCN* oncogene

Table 5.06 The International Neuroblastoma Risk Group (INRG) consensus pretreatment classification schema {536}

INRG stage	Patient age (months)	Histological category	Grade of tumour differentiation	*MYCN* status	Unbalanced 11q aberration	Ploidy	Pretreatment risk group
L1		GN maturing or GNB intermixed					Very low
		Any except GN maturing or GNB intermixed		Unamplified			Very low
				Amplified			High
L2		GN maturing or GNB intermixed					Very low
	< 18	Any except GN maturing or GNB intermixed		Unamplified	No		Low
					Yes		Intermediate
	≥ 18	GNB nodular or neuroblastoma	Differentiating	Unamplified	No		Low
					Yes		Intermediate
			Poorly differentiated or undifferentiated	Unamplified	(Any)		Intermediate
	Any age			Amplified			High
M	< 18			Unamplified		Hyperdiploid	Low
	< 12			Unamplified		Diploid	Intermediate
	12 to < 18			Unamplified		Diploid	Intermediate
	< 18			Amplified			High
	≥ 18						High
MS	< 18			Unamplified	No		Very low
					Yes		High
				Amplified			High

GN, ganglioneuroma; GNB, ganglioneuroblastoma.
Source: Cohn SL, Pearson AD, London WB, Monclair T, Ambros PF, Brodeur GM, et al. (2009). The International Neuroblastoma Risk Group (INRG) classification system: an INRG Task Force report {536}. Reprinted with permission. ©2009 American Society of Clinical Oncology. All rights reserved.

amplification) play a critical role in activating downstream molecular targets through E-box gene sequence, leading to a poor prognosis {197,681}.

Augmented expression of MYC family proteins

In addition to *MYCN* oncogene amplification and MYCN protein overexpression, MYC protein overexpression has been reported as a newly identified prognostic factor {2933,2934}. MYC family–driven neuroblastoma, defined by augmented expression of MYC protein (detected in ~10% of neuroblastomas of the undifferentiated and poorly differentiated subtypes) and/or MYCN protein (detected in ~20% of neuroblastomas of the same subtypes), is highly aggressive and often associated with prominent nucleolar formation, which is considered to be a putative site of MYCN/MYC RNA synthesis and accumulation {2934}. Due to the presence of prominent nucleoli, MYC family–driven neuroblastoma can be morphologically distinguished from other conventional neuroblastomas, which have so-called salt-and-pepper nuclei. Also included in the group of MYC family–driven neuroblastoma is large cell neuroblastoma, which is histologically defined, rare, and the most aggressive tumour {2800}. Neuroblastic cells are characterized by slightly enlarged and uniquely open nuclei containing one to several prominent nucleoli. Their so-called euchromatin-rich open nuclei suggest stemness of the tumour cells, and the prominent nucleolar formation is associated with overexpression of either MYCN or MYC {1210}.

Chromosomal loss or gain

Chromosomal alterations (i.e. 1p deletion, 11q deletion, and 17q gain) were tested for in neuroblastomas without *MYCN* amplification; 11q deletion and 17q gain were associated with poor survival in univariate analysis. A segmental profile (i.e. the presence of multiple chromosomal alterations rather than single genetic alterations) adds prognostic information in addition to patient age and clinical stage in multivariate analysis {1013}.

Risk grouping

Risk grouping systems incorporate a combination of predictive factors, such as clinical stage, patient age at diagnosis, histopathology, and genetic and molecular properties.

The COG neuroblastoma risk grouping system (Table 5.05, p. 201) has been used for patient stratification and protocol assignment in clinical trials {2114,2963}. Patients in the low-risk group are often followed by observation (with no chemotherapy or radiation therapy) after surgery or even biopsy alone. Intermediate-risk patients are treated with surgery and non-aggressive chemotherapy. High-risk patients are treated with intensive chemotherapy, surgery, radiation therapy, bone marrow / haematopoietic stem cell transplantation, and biological therapies. The reported 5-year survival rates for non–high-risk and high-risk patients are 90% and 50%, respectively {2114}.

The estimated 5-year event-free survival rates by pretreatment risk group as defined in the INRG classification system (Table 5.06) are > 85% for very-low–risk patients, > 75% to 85% for low-risk patients, 50–75% for intermediate-risk patients, and < 50% for high-risk patients {536}. However, this classification system has not been widely adopted.

Composite phaeochromocytoma

Tischler A.S.
de Krijger R.R.
Kimura N.
Komminoth P.
Lloyd R.V.

Definition

A tumour consisting of phaeochromocytoma combined with a developmentally related neurogenic tumour such as ganglioneuroma, ganglioneuroblastoma, neuroblastoma, or peripheral nerve sheath tumour.

ICD-O code   8700/3

Synonyms

Compound adrenal medullary tumour; mixed adrenal medullary tumour; mixed neuroendocrine–neural tumour

Epidemiology

Composite features can be found in 3–9% of all phaeochromocytomas {1532,1628}. Ganglioneuroma is present in 70–80% of composite cases, ganglioneuroblastoma in 10–20%, and undifferentiated neuroblastoma and malignant peripheral nerve sheath tumour extremely rarely {132,439, 1348}. Composite phaeochromocytomas usually occur in adults, with a median patient age of 40–50 years (range: 5–82 years) and equal frequency in males and females {1348,1532}.

Localization

Composite phaeochromocytomas arise in the adrenal medulla. Approximately 7% of cases are bilateral {1348}.

Clinical features

The signs and symptoms are generally the same as with ordinary phaeochromocytomas. Heterogeneity in imaging sometimes suggests composite features {1532}. Levels of catecholamines vary {1348}. Occasional cases are associated with the syndrome of watery diarrhoea, hypokalaemia, and achlorhydria (WDHA syndrome, also called Verner–Morrison syndrome), caused by production of VIP {1348,1532,1662}.

Composite phaeochromocytomas can metastasize by lymphatic and haematogenous routes to lymph nodes, lung, bone, and liver, and may seed the omentum and diaphragm {1985,2430}. The risk of metastasis is low overall but is difficult

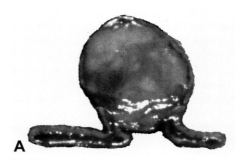
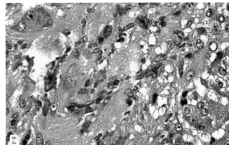

Fig. 5.30 Composite phaeochromocytoma. **A** Composite phaeochromocytoma (dark-grey areas) with ganglioneuroma (pale-grey areas). The heterogeneous gross appearance provides an important clue to the composite nature of the tumour. **B** An area of tumour showing neoplastic chromaffin cells (at right), ganglion cells (at left), neurons (at right), and an intervening Schwann cell–rich stroma.

to estimate due to tumour rarity; insufficient follow-up; and probable underreporting of phaeochromocytomas with small, incidentally discovered composite areas. When metastases occur, they usually arise from tumours containing ganglioneuroblastoma, neuroblastoma, or malignant peripheral nerve sheath tumour {1348}. These components can metastasize alone or together with phaeochromocytoma {1941}. Less often, phaeochromocytoma metastasizes alone {1532}, or two components metastasize independently {439}. Pure primary phaeochromocytomas that metastasize as composite tumours containing ganglioneuroma {1357} or malignant peripheral nerve sheath tumour {439} have also been reported.

Macroscopy

Macroscopic examination sometimes reveals patchy, firm, pale areas corresponding to ganglioneuroma or to necrotic and haemorrhagic areas of ganglioneuroblastoma or neuroblastoma {309, 1532}. Usually, composite features are first noted microscopically.

Microscopy

The diagnosis of composite phaeochromocytoma requires complete histoarchitecture of the additional tumour type. Scattered neuron-like cells can be present in typical phaeochromocytomas and are not sufficient. The first diagnostic

clue is often provided by stromal features, which can include bundles of spindle-shaped Schwann cells and axon-like processes, patchy areas with unusually prominent sustentacular cells, or hyalinization {2780}.

Immunohistochemically, the components of composite phaeochromocytomas resemble their counterparts in normal tissue or in pure tumours of the same type {2783}. Therefore, staining patterns help to identify neuroblastomatous foci {885} and to distinguish immature neurons from neoplastic chromaffin cells of the same size. Schwann cells and sustentacular cells stain for S100, whereas axon-like processes stain for NFPs. Phaeochromocytoma cells contain many secretory granules and stain strongly for chromogranin A and synaptophysin, whereas neurons contain relatively sparse granules and show weak or focal staining, often in a linear or punctate pattern corresponding to cell processes {885,2783}. Additional markers associated with neuronal differentiation are strong expression of RET protein {2193} and VIP {2783}. However, tumours causing clinical signs of excess VIP are divided between composite phaeochromocytomas in which immunoreactive VIP is localized to neuronal cells {2050} and pure phaeochromocytomas without obvious neuronal morphology {1260}, with the latter suggesting an intermediate phenotype.

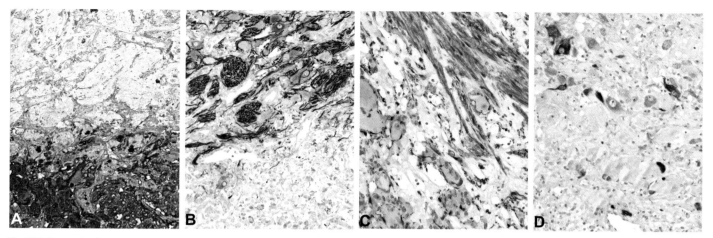

Fig. 5.31 Composite phaeochromocytoma. **A** Strong immunoreactivity for chromogranin A indicates areas of phaeochromocytoma. **B** Strong immunoreactivity for NFP indicates areas of ganglioneuroma. **C** S100 is expressed in both Schwann cells and sustentacular cells. **D** RET is most strongly expressed in subsets of neurons.

Genetic profile

Reduced expression of neurofibromin has been reported in Schwann cells and sustentacular cells of composite phaeochromocytomas in patients with or without evidence of neurofibromatosis, suggesting possible somatic *NF1* mutations {1379}. *MYCN* was not amplified in the neuroblastic component of the few cases studied {548}.

Genetic susceptibility

Approximately 17% of all reported composite phaeochromocytomas have involved patients with neurofibromatosis type 1, and as many as 50% of phaeochromocytomas associated with neurofibromatosis type 1 are bilateral {1348}. Two patients with multiple endocrine neoplasia type 2A have been reported {309,1756}. Other isolated associations have included vertebral and hepatic haemangiomas {225} and a renal angiomyolipoma {1471}.

Prognosis and predictive factors

Composite phaeochromocytomas confined to the adrenal gland and completely excised do not usually metastasize or recur. Even an extensive neuroblastic component is usually compatible with surgical cure {903}. Nonetheless, all patients require long-term follow-up because the clinical course is unpredictable. One case recurred locally after 15 years {1985}.

Composite paraganglioma

Tischler A.S.
de Krijger R.R.
Kimura N.

Definition

A tumour consisting of paraganglioma combined with a developmentally related neurogenic tumour such as ganglioneuroma, ganglioneuroblastoma, neuroblastoma, or peripheral nerve sheath tumour.

ICD-O code   8693/3

Synonyms

Composite extra-adrenal phaeochromocytoma; compound paraganglioma; ganglioneuromatous paraganglioma; mixed neuroendocrine–neural tumour

Epidemiology

Composite paragangliomas are extremely rare tumours, approximately one tenth as frequent as composite phaeochromocytomas. They have been reported in patients aged 15 months {1889} to 81 years {1537}, with a slight female predominance. All reported cases have consisted of paraganglioma with ganglioneuroma, except for a few examples with neuroblastoma {1889} or ganglioneuroblastoma {1373}.

Localization

The most common anatomical sites are the urinary bladder {467,1537} and the retroperitoneum {1185}. Other locations are the cauda equina/filum terminale and (very rarely) the posterior mediastinum {634}. Composite features have

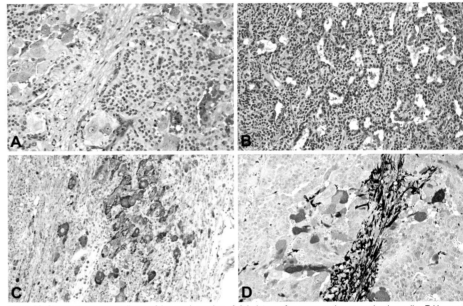

Fig. 5.32 Composite paraganglioma of the cauda equina. **A** Admixture of neurons and neuroendocrine cells. **B** Unusual rosette-like pattern in a neuroendocrine area of the tumour. Classic paraganglioma architecture is not present. **C** Strong immunoreactivity for chromogranin A in neuroendocrine cells and weaker immunoreactivity in neuronal cell bodies and processes. **D** Strong immunoreactivity for S100 in Schwann cells and sustentacular cells; weak immunoreactivity in some neurons. Tyrosine hydroxylase expression could not be definitively assessed.

not been reported in head and neck paragangliomas.

Clinical features

One reported case was associated with the syndrome of watery diarrhoea, hypokalaemia, and achlorhydria (WDHA syndrome) {1185}. The others were either clinically silent or associated with catecholamine-related signs. Local lymph nodes were involved in one case {1889}. There have been no reported recurrences.

Macroscopy

The macroscopic features are the same as those of composite phaeochromocytomas.

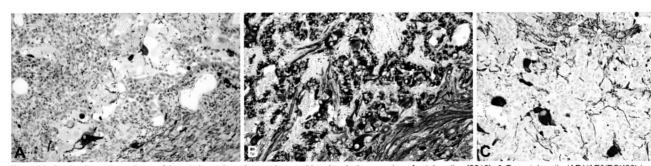

Fig. 5.33 Composite paraganglioma of the cauda equina: aberrant immunohistochemical expression of cytokeratins {2516}. **A** Pancytokeratin (AE1/AE3/PCK26) immunoreactivity is present in the neuronal processes and cell bodies of some neurons, and is present in a perinuclear dot-like pattern in neuroendocrine cells. **B** Strong immunoreactivity for low-molecular-weight cytokeratins (CAM 5.2) is seen in the neuroendocrine cells, neuronal processes, and cell bodies of some neurons. **C** Immunoreactivity for NFPs is present only in neuronal processes and in the processes of some neurons.

Microscopy

The histopathology is the same as that of composite phaeochromocytoma, except in cauda equina paragangliomas, which can show extensive expression of keratins {2216,2516}. In some cases, keratin expression can blur the distinction between composite paraganglioma and gangliocytic paraganglioma {634}, which is more closely related to neuroendocrine tumours of the gastrointestinal tract.

Keratin expression is not incompatible with paraganglionic origin per se {484, 515,883}, but must be carefully interpreted in the context of clinical findings, morphology, and other markers.

There has been one reported case of a pigmented composite paraganglioma in the urinary bladder, with neuromelanin-like pigment localized to the paraganglioma component {717}.

Genetic profile

MYCN amplification, gain of 17q, or loss of 1p/11q were not present in one case studied {1889}.

Prognosis and predictive factors

No metastatic cases have been reported.

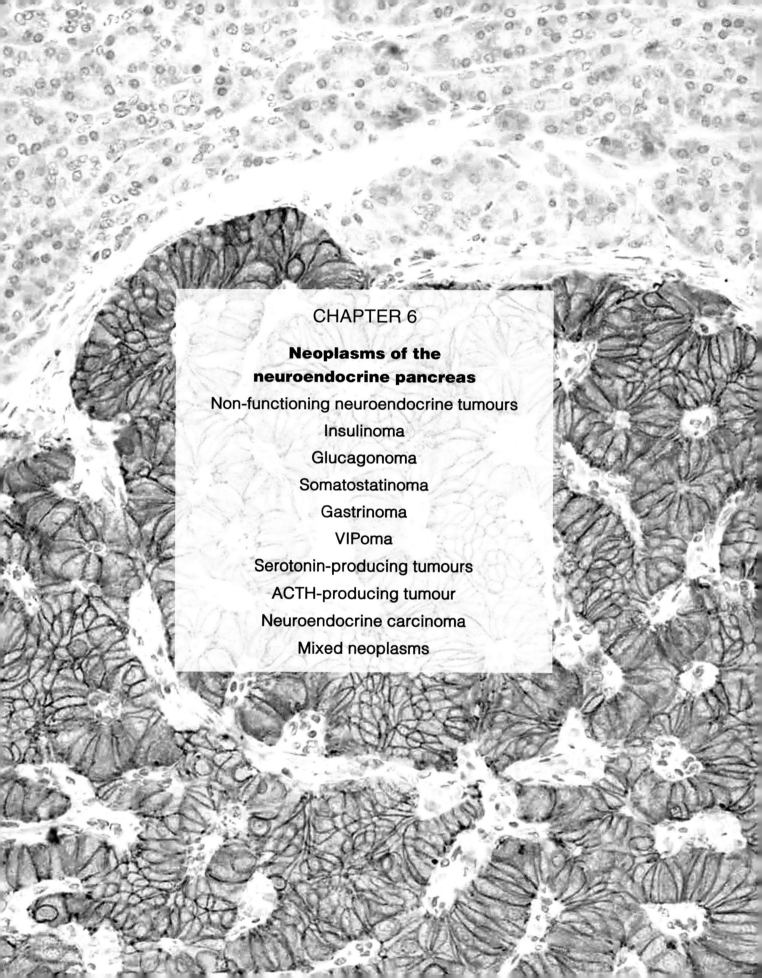

CHAPTER 6

Neoplasms of the neuroendocrine pancreas

WHO classification of neoplasms of the neuroendocrine pancreas

Non-functioning (non-syndromic) neuroendocrine tumours

Pancreatic neuroendocrine microadenoma	8150/0
Non-functioning pancreatic neuroendocrine tumour	8150/3

Insulinoma	8151/3
Glucagonoma	8152/3
Somatostatinoma	8156/3
Gastrinoma	8153/3
VIPoma	8155/3

Serotonin-producing tumours with and without carcinoid syndrome

Serotonin-producing tumour	8241/3

ACTH-producing tumour with Cushing syndrome

ACTH-producing tumour	8158/3*

Pancreatic neuroendocrine carcinoma (poorly differentiated neuroendocrine neoplasm)

Neuroendocrine carcinoma (poorly differentiated neuroendocrine neoplasm)	8246/3 [a]
Small cell neuroendocrine carcinoma	8041/3
Large cell neuroendocrine carcinoma	8013/3

Mixed neuroendocrine–non-neuroendocrine neoplasms — 8154/3
  Mixed ductal–neuroendocrine carcinomas
  Mixed acinar–neuroendocrine carcinomas

---

[a] This ICD-O code should not be used for well-differentiated G3 pancreatic neuroendocrine tumours, which are coded using the functioning or non-functioning pancreatic neuroendocrine tumour codes.

The morphology codes are from the International Classification of Diseases for Oncology (ICD-O) {898A}. Behaviour is coded /0 for benign tumours; /1 for unspecified, borderline, or uncertain behaviour; /2 for carcinoma in situ and grade III intraepithelial neoplasia; and /3 for malignant tumours. The classification is modified from the previous WHO classification, taking into account changes in our understanding of these lesions.
* This new code was approved by the IARC/WHO Committee for ICD-O.

TNM classification of tumours of the neuroendocrine pancreas (G1+G2)*

T – Primary Tumour

TX	Primary tumour cannot be assessed
T0	No evidence of primary tumour
T1	Tumour limited to pancreas**, less than 2 cm in greatest dimension
T2	Tumour limited to pancreas**, 2 cm or more but less than 4 cm in greatest dimension
T3	Tumour limited to pancreas**, 4 cm or more in greatest dimension or Tumour invading duodenum or bile duct.
T4	Tumour perforates visceral peritoneum (serosa) or other organs or adjacent structures

N – Regional Lymph Nodes

NX	Regional lymph nodes cannot be assessed
N0	No regional lymph node metastasis
N1	Regional lymph node metastasis

M – Distant Metastasis

M0	No distant metastasis
M1	Distant metastasis
M1a	Hepatic metastasis only
M1b	Extrahepatic metastasis only
M1c	Hepatic and extrahepatic metastases

Stage

Stage	T	N	M
Stage I	T1	N0	M0
Stage II	T2, T3	N0	M0
Stage III	T4	N0	M0
	Any T	N1	M0
Stage IV	Any T	Any N	Any M

Note: For any T, add (m) for multiple tumours.

---

* The TNM classification of PanNECs follows the criteria for classifying ductal adenocarcinomas.

** This includes invasion of the peripancreatic adipose tissue.

Adapted from: TNM Classification of Malignant Tumours, 8th Edition (2016). {323}

Introduction

Klöppel G.   Komminoth P.
Couvelard A.   Osamura R. Y.
Hruban R. H.   Perren A.
Klimstra D. S.   Rindi G.

Pancreatic neuroendocrine neoplasms (PanNENs) have significant neuroendocrine differentiation, with expression of synaptophysin and usually also chromogranin A. They include malignant well-differentiated neuroendocrine neoplasms (NENs), which are called pancreatic neuroendocrine tumours (PanNETs), and poorly differentiated NENs, which are called pancreatic neuroendocrine carcinomas (PanNECs).

Epidemiology

The relative frequency of NENs among the pancreatic tumours is 2–5%, and their incidence is estimated to be < 1 case per 100 000 person-years {884,1069}, although autopsy studies that also take into account tumours measuring < 5 mm suggest a much higher incidence {1381} (see *Non-functioning neuroendocrine tumours*, p. 215). PanNENs show no significant sex difference and occur in a wide age range, with the highest incidence found in patients aged 30–60 years. The incidence of well-differentiated PanNENs has steadily increased over the past 40 years {300,884,1119}, probably due to continual improvements in diagnostics.

Clinical features

PanNETs are generally slow-growing, with overall survival rates of 33% at 5 years, 17% at 10 years, and 10% at 20 years {884}. Surgical resection markedly improves these survival rates (see *Non-functioning neuroendocrine tumours*, pp. 215 and 218). In contrast, patients with fast-growing PanNECs rarely survive 1 year {173}. PanNETs are divided into functioning and non-functioning neoplasms. Tumours associated with clinical syndromes caused by abnormal secretion of hormones are considered functioning (syndromic) PanNETs and include insulinomas, gastrinomas, glucagonomas, VIPomas, and other less common tumours. Non-functioning (non-syndromic) tumours are not associated with a clinical hormone hypersecretion syndrome, but may secrete peptide hormones and biogenic substances, such

as pancreatic polypeptide and chromogranins, which are either secreted at levels insufficient to cause symptoms or do not give rise to a clinical syndrome. Non-functioning tumours are discovered incidentally or become clinically apparent due to their large size, invasion of adjacent organs, or metastasis. Tumours with a diameter of < 5 mm, the minimum size for detection by imaging, are typically non-functioning and are designated neuroendocrine microadenomas. In the past, functioning PanNETs accounted for 60–85% of all PanNENs, with insulinomas being the most frequent type (accounting for as many as 70% of cases), followed by gastrinomas, glucagonomas, VIPomas, and other functioning PanNETs such as PanNETs producing serotonin (p. 233), adrenocorticotropic hormone (ACTH) (p. 234), growth hormone-releasing hormone (GHRH) {930}, parathyroid hormone-related peptide (PTHrP) {1305A}, and cholecystokinin (CCK) {2266A}. However, recent data show that non-functioning PanNETs now account for > 60% of all PanNENs {821,821A}.

Genetic syndromes

In 10–20% of cases, well-differentiated PanNENs are associated with genetically

determined hereditary syndromes such as multiple endocrine neoplasia type 1, von Hippel–Lindau syndrome (VHL), neurofibromatosis type 1, tuberous sclerosis, and glucagon cell hyperplasia and neoplasia {795,2580}. Germline mutations in DNA repair genes (*MUTYH*, *CHEK2* and *BRCA2*) have been described in patients with apparently sporadic PanNETs {2440A}. PanNECs do not show these associations {795}.

Molecular genetics

In PanNETs, the *MEN1* gene is somatically inactivated in 45% of cases. This gene codes for menin, a tumour suppressor protein with diverse functions. *DAXX* and *ATRX* are also frequently targeted in PanNETs, with 45% of cases having a mutation in one of the two genes. The DAXX and ATRX proteins function in chromatin remodelling at telomeric and pericentromeric regions, and mutations of the encoding genes are strongly associated with the alternative lengthening of telomeres pathway for telomere maintenance, as well as with chromosomal instability. About 15% of PanNETs have alterations in mTOR pathway genes such as *TSC2*, *PTEN*, and *PIK3CA*. The mTOR pathway is important because it is

Table 6.01 2017 WHO classification and grading of pancreatic neuroendocrine neoplasms (PanNENs)

Classification/grade	Ki-67 proliferation index [a]	Mitotic index [a]
Well-differentiated PanNENs: pancreatic neuroendocrine tumours (PanNETs)		
PanNET G1	< 3%	< 2
PanNET G2	3–20%	2–20
PanNET G3	> 20%	> 20
Poorly differentiated PanNENs: pancreatic neuroendocrine carcinomas (PanNECs)		
PanNEC (G3)	> 20%	> 20
Small cell type		
Large cell type		
Mixed neuroendocrine–non-neuroendocrine neoplasm		

[a] The Ki-67 proliferation index is based on the evaluation of ≥ 500 cells in areas of higher nuclear labelling (so-called hotspots). The mitotic index is based on the evaluation of mitoses in 50 high-power fields (HPF; 0.2 mm² each) in areas of higher density, and is expressed as mitoses per 10 high-power fields (2.0 mm²). The final grade is determined based on whichever index (Ki-67 or mitotic) places the tumour in the highest grade category. For assessing Ki-67, casual visual estimation (eyeballing) is not recommended; manual counting using printed images is advocated {2267}.

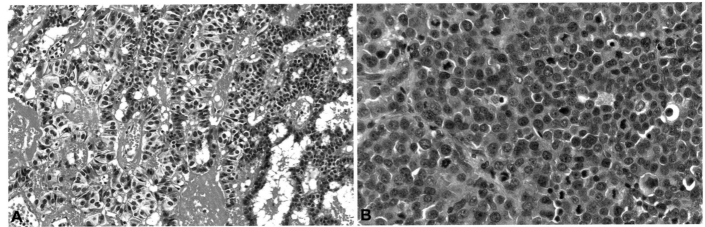

Fig. 6.01 Pancreatic neuroendocrine neoplasm (NEN). **A** Neuroendocrine tumour (well-differentiated NEN). **B** Neuroendocrine carcinoma (poorly differentiated NEN), large cell type.

a potential therapeutic target. There are also PanNETs that show *HIF1A* and *VHL* alterations {704,795,1261,2132,2440A, 2467,2538,2580}.

The genetic alterations in PanNECs differ considerably from those in Pan-NETs. Genes involved in the cell cycle, such as *TP53*, *RB1*, and *CDKN2A* (also called *P16*), are somatically targeted in PanNECs, whereas *MEN1*, *ATRX*, and *DAXX* are not {3031}.

Germline alterations in *MEN1*, *VHL*, *NF1*, and *GCGR*, respectively, are found in familial PanNETs associated with multiple endocrine neoplasia type 1, VHL, neurofibromatosis type 1, and glucagon cell hyperplasia and neoplasia. Some of these PanNETs have distinctive morphologies. Mutations in *VHL* result in dysregulation of the hypoxia-inducible factor pathway, and PanNETs that arise in patients with VHL can have clear-cell morphology {1149}. Alterations in *GCCR* alter glucagon receptor signalling and lead to glucagon cell hyperplasia and subsequent neoplasia, but the mechanism through which these alterations occur is

not yet clear {2580}. Some patients with clinically sporadic PanNETs have been found to have germline mutations in DNA repair genes {2440A}.

Updated WHO classification

New features

The 2010 *WHO classification of tumours of the digestive system* {2293} divided NENs of the gastrointestinal tract, including PanNENs, into two groups based on their morphology and proliferation rate: (1) well-differentiated NENs, called neuroendocrine tumours (NETs), and (2) poorly differentiated NENs, called neuroendocrine carcinomas (NECs). PanNETs were graded according to their proliferative activity into either grade 1 (G1) neuroendocrine tumours (NETs) (< 2 mitoses per 10 high-power fields and Ki-67 proliferation index ≤ 2%) or grade 2 (G2) NETs (2–20 mitoses per 10 high-power fields or Ki-67 proliferation index of 3–20%). PanNECs were classified as grade 3 (G3) tumours (> 20 mitoses per 10 high-power fields or Ki-67 proliferation index > 20%) and were further

subclassified as small cell carcinoma or large cell carcinoma.

The 2010 WHO classification was functional and effectively stratified PanNEN survival, but in the years since its publication, some PanNENs with the histological features of PanNET have been found to have a Ki-67 proliferation index > 20%. This is particularly common in liver metastases developing during the course of the disease. Per the 2010 WHO criteria, these tumours would be classified as PanNEC. Although these tumours appear to have a somewhat worse prognosis than do G2 NETs, their behaviour is still less aggressive than that of PanNECs {174,1123}. They show the features associated with PanNETs (i.e. hormone expression and hormonal syndromes) and they appear to lack the genetic abnormalities found in true NECs (i.e. changes in expression and mutation of *TP53* and *RB1*) {173,3031}. Furthermore, a study in patients with PanNECs as defined by the 2010 WHO classification showed that patients with neoplasms with a Ki-67 proliferation index < 55% had a

Table 6.02 Comparison of the WHO classifications of pancreatic neuroendocrine neoplasms (NENs)

WHO 1980	WHO 2000/2004	WHO 2010	WHO 2017
Islet cell tumour (adenoma/carcinoma)	Well-differentiated endocrine tumour/carcinoma (WDET/WDEC)	NET G1/G2	NET G1/G2/G3 (well-differentiated NEN)
Poorly differentiated endocrine carcinoma	Poorly differentiated endocrine carcinoma / small cell carcinoma (PDEC)	NEC (G3), large cell or small cell type	NEC (G3), large cell or small cell type (poorly differentiated NEN)
	Mixed exocrine–endocrine carcinoma (MEEC)	Mixed adenoneuroendocrine carcinoma	Mixed neuroendocrine– non-neuroendocrine neoplasm
Pseudotumour lesions	Tumour-like lesions (TLLs)	Hyperplastic and preneoplastic lesions	

NEC, neuroendocrine carcinoma; NET, neuroendocrine tumour.

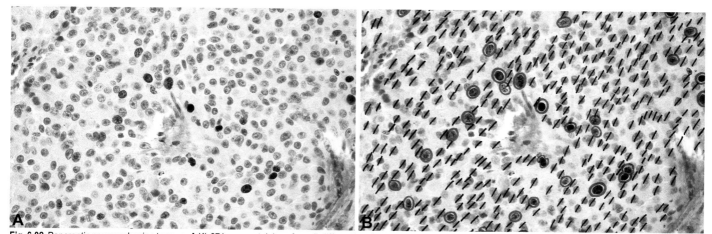

Fig. 6.02 Pancreatic neuroendocrine tumour. **A** Ki-67 immunostaining of a well-differentiated neuroendocrine neoplasm. **B** The Ki-67 proliferation index at this hotspot was 6.9%, qualifying the tumour as G2. The counting was performed manually on this image-captured print by crossing out (in black) the negative cells (475 cells) and circling (in red) the positive nuclei (35 nuclei). The index value was then calculated: 35 positive nuclei / 510 cells total = 6.9% {2267}.

lower response rate, but better survival, than did patients with neoplasms with a Ki-67 proliferation index ≥ 55% when treated with first-line platinum-based chemotherapy as used for the treatment of poorly differentiated NENs {2619}.

Therefore, the new WHO classification presented in this volume includes a new tumour category of PanNET G3. These tumours retain a well-differentiated histological pattern, with only low immunohistochemical expression of p53 or loss of RB, but show a Ki-67 proliferation index > 20%. No upper limit has been defined for the mitotic index or the Ki-67 proliferation index of G3 NET, but the values are usually ≤ 20 mitoses per 10 high-power fields and ≤ 55%, respectively. G3 PanNETs may contain lower-grade components or they may be found as metastases in patients with a prior G1 or G2 PanNET. PanNECs (G3) retain their Ki-67 proliferation index lower cut-off point of 20%, but show a poorly differentiated histology (of either small cell or large cell type), often express p53 or lack RB, lack expression of ISL1, and retain expression of DAXX and ATRX {12,3031}.

Studies in large patient cohorts have shown that the subgroups of patients with G1 or G2 tumours have a significantly higher risk of progression when 5% is used as the Ki-67 proliferation index cut-off point instead of 2% {2144,2294,2441}. However, there is insufficient evidence of differences in clinical management based on this higher cut-off point to justify changing it at this time.

Another change in the current classification concerns the terminology used for the mixed neoplasms. Because these neoplasms are occasionally well differentiated and can contain a non-neuroendocrine component other than adenocarcinoma, the term "mixed neuroendocrine–non-neuroendocrine neoplasm (MiNEN)" has been introduced to replace the previous term ("mixed adenoneuroendocrine carcinoma").

The category of hyperplastic and preneoplastic lesions included in the 2010 WHO classification has been abolished, because PanNEN precursor changes have not been clearly identified in association with sporadic neoplasms; they have only been well described in the settings of multiple endocrine neoplasia type 1, VHL {2624}, and glucagon cell hyperplasia and neoplasia (previously called glucagon cell adenomatosis) {795,1414,2580}.

The WHO 2017 classification staging of PanNENs follows the eighth edition of the American Joint Committee on Cancer (AJCC) {72A} / Union for International Cancer Control (UICC) TNM staging system (p. 210) {323} and corresponds to the European Neuroendocrine Tumour Society (ENETS) TNM classification {2294}.

Definition of pancreatic neuroendocrine tumour

PanNET is a well-differentiated NEN of low, intermediate, or high grade, composed of cells showing minimal to moderate atypia, displaying organoid patterns, lacking necrosis, and expressing general markers of neuroendocrine differentiation (diffuse and intense synaptophysin and usually also chromogranin A staining) and hormones (usually intense but not necessarily diffuse), either orthotopic or ectopic to the pancreas. On the basis of their proliferative activity, PanNETs are graded as G1 (< 2 mitoses per 10 high-power fields and a Ki-67 proliferation index < 3%), G2 (2–20 mitoses per 10 high-power fields or a Ki-67 proliferation index of 3–20%), or G3 (> 20 mitoses per 10 high-power fields or a Ki-67 proliferation index > 20%) (see Table 6.01, p. 211). In cases with an associated clinical hormonal syndrome, PanNETs can be further categorized as insulinoma, glucagonoma, somatostatinoma, gastrinoma, VIPoma, serotonin-producing tumour (with or without carcinoid syndrome), ACTH-producing tumour, etc.

Definition of pancreatic neuroendocrine carcinoma

PanNEC is a poorly differentiated high-grade NEN, composed of highly atypical small cells or intermediate to large cells expressing the general markers of neuroendocrine differentiation (diffuse or faint synaptophysin and faint or focal chromogranin A staining) and rarely hormones, and lacking expression of exocrine enzyme markers (i.e. trypsin, chymotrypsin, etc.). On the basis of their proliferative activity (> 20 mitoses per 10 high-power fields or a Ki-67 proliferation index > 20%), PanNECs are considered high-grade (G3) neoplasms (see Table 6.01, p. 211). The TNM classification of PanNECs follows the criteria for classifying ductal adenocarcinomas.

Definition of mixed neuroendocrine–non-neuroendocrine neoplasm

MiNEN is a mixed neoplasm with a neuroendocrine component combined with a non-neuroendocrine component (typically ductal adenocarcinoma or acinar cell carcinoma). Both components are usually high-grade (G3), but occasionally one or both components may be G1 or G2. Therefore, when the components are morphologically distinguishable, they should be individually graded, using the respective grading systems for each. For a tumour to qualify as MiNEN, each component should account for ≥ 30% of the tumour cell population. Non-neuroendocrine carcinomas with scattered neuroendocrine cells by immunohistochemistry do not fulfil this criterion; the presence of focal (< 30%) neuroendocrine differentiation can be mentioned, but does not affect the diagnostic categorization. MiNEN is a conceptual category rather than a discrete entity; individual diagnoses indicating the specific cellular components should be applied (i.e. mixed acinar–neuroendocrine carcinoma, mixed ductal–neuroendocrine carcinoma, etc.); see *Mixed neuroendocrine–non-neuroendocrine neoplasms* (p. 238).

Reporting of pancreatic neuroendocrine neoplasms

In the diagnosis, PanNENs should be classified as NET or NEC on the basis of histology and immunohistochemistry, and graded G1, G2, or G3. For resection specimens, the TNM stage (based on macroscopic assessment of site, size, and metastasis) should be reported. It is recommended to include a comment on the probable clinical behaviour of the tumour. Endocrine function assessment should be provided upon specific clinical request. See the sections that follow for the tumour-type–specific requirements.

Risk of tumour progression

The criteria that predict the probable risk of tumour progression of PanNEN are summarized in the TNM classification table on p. 210 and the grading table on p. 211. Although the listed criteria have a high probability and statistical significance (in particular Ki-67 proliferation index {2144, 2294}) for predicting the behaviour of a given PanNEN {2465}, establishing the final outcome of a PanNEN often requires long clinical follow-up, particularly of a PanNET, because metastasis may not occur until many years after resection of the primary. Prognostic immunohistochemical markers other than Ki-67 (e.g. CK19, KIT, CD99, CD44, and p27) have been reported {669,2465} (see also *Nonfunctioning neuroendocrine tumours*, p. 215), but have not been validated in a large cohort. Prognostic molecular markers for most PanNENs are not yet available.

Non-functioning (non-syndromic) neuroendocrine tumours

Klimstra D. S.
Klöppel G.
Couvelard A.
Hruban R. H.
Komminoth P.

La Rosa S.
Osamura R. Y.
Perren A.
Rindi G.

Definition

Non-functioning pancreatic neuroendocrine tumour (NF-PanNET) is a nonfunctioning well-differentiated pancreatic neuroendocrine neoplasm (NEN) that occurs in patients who have no paraneoplastic symptoms attributable to abnormal secretion of hormones or bioamines by the tumour cells. The term "non-syndromic" is in fact more accurate than "non-functioning", but is not widely used. NF-PanNETs measuring < 5 mm are called pancreatic neuroendocrine microadenomas, and are considered to be biologically benign. Multifocal occurrence of microadenomas, as can occur in multiple endocrine neoplasia type 1 (MEN1), is called microadenomatosis. The terms "insulinoma", "glucagonoma", etc. are reserved for clinically functioning (syndromic) PanNETs.

ICD-O codes

Pancreatic neuroendocrine
   microadenoma (< 0.5 cm)   8150/0
Non-functioning pancreatic
   neuroendocrine tumour   8150/3

Synonyms

Former terms for NF-PanNET include non-functioning pancreatic endocrine tumour, non-functioning pancreatic endocrine neoplasm, islet cell tumour, and low-grade endocrine carcinoma of the pancreas. The last term in particular is not recommended, due to potential confusion with poorly differentiated pancreatic neuroendocrine neoplasms, which are called pancreatic neuroendocrine carcinomas (PanNECs).

Epidemiology

The prevalence of clinically relevant sporadic NF-PanNETs differs substantially from that of incidental microadenomas that do not come to clinical attention. In autopsy studies, the prevalence of microadenomas is 1–10%, depending on the amount of pancreatic tissue examined {1182,1381}. Clinically relevant NF-PanNETs are much less common; their reported incidence is approximately 0.2–2 cases per 100 000 person-years {1068, 2607}, and seems to have increased steadily over the past 40 years {1564}. Historically, NF-PanNETs were reported to constitute only a third of all PanNETs {334,1347,1416}; however, in the era of enhanced diagnostic imaging, their relative frequency has increased to as high as 70–80% of PanNETs {821A,855,2294, 2441}. An estimated 30–75% of patients with MEN1 have clinical evidence of a PanNET, and pancreatic involvement is found in nearly 100% of cases at autopsy {1720}. In these patients, a high proportion of individual tumours are non-functioning {1050}, but most patients with MEN1 with pancreatic involvement have at least one functioning PanNET {1418,

1565} (see *Multiple endocrine neoplasia type 1*, p. 243).

Sporadic clinically detected NF-PanNETs can occur at any age but are rare in childhood {2556}. The patient age range is 12–79 years, with a mean patient age of 50–55 years {855,1074,1347,2294,2441, 2862}. The sexes are about equally affected, with a male-to-female ratio of 1:1.15.

Etiology

NF-PanNETs are associated with a variety of hereditary syndromes (see *Genetic susceptibility* below, as well as the *Introduction* section of Chapter 7, p. 242, *Multiple endocrine neoplasia type 1*, p. 243, and *Multiple endocrine neoplasia type 4*, p. 253). There are no known etiological factors for sporadic NF-PanNETs.

Localization

Approximately two thirds of surgically resected NF-PanNETs occur in the head of the pancreas {1347,2862}. Perhaps because these tumours are hormonally silent, the cases most likely to cause symptoms due to duct obstruction are those in the head of the gland, whereas tumours in the tail are more likely to be detected incidentally.

Clinical features

NF-PanNETs can produce symptoms due to local spread, such as abdominal pain, nausea, and duodenal or biliary

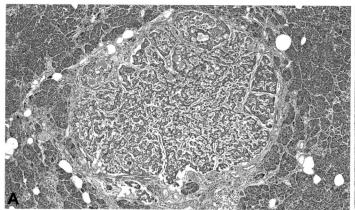
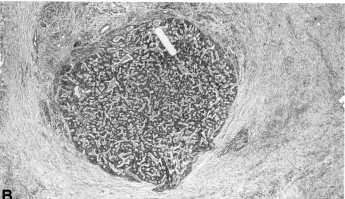

Fig. 6.03 Neuroendocrine microadenoma. **A** Microscopically, the tumour is circumscribed but unencapsulated and has a nesting and trabecular architecture. **B** Immunostaining for glucagon.

Table 6.03 Differential diagnostic considerations for non-functioning pancreatic neuroendocrine tumours

Entity	Architecture	Cytomorphology	Immunophenotype
Pancreatic neuroendocrine carcinoma {174}	Infiltrative, necrotic	Small cell or large cell cytology, diffuse or nested pattern, > 20 mitoses per 10 high-power fields, desmoplastic stroma, may have an adenocarcinoma component	Chromogranin and synaptophysin (weak or +), p53 (+), RB (lost), DAXX and ATRX (retained), Ki-67 proliferation index (usually > 50%)
Acinar cell carcinoma {1511,1514, 3007}	Solid and acinar patterns	Granular eosinophilic cytoplasm, prominent nucleoli	Trypsin, chymotrypsin, and BCL10 (+); chromogranin and synaptophysin (focal)
Pancreatoblastoma {1511,1514, 3007}	Solid and acinar patterns, lobulated	Acinar cytomorphology, squamoid nests, hypercellular stromal bands	Trypsin, chymotrypsin, and BCL10 (+); chromogranin and synaptophysin (focal)
Solid-pseudopapillary neoplasm {1407,2718,2739}	Solid and cystic with degenerative changes	Loosely cohesive cells, pseudopapillae, cytoplasmic vacuoles, hyaline globules, foamy histiocytes, nuclear grooves	Vimentin, CD10, CD56, alpha-1-antitrypsin, and beta-catenin (+); keratin and synaptophysin (focal); trypsin, chymotrypsin, and chromogranin (−)
Ductal adenocarcinoma	Infiltrative, sclerotic	Individual mucin-producing glands, desmoplastic stroma, substantial mitotic activity	Chromogranin and synaptophysin (− or focal)

obstruction, although jaundice is less common than with ductal adenocarcinomas due to the less-infiltrative growth pattern of PanNETs {1182,1489}. Some NF-PanNETs remain clinically silent while localized, coming to clinical attention only once metastases are present. When tested, they may be found to be associated with elevated serum levels of hormones such as pancreatic polypeptide, somatostatin, and glucagon, although hormonal symptoms are absent.

NF-PanNETs can be visualized by cross-sectional imaging (CT and MRI) or by endoscopic ultrasound, which is commonly used to guide preoperative biopsies. NF-PanNETs are characteristically very vascular lesions on imaging. Functional imaging, including somatostatin receptor scintigraphy (octreotide scan and DOTA-TOC scan), is increasingly used to establish the neuroendocrine nature of lesions suspected to be NF-PanNETs, and to locate occult pancreatic primaries that present with metastatic disease {1489}. NF-PanNETs are staged using the eighth edition of the American Joint Committee on Cancer (AJCC) {72A} / Union for International Cancer Control (UICC) TNM staging system (p. 210) {323}, which is based on a system first proposed by the European Neuroendocrine Tumour Society (ENETS) in 2006 {2295}.

Macroscopy

Because microadenomas are by definition < 0.5 cm, most examples are not grossly detectable. Those that are identified on macroscopic examination of the pancreas appear as circumscribed but unencapsulated red to tan soft nodules. NF-PanNETs are on average 2–5 cm in diameter {1489} and can exhibit a wide variety of gross appearances {1182}. Some examples are sharply circumscribed and partially or entirely surrounded by a fibrous capsule. The consistency is often soft and fleshy and the tumours vary from reddish-tan to yellow. Other examples have a more pronounced fibrous consistency, and gross lobulation can occur. Larger NF-PanNETs are more heterogeneous and may have an infiltrative appearance. Areas of gross necrosis are uncommon, but cystic change can occur, usually with a single, central unilocular cyst surrounded by a rim of neoplastic tissue {1445,1617,2576}.

NF-PanNETs grow initially by direct extension into local structures, including peripancreatic soft tissues and the spleen for tumours in the tail of the gland, and the common bile duct and/or duodenum for tumours in the head. Tumour thrombi within large veins may be found. Metastases occur both to regional lymph nodes and to the liver; distant metastases are usually limited to the later stages of the disease and can involve a wide variety of sites, including lung and bone {1182,1347,1489,2862}.

Microscopy

NF-PanNETs have organoid growth patterns that are typical of well-differentiated NENs and not substantially different from those of most types of functioning

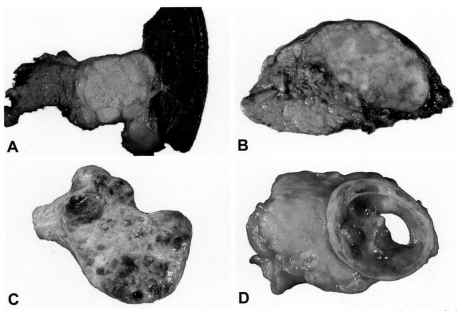

Fig. 6.04 Non-functioning pancreatic neuroendocrine tumour. **A** Gross appearance of a circumscribed example in the pancreatic tail. **B** Variegated, pinkish-tan to white cut surface lacking necrosis. **C** An example with a strikingly heterogeneous, red hypervascular cut surface. The yellow regions correspond to lipid-rich, clear-cell features microscopically. **D** Tumour with central cystic change producing a unilocular cyst.

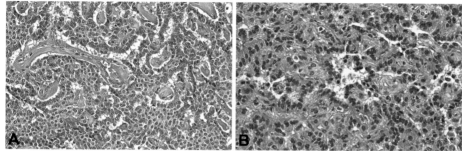

Fig. 6.05 Non-functioning pancreatic neuroendocrine tumour. **A** Nesting (solid) and trabecular architecture. **B** An example with a pseudoglandular pattern.

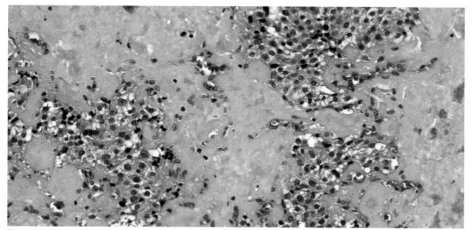

Fig. 6.06 Non-functioning pancreatic neuroendocrine tumour with extensive stromal sclerosis.

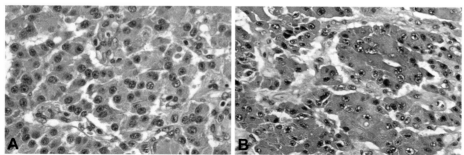

Fig. 6.07 Non-functioning pancreatic neuroendocrine tumour. **A** Round to oval nuclei with coarsely clumped chromatin and granular cytoplasm. **B** An example with prominent, enlarged, and irregular nuclei with large nucleoli. No mitoses are identifiable.

PanNETs {585,1182,2538}. The spectrum includes a nesting (solid) growth pattern, trabecular and gyriform patterns, and a (pseudo)glandular pattern. Intratumoural heterogeneity is rare in small tumours and relatively common in larger neoplasms {1416,1417}. The stromal component varies considerably, from simple, fine, capillary-sized vessels between neoplastic cell nests to broad areas of dense, hyalinized collagen. Some tumours exhibit amyloid-like stroma, and stromal calcifications (sometimes including psammoma bodies) may be found. Desmoplastic stroma is uncommon.
Most cells are cuboidal and have eosino-

philic or slightly basophilic, finely granular cytoplasm. The nuclei are generally round to oval, with minimal atypia and coarsely clumped (so-called salt-and-pepper) chromatin; they are centrally located but may be polarized, particularly in trabecular tumours. Rarely, eccentric nuclei can be found, imparting a rhabdoid configuration to the cells {2149}. Also uncommon are nuclear irregularities, including enlarged nuclei and irregular nuclear membranes {3096}; prominent nucleoli may also be found. NF-PanNETs usually have no necrosis, but large, infarct-like areas can occasionally be found. In most NF-PanNETs,

mitoses are rare. G1 tumours have < 2 mitoses per 10 high-power fields, G2 tumours have < 20 mitoses per 10 high-power fields, and G3 tumours have no limit on mitotic rate but generally have no more than 30-40 mitoses per 10 high-power fields.
In some NF-PanNETs, small pancreatic ductules and islets are found between nests of neoplastic cells; rarely, acinar cells are present as well {1312,2847}. These are entrapped structures and have been proven to be non-neoplastic. True glandular differentiation can occur in NF-PanNETs, with lumina formed within nests of neoplastic cells {1182}. In contrast to entrapped ductules, these lumina are lined by cells cytologically indistinguishable from the surrounding neoplastic cells.
A number of morphological variants of NF-PanNETs have been described. Oncocytic PanNETs have cells with copious granular eosinophilic cytoplasm due to abundant mitochondria {415,2229, 2892}. In many oncocytic NF-PanNETs, the nuclei are enlarged and moderately atypical, frequently with prominent nucleoli. Pleomorphic PanNETs show marked nuclear pleomorphism, with very large irregular and atypical nuclei, but generally abundant cytoplasm {3096}. These tumours are frequently confused with higher-grade lesions such as anaplastic carcinomas or ductal adenocarcinomas. Their proliferation rate is not elevated and the pleomorphic nuclei have no adverse prognostic significance {3096}.
Clear cell NF-PanNETs show innumerable vacuoles in the cytoplasm (scalloping the nucleus), as a result of cytoplasmic lipid accumulation. Such tumours have been reported particularly commonly in patients with von Hippel–Lindau syndrome (VHL), and may be confused with metastatic renal cell carcinoma {1149}, although clear-cell features also occur in sporadic NF-PanNETs and may be only a focal finding {2575}. Some NF-PanNETs, particularly those that express serotonin, have dense stromal sclerosis and are composed of small nests and tubules. These tumours often arise adjacent to the main duct, causing secondary duct obstruction and dilatation and mimicking an intraductal papillary mucinous neoplasm {1345,1780}. NF-PanNETs with a paraganglioma-like pattern are often immunoreactive for somatostatin. Cystic NF-PanNETs with a trabecular and

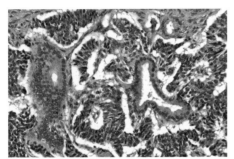

Fig. 6.08 Non-functioning pancreatic neuroendocrine tumour with entrapped non-neoplastic ductules.

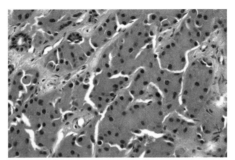

Fig. 6.09 Oncocytic non-functioning pancreatic neuroendocrine tumour with abundant granular eosinophilic cytoplasm.

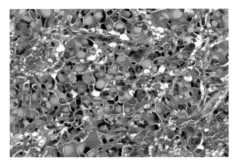

Fig. 6.10 Pleomorphic non-functioning pancreatic neuroendocrine tumour with pleomorphic nuclei and rhabdoid-like cytoplasmic inclusions.

reticular pattern are usually glucagon positive {1445}.

Immunophenotype
NF-PanNETs express synaptophysin and chromogranin A as specific markers of general neuroendocrine differentiation. NF-PanNETs also express neuron-specific enolase, CD56, and CD57; however, these markers are also positive in some non-neuroendocrine tumours, and are not considered sufficiently specific to demonstrate neuroendocrine differentiation {1126,1182,1656,1923,2538}. Synaptophysin staining is generally diffuse and strong, and there is apical positivity for chromogranin A. In PanNETs with few neurosecretory granules, chromogranin expression is focal and less intense. Although NF-PanNETs are not associated with clinical syndromes, it is common for immunohistochemical labelling to demonstrate peptide hormones in highly variable proportions of the tumour cells. About 40% of the tumours are multihormonal {1312}. The hormones most often expressed are somatostatin, pancreatic polypeptide, and glucagon {1150, 1312,2607}. Only rarely does an entire tumour fail to stain for any hormone. In some tumours in which one hormone predominates, characteristic histological patterns may occur. Glucagon-positive NF-PanNETs frequently demonstrate cystic changes {1445}. Somatostatin-positive NF-PanNETs may show a paraganglioma-like pattern and/or glandular structures with psammoma bodies {929}. Serotonin-positive NF-PanNETs with trabecular pattern and dense stromal sclerosis often arise in a periductal location {1780}. Microadenomas are more likely to show diffuse expression of a single peptide, most often glucagon or pancreatic polypeptide {84,2607}.

Many NF-PanNETs, particularly those that show gland formation, also express glycoproteins, including CEA and CA19-9 {1150,1182,1305}. Focal acinar differentiation may also be seen, generally in single, widely scattered cells that label with antibodies to trypsin or chymotrypsin {1305,3058}. NF-PanNETs express the transcription factor ISL1, which may be useful to support pancreatic origin for a metastatic neuroendocrine tumour of unknown primary {12,1029}. Less useful for determining the site of origin are PDX1, PAX8, and CDX2 {28,1135, 1525}. Immunolabelling for DAXX and ATRX reveals loss of expression in 45% of NF-PanNETs {1261,1736}. There is generally no significant overexpression of p53 or loss of expression of RB or SMAD4 {2538,3031}. The somatostatin receptors SSTR1, SSTR2A, SSTR3, SSTR4, and SSTR5 can be expressed by PanNETs; SSTR2A expression is particularly strong and correlates with molecular imaging {2890}. Other immunohistochemical markers of interest include CK19, KIT (also known as CD117 and c-KIT), CD99, CD44, p27, progesterone receptor, and

PTEN; abnormal expression of each of these markers has been linked to prognosis. However, none of these markers is in current widespread use for clinical management {669,1150,1213,2872,2965, 3101}. NF-PanNETs in patients with VHL typically express HIF1A and CAIX, as do foci of islet cell hyperplasia not identifiable on routinely stained sections in these patients {557,2151}.

The Ki-67 proliferation index is used for grading NF-PanNETs {1405,1489,2295} (see the *Introduction*, p. 211). Heterogeneity of Ki-67 labelling is common, and the regions of highest labelling (so-called hotspots) should be used to define the grade {174,2724}. Grade heterogeneity may be found synchronously within different regions of an individual tumour or among different metastatic sites, or a higher-grade metastasis may develop later in the course of disease progression. There is no upper limit of the Ki-67 proliferation index in NF-PanNETs, but the value is < 50% in most cases, and higher values are more suggestive of a poorly differentiated NEN (PanNEC) {174, 2620}.

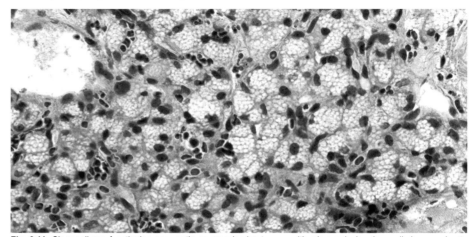

Fig. 6.11 Clear cell non-functioning pancreatic neuroendocrine tumour with microvesicular clear-cell changes due to numerous cytoplasmic lipid vacuoles.

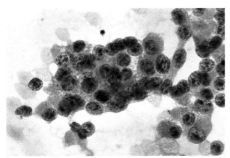

Fig. 6.12 Non-functioning pancreatic neuroendocrine tumour. Cytology shows loosely cohesive cells with plasmacytoid cytoplasm and coarsely granular chromatin.

Cytology

Cytological evaluation of NF-PanNETs is based predominantly on fine-needle aspiration of primary tumours (performed using endoscopic ultrasound) or of liver metastases {1142}. Aspirates from PanNETs are usually highly cellular with a clean background {1182}. The neoplastic cells are found in loosely cohesive clusters and individually. A plasmacytoid configuration is characteristic. The nuclei, which are uniform and round to oval, contain coarsely granular chromatin. Mitotic figures are not usually seen, and the grading of NF-PanNETs on the basis of cytological specimens is not well established {830,2882}.

Ultrastructure

The ultrastructural features of NF-PanNETs resemble those of other PanNETs {1182}. Variable numbers of membrane-bound electron-dense neurosecretory granules are found, either non-polarized within the cytoplasm or oriented near the basal surfaces facing the capillaries. The granule morphology is usually non-specific, but the characteristic granule types of alpha cells or delta cells may also be found in some NF-PanNETs. Ultrastructural assessment currently has a limited role in the diagnostic evaluation of NF-PanNETs.

Differential diagnosis

The differential diagnosis includes PanNEC, acinar cell carcinoma, pancreatoblastoma, solid pseudopapillary neoplasm, ductal adenocarcinoma, and mixed pancreatic carcinomas (Table 6.03, p. 216) {1182}. Most of these tumours have a solid, hypercellular low-power appearance, and they may have a nesting growth pattern {1404}. PanNECs share neuroendocrine differentiation with NF-PanNETs and are also typically non-functioning {173,174, 3031}. There are small cell and large cell subtypes of PanNEC (see *Pancreatic neuroendocrine carcinoma*, p. 235); both commonly show necrosis and apoptosis, and although there may be a nesting growth pattern, the tumour cells are often arrayed in sheets and lack the more complex organoid patterns seen in PanNETs. By definition, the proliferation rate of PanNECs is > 20 mitoses per 10 high-power fields and the Ki-67 proliferation index is > 20%; most PanNECs have a very high Ki-67 proliferation index (> 50%), and in small cell carcinomas, the Ki-67 proliferation index is often > 80% {174}. The range of Ki-67 proliferation index values observed in PanNECs overlaps with that of G3 PanNETs, making the distinction difficult, especially in cases with large cell morphology. G3 PanNETs may contain foci of lower-grade PanNET, pointing to the correct diagnosis, or there may be a clinical history of a prior G1 or G2 PanNET (e. g. when G3 liver metastases are subsequently detected). Immunolabelling can be helpful, because PanNETs may show loss of DAXX or ATRX expression, whereas PanNECs often exhibit strong overexpression of p53 (or complete loss in case of a *TP53* deletion) or loss of RB, SMAD4 or SSTR2A {1445A}.

Both acinar cell carcinoma and pancreatoblastoma have substantial acinar differentiation; however, both may also have neuroendocrine differentiation in a smaller proportion of the cells, so labelling for neuroendocrine markers may be patchy. Solid-pseudopapillary neoplasms also have many close similarities with NF-PanNETs, but have a distinct immunoprofile (with nuclear labelling for beta-catenin, positivity for vimentin etc.). The distinction of PanNETs from ductal adenocarcinoma is generally not difficult, but some PanNETs show widespread gland formation, stromal sclerosis, or nuclear pleomorphism, mimicking an adenocarcinoma. PanNETs do not generally contain intracellular mucin, and the glands are usually found within larger nests of cells, in contrast to the individual infiltrating glands (each surrounded by desmoplastic stroma) seen in ductal adenocarcinomas.

Some of the morphological variants of PanNET bear resemblance to other neoplasms, based on their distinctive morphological features. Clear cell PanNETs resemble renal cell carcinomas, and oncocytic PanNETs resemble hepatocellular carcinoma or adrenal cortical carcinoma {1149,2892}.

Microadenomas can be difficult to distinguish from enlarged non-neoplastic islets. Immunohistochemical staining for islet peptides is helpful, because microadenomas lose the normal proportions and distribution of peptide cell types seen in non-neoplastic islets {84,1182}.

Genetic profile

The genetic features of NF-PanNETs are similar to those described for PanNETs in general (see the *Introduction*, p. 211). Most of the histological variants have no demonstrated distinctive genetic features, although the reported association between the clear-cell phenotype and VHL suggests the presence of *VHL* abnormalities in that subset {1149}.

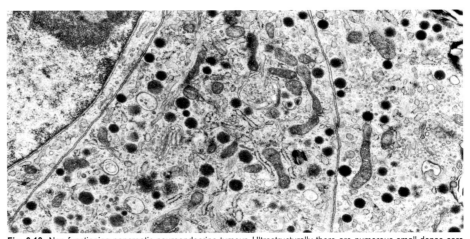

Fig. 6.13 Non-functioning pancreatic neuroendocrine tumour. Ultrastructurally there are numerous small dense-core neurosecretory granules dispersed in the cytoplasm.

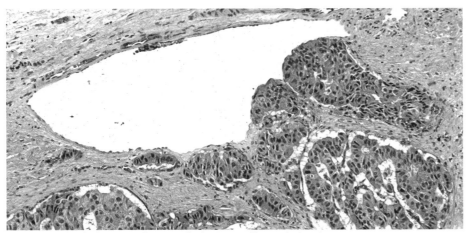

Fig. 6.14 Non-functioning pancreatic neuroendocrine tumour with vascular invasion.

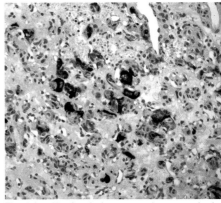

Fig. 6.15 Non-functioning pancreatic neuroendocrine tumour with a paraganglioma-like pattern of immunolabelling for somatostatin.

Genetic susceptibility

NF-PanNETs occur in patients with MEN1 {799,1418,2172} (see *Multiple endocrine neoplasia type 1*, p. 243), VHL {1149,1192} (see *Von Hippel–Lindau syndrome*, p. 257), tuberous sclerosis {2867}, neurofibromatosis type 1 (see *Neurofibromatosis type 1*, p. 266), and glucagon cell hyperplasia and neoplasia {2580,3117} (see *Glucagon cell hyperplasia and neoplasia*, p. 282). In these patients, the specific genetic abnormalities underlying the syndrome are involved in the etiology of the PanNETs.

Prognosis and predictive factors

Microadenomas are considered to be benign {2607}, but it is unknown whether a subset of these tumours may progress to clinically relevant malignant PanNETs. Approximately 55–75% of all other NF-PanNETs are associated with evidence of malignant behaviour (i. e. extrapancreatic spread, metastasis, or recurrence) {1347, 2294,2862}. Following surgical resection of NF-PanNETs, the reported 5-year survival rate is 65–86%, and the 10-year survival rate is 45–68% {855,1074,1150, 2294}. Some patients die of disease > 10 years after surgery. A substantial proportion (≥ 25% {2294}) of patients with NF-PanNETs initially present with distant metastases, perhaps because there is no paraneoplastic syndrome to draw clinical attention to the tumour early in its course. Once distant metastases occur, cure is highly unlikely, although tumour progression often occurs slowly. Most patients with metastatic PanNETs survive for several years; the median survival after recurrence is 2.3 years {1074}. The 5-year survival rate with metastatic PanNETs is 59%, and the 10-year survival rate is 36% {1350}.

Table 6.04 Prognostic factors for non-functioning pancreatic neuroendocrine tumours

Factor	Method of assessment	In routine use?	References
Tumour size	Gross evaluation	Yes	{1050,1489,2367}
Invasiveness (vascular invasion, extrapancreatic invasion)	Microscopic evaluation	Yes	{1489}
Necrosis	Microscopic evaluation	No	{1150}
Stage	Microscopic evaluation and clinical/radiographical evaluation	Yes	{2294}
Grade	Microscopic evaluation and immunohistochemistry	Yes	{855,1405,2143,2294,2441,2465}
Mitotic rate	Microscopic evaluation	Yes	{855,1405,2143,2294,2441,2465}
Ki-67 proliferation index	Immunohistochemistry	Yes	{855,1405,2143,2294,2441,2465, 2900,3057}
PTEN loss	Immunohistochemistry	No	{799}
Progesterone receptor loss	Immunohistochemistry	No	{799,2872}
Aneuploidy	Flow cytometry	No	{1346}
Increased fractional allelic loss	High-resolution allelotyping	No	{2290}
Upregulated CD44 isoform expression	Immunohistochemistry	No	{1213}
CK19 expression	Immunohistochemistry	No	{56,669,3102}
KIT (also known as CD117 and c-KIT) expression	Immunohistochemistry	No	{3102}
p27 expression	Immunohistochemistry	No	{2232}
Loss of heterozygosity of 1p, 3p, 6q, 17p, 22q, and X	Comparative genomic hybridization	No	{154,155,517,732,2183,2987}

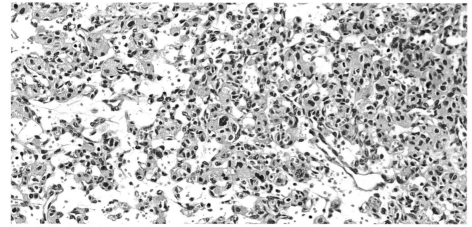

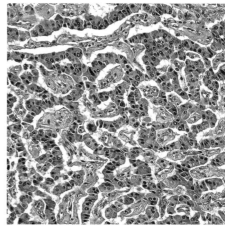

Fig. 6.16 Non-functioning pancreatic neuroendocrine tumour with a paraganglioma-like pattern.

Fig. 6.17 Non-functioning pancreatic neuroendocrine tumour with a gyriform architecture.

A number of factors have been shown to predict the prognosis of NF-PanNETs (Table 6.04). Tumour size is an important prognostic factor, with tumours < 2 cm uncommonly demonstrating clinical aggressiveness, whereas larger tumours have an increasing risk for metastases {1050,1489}. Small (< 2 cm), low-grade NF-PanNETs have very indolent biology, to the extent that some investigators have suggested that asymptomatic cases can be closely followed radiographically rather than resected {2367}. The likelihood of metastasis also increases with extent of invasive growth (especially vascular invasion), necrosis, status of regional lymph nodes {1150,1489}, and tumour grade {2465}.

The most significant histological factor predictive of outcome is proliferation rate. The grading system based on mitotic rate and Ki-67 proliferation index, first proposed by the European Neuroendocrine Tumour Society (ENETS) and then endorsed in 2010 by WHO {1405,2295}, is now in widespread use and is a well-established prognosticator {855,1636, 2144,2294,2441,2900,3057} (see the *Introduction*, p. 211). Abundant data demonstrate the prognostic stratification of G1 and G2 NF-PanNETs, both in the setting of a resected primary tumour and for metastatic disease, although the accuracy of Ki-67 proliferation index assessment based on biopsies of metastases has been questioned, due to the heterogeneity of the hotspots of highest proliferative activity, which may not be sampled in a limited specimen {3057}. Both G1 and G2 tumours are prognostically

distinct from PanNECs in the ENETS/ WHO system {174,2294,2619}. However, the finding that NF-PanNETs can have a Ki-67 proliferation index > 20% has led to the creation of a well-differentiated G3 PanNET category (see the *Introduction* section, p. 211). This group is somewhat more aggressive than G2 PanNETs but not as rapidly progressive as PanNECs. The 5-year survival rate associated with G3 PanNETs is 29%, versus 62% for G2 PanNETs and 16% for PanNECs {174}.

Abnormal peptide secretion (excluding insulin secretion) is an adverse prognostic factor for PanNETs overall, but within the subset of NF-PanNETs, immunoexpression of a secreted peptide in the absence of a clinical syndrome has no impact on survival {1150}. Nuclear pleomorphism is not a powerful predictor either, with the pleomorphic variant having no adverse effect on prognosis {3096}. The histological variants of NF-PanNETs are not prognostically significant in general, although cystic PanNETs frequently lack adverse prognostic factors and often

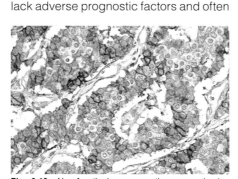

Fig. 6.18 Non-functioning pancreatic neuroendocrine tumour. Immunoreactivity for SSTR2A, with strong membrane staining qualifying the tumour for SSTR2A immunohistochemical score 2 (out of 3) {2890}.

present at a lower stage {1617,2576}, and oncocytic NF-PanNETs appear to be aggressive {2892}.

Other factors reportedly predictive of more aggressive behaviour include loss of PTEN expression {798} or loss of nuclear DAXX/ATRX {1736}; aneuploidy {1346}; increased fractional allelic loss {2290}; upregulated CD44 isoform expression {1213}; and immunohistochemical expression of CK19 {669}, p27, KIT (also known as CD117) {3102}. Maintained progesterone receptor expression is a favourable prognostic finding {798, 2872}. Loss of heterozygosity of several chromosomal loci has also been reported to correlate with adverse prognosis, including 1p {732}, 3p {154,517}, 6q {155}, 17p {1050}, 22q {2987}, and X {2183}. It has proven difficult to incorporate these numerous parameters into a final prognostic classification system.

Biomarkers predictive of therapeutic response are emerging for NF-PanNETs. Immunolabelling for SSTR2A can be used to identify patients who will benefit from treatment with somatostatin analogues {2890}. The status of MGMT immunoexpression or promoter methylation may predict sensitivity of the tumour to temozolomide {1490,2466,2538,2922}. Targeting the PI3K/AKT/mTOR signalling pathway is effective in some patients with NF-PanNETs, and the status of this pathway as assessed by mutation analysis or immunohistochemistry may help to guide treatment {2538,3060}. However, the optimal means of assessing this pathway pathologically is yet to be determined.

Insulinoma

Perren A.
Anlauf M.
Klimstra D. S.
Klöppel G.
Komminoth P.
La Rosa S.

Öberg K.
Scarpa A.
Scoazec J.-Y.
Speel E. J. M.
Zamboni G.

Definition

Insulinoma is a functioning well-differentiated pancreatic neuroendocrine neoplasm composed of insulin-producing and proinsulin-producing cells, with uncontrolled insulin secretion causing a hypoglycaemic syndrome.

ICD-O code   8151/3

Synonyms

"Insulin-producing pancreatic endocrine tumour", "insulin-producing islet cell tumour", and "beta cell tumour" are related terms that do not take functional status into account.

Epidemiology

Insulinomas have an estimated annual incidence of 0.4 cases per 100 000 population {2506}. They are the most common functioning pancreatic neuroendocrine neoplasms and account for about 20% of resected pancreatic neuroendocrine neoplasms {1227}. Peak incidence occurs in the sixth decade of life, but patients of any age can be affected {1796}, although these tumours are rare in children and young adults, with < 1% of cases occurring in patients aged < 30 years {1796}. Women seem to be affected slightly more commonly than men. About 10% of insulinomas develop metastases, which are more common in men {1988,2506}.

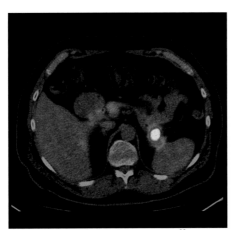

Fig. 6.19 Insulinoma in the pancreatic tail. ⁶⁸Ga-DOTA-exendin-4 PET/CT 2.5 hours after injection.

Multiple insulinomas are seen in about 10% of cases, most often in association with multiple endocrine neoplasia type 1 (MEN1), but also (rarely) in the setting of insulinomatosis {80}.

Etiology

There are no known etiological factors for sporadic solitary insulinomas. There may be an association with diabetes, but unlike for ductal adenocarcinoma, there is no association with smoking {1067}. Multiple insulinomas are usually associated with the inherited familial syndrome of MEN1.

Localization

Almost all insulinomas are found in the pancreas, where they are evenly distributed {1796} or may show a slight predominance in the head and tail regions {2505}. Extrapancreatic insulinomas, which are extremely rare, have been described in the duodenal wall, ileum, jejunum, and splenic hilum {5,1428,1515,2142,2513}.

Clinical features

Hyperinsulinaemic hypoglycaemia leads to autonomic and neuroglycopenic symptoms. Adrenergic symptoms include palpitations and tremor; cholinergic symptoms include sweating, hunger, and paraesthesias. The neuroglycopenic symptoms include severe weakness and a wide variety of psychiatric and neurological manifestations; the most common

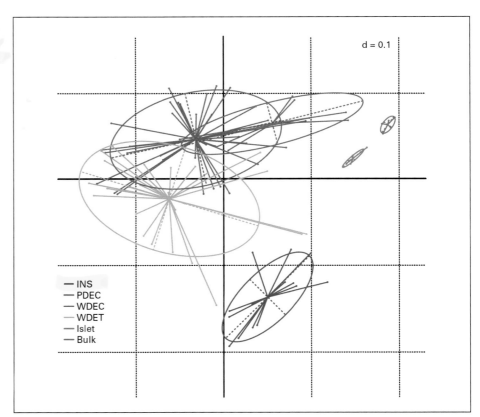

Fig. 6.20 Bidimensional projection of the expression profiles of pancreatic neuroendocrine tumours (PanNETs) and normal samples by correspondence analysis: insulinomas (INS) differ from other PanNETs (poorly differentiated neuroendocrine carcinoma [PDEC], well-differentiated neuroendocrine carcinoma [WDEC], and well-differentiated neuroendocrine tumour [WDET]), normal islets (Islet), and normal bulk tissue (Bulk). From: Missiaglia E et al. J Clin Oncol. 28:245–55 (2010) {1856}. Reprinted with permission. © (2010) American Society of Clinical Oncology.

are confusion, agitation, slow reaction pattern, blurred vision, seizures, transient loss of consciousness, and hypoglycaemic coma {1031}. The diagnosis is based on the Whipple triad: hypoglycaemic symptoms, plasma glucose levels < 2.2 mmol/L (< 40 mg/dL), and symptom relief following glucose administration. The best diagnostic test is prolonged fasting (48–72 hours) with measurement of blood glucose, serum insulin, C-peptide, and proinsulin {2504}. The tumours are usually detected by CT, MRI, endoscopic ultrasound, and/or 68Ga-DOTATOC/DOTATATE PET {788,1415, 2680}. Recently, radiolabelled GLP1R scintigraphy has been introduced as a sensitive method for localizing small insulinomas {513}. Metastatic insulinoma can change hormone production during the course of the disease, starting to produce gastrin or glucagon, with the related symptoms {909}.

Macroscopy

Insulinomas usually present as solitary, round, well-demarcated tumours, with greyish-white to yellowish-tan or occasionally haemorrhagic cut surfaces. About 80% of insulinomas are much smaller (1–2 cm in diameter) than other functioning pancreatic neuroendocrine tumours (PanNETs), making their diagnosis by morphological and/or functional imaging sometimes difficult. An estimated 1.6% of insulinomas are < 1 cm in diameter {1796}. Insulinomas that metastasize are typically > 2 cm, with a mean diameter of 3 cm {200}.

Microscopy

Insulinomas are typically well-differentiated PanNETs with a Ki-67 proliferation index < 2%. Malignant insulinomas are often G2 neuroendocrine tumours. In rare cases, the Ki-67 proliferation index can be > 20% {2932}. The growth pattern is either trabecular or solid. There is sometimes a tubuloacinar growth pattern with psammoma bodies, as is seen in somatostatin-producing PanNETs. Occasionally there are entrapped non-neoplastic ducts and intense sclerosis. Stromal deposits of islet amyloid polypeptide (also called amylin) are specific to insulinomas, but occur in only about 5% of cases. The tumour cells are in close contact with a fine network of endothelial cells. The cytological features are the same as those of other PanNETs. Mitotic figures are rare.

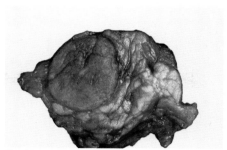

Fig. 6.21 Insulinoma. Resection specimen showing a well-circumscribed tumour measuring 1.0 cm.

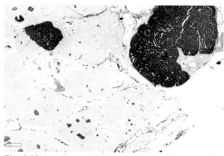

Fig. 6.22 Insulinomatosis with two microadenomas. Immunolabelling for insulin.

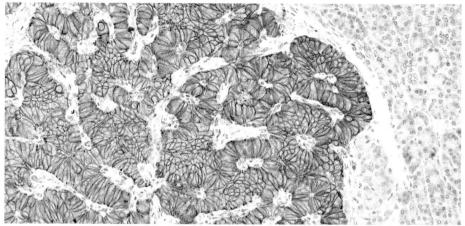

Fig. 6.23 Insulinoma. Immunostaining showing membrane labelling for GLP1R, the receptor used for exendin PET.

Immunophenotype

Like the cells of other PanNETs, insulinoma tumour cells stain for synaptophysin and chromogranin A, as well as ISL1. Insulin is expressed in most of the tumour cells, but with varying intensity. In some well-differentiated trabecular insulinomas, insulin staining shows an apical concentration, whereas proinsulin staining shows a perinuclear Golgi pattern {2349}. In other insulinomas, this special intracellular distribution of insulin and proinsulin is lost. About half of all insulinomas include scattered non-insulin cells staining for glucagon, pancreatic polypeptide, somatostatin, and/or other hormones. This is particularly common in malignant insulinomas. The demonstration of insulin is not mandatory for the diagnosis of insulinoma. However, if multiple PanNETs are present in the setting of a hypoglycaemic syndrome, it is

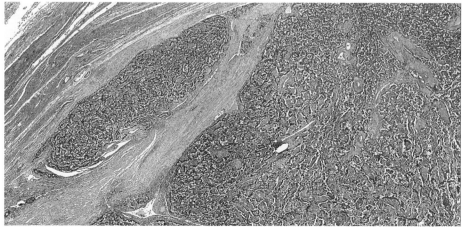

Fig. 6.24 Insulinoma with venous invasion. Liver metastases were also present.

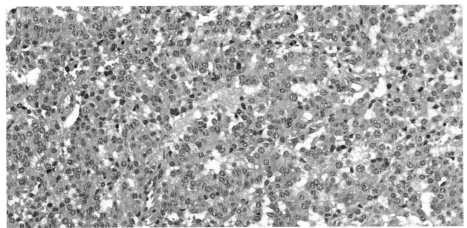
Fig. 6.25 Insulinoma showing a solid and trabecular pattern.

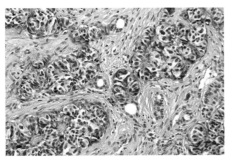
Fig. 6.26 Insulinoma showing peripheral immunolabelling for insulin.

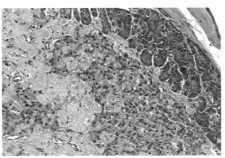
Fig. 6.27 Insulinoma with stromal amyloid deposition.

important to stain for insulin to identify the insulinoma(s), because the largest of multiple PanNETs is not always the tumour responsible for the clinical syndrome {84}. Insulin staining is required for the diagnosis of insulinomatosis {80}, to confirm that all the tumours (macrotumours and microadenomas) are positive for insulin, which is not the case in microadenomatosis associated with MEN1 or von Hippel–Lindau syndrome; in those settings, many tumours are positive for glucagon, pancreatic polypeptide, or somatostatin (or are multihormonal), but only individual tumours may stain for insulin.

Genetic profile
Insulinomas share many mutation events with other PanNETs (e.g. mutations in *MEN1*, *DAXX*, *ATRX*, *PTEN*, and *TSC2*). Somatic *MEN1* mutations and loss of heterozygosity are detected in about 20% of insulinomas {556,1019,3124}. *DAXX* and *ATRX* mutations are associated with alternative lengthening of telomeres, chromosomal instability, and adverse outcome in insulinomas {1736}. However, at the RNA level, insulinomas cluster separately from non-functioning PanNETs {1856}. Recently, a novel recurrent mutation in *YY1* (encoding the YY1 transcription factor) was reported in 30% of sporadic insulinomas.

This Thr372Arg mutation was associated with later onset of insulinoma in various cohorts of patients {379,1613}. *YY1* is a downstream effector of the mTOR pathway and is required for rapamycin-mediated repression of mTOR activity {588}. The expression of miR-204 in well-differentiated insulinomas has been found to be related to the immunohistochemical expression of insulin, whereas miR-21 overexpression has been found to be associated with a higher proliferation index and the presence of liver metastases. One of the targets of miR-21 is *PTEN*, which further supports the central role of the mTOR pathway in the pathogenesis of PanNETs {2320}.

Genetic susceptibility
Insulinomas are associated with MEN1 in about 5% of cases, and very rarely with tuberous sclerosis type 2 {1796}.

Prognosis and predictive factors
As is the case for other PanNETs, the most important prognostic markers for insulinomas are proliferation index and tumour size {1415}. Insulinomas < 2 cm are associated with a 10-year survival rate of close to 100%, whereas insulinomas > 2 cm very often metastasize, and are associated with a 10-year survival rate of about 30%. Along with CK19 expression as a marker of adverse outcome, molecular alterations consistent with chromosomal instability, chromosome 3p or 6q loss, and chromosome 12q gain have been described as the most powerful predictors of disease-free and overall survival for insulinomas {1272,2622}.

Glucagonoma

Couvelard A.
Klöppel G.
Öberg K.
Scoazec J.-Y.
Sipos B.

Definition
Glucagonoma is a functioning well-differentiated pancreatic neuroendocrine neoplasm composed of glucagon-producing and preproglucagon-derived peptide–producing cells, with uncontrolled glucagon secretion causing glucagonoma syndrome.

ICD-O code   8152/3

Epidemiology
Glucagonoma accounts for 1–2% of all pancreatic neuroendocrine tumours (PanNETs) and is the fourth most common functioning PanNET, after insulinoma, gastrinoma, and VIPoma {1255, 3035,3059}. Its annual incidence is approximatively 1 case per 20 million population. The average patient age at diagnosis is 52.5 years and the male-to-female ratio is 1:1 {570,2603,3035}.

Etiology
There are no known etiological factors for sporadic solitary glucagonomas. Rarely, a glucagonoma occurs in association with multiple endocrine neoplasia type 1 {1255,2603}.

Localization
All glucagonomas are localized in the pancreas, where they predominantly involve the tail {570}.

Clinical features
The clinical diagnosis of glucagonoma includes the typical triad of a skin rash called necrolytic migratory erythema, worsening or onset of diabetes mellitus, and weight loss. The necrolytic migratory erythema is usually located in the groin and migrates to the limbs, buttocks, and perineum. In addition to a skin rash, there may be angular stomatitis and cheilitis and atrophic glossitis. Other features of the syndrome are glucose intolerance (with diabetes mellitus seen in as many as 95% of patients), weight loss (in 50–60%), amino acid deficiency (in 50%), normochromic normocytic anaemia, and (in late-stage disease) widespread venous thrombosis with pulmonary embolism {570,2629,2982}. The diagnosis is established by markedly elevated plasma glucagon levels. The tumours are usually detected by CT, MRI, ultrasound, octreotide scan, and/or 68Ga-DOTATATE PET/CT. The liver is the most common site for metastases, followed by regional lymph nodes, bone, adrenal gland, kidney, and lung. The prevalence of metastatic disease at the time of diagnosis is 50–100% {2629,2679,2982,3035}.

Macroscopy
Glucagonomas are usually solitary, round, well-demarcated large tumours, 3–7 cm in size {2982,3035}. Like most PanNETs, they are well demarcated from the adjacent pancreas, but in some cases can infiltrate the pancreatic parenchyma. They can be cystic {335,1445}.

Microscopy
Glucagonomas are well-differentiated G1 or G2 neuroendocrine tumours with densely packed trabecular formations and a scant stromal reaction. The cytological features are the same as those of other PanNETs. Mitotic figures are rare. No poorly differentiated glucagonoma has been described.

Immunophenotype
The tumour cells express synaptophysin, chromogranin A, ISL1, and glucagon {2982}. They may also stain for pancreatic polypeptide. Multiple glucagon-positive microadenomas and macrotumours in conjunction with a glucagon cell hyperplasia of many islets characterize glucagon cell hyperplasia and neoplasia, a disease associated with germline glucagon receptor mutations (see *Glucagon cell hyperplasia and neoplasia*, p. 282) {2580,3117}. Multiple microadenomas that are commonly positive for glucagon but may also stain for pancreatic polypeptide, somatostatin, or insulin are typical of multiple endocrine neoplasia type 1 (see *Multiple endocrine neoplasia type 1*, p. 243).

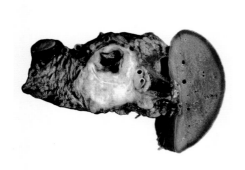

Fig. 6.28 Glucagonoma (5 cm) in the pancreatic tail with a cystic, haemorrhagic cut surface.

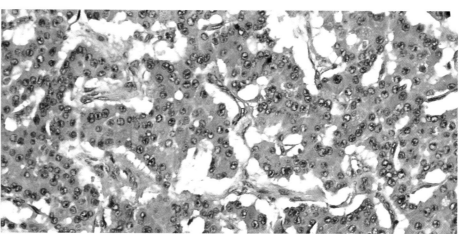

Fig. 6.29 Glucagonoma with a trabecular pattern.

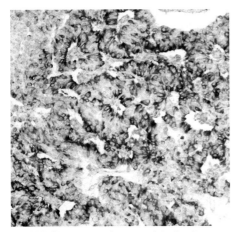

Fig. 6.30 Glucagonoma. Immunostaining for glucagon.

Genetic susceptibility

Most glucagonomas are sporadic. A small subset may occur in multiple endocrine neoplasia type 1.

Prognosis and predictive factors

Glucagonomas are slow-growing tumours, usually presenting at a late stage {2982}. Their prognosis depends on grade and stage {252,1363,3059}, although in a recent series, the Ki-67 proliferation index was not found to be of prognostic relevance {1382}. At diagnosis, most are locally advanced and 70–90% are metastatic {756,1382,2603, 2982}. Recent data show that 70% of patients survive 5 years and the mean time to death after diagnosis is > 6 years {756, 1382}. Death is usually related to tumour growth rather than to tumour-related functional complications such as diabetes {1382,2982}.

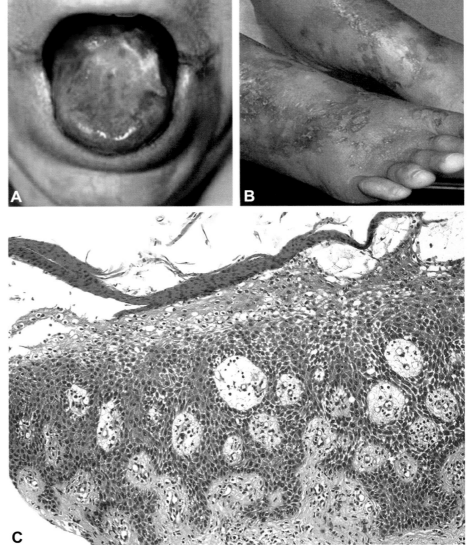

Fig. 6.31 Glucagonoma syndrome with glossitis (**A**), necrolytic migratory erythema (**B**) showing superficial epidermal clefts, necrolysis in the upper epidermis, vacuolated keratinocytes, and mild perivascular lymphocytic infiltration (**C**).

Somatostatinoma

La Rosa S.
Komminoth P.
Öberg K.
Perren A.

Definition
Somatostatinoma is a functioning well-differentiated pancreatic neuroendocrine neoplasm composed of somatostatin-producing cells, with uncontrolled somatostatin secretion causing somatostatinoma syndrome (diarrhoea, hyperglycaemia and overt diabetes, gallstones, and hypochlorhydria). Tumours composed either exclusively or predominantly of somatostatin-immunoreactive cells but lacking the symptoms of somatostatinoma syndrome, as is observed with ampullary neuroendocrine tumours (NETs), should be called somatostatin-producing NETs rather than somatostatinomas.

ICD-O code   8156/3

Epidemiology
Pancreatic somatostatinomas are extremely rare. They account for < 1% of functioning pancreatic NETs (PanNETs) and their annual incidence has been estimated to be 1 case per 40 million population. They occur more frequently in women and arise in middle-aged to older patients, with an average patient age at diagnosis of 55 years (range: 30–74 years) {1431,2605}.

Etiology
The etiology and pathogenesis of sporadic somatostatinomas are unknown. A minority of non-functioning somatostatin-expressing PanNETs are associated with neurofibromatosis type 1 {2749}, multiple endocrine neoplasia type 1 {929,2605}, or von Hippel–Lindau syndrome {1721}. No other risk factors are known.

Localization
Somatostatinomas can arise anywhere in the pancreas, but are most commonly located in the head {1431}.

Clinical features
The somatostatinoma syndrome is associated with high serum somatostatin levels. The syndrome comprises diarrhoea (secondary to a decrease of pancreatic enzymes and bicarbonate secretion), hyperglycaemia and diabetes (resulting from insulin inhibition), gallstones (due to cholecystokinin inhibition), and hypochlorhydria (due to inhibition of acid secretion). However, these symptoms are rarely seen simultaneously, and it is frequently difficult to clearly differentiate between symptoms caused by high plasma somatostatin levels and symptoms caused by tumour localization or tumour burden. For these reasons, and because no case of somatostatinoma syndrome showing the full clinical spectrum has been reported in recent years, the existence of full-blown somatostatinoma syndrome has been questioned {929,1690}. Localization is determined by CT, MRI, angiography, octreotide scan, or ^{68}Ga-DOTATOC PET/CT {1474}.

Most non-functioning pancreatic or ampullary somatostatin-producing tumours present with local mass effects and are detected incidentally. The symptoms, which are non-specific, include abdominal pain, weight loss, jaundice, nausea, and vomiting {929}.

Macroscopy
Somatostatinoma is a large, solitary, well-circumscribed but not encapsulated, greyish-white to yellowish-tan tumour, with an average size of 5–6 cm.

Microscopy
Somatostatinomas have no distinctive histological features compared with other PanNETs, except for an occasional paraganglioma-like pattern. The tumour cells are cuboidal to round, with eosinophilic cytoplasm and uniform nuclei. They form trabecular, solid, or acinar patterns. Unlike duodenal somatostatin-producing NETs, pancreatic somatostatinomas usually do not show a tubuloacinar pattern with psammoma bodies. Vascular and perineural invasion are frequent, but extensive necrosis is typically absent. The Ki-67 proliferation index and mitotic count have rarely been reported in the literature, but the available information indicates that most cases are G2 NETs.

Immunophenotype
The tumour cells are positive for synaptophysin. Chromogranin A is less consistently expressed and may even be absent. Somatostatin is expressed in most tumour cells, with various degrees of intensity. Most tumours also contain scattered cells immunoreactive for other hormones, such as pancreatic polypeptide, calcitonin, gastrin, adrenocorticotropic hormone, glucagon, and insulin.

Ultrastructure
The tumour cells contain two types of membrane-bound secretory granules. Most of the granules are large (250–450 nm in diameter), round, and moderately electron-dense, resembling those of normal islet delta cells. The second type of granules are smaller (150–300 nm in diameter) and have dense cores surrounded by a thin peripheral halo {1514}.

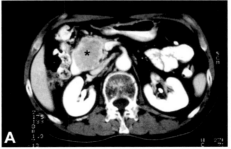
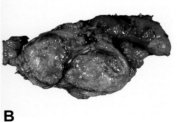

Fig. 6.32 Somatostatinoma. **A** CT image showing a large mass in the pancreatic head (asterisk). **B** Macroscopy showing a circumscribed, yellowish-tan, haemorrhagic tumour.

Genetic profile

The genetics of sporadic pancreatic somatostatinomas are not well studied, but there are no known genetic differences compared with non-functioning PanNETs.

Genetic susceptibility

Patients with neurofibromatosis type 1 are at risk for ampullary somatostatin-producing tumours {929}. Patients with multiple endocrine neoplasia type 1 are at risk for both ampullary and pancreatic somatostatin-producing tumours {2356}. Activating somatic mutations in *EPAS1* (also called *HIF2A*) were recently described in patients with polycythaemia and multiple paragangliomas, including duodenal and pancreatic somatostatin-producing tumours {3049}.

Prognosis and predictive factors

The overall 5-year survival rate has been estimated to be 75.2%, ranging from 60–100% in patients with localized disease to 15–60% in those with metastatic disease. Large tumour size (> 3 cm) and lymph node involvement are poor prognostic markers.

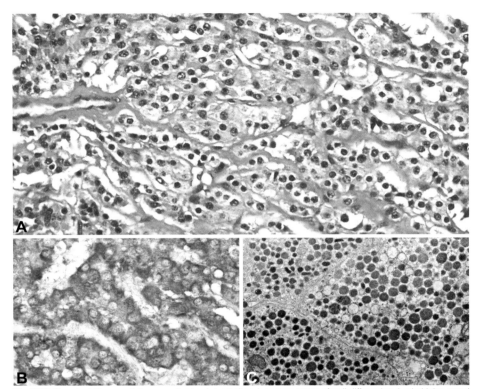

Fig. 6.33 Somatostatinoma. **A** An example showing a trabecular arrangement of well-differentiated cuboidal to round cells with eosinophilic cytoplasm and uniform nuclei. **B** Immunolabelling for somatostatin in almost all cells. **C** Ultrastructurally, the tumour cells contain large (250–450 nm), round, and moderately electron-dense secretory granules resembling those of normal islet delta cells.

Gastrinoma

Rindi G.
Anlauf M.
Öberg K.
Perren A.

Definition

Gastrinoma is a functioning well-differentiated pancreatic neuroendocrine neoplasm (PanNEN) composed of gastrin-producing cells (G cells), with uncontrolled gastrin secretion causing Zollinger–Ellison syndrome (ZES).

ICD-O code   8153/3

Epidemiology

Gastrinomas of all sites have an estimated annual incidence of 0.05–0.2 cases per 100 000 population overall {1255, 1472}, but those arising in the pancreas are much rarer. ZES, which is the second most common hormonal syndrome, is observed in as many as 20% of all cases of functioning neuroendocrine tumours. Patients with sporadic pancreatic gastrinomas are usually in their fifth to sixth decade of life; younger than patients with non-functioning pancreatic neuroendocrine tumours (PanNETs). The male and female distributions are equal {1255, 2294}. The rare cases of pancreatic gastrinoma that occur in the setting of a genetic syndrome, most frequently multiple endocrine neoplasia type 1 (MEN1), usually arise in patients about a decade younger {971,1255}. Most patients (> 90%) with MEN1 who are affected by gastrinomas have primary tumours located in the duodenum {81,83} (see *Multiple endocrine neoplasia type 1*, p. 243).

Etiology

With the exception of MEN1, there are no known gastrinoma-specific etiological factors. In general, the risk factors for PanNENs overlap with those for pancreatic exocrine cancers, and include cigarette smoking and alcohol consumption, as well as family history of cancer and diabetes {1591}.

Localization

Gastrinomas have no preferential location in the pancreas {525,698,1255,1472}.

Clinical features

Patients have elevated fasting gastrin levels (> 150 pg/L) and gastric acid hypersecretion {1255,1472}. When the results of fasting serum gastrin and acid secretory studies are borderline or non-diagnostic in patients for whom there is clinical suspicion of ZES, provocative testing of fasting serum gastrin can be performed by intravenous secretin (2 mg/kg). Serum chromogranin A levels are also increased in as many as 90% of gastrinoma cases. Gastric acid hypersecretion causes duodenal ulcer, gastro-oesophageal reflux disease, diarrhoea, nausea, vomiting, and abdominal pain. The widespread use of proton pump inhibitors can mask symptoms, resulting in a diagnosis time lag of > 5 years {970,1255}. Diagnosis may require patients to be off proton pump inhibitor therapy for 48 hours before testing in a specialized setting, given the potential complication induced by the elevated acid output rebound. Like other pancreatic masses, gastrinomas can be imaged by ultrasonography, CT, MRI, and somatostatin receptor scintigraphy {1255,1472}. Endoscopic ultrasound with related fine-needle aspiration biopsy and fine-needle tissue acquisition is used for preoperative diagnosis, and intraoperative ultrasound is used for intraoperative tumour localization {1255,1472}.

Macroscopy

The tumours are usually 2–3 cm in size {698,1255,1472}. At gross examination, gastrinomas do not differ from the other PanNETs; they are usually compact in texture and have fairly well-circumscribed margins. Pancreatic gastrinomas

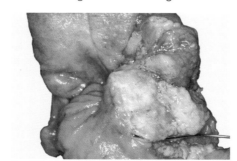

Fig. 6.34 Pancreatic gastrinoma. Macroscopy showing a large tumour in the head of the pancreas.

can invade locally, spread to local lymph nodes (which occurs in 40–75% of cases), and metastasize to the liver (in 8–20%) and distant sites including bone {1255,1472}. Gastrinomas that present as a tumour adjacent to the pancreas or with predominantly peripancreatic lymph node involvement are much more likely to be duodenal rather than pancreatic primaries.

Microscopy

Gastrinomas are usually G1 or G2 neuroendocrine tumours and display trabecular, glandular, or mixed structures (B type, C type, or mixed type histology as described by Soga and Tazawa in 1971 {2602}). At the tumour periphery, the margins can be expansive or focally infiltrative. The stroma is typically delicate and only in large tumours may be prominent. Lymphovascular invasion may be observed. Evident mitotic activity and necrosis are unusual; when present, they are associated with higher grade disease.

Immunophenotype

Gastrinomas are diffusely positive for neuroendocrine markers. Positive gastrin immunohistochemistry is required to positively identify the pancreatic tumour as the source of unregulated gastrin responsible for the concurring gastrinoma syndrome. Gastrin-positive cells may constitute either the prevalent tumour cell population or only a minor tumour cell subset; the proportion of gastrin-producing cells is irrelevant for the concurrent clinical syndrome. Additional hormones that may be found in the tumour cells include insulin, glucagon, pancreatic polypeptide, ghrelin, and serotonin. Hormone hypersecretion with consequent change in the associated clinical syndrome may occur {618,1733}. As is the case in other PanNETs, the pancreas lineage–related transcription factors PDX1 and ISL1 may be expressed in pancreatic and duodenal gastrinomas {12,842,1135,2627}. CDX2 expression, previously thought to be restricted to the tubular digestive tract, may also occur in pancreatic and duodenal gastrinomas {1135,2627}. Membranous SSTR2A expression can usually be demonstrated by immunohistochemistry {1455,1487}, and correlates with in vivo somatostatin receptor imaging and prognosis {1288,2610,2890}.

Genetic profile

The few data available about the genetic profile of pancreatic gastrinomas mostly pertain to the *MEN1* gene (see the *Introduction*, p. 211), as is the case for other PanNETs. Of great interest is the recent finding that specific *MEN1* mutations leading to abnormal menin interaction with FOXN3 (also known as CHES1), which is encoded by *FOXN3* (previously called *CHES1*), may be associated with a higher risk of aggressive behaviour {165}.

Genetic susceptibility

Most pancreatic gastrinomas are sporadic. A minor subset may occur in the setting of familial predisposing conditions such as MEN1 and rarely neurofibromatosis type 1, neurofibromatosis type 2 {1581,1751}, or tuberous sclerosis {2485}. Gastrinomas in patients with MEN1 or ZES usually develop in the duodenum {1255,1472}.

Prognosis and predictive factors

Grading and staging are the most important prognostic parameters for pancreatic gastrinomas, as they are for all PanNENs. Patients with functioning PanNEN other than insulinoma have the same disease-specific survival rates as patients with non-functioning neuroendocrine neoplasms {2294}. Pancreatic gastrinomas found to express SSTR2A, either in histological samples or in vivo by imaging procedures, usually qualify for treatment with somatostatin analogues {387,2297} and somatostatin receptor–targeted radiotherapy {733}.

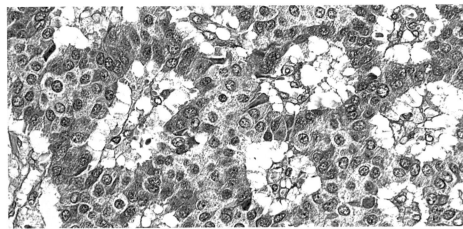

Fig. 6.35 Gastrinoma with a trabecular and pseudoglandular pattern.

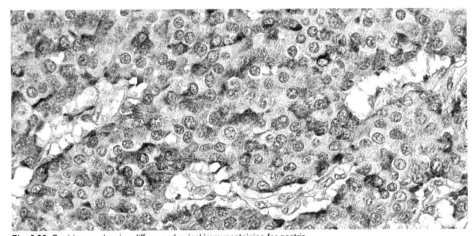

Fig. 6.36 Gastrinoma showing diffuse and apical immunostaining for gastrin.

Pancreatic neuroendocrine carcinoma (poorly differentiated neuroendocrine neoplasm)

Adsay N. V.
Klimstra D. S.
Klöppel G.
Öberg K.
Papotti M.
Rindi G.
Scarpa A.

Definition

Pancreatic neuroendocrine carcinoma (PanNEC) is a poorly differentiated, high-grade pancreatic neuroendocrine neoplasm composed of highly atypical small cells or large to intermediate-sized epithelial cells showing neuroendocrine differentiation and lacking evidence of acinar or ductal/glandular lineage. PanNECs show brisk mitotic activity, a Ki-67 proliferation index > 20%, and usually necrosis {173,174,1123,2620}.

ICD-O codes

Neuroendocrine carcinoma (poorly differentiated neuroendocrine neoplasm)
8246/3 [a]

Small cell neuroendocrine carcinoma
8041/3

Large cell neuroendocrine carcinoma
8013/3

[a] This ICD-O code should not be used for well-differentiated G3 pancreatic neuroendocrine tumours, which are coded using the functioning or non-functioning pancreatic neuroendocrine tumour codes.

Synonyms

This entity was classified under the heading of "poorly differentiated neuroendocrine carcinoma" in the 2004 WHO classification and the subsequent literature {173,174,1123,2620}; however, with the revised definition of neuroendocrine carcinoma (NEC) provided in the current edition, the category of NEC is now specifically defined as being poorly differentiated; therefore, the term "poorly differentiated" is no longer warranted as part of the name. In the 2010 *WHO classification of tumours of the digestive system*, this group of tumours was included under the heading "neuroendocrine carcinoma (NEC)", defined as high-grade (G3) on the basis of a high mitotic rate (> 20 mitoses per 10 high-power fields) and a Ki-67 proliferation index > 20% {173,174, 1123,2620}.

Epidemiology

PanNECs are rare, accounting for < 1% of pancreatic tumours overall and no more than 2–3% of neuroendocrine neoplasms of this organ {174,1069,1212,1981,2277}. They typically occur in patients in their sixth to seventh decade of life {173,1123, 1594,2620}, but can also affect younger patients. They are slightly more common in men {173}.

Etiology

Like their counterparts in other organs, PanNECs have been reported to be associated with cigarette smoking {481}, but this finding requires confirmation.

Localization

The tumours occur twice as frequently in the head of the pancreas as elsewhere within the organ {173}.

Clinical features

The presentation of PanNECs is similar to that of exocrine pancreatic cancers, including back pain, jaundice, and non-specific abdominal symptoms {173,174, 1123,1392,1594,2620}. Hormonal hypersecretion is seldom noted {561,2406}, and increased serum chromogranin A does not seem to be a feature. Serum CA19-9 may be elevated. Serum neuron-specific enolase levels are increased in some cases. Somatostatin receptor scintigraphy (octreotide scan and DOTATOC scan) is often negative due to lack of expression of SSTR2A and SSTR5. The FDG-PET, however, is usually positive. The vast majority (> 90%) of patients already have metastases at the time of diagnosis.

Macroscopy

PanNECs are relatively large (measuring up to 18 cm; mean: 4 cm), solid, compact tumours that often exhibit vague nodularity and focal haemorrhagic necrosis {173}. They tend to be better demarcated than pancreatic ductal adenocarcinomas.

Microscopy

The histology is fairly similar to that of their counterparts in other organs {173, 174,2268,2665,2888}. The large cell type, which is more common (accounting for 60% of cases) {173,174}, is characterized by organoid, nesting, or solid sheet-like patterns, with relatively uniform round or polygonal cells containing amphophilic cytoplasm, large nuclei, vesicular chromatin, and in most cases prominent nucleoli. The small cell type has a more diffusely infiltrative growth pattern, with cells showing scant cytoplasm, round

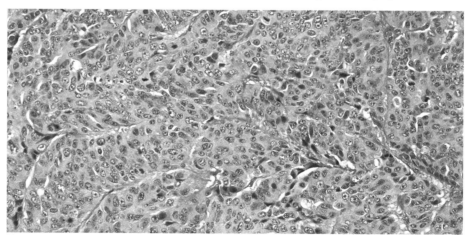

Fig. 6.43 Pancreatic neuroendocrine carcinoma (poorly differentiated neuroendocrine neoplasm), large cell type. Diffuse growth of relatively monotonous cells with a nested/organoid pattern compartmentalized by delicate vasculature, indicating neuroendocrine differentiation, which was confirmed by synaptophysin staining. Cytological atypia and prominent mitotic activity indicate the high-grade (poorly differentiated) nature of this carcinoma.

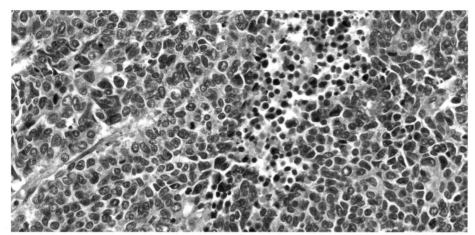

Fig. 6.44 Pancreatic neuroendocrine carcinoma (poorly differentiated neuroendocrine neoplasm), small cell type. The cells have high-grade cytology, with minimal cytoplasm and a high N:C ratio. Mitotic activity is brisk and necrosis is readily evident.

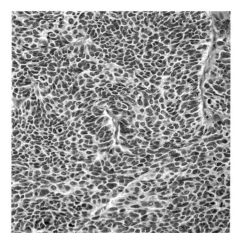

Fig. 6.45 Pancreatic neuroendocrine carcinoma (poorly differentiated neuroendocrine neoplasm), small cell type. Characteristic fusiform cytology with moulding is apparent.

or elongated nuclei, finely granular chromatin, inconspicuous nucleoli, and focal nuclear moulding. Foci of necrosis are easily identifiable in both types, and may create a so-called peritheliomatous or pseudopapillary-like pattern {173}. Mitoses are abundant (> 20 mitoses per 10 high-power fields by definition) and the mitotic rate is typically very brisk, commonly with > 40–50 mitoses per 10 high-power fields. Similarly, the Ki-67 proliferation index is > 20% by definition, but in most cases it is > 50% and is commonly > 60–80%, particularly in the small cell type {173,174,2620}. Poorly differentiated neuroendocrine cells (possibly different from small cell or large cell NEC cells) may be found in association with non-neuroendocrine carcinoma types, usually tubular-type ductal adenocarcinoma or acinar cell carcinoma {173} (see

ACTH-producing tumour with Cushing syndrome, p. 234).

Immunohistochemistry and differential diagnosis
Like their counterparts in other organs, PanNECs are largely defined and recognized by their morphological characteristics. However, due to the poorly differentiated nature of these tumours, immunohistochemical confirmation is also crucial and is required in all cases. Synaptophysin should be positive in all cases; the diagnosis must be questioned if this marker is negative within a given tumour. However, synaptophysin positivity may vary in intensity from case to case and is often dot-like or may be only focal {173}. Chromogranin A is a good and specific marker, but can be scant or even negative in some cases due to

the scarcity of neurosecretory granules in the tumour cells. Although CD56 is not a specific neuroendocrine marker, membranous cell labelling in conjunction with synaptophysin positivity contributes greatly to the recognition of PanNECs. Neuron-specific enolase may also be positive, but due to the non-specificity of the antiserum, it should always be interpreted in conjunction with synaptophysin and chromogranin A. Some PanNECs, especially of the small cell type, have minimal cytoplasm and demonstrate a dot-like pattern of cytokeratin immunolabelling {2535}. SSTR2A staining is negative in approximately 90% of cases {1445A}, correlating with the fact that radiolabelled somatostatin analogues cannot be used to diagnose or treat most PanNECs {2043,2620}. Good markers for small and large cell PanNECs are diffuse

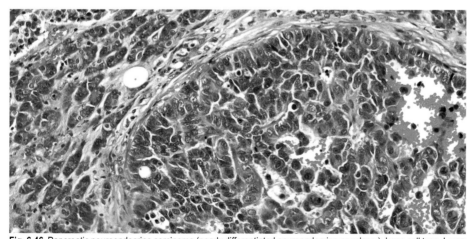

Fig. 6.46 Pancreatic neuroendocrine carcinoma (poorly differentiated neuroendocrine neoplasm), large cell type. Large nuclei with prominent nucleoli and moderate cytoplasm.

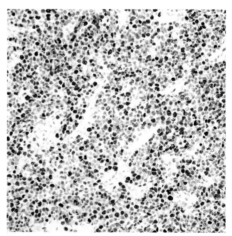

Fig. 6.47 Pancreatic neuroendocrine carcinoma (poorly differentiated neuroendocrine neoplasm), large cell type. Ki-67 immunostaining shows diffuse nuclear labelling, with a Ki-67 proliferation index > 80%.

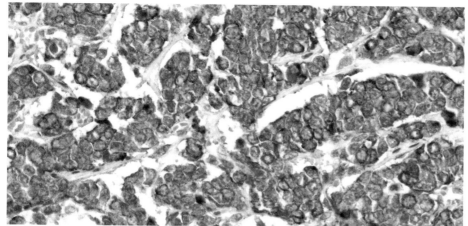

Fig. 6.48 Pancreatic neuroendocrine carcinoma (poorly differentiated neuroendocrine neoplasm), large cell type. Synaptophysin staining shows diffuse labelling with focal, punctate positivity in rare cells.

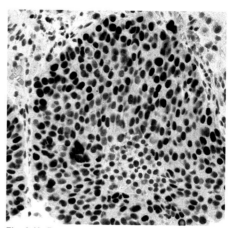

Fig. 6.49 Pancreatic neuroendocrine carcinoma (poorly differentiated neuroendocrine neoplasm), large cell type, showing diffuse and strong immunolabelling for p53.

(>20%) and strong nuclear expression of p53 or complete loss of RB expression. These markers are particularly helpful in distinguishing PanNECs from G3 pancreatic neuroendocrine tumours (NETs) {2722,2724} (see the *Introduction*, p. 211, and *Non-functioning neuroendocrine tumours*, p. 215).

One of the most important mimics of PanNEC, especially of the large cell type, is acinar cell carcinoma {173}, especially acinar cell carcinomas with a solid pattern and focal positivity for synaptophysin and chromogranin. Immunostaining for trypsin, chymotrypsin, or BCL10 is then required to diagnose these tumours as acinar cell carcinoma or mixed acinar–neuroendocrine carcinoma. The Ki-67 proliferation index is generally lower in acinar cell carcinomas than in PanNECs. Diagnosing a PanNEC without first excluding the possibility of an acinar cell neoplasm carries a risk of misdiagnosis {173}.

Distinguishing between a primary PanNEC and a metastasis to the pancreas from a small cell carcinoma, especially of the lung, can be almost impossible, and requires clinical correlation {7}. Immunohistochemical staining for organ-related transcription factors such as TTF1, CDX2, and ISL1 may not be helpful, because these markers can be found in NECs of any location {12,2870}.

Immunohistochemical staining is helpful for identifying so-called small blue cell tumours of young adulthood, such as primitive neuroectodermal tumour and desmoplastic small round cell tumour, which can occur in the pancreas and can mimic PanNEC {260,1919}. Each of these tumours has its own relatively specific immunoprofile. Molecular genetic analysis may also be indicated in some cases.

Genetic profile

Specific genetic alterations that are common in well-differentiated NETs (e. g. *MEN1*, *ATRX*, and *DAXX* mutations) or pancreatic ductal adenocarcinoma (e. g. *KRAS* and *SMAD4* mutations) {3031} are not typical features of PanNEC {187, 2137}. Instead, PanNECs are characterized by mutations of *TP53* and inactivation of the RB/p16 pathway (determined either by mutations in *RB1* or loss of expression of p16) {995,3031}. Overexpression of BCL2 has been identified in some cases, with resulting activation of oncogenic pro-survival and anti-apoptotic pathways {3031}. The roles of the epigenetic and microRNA expression modifications {1053,2320} and the increased CDK4/CDK6 expression {2723} that have been identified in NETs have yet to be determined in PanNECs.

In terms of molecular targets for therapy, the current literature suggests that PanNECs may not be good candidates for somatostatin receptor analogue therapy. There is emerging evidence that primary PanNECs, like NECs of other sites, may warrant platinum-based therapy instead {174,1123,2620}.

Genetic susceptibility

The syndromes associated with well-differentiated NETs, such as multiple endocrine neoplasia type 1 and von Hippel–Lindau syndrome, do not seem to be associated with PanNECs. One case with *BRCA1* mutation was noted in a study of 44 PanNECs {173}, a frequency similar to that seen in pancreatic ductal adenocarcinomas.

Prognosis and predictive factors

PanNECs are highly aggressive malignant neoplasms {173,174,1123,1594, 2620}. Metastasis is present in the vast majority of cases at the time of diagnosis. Even in resected cases and with platinum-based therapy, the median survival is very short (< 1 year), and < 25% of patients survive beyond 2 years. Survival with large cell PanNECs seems to be only very slightly better than with the small cell type. PanNECs with other carcinoma components (e. g. ductal adenocarcinoma) appear to behave aggressively, which underscores the importance of recognizing the PanNEC component in such cases.

Mixed neuroendocrine–non-neuroendocrine neoplasms

Ohike N.
Adsay N. V.
La Rosa S.
Volante M.
Zamboni G.

Definition

Mixed neuroendocrine–non-neuroendocrine neoplasms of the pancreas are carcinomas with components of both a non-neuroendocrine carcinoma (typically adenocarcinoma) and a neuroendocrine neoplasm. Each of these components should account for ≥ 30% of the tumour cell population. Usually, both components are high-grade (G3) carcinomas, but occasionally one or both components are low-grade malignant. Therefore, when the components can be morphologically distinguished, they should be graded individually, using the respective grading systems specific to each. On the basis of the cell types identified, mixed neuroendocrine–non-neuroendocrine neoplasms can be subclassified as mixed ductal–neuroendocrine carcinomas, mixed acinar–neuroendocrine carcinomas, or mixed acinar–ductal–neuroendocrine carcinomas.

ICD-O code   8154/3

Synonym

Mixed adenoneuroendocrine carcinoma

Mixed ductal–neuroendocrine carcinomas

Epidemiology, localization, and clinical features

These carcinomas account for approximately 0.5% of all ductal adenocarcinomas {1411,2046}, with which they share demographic characteristics, pancreatic head localization, and clinical symptoms. In one reported case, the patient developed Zollinger–Ellison syndrome {2738}.

Macroscopy

The solid tumours are 2–10 cm in diameter and typically metastasize to the lymph nodes and liver.

Microscopy

There are two histopathological patterns. One pattern consists of intermingled

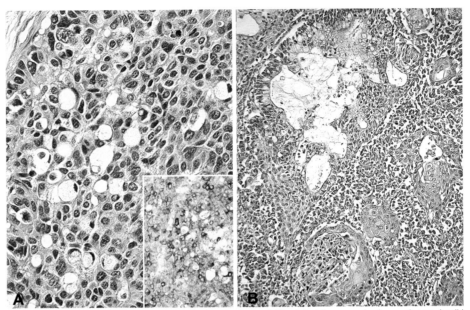

Fig. 6.50 Mixed neuroendocrine–non-neuroendocrine neoplasm. **A** Mixed ductal–neuroendocrine carcinoma. A solid neuroendocrine component positive for chromogranin A (inset) is admixed with goblet cells. **B** Carcinoma with ductal and squamous differentiation mixed with a poorly differentiated neuroendocrine neoplasm.

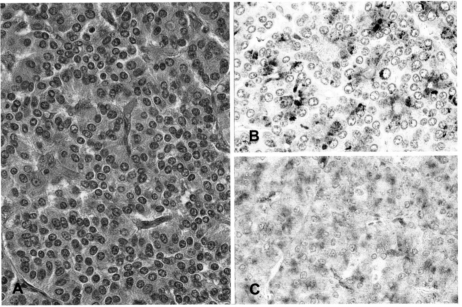

Fig. 6.51 Mixed neuroendocrine–non-neuroendocrine neoplasm. **A** Solid growth pattern with focal acinar structures. **B** Immunopositivity for trypsin. **C** Immunopositivity for synaptophysin.

neoplastic ductal and neuroendocrine cells forming glandular, cribriform, solid, and/or trabecular structures and often showing intracellular (i.e. signet-ring cell–like or goblet cell–like) or extracellular mucin accumulation. High-grade pancreatic intraepithelial neoplasia may also be observed. The other pattern consists

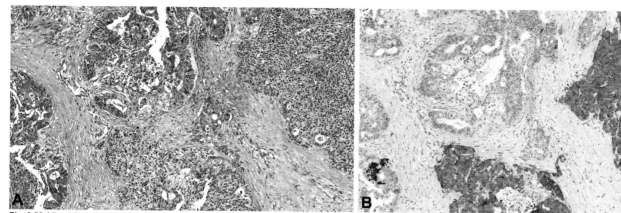

Fig. 6.52 Mixed ductal–neuroendocrine carcinoma. **A** Periodic acid–Schiff (PAS) staining shows tumour tissue composed of a ductal adenocarcinoma component and neuroendocrine carcinoma of the large cell type. **B** In the same tumour tissue, immunostaining for synaptophysin reveals the neuroendocrine component.

of a ductal adenocarcinoma component that combines (but does not intermingle) with a usually poorly differentiated neuroendocrine neoplasm.

Immunophenotype
Positive periodic acid–Schiff (PAS) reactivity and positivity for CEA and MUC1 indicate ductal differentiation. Positivity for synaptophysin and chromogranin A indicates neuroendocrine differentiation.

Ultrastructure
The tumour cells contain mucin and/or neurosecretory granules.

Differential diagnosis
Mixed ductal–neuroendocrine carcinomas must be distinguished from ductal adenocarcinomas showing cords and nests (i.e. islets) of non-neoplastic neuroendocrine cells intimately attached to well-differentiated neoplastic duct-like glands. Other differential diagnoses are pancreatic neuroendocrine tumours with entrapped normal ductal structures and islets, and pancreatic neuroendocrine carcinomas that are located next to (but clearly separated from) a ductal adenocarcinoma or an intraductal papillary mucinous neoplasm {174}. Some intraductal papillary mucinous neoplasms contain single neuroendocrine cells, which are usually absent in an associated invasive component.

Prognosis and predictive factors
Resectability is the most important prognostic factor, but even when total resection is achieved, patients rarely survive beyond 3 years.

Mixed acinar–neuroendocrine carcinomas

Epidemiology, localization, and clinical features
These carcinomas are rare, accounting for 15–20% of all acinar cell carcinomas {1406,1511}, with which they share the typical patient age distribution, but not the overall male predominance {1406, 1511,2047}. They are evenly distributed within the pancreas, and the presenting symptoms are usually non-specific. Serum levels of alpha-fetoprotein and chromogranin A may be elevated.

Macroscopy
These carcinomas typically form a large (4–8 cm) nodular mass with a fleshy, focally necrotic cut surface. Intraductal spread can occur. Large liver metastases are common.

Microscopy
The histology of these tumours often resembles that of acinar cell carcinoma, with the neuroendocrine differentiation of single cells or groups of cells revealed only by immunohistochemistry. However, a few tumours show histologically discernible acinar and neuroendocrine components, which form closely connected sheets and nests.

Immunophenotype
In most cases, the tumours are diffusely positive for trypsin, chymotrypsin, and BCL10 {1513} and also contain intermingled cells that are positive for synaptophysin and chromogranin A. Double staining may reveal amphicrine cells.

Rarely, the trypsin-positive cells and the cells positive for synaptophysin and chromogranin form distinct compartments within the tumour tissue. Carcinomas with only scattered neuroendocrine cells (i.e. accounting for < 30% of the tumour cells) do not qualify as mixed carcinoma and should be called acinar cell carcinoma with focal neuroendocrine differentiation.

Ultrastructure
The cells contain large electron-dense zymogen granules (250–900 nm in size) and/or small neurosecretory granules (100–300 nm in size).

Differential diagnosis
Neuroendocrine tumours can occasionally entrap normal acinar cells, but they otherwise stain diffusely for neuroendocrine markers. Pancreatoblastomas, distinguished by squamoid nests, may contain neuroendocrine cells. In mixed acinar–ductal–neuroendocrine carcinomas, both exocrine components should be clearly identifiable.

Genetic profile and susceptibility
The tumours seem to have the same genetic changes seen in acinar cell carcinomas, including APC/beta-catenin pathway alterations and *BRAF* gene fusions {498,908}. No associations with genetic syndromes have been documented.

Prognosis and predictive factors
After tumour resection, the reported 5-year survival rate is 40%, similar to the rate associated with pure acinar cell carcinomas {1511,1675}.

CHAPTER 7

Inherited tumour syndromes

Multiple endocrine neoplasia

Hyperparathyroidism–jaw tumour syndrome

Von Hippel–Lindau syndrome

Familial paraganglioma–
phaeochromocytoma syndromes

Neurofibromatosis type 1

Carney complex

McCune–Albright syndrome

Familial non-medullary thyroid cancer

Non-syndromic familial thyroid cancer

Werner syndrome and Carney complex

DICER1 syndrome

Glucagon cell hyperplasia and neoplasia

Introduction

Klöppel G.
Lloyd R.V.

This chapter is devoted to the epidemiological, clinical, morphological, and genetic characteristics of inherited tumour syndromes that involve the endocrine organs. These syndromes are varied and complex, and often involve non-endocrine organs and tissues in addition to endocrine glands. All entities included in the previous edition are discussed and have been updated, and three new syndromes have been added since the previous edition: multiple endocrine neoplasia type 4, *DICER1* syndrome, and glucagon cell hyperplasia and neoplasia. All the neoplastic lesions, syndromes, and genetic changes related to the affected endocrine organs are listed in Table 7.01.

Table 7.01 Endocrine organ involvement and genetic changes in inherited tumour syndromes

Organ	Neoplastic lesion(s)	Syndromes	Genes
Pituitary gland	Adenoma; pituitary blastoma in *DICER1* syndrome	Multiple endocrine neoplasia type 1	*MEN1*
		Multiple endocrine neoplasia type 4	*CDKN1B*
		Carney complex	*PRKAR1A*
		McCune–Albright syndrome	*GNAS*
		DICER1 syndrome	*DICER1*
Thyroid gland	Papillary carcinoma (rarely, follicular carcinoma)	Familial non-medullary thyroid cancer, including Cowden syndrome, familial adenomatous polyposis, non-syndromic familial thyroid cancer, Werner syndrome, Carney complex and *DICER1* syndrome	Various, *DICER1*
	Medullary carcinoma	Multiple endocrine neoplasia type 2	*RET*
Parathyroid glands	Microadenomatosis	Multiple endocrine neoplasia type 1	*MEN1*
		Multiple endocrine neoplasia type 2A	*RET*
		Multiple endocrine neoplasia type 4	*CDKN1B*
		Hyperparathyroidism–jaw tumour syndrome	*CDC73* (also called *HRPT2*)
Paraganglia	Paraganglioma	Paraganglioma–phaeochromocytoma syndromes, Carney–Stratakis syndrome (paraganglioma and gastrointestinal stromal tumour)	*SDHA, SDHB, SDHC, SDHD, TMEM127, MAX, FH, MDH2*
		von Hippel–Lindau syndrome	*VHL*
		Multiple endocrine neoplasia type 2A	*RET*
		Neurofibromatosis type 1	*NF1*
		Paraganglioma–polycythaemia syndrome	*EGLN2, EGLN1*
		Pacak–Zhuang syndrome	*EPAS1*
Adrenal glands	Adrenal cortical neoplasm*	Multiple endocrine neoplasia type 1	*MEN1*
		Carney complex	*PRKAR1A*
	Phaeochromocytoma	Multiple endocrine neoplasia type 2	*RET*
		von Hippel–Lindau syndrome	*VHL*
		Paraganglioma–phaeochromocytoma syndrome	*SDHA, SDHB, SDHC, SDHD, TMEM127, MAX, FH, MDH2*
		Neurofibromatosis type 1	*NF1*
		Paraganglioma–polycythaemia syndrome	*EGLN2, EGLN1*
		Pacak–Zhuang syndrome	*EPAS1*
Pancreas	Microadenomatosis and neuroendocrine tumour	Multiple endocrine neoplasia type 1	*MEN1*
		von Hippel–Lindau syndrome	*VHL*
		Neurofibromatosis type 1	*NF1*
		Multiple endocrine neoplasia type 4	*CDKN1B*
		Glucagon cell hyperplasia and neoplasia	*GCGR*
		Tuberous sclerosis	*TSC1, TSC2*
Duodenum	Neuroendocrine tumour	Neurofibromatosis type 1	*NF1*
		Multiple endocrine neoplasia type 1	*MEN1*
		Pacak–Zhuang syndrome	*EPAS1*
Ovary	Sertoli cell tumour	*DICER1* syndrome	*DICER1*

* See also *Adrenal cortical adenoma* (p. 163) and *Adrenal cortical carcinoma* (p. 169) in Chapter 4.

Multiple endocrine neoplasia type 1

Komminoth P.
Klöppel G.
Korbonits M.
Mete O.
Scoazec J.-Y.
Stratakis C. A.

Definition

Multiple endocrine neoplasia type 1 (MEN1) is an autosomal dominant disease caused by germline *MEN1* mutations leading to the development of multifocal neoplastic endocrine lesions of the parathyroid glands, endocrine pancreas, duodenum, anterior pituitary, and less commonly also of the stomach, adrenal cortex, thymus, and lungs. In addition, various non-endocrine lesions may occur in the skin, CNS, and soft tissues.

Synonyms

Werner syndrome; multiple endocrine adenomatosis type 1; familial Zollinger–Ellison syndrome (all obsolete)

Incidence and prevalence

In most populations, the prevalence is estimated to be between 1 case per 40 000 and 1 case per 20 000 population. About 10% of patients have germline *MEN1* mutations arising de novo, with no family history {171,2745}.

Age distribution and penetrance

MEN1 is inherited as an autosomal dominant trait with age-related penetrance and variable expression {2745}. Both sexes are equally affected, with no geographical, racial, or ethnic differences. Primary hyperparathyroidism is clinically present in ≥ 50% of patients by the age of 20 years {2484}. The penetrance is high, with clinical evidence of MEN1 found in 43% of affected gene carriers by the age of 20 years, 85% by 35 years, and 94% by 50 years in one series {2818}. In other series, a penetrance of 100% has been observed by the age of 60 years {171}. The great majority (90%) of individuals with MEN1 have an affected parent, although the onset of symptoms can vary considerably, even within the same family.

Diagnostic criteria

The diagnosis of MEN1 should be considered in individuals with newly diagnosed MEN1-associated lesions (see Table 7.02) who meet the criteria commonly related to inherited cancers (e.g. age < 50 years, positive family history, multifocal or recurrent neoplasia, two or more endocrine organs or systems affected).

Specific tumours and lesions

Hyperparathyroidism

Age distribution and penetrance
Parathyroid involvement affects all age groups, with equal sex distribution, and occurs in approximately 90–95% of patients with MEN1 {2457,2745,2818}. The cumulative proportion of patients who develop biochemical evidence of hyperparathyroidism increases with patient age. Among individuals aged < 40 years with primary hyperparathyroidism, the incidence of MEN1 has been estimated to be 5–13% {2745}.

Clinical features
Primary hyperparathyroidism is the first clinical manifestation of MEN1 in most patients {2745}. Patients usually present with multiglandular parathyroid disease rather than solitary adenoma, a common feature in sporadic primary hyperparathyroidism {688,708,2457,2745}. With the advent of routine serum calcium testing, most patients with MEN1 with hyperparathyroidism are asymptomatic and lack the classic symptoms associated with longstanding or severe hypercalcaemia; i. e. the so-called moans (gastrointestinal conditions), stones (nephrolithiasis-related conditions), bones (bone pain and bone-related conditions), and groans (psychological and/or CNS-related conditions) symptoms {708}.

Table 7.02 Frequency and clinical features of various organ changes in multiple endocrine neoplasia type 1

Organ changes	Frequency	Clinical features
Parathyroid gland	≥ 90%	Primary hyperparathyroidism
Microadenomatosis		
Endocrine pancreas	30–75%	
Multiple non-functioning microadenomas		
Non-functioning macrotumours		
Functioning macrotumours		
Insulinoma	10–30%	Hypoglycaemia syndrome
Others	Rare	
Duodenum		
Multiple gastrinomas	50–80%	Zollinger–Ellison syndrome
Pituitary gland	30–40%	
Adenoma	70%	Clinically silent, local symptoms, pituitary insufficiency
Lactotroph adenoma	Frequent	Amenorrhoea, galactorrhoea
Somatotroph adenoma	9%	Acromegaly
Corticotroph adenoma	4%	Cushing syndrome
Others	Rare	
Other lesions		
Neuroendocrine tumours (thymus, stomach, lung, intestinal)	5–10%	
Skin (facial angiofibromas, collagenoma, pigment lesions)	40–80%	
Adrenal cortical hyperplasia/tumour	20–45%	
Lipoma	10%	
Spinal ependymoma	Rare	
Soft tissue tumours	Rare	

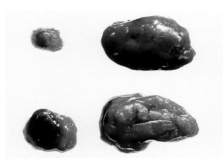

Fig. 7.01 Multiple endocrine neoplasia type 1 (MEN1). Micronodular adenomatosis of parathyroid glands. Macroscopic aspect of the parathyroid glands.

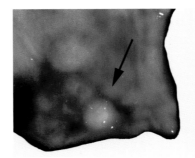

Fig. 7.02 Multiple endocrine neoplasia type 1 (MEN1). Endoscopic view of a small neuroendocrine tumour in the duodenum of a patient with MEN1.

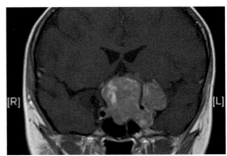

Fig. 7.03 Multiple endocrine neoplasia type 1 (MEN1). T1-weighted MRI showing a large pituitary tumour in an 11-year-old boy with MEN1.

Pathology

Multiglandular parathyroid disease is the hallmark {688,2457,2745}. Although the finding of multiple abnormal parathyroid glands generally results in a diagnosis of parathyroid hyperplasia, recent molecular data suggest that MEN1-associated multiglandular parathyroid lesions are composed of multiple monoclonal proliferations, constituting multiple multiglandular microadenomas {708,728,896}. Because multiglandular parathyroid involvement can be asymmetrical and asynchronous, most patients with MEN1 are not subjected to the more common restricted surgical procedure {2171,2473}. Prophylactic partial thymectomy is also considered by experienced surgeons, given mediastinal recurrence due to ectopic or supernumerary parathyroid glands in as many as 12% of cases {596,2171,2473}. As a consequence, surgical pathologists are often asked to evaluate multiple specimens during the full neck and mediastinal exploration of a patient with MEN1. Therefore, the role of the diagnostician during the intraoperative consultation for MEN1-associated hyperparathyroidism typically involves the distinction of the parathyroid glands from other structures that could be mistaken for a parathyroid gland by the surgeon {708}.

The individual glands are variably involved, but all are usually more or less grossly enlarged (> 6–8 mm) and increased in weight (> 40–60 mg). Histologically, they show multinodular proliferations composed primarily of chief cells, followed by oncocytic and/or clear cells {708}. Unlike most sporadic parathyroid adenomas, MEN1-associated parathyroid proliferations lack the characteristic atrophic rim of non-lesional parathyroid tissue. Rim-like areas can occur in some glands; however, these regions are cellular rather than atrophic. Rarely, cystic change can occur {2709}. Nuclear atypia, necrosis, and prominent mitotic figures are uncommon. Glands may show stromal fibrosis and even irregular borders that can mimic the morphological features associated with parathyroid hyperplasia related to longstanding chronic renal failure or lithium exposure, atypical parathyroid adenoma, and reactive changes associated with previous manipulations (e.g. fine-needle aspiration and ethanol ablation) {64,708,709}. Almost all MEN1-associated parathyroid neoplasms behave as benign tumours; carcinomas are extremely rare {646, 2572}, and their diagnosis requires the unequivocal demonstration of invasion into adjacent organs, vessels, or perineural space, and/or presence of metastases {649,708,709}. The parathyroid changes in multiple endocrine neoplasia type 4 are histologically indistinguishable from those of MEN1. Patients presenting with MEN1-like changes but lacking germline *MEN1* mutation should therefore be tested for *CDKN1B* mutation {2745}.

Pituitary tumours

Age distribution and penetrance
Pituitary tumours occur in about 30–40% (range: 10–50%) of patients with MEN1 {2746,2865}. Recent data derived from regular screening of 323 patients with MEN1 aged > 16 years suggest a penetrance of 38% {631}. Patients with MEN1 with pituitary adenomas tend to be younger (mean patient age ± standard deviation: 35.1 ± 14.8 years) than patients with sporadic tumours (mean patient age: 40 years) {9,631,2865}. The youngest reported patient age at presentation is 5 years {831}.

Clinical features
Women, especially young women, are more commonly affected than men, with women accounting for 76% of patients aged < 21 years and 63% aged > 16 years {1022,1023}; but men have more macroadenomas, especially at young ages {1023}. A pituitary adenoma is the first manifestation of MEN1 in 17% (range: 10–25%) of patients {312,2865}, with 21% of such patients aged < 21 years {1023}. Lactotroph adenomas are most common, followed by

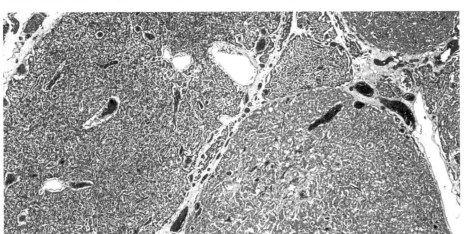

Fig. 7.04 Multiple endocrine neoplasia type 1 (MEN1). Micronodular adenomatosis of parathyroid glands. Microscopic aspect of a parathyroid gland of a patient with MEN1.

non-functioning adenomas (accounting for 15% of cases), somatotroph adenomas (9%), corticotroph adenomas (4%), and thyrotroph adenomas {631,2865}. Reports of gonadotroph carcinoma are exceptional {212}.

The data on treatment response are conflicting. Earlier and paediatric reports suggest that the response of functioning pituitary adenomas to pharmacotherapy and/or surgery is suboptimal {921,1023, 2394,2865}, but data from the cohort of adult patients with MEN1 in the Netherlands suggest a good response of lactotroph adenomas to dopamine agonist therapy {631}.

Pathology
The frequency of surgically resected MEN1-associated functioning adenomas (72%) is similar to that of non-associated cases (64%), but MEN1-associated adenomas are more often multiple (i.e. in 4–5% of cases vs 0.1%) and multihormonal (i.e. in 10–39% of the cases), with prolactin and growth hormone being most frequently detected {631,2813, 2865}. Most (76–85%) of the tumours are macroadenomas, which are significantly larger and often more invasive, and have a higher Ki-67 proliferation index, than in sporadic cases {921,2813,2865}. MEN1 tumours show more S100-positive folliculostellate cells than do sporadic adenomas. Somatotroph or mammosomatotroph hyperplasia has been described, but is not common; in some cases it is due to an ectopic GHRH-secreting neuroendocrine tumour (NET), often in the pancreas {386,2813}. It is important to note that multiple adenomas and pituitary hyperplasia have also been described in other conditions {196,1209,1593,2879}. In an invasive tumour from a very young patient with MEN1, overexpression of genes related to tumorigenesis (*TPD52*, *FOS*, and *SHC1*) and cell growth (*GNAS*, *FOSB*, and *SRF*) and loss of E-cadherin function were detected {831}. No genotype–phenotype correlation has yet been found.

Duodenal and pancreatic lesions
Age distribution and penetrance
The incidence of MEN1-associated duodenal and pancreatic NETs (PanNETs) at clinical manifestation peaks at 40–60 years, but patients of any age can be affected. The sex distribution is even. MEN1-associated Zollinger–Ellison

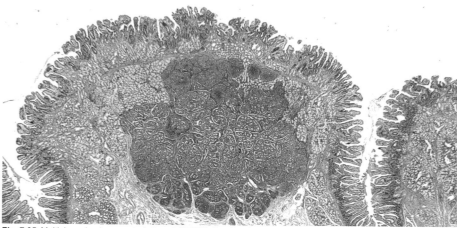
Fig. 7.05 Multiple endocrine neoplasia type 1 (MEN1). Duodenal neuroendocrine tumour in a patient with MEN1, showing a submucosal location.

syndrome (ZES) accounts for 20–30% of all ZES cases, and patients with MEN1-associated ZES are generally about a decade younger than those with sporadic disease {82,698}. In an autopsy study, the penetrance of pancreatic tumours was nearly 100% {1720}.

Clinical features
Clinical manifestations of duodenal and/or PanNETs are observed in approximately 40% of patients with MEN1. When assessed by clinical screening methods, the manifestation rate is 30–75% {2745}. ZES is the most common hormonal syndrome (present in 60% of cases), followed by hyperinsulinaemic hypoglycaemia and other very rare syndromes such as GHRH syndrome and glucagonoma syndrome; for more detailed descriptions of the syndromes and their diagnosis, see the corresponding sections.

Pathology
In almost all patients with MEN1 with ZES, the source of gastrin excess is multicentric NETs {698,1256,1413,2178}, typically in the mucosa and submucosa

of the upper duodenum, and sometimes at the margin of an ulcer. The tumours are usually < 1 cm and are therefore difficult to detect {81}. In as many as 80% of cases, the tumours give rise to large periduodenal and/or peripancreatic lymph node metastases, which were formerly interpreted as gastrinoma primaries. Liver metastases are rare (affecting only 3–4% of patients with MEN1) and occur late in the course of the disease. Histologically, they are well differentiated (grade 1), show a trabecular to pseudoglandular pattern, and stain mainly for gastrin. Rarely, somatostatin-positive tumours also develop in the duodenum. These tumours are associated with focal hyperplastic changes of gastrin and somatostatin cells in the duodenal crypts and Brunner glands, from which they arise as small monoclonal nodules {83}. Diffuse microadenomatosis associated with one or several macrotumours (> 0.5 cm) is a distinctive feature of the pancreas in MEN1 {84}. Lymph node and liver metastases are rare. The criteria that define the risk for metastasis are probably the same as in sporadic PanNETs.

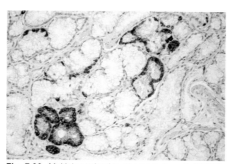
Fig. 7.06 Multiple endocrine neoplasia type 1 (MEN1). Somatotropin cell hyperplasia labelled immunohistochemically in the duodenum of a patient with MEN1.

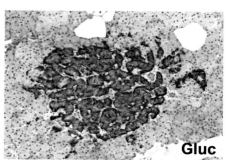
Fig. 7.07 Multiple endocrine neoplasia type 1. Pancreatic microadenoma with glucagon immunostaining.

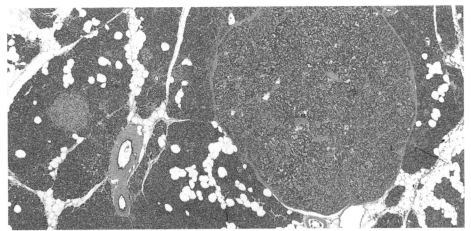

Fig. 7.08 Multiple endocrine neoplasia type 1 (MEN1). Microscopic appearance of the pancreas of a patient with MEN1, showing two microadenomas.

Most of the multiple NETs have a trabecular–pseudoglandular pattern, occasionally with blurred outlines and highly sclerotic stroma. Eosinophilic and clear cells may intermingle. In addition, it has been found that the tiny monohormonal glucagon cell proliferations that appear to originate from islets with a hyperplastic glucagon cell component are composed of monoclonal cells characterized by loss of heterozygosity of 11q13, which is obviously required to transform the hyperplastic cells into neoplastic proliferations {2155}. Islet hyperplasia and endocrine cell budding from ducts are not features {1418}. Severe obstructive pancreatitis due to duct stenosis by macrotumours may occur. Immunostaining reveals that many tumours are multihormonal, typically with one hormone prevailing {84,1565}. Most common is the expression of glucagon, followed by pancreatic polypeptide, insulin, and somatostatin. Rarely, other hormones (e. g. calcitonin) may also be found {177}. Glucagon-positive tumours may be cystic {1445}. Gastrin is virtually never expressed. In cases of a MEN1-related hypoglycaemic syndrome, one macrotumour (occasionally with amyloid)

is usually found to express insulin and to be the source of the insulin excess. Very rarely a macrotumour may express a non-pancreatic hormone; for example, GHRH causing acromegaly {84}, glucagon causing glucagonoma syndrome {1255,2603}, or VIP causing the syndrome of watery diarrhoea, hypokalaemia, and achlorhydria (WDHA syndrome, also called Verner–Morrison syndrome) {904}.

Other component features

Adrenal cortical lesions

Adrenal cortical lesions are observed in 20–45% of patients with MEN1 and encompass hyperplastic as well as tumorous lesions {166,346,971,1548}. The tumours are often bilateral, ≤ 3 cm, and non-functioning {1548,2918}. Adrenal cortical carcinomas seem to be rare and may also be found bilaterally {1040}. Isolated cases with hyperaldosteronism or Cushing syndrome have been reported {194,1548,3073}.

In a recent study from France, adrenal lesions from 715 patients with MEN1 were compared with sporadically occurring adrenal tumours {941}. The

MEN1-associated tumours were more often associated with symptoms of primary hyperaldosteronism and included more adrenal cortical carcinomas (13.8% vs 1.3%), but no genotype–phenotype correlations have yet been found {941}. ^{68}Ga-DOTATATE PET/CT is helpful in detecting MEN1-associated lesions, with a sensitivity of 62.5% and specificity of 100% in adrenal glands {1557}.

Cutaneous lesions

Cutaneous lesions are present in 40–80% of patients with MEN1 {610}, with collagenomas and facial angiofibromas being most common {610,2388}. Among the less common lesions are nodular lipomas (which are usually multicentric and show no recurrence after surgery), café-au-lait spots, confetti-like hypopigmented macules, and multiple gingival papules {610}. Careful attention to cutaneous lesions in patients with endocrine tumours can facilitate the early diagnosis of MEN1 {105}.

Primary malignant melanomas have been observed in a small series of patients with MEN1, and a nonsense mutation in exon 7 (Q349X) has been identified in one sporadic melanoma, indicating that alterations of the *MEN1* gene might be involved in the tumorigenesis of a small subgroup of melanomas {2023}.

Thymic and bronchial lesions

These tumours are observed in about 5–10% of patients with MEN1 {632,2170}. Thymic NETs (carcinoids) occur predominantly in males {1022,2387}, may produce ACTH, and have a poor prognosis {632,960,1606,2573,2736}. They account for approximately 25% of all thymic carcinoids. Local invasion, recurrence, and distant metastasis are common, with no known effective treatment.

Bronchial carcinoids (typical and atypical) also belong to the MEN1 tumour

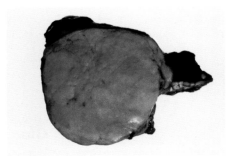

Fig. 7.09 Multiple endocrine neoplasia type 1 (MEN1). Adrenal cortical adenoma in a patient with MEN1.

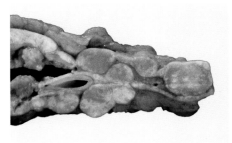

Fig. 7.10 Macroscopic view of adrenal cortical nodular hyperplasia in a patient with MEN1.

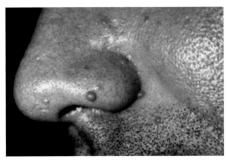

Fig. 7.11 Multiple endocrine neoplasia type 1 (MEN). Facial angiofibromas in a patient with MEN1.

spectrum {715,1933,2573}. They are usually non-functioning. In a recent study in 75 patients with MEN1 with a mean patient age of 47 years, equal sex distribution, and known parathyroid and pancreatic–duodenal disease, CT screening revealed typical carcinoids (most with a Ki-67 proliferation index < 2%) in 6.7% of the cases. The resected tumours were frequently associated with neuroendocrine precursor lesions (so-called tumourlets and multifocal intrabronchial neuroendocrine cell hyperplasia similar to the changes described in diffuse idiopathic pulmonary neuroendocrine cell hyperplasia) {164}. When the CT images of these patients were re-evaluated for tiny (≥ 3 mm) pulmonary nodules, the prevalence for these changes was found to be 30%, suggesting that pulmonary neuroendocrine precursor lesions may be common in MEN1.

Gastric lesions
Multiple NETs (type 2 gastric NETs) associated with enterochromaffin-like cell hyperplasia are found in the fundic mucosa of 23–29% of patients with MEN1-associated ZES {224,287}. Tumours that are small (< 1 cm) usually have a good prognosis after complete endoscopic removal {287}; larger tumours may metastasize and require surgical management {659, 2458}, but tumour-related deaths are exceptional {2025}.

CNS lesions
Spinal ependymomas have been rarely observed in patients with MEN1 and typically occur in infratentorial cervical or lumbar regions {907}. They are rapidly symptomatic and require surgery. Uncommon forms of meningioma and astrocytoma can also occur in the context of MEN1 {359}.

Soft tissue and breast lesions
Among the tumours that have been described in patients with MEN1 are leiomyoma and renal angiomyolipoma {502, 1211,1790,2904}, gastrointestinal stromal tumour {1750}, large visceral and intrathoracic lipomas {2667}, and aggressive malignant peripheral nerve sheath tumour arising from an adrenal ganglioneuroma {2200}. Breast cancer has been found in 6% of females with MEN1 {1258}, and

animal studies have also demonstrated an increased incidence of breast cancer {2498}. However, because the frequency of breast cancer is so high in general, further data are needed to confirm an association with MEN1 {319,705}.

Other lesions
Thyroid lesions, which were previously suggested to be part of the syndrome, are now thought to be coincidental findings, because newer studies have shown that the prevalence of thyroid lesions among patients with MEN1 is no higher than the prevalence among individuals without MEN1 {1660}. Other lesions and features that have rarely been reported in MEN1 gene carriers include bilateral granulosa cell tumours {1070}, phaeochromocytoma {663}, paraganglioma {1244}, hibernoma {1121}, small body height (especially in women) {1670}, and mediastinal seminoma {2714}.

Genetics
Chromosomal location, gene structure, gene expression, and function
The MEN1 gene is located on chromosome 11q13, in a gene-dense region of the genome {2744}. MEN1 codes for menin, a protein with a multitude of functions and interactions and a known tumour suppressor. Menin has multiple domains and interacting partners, ranging from transcription factors to histone deacetylase complexes {14}. The crystal structure of menin identifies it as a scaffold protein (which may be one of the reasons why so many interacting molecular partners have been found) that may associate with the cell membrane and organelles and may be active in the nucleus, where it regulates gene transcription {1116}. A well-known protein–protein interaction of menin is its interaction with the mixed-lineage leukaemia protein, through which a substantial part of its role in the regulation of cellular growth and proliferation is exerted {2756}.

MEN1 mutations and genotype–phenotype correlations
MEN1 is inherited as an autosomal dominant trait or occurs de novo. In MEN1, all somatic cells have an inactivating mutation in one MEN1 allele, predisposing the patient to the development of tumours

associated with the condition, but the neoplasms do not develop until loss of heterozygosity of the normal MEN1 allele occurs at the tissue level. Therefore, loss of heterozygosity is essential for tumorigenicity, although other factors are also at play {1027}.

The tissue-specific factors that determine the expression of MEN1 mutations in some organs and not others range from menin expression levels and interacting proteins, such as the mixed-lineage leukaemia protein, to the presence (or absence) of other genes that regulate cell growth and proliferation, such as CDKN1B (also called P27) {2548,2693}. MEN1 mutations occur throughout the entire length of the gene, with no hotspots; therefore, there are no significant genotype–phenotype correlations, with few exceptions. Overall, frameshift changes account for approximately 40% of the reported MEN1 defects, and nonsense and missense mutations for only 20% and 25% of the defects, respectively. The remaining defects are splice-site and in-frame alterations and large gene deletions, the latter of which may also include several other genes on 11q13 {14}.

Prognosis and predictive factors
Patients with MEN1 are at increased risk of premature death, usually related to the disease and its complications {638, 1024,1228}. The main causes of death are thymic tumours (mostly occurring in male patients) and PanNETs, along with rare cases of aggressive adrenal tumours {638,1024,1228}. Female sex, family history of MEN1, and recent diagnosis are associated with a lower risk of death {1024}. At the tumour level, the prognostic factors are the same as those for sporadic tumours; tumour size and histological grade are the most important parameters {1228}. Patients with small duodenal NETs have a 15-year survival rate of nearly 100%.

Recent studies suggest the existence of high-risk MEN1 mutations. Mutations affecting the JUND interacting domain may be associated with an increased risk of death {2754}, and mutations affecting the FOXN3 (previously known as CHES1) interacting domain with an increased risk of aggressive PanNETs {165}. However, these findings require further validation.

Multiple endocrine neoplasia type 2

LiVolsi V.
DeLellis R.
Komminoth P.
Mete O.
Mulligan L.

Schmid K. W.
Waguespack S. G.
Elisei R.
Eng C.

Definition

Multiple endocrine neoplasia type 2 (MEN2) is an autosomal dominant tumour syndrome caused by activating (gain-of-function) germline mutations in the *RET* gene. Classic MEN2A is characterized by medullary thyroid carcinoma (MTC), usually in association with phaeochromocytoma and/or parathyroid neoplasia causing hyperparathyroidism {2639}. Variants include MEN2A with cutaneous lichen amyloidosis, MEN2A with Hirschsprung disease, and familial MTC {881,1016,2976}. MEN2B, which is rare, is characterized by early-onset MTC; a high risk of phaeochromocytoma; and a pathognomonic physical appearance that includes a Marfanoid body habitus, oral mucosal neuromas, intestinal ganglioneuromatosis, and medullated corneal nerve fibres {2917}.

Synonyms

Multiple endocrine neoplasia type 2A: Sipple syndrome {146,2976}
Multiple endocrine neoplasia type 2B: Wagenmann–Froboese syndrome; mucosal neuroma syndrome; multiple endocrine neoplasia type 3 {2354}

Incidence and prevalence

The true annual incidence rates of MEN2A and MEN2B are unknown, but they are estimated to be 1 case per 1 973 500 population and 1 case per 38 750 000 population, respectively {2976}. The prevalence of MEN2 is believed to be about 1 case per 30 000 population {881}. The female-to-male ratio of MEN2 is about 1:1; in some studies, a slight female predominance has been reported.

Diagnostic criteria

The diagnosis of MEN2 can be made on the basis of the identification of a germline DNA variant in the *RET* gene that is known to be a pathogenic MEN2-causing mutation (see Fig. 7.17, p. 251). *RET* mutation analysis should be performed on any patient diagnosed with MTC {1969} (regardless of patient age) and/or in the absence of accompanying disease features or family history, in order to identify index patients (probands) and to facilitate timely diagnosis and therapy for at-risk relatives.

The clinical diagnosis of MEN2 (prior to confirmation with genetic testing) should be highly suspected in any patient with (1) at least two of the tumours associated with MEN2, (2) a diagnosis of MTC and one or more close relatives with MTC or another MEN2-defining tumour, or (3) a diagnosis of MTC with clinical features of MEN2B. Note that primary hyperparathyroidism is not part of MEN2B. Cases with MTC as their only feature were previously classified as familial MTC; however, recent recommendations suggest including these cases as variant forms within the spectrum of MEN2A {2976}.

Specific tumours and lesions

Medullary thyroid carcinoma

Age distribution and penetrance
Approximately 30% of MTCs are associated with germline *RET* mutations manifesting as MEN2A (including familial MTC as a variant) or MEN2B {146,839,1822, 2976}. Most individuals with MEN2 develop MTC, with age-related and mutation-specific penetrance {839,2976}. MTCs occurring in MEN2B are associated with early onset (as early as the first year of life), whereas cases occurring in MEN2A are often late-onset {2976}.

Clinical features

MTC is usually the first clinical manifestation of MEN2. There is a well-described age-related progression of malignant disease, starting with C-cell hyperplasia {146,1822,2917}. The cervical lymph nodes, lungs, liver, and bone are the most common sites of metastatic disease. In MEN2A, metastases usually occur years after the onset of MTC; in MEN2B, they may already be present at the time of diagnosis {1702}.

MTC presents either with clinical disease (palpable thyroid nodule and/or palpable lymphadenopathy) or with subclinical disease identified only after clinical testing or early thyroidectomy performed on a patient with a pathogenic *RET* mutation. Symptomatic patients may have diarrhoea {573}, or rarely develop ectopic

Table 7.03 Syndromes associated with heritable medullary thyroid carcinoma: the three phenotypes of multiple endocrine neoplasia type 2 (MEN2)

	MEN2A	MEN2B	Familial medullary thyroid carcinoma
MIM number (www.omim.org)	171400	162300	155240
Relative frequency	35–40%	5–10%	50–60%
Mean patient age at clinical presentation	25–35 years	10–20 years	45–55 years
Commonly involved *RET* codons	634, 609, 611, 618, 620, 630, 631	918, 883	768, 790, 791, 804, 649, 891, 609, 611, 618, 620, 630, 631
Medullary thyroid carcinoma	> 90%	> 90%	> 90%
Phaeochromocytoma	30–50%	50%	–
Hyperparathyroidism	15–30%	–	–
Interscapular cutaneous lichen amyloidosis	10–15%	–	–
Neuromas of lips, tongue, conjunctiva; medullated corneal nerves; intestinal ganglioneuromatosis	–	98–100%	–
Marfanoid habitus	–	98–100%	–
Musculoskeletal abnormalities (pes cavus, pectus excavatum, scoliosis, etc.); urinary tract ganglioneuromatosis and malformations	–	Variable	–

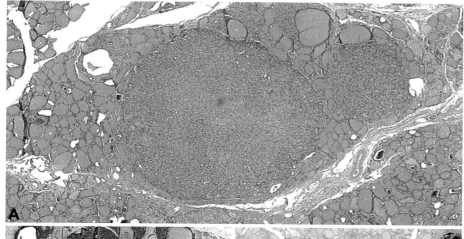

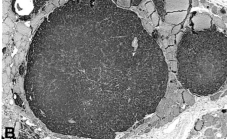
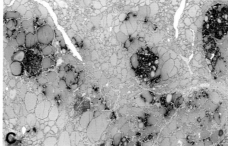

Fig. 7.12 Multiple endocrine neoplasia type 2 (MEN2). C-cell hyperplasia-to-neoplasia progression sequence. **A** C-cell hyperplasia and carcinoma in MEN2 with (**B**) matching immunohistochemistry for calcitonin. **C** In the same case, the contralateral lobe also shows C-cell hyperplasia immunolabelling for calcitonin.

Cushing syndrome due to ACTH or CRH secretion {153,512,707}. In patients with de novo MEN2B, MTC is usually diagnosed at more-advanced stages, because there is often a failure to recognize the MEN2B phenotype in young patients {317,3009}. Calcitonin and CEA are excellent tumour markers for MTC. Patients with clinical MTC show elevated calcitonin and CEA levels, but basal calcitonin levels can be normal with microscopic MTC {1616,2140}.

Pathology
C-cell hyperplasia-to-neoplasia progression is the hallmark of inherited forms of MTC {146,1822}. The diagnosis of C-cell hyperplasia is suggested when > 6–8 C cells per cluster in several foci with > 50 C cells per low-power field are identified {1646,1822}. Primary C-cell hyperplasia is usually obvious on H&E-stained slides; therefore, counting is often unnecessary. Primary C-cell hyperplasia can be recognized on the basis of an expansile intrafollicular C-cell proliferation with varying degrees of dysplasia, comparable to that present in the associated invasive tumours {47,1482,2157}. The earliest manifestation of invasive

carcinoma is characterized by extension of C cells through the basement membrane of expanded C cell–filled follicles into the surrounding thyroid interstitium {652}; collagen IV staining can be used to confirm this observation {1787}. The transition to invasive carcinoma is associated with loss of the organoid arrangement of C cell–filled follicles and the appearance of a desmoplastic stromal reaction surrounding groups of infiltrating tumour cells.

A subset of patients with apparently sporadic medullary microcarcinomas identified on the basis of abnormal pentagastrin-induced stimulation testing have associated primary C-cell hyperplasia in the absence of germline *RET* mutations {1319,1320,1321}. There is evidence to support the interpretation that primary C-cell hyperplasia in MEN2 syndromes and in some sporadic microcarcinomas constitutes thyroid intraepithelial neoplasia of C cells {405,678,1319}.

So-called physiological C-cell hyperplasia is characterized by the presence of ≥ 50 C cells per low-power (100× magnification) microscopic field {40}. The C cells (which must be identified by immunoperoxidase staining) are typically

clustered in the upper two thirds of the lateral lobes, but some experts also diagnose C-cell hyperplasia when parafollicular C cells are identified beyond their normal geographical distribution {1822, 3089}. Physiological C-cell hyperplasia can be observed in association with sporadic MTCs {2373} and other thyroid tumour types {45}, Hashimoto thyroiditis, hypothyroidism, hypergastrinaemic and hypercalcaemic states {1060,1646,1822}, and *PTEN* hamartoma tumour syndrome {1563}. Unlike primary C-cell hyperplasia, physiological C-cell hyperplasia does not appear to be a precursor of MTC.

Phaeochromocytoma
Age distribution and penetrance
Approximately 40–60% of patients with MEN2 develop a phaeochromocytoma, with age-related and mutation-specific penetrance. The adrenal involvement is often diagnosed in patients aged 30–40 years {1383}.

Clinical features
Phaeochromocytomas are often preceded by MTC in the MEN2 syndromes {51}. Therefore, patients may present with a relevant family history {2077}. At-risk individuals should undergo yearly screening via measurement of either plasma free metanephrines or urinary fractionated metanephrines {1587}. Unlike cases associated with the hypoxia pathway tumours, MEN2 cases present with either an adrenergic or a mixed adrenergic and noradrenergic secretory phenotype {748, 1383,1829,2785}. Life-threating events, including stroke and myocardial infarction with multiple microinfarcts, can also occur {1726,2289}. Exceptionally, rare examples of extra-adrenal paragangliomas have been described in MEN2.

Pathology
The adrenal medullary hyperplasia-to-neoplasia progression sequence leading to bilateral and multifocal phaeochromocytomas is the hallmark of MEN2-related phaeochromocytoma {1383,1457,1822}. The normal medulla is located in the apex and corpus of the adrenal gland and accounts for less than one third of the gland's thickness {1822,1829}. The diagnosis of adrenal medullary hyperplasia is rendered when the adrenal medulla exceeds one third of the gland's thickness in the absence of cortical atrophy and/or when medulla is noted in the tail of

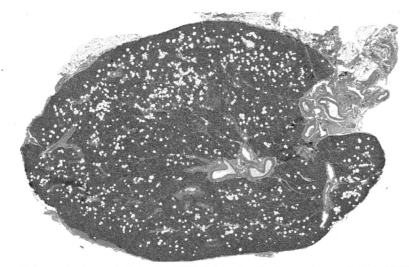

Fig. 7.13 Multiple endocrine neoplasia type 2A (MEN2A). A parathyroid adenoma from a patient with MEN2A. The enlarged gland weighed 0.70 g and measured 8 × 5 × 4 mm. After removal of the gland, the intraoperative parathyroid hormone level returned to normal.

the gland {1822,1829}. The term "nodular hyperplasia" is no longer recommended {1136,1457,1822,1829}. At the molecular level, such lesions do not represent hyperplasia in MEN2; therefore, the term "microphaeochromocytoma" was introduced {1457}. The morphological and immunohistochemical findings of MEN2-related phaeochromocytomas are indistinguishable from sporadic presentations {2090,2784}. Composite phaeochromocytomas have also been reported in association with MEN2 (see *Phaeochromocytoma*, p. 183) {2090}. No single parameter predicts malignant behaviour; malignancy is defined when metastasis occurs {1829,2077,2090,2781}. However, phaeochromocytomas can sometimes express calcitonin or calcitonin gene–related peptide {1138}. In such cases,

positivity for tyrosine hydroxylase and negativity for cytokeratin and CEA can be used to distinguish phaeochromocytoma from metastatic medullary carcinoma.

Hyperparathyroidism

Age distribution and penetrance
Approximately 20–30% of patients with MEN2A present with hyperparathyroidism {51}, whereas MEN2B is not associated with parathyroid disease. Hyperparathyroidism related to MEN2 shows high interfamilial variability as well as age-related and mutation-specific penetrance, predominantly clustering in individuals with the codon 634 *RET* mutations {51,2479}. Parathyroid disease affects adults, usually aged > 30 years {51, 1701,2479,2833}.

Clinical features
Hyperparathyroidism has been rarely reported to be the initial presentation of MEN2A {1707,1831}. Like individuals with sporadic hyperparathyroidism, most patients are diagnosed with asymptomatic biochemical hyperparathyroidism {51, 708,2479}.

Pathology
An individual gland measuring > 6–8 mm and weighing > 40–60 mg is considered an abnormal parathyroid gland {708} (see *Parathyroid adenoma*, p. 153). An enlarged parathyroid gland surrounded by an atrophic rim is often considered evidence of adenoma if the removal of the gland results in biochemical cure {708}, whereas the identification of multiple enlarged cellular parathyroid glands has been linked to parathyroid hyperplasia {708}. However, at the molecular level, parathyroid hyperplasia corresponds to multiglandular adenomas in the background of an underlying genetic predisposition {708,728,896}. The role of the surgical pathologist during the intraoperative consultation for MEN2-related hyperparathyroidism is to identify tissue as parathyroid and to define an abnormal gland {708}. MEN2-related hyperparathyroidism is associated with benign parathyroid proliferations; however, a single case of parathyroid carcinoma has also been reported in this syndrome {1254}.

Other component features
Hirschsprung disease
Hirschsprung disease is a congenital disease characterized by the complete absence of neuronal ganglion cells (aganglionosis) in the myenteric (Auerbach) and submucosal (Meissner) plexuses in variable lengths of the gastrointestinal tract, primarily the rectosigmoid colon. MEN2A with Hirschsprung disease is primarily associated only with mutations in *RET* exon 10, primarily codon 620, affecting cysteine residues {574}.

Cutaneous lichen amyloidosis
Cutaneous lichen amyloidosis is a skin disorder associated with intense pruritus and secondary skin changes and dermal amyloid deposition that arises as a consequence of repeated scratching. It is typically located in the interscapular region of the back and is primarily associated with codon 634 mutations {697, 2864}.

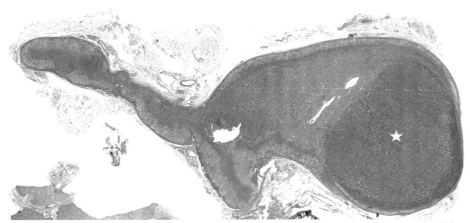

Fig. 7.14 Multiple endocrine neoplasia type 2A (MEN2A). Phaeochromocytoma (asterisk) arising in adrenal medullary hyperplasia.

Hyperparathyroidism–jaw tumour syndrome

Lloyd R. V.
Arnold A.
Gill A.
Morreau H.

Definition

Hyperparathyroidism–jaw tumour syndrome (HPT-JT) is an autosomal dominant tumour disorder associated with mutations of *CDC73* (previously called *HRPT2*). It is characterized by parathyroid adenoma or carcinoma and fibro-osseous lesions of the mandible and maxilla.

Synonym

Familial cystic parathyroid adenomatosis

Incidence and prevalence

HPT-JT is rare, but the exact incidence and prevalence rates are unknown. Germline mutations in *CDC73* are found in < 1.5% of patients with hyperparathyroidism aged < 45 years {2632}, and somatic or germline mutations in < 0.8% of unselected parathyroid adenomas {1476}.

Age distribution and penetrance

About 70–80% of patients develop hyperparathyroidism, usually by the age of 40 years, with a slightly lower penetrance in females {412,1203,1797,2735}. The median patient age at presentation with hyperparathyroidism is in the third to fourth decade of life (reported range: 7–65 years) {321,879,1797}. Jaw tumours were initially reported to occur in nearly a third of all patients with HPT-JT, but the penetrance has since been shown to be substantially lower, with jaw tumours occurring in as few as 5.9–12.5% of known *CDC73* mutation carriers {1203,1749, 2421,2936}.

Diagnostic criteria

The parathyroid tumours are usually single, but may be multiple, presenting simultaneously or asynchronously. Parathyroid carcinoma is the cause of hypercalcaemia in 15–37.5% of cases, although the diagnosis of carcinoma is commonly not made until recurrence {321,1203,1797,2421}. Given the extreme rarity of parathyroid carcinoma in all other settings, the high lifetime risk of parathyroid carcinoma is an important clue to the diagnosis {412}. In most families, parathyroid tumours are the only lesions at presentation {1203,2421}, but when jaw tumours are present in an individual or kindred, the diagnosis is strongly suggested {1203,1797,2421}.

It has been suggested that as many as 15% of patients develop a variety of renal lesions; these are usually simple cysts, but there have also been reports of occasional adenomas, hamartomas, Wilms tumours, and carcinomas {321,1103,1797}. However, simple cysts are not uncommon in the general population, and the strength of the association with renal pathology has been questioned {879,1436, 1749,2936}.

About 60–75% of female patients have been reported to develop uterine pathology, usually lesions that are also common in the general population: most frequently benign leiomyomas, but also endometrial hyperplasia, polyps, adenomyosis, and adenofibromas {306,1749,1797}. Two cases of uterine adenosarcoma have been reported {1797}.

Specific tumours and lesions

Hyperparathyroidism

Clinical features

Patients with HPT-JT can present with severe hypercalcaemia, and a few present with hypercalcaemic crisis {321, 1203,1749}. Parathyroid carcinoma is extremely rare in the general population and in other hereditary syndromes associated with hypercalcaemia, and therefore serves as an important clue to the diagnosis of HPT-JT. About 20–30% of patients with apparently sporadic parathyroid carcinomas in fact have germline mutations in *CDC73*, indicating occult HPT-JT {435,2523}.

Pathology

Hyperparathyroidism is usually caused by a single adenoma or carcinoma {879, 1203}; however, synchronous tumours can be found in as many as a third of patients when specifically sought, and multiglandular involvement at long-term follow-up (over decades) occurs in the majority of patients in some series {1203, 1237,1797,2421}. Cystic change was originally described as a common feature {412}, but is found in only a quarter (or fewer) of the parathyroid tumours {2421}. The incidence of parathyroid carcinoma is considerable, with a lifetime risk of 15–24% in most series {321,412,1797, 2421} and as high as 37.5% in one report {1797}. The diagnosis of parathyroid carcinoma in HPT-JT is based on the standard criteria of extensive local invasion and/or metastasis. Given the known high risk of malignancy, the glands should be extensively sampled during pathological analysis after resection {974}. In unequivocal carcinoma, germline and

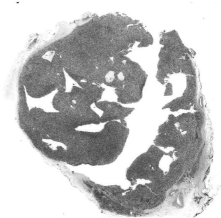

Fig. 7.19 Hyperparathyroidism–jaw tumour syndrome-related parathyroid adenoma, with prominent cystic spaces.

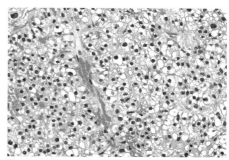

Fig. 7.20 Hyperparathyroidism–jaw tumour syndrome-related parathyroid adenoma. The tumour consists mainly of uniform chief cells, with rare pleomorphic cells in the background. There is no significant mitotic activity, fibrous bands, or invasion.

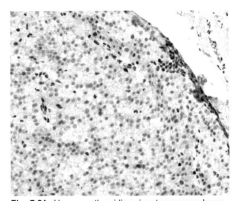

Fig. 7.21 Hyperparathyroidism–jaw tumour syndrome–related parathyroid adenoma. The chief cells show loss of immunostaining for CDC73 (also called parafibromin); whereas the stromal cells and endothelial cells stain positively.

somatic *CDC73* mutations can be found in 67–100% of cases (most commonly in those with distant metastasis); whereas the mutation rate in adenomas is 0–4%. Adenomas and carcinomas arising in the setting of HPT-JT usually demonstrate negative immunohistochemical staining for CDC73 (also called parafibromin) and positive staining for PGP9.5 {977,1176}. CDC73 immunohistochemistry should be interpreted with care; a significant result requires both the loss of nuclear expression in all neoplastic cells and preserved expression in endothelial, stromal, and non-neoplastic parathyroid tissue {977, 1797,2998}. Furthermore, some *CDC73* mutations, particularly point mutations, are not associated with loss of CDC73 expression, and therefore normal immunohistochemistry does not exclude the diagnosis of HPT-JT {977,1797,2998}.

Jaw tumours
Clinical features
Jaw tumours show a variable rate of growth, with some growing slowly and others more rapidly. Radiographical features include a well-demarcated, usually radiolucent unilocular lesion in the mandible or maxilla {2175,2939}. Multifocal lesions can occur {431,2939,2949}.

Pathology
Although the terminology used is not uniform, the tumours are usually classified as ossifying fibromas {2175,2939}. They are composed of a relatively avascular cellular fibroblast-rich stroma, sometimes with a prominent storiform pattern admixed with bone trabeculae and/or cementum-like spherules. The histological appearance is different from that of osteitis fibrosa cystica associated with sporadic primary hyperparathyroidism, which (unlike jaw tumours) tends to resolve slowly after correction of the hyperparathyroidism {2175,2939}.

Genetics
Chromosomal location
The *CDC73* gene is mapped to 1q25-q31 {2688}.

Gene structure
The *CDC73* gene contains 17 exons spanning 18.5 kb of genomic distance and predicted to express a 2.7 kb transcript. It encodes the 531 amino acid protein CDC73 {412}.

Gene expression
CDC73 is ubiquitously expressed in many organs, including the brain, lungs, kidneys, liver, pancreas, and skeletal muscle {412}.

Gene function
CDC73 functions as a bona fide tumour suppressor gene. CDC73 is involved in the regulation of p53 and is a component of the PAF protein complex, which controls RNA polymerase II–mediated general transcription {431,1264}.

Mutation spectrum
More than 129 coding-inactivating mutations and genomic deletions have been detected in the *CDC73* gene. Approximately 80% of the mutations occur in hotspots in exons 1, 2, and 7 {1743}. Most of the coding alterations are frameshift and nonsense mutations, predicting a truncated protein {431,2131,2539}. Large-scale deletions are not uncommon, and account for as many as a third of all pathogenic mutations {321}.

Genotype–phenotype correlations
To date, no genotype–phenotype correlations have been reported {1458}.

Prognosis and predictive factors
Most patients with a diagnosis of parathyroid adenoma can be cured by surgery, but about a quarter of cases recur in the same or other glands {1203,1797}, and some studies have reported recurrence in the majority of patients over prolonged follow-up {2421,2560}.

Adenomas should be treated surgically, with a low threshold for progressing from simple excision to wider en bloc resection if the operative features suggest malignancy. The extent of surgery, specifically whether bilateral exploration should be the routine approach in HPT-JT, remains controversial and can depend on the experience of the surgical group {1203,1797,2421}.

There have been isolated case reports of unequivocally histologically benign apparent adenomas that have metastasized in the setting of HPT-JT, although this is a very rare event {974,2421}. However, it is worth noting that in some patients with HPT-JT, newly presenting metastatic disease may not necessarily have come from the originally recognized adenoma, but may instead have originated from a separate primary tumour in a different parathyroid gland. Long-term follow-up is indicated for all patients.

Ossifying fibromas of the jaw are usually benign, but may be locally infiltrative and recurrent {431,2949}.

Fig. 7.22 Hyperparathyroidism–jaw tumour syndrome–related ossifying fibroma, with scattered irregular trabeculae of bone separated by a bland and relatively avascular stroma.

Von Hippel–Lindau syndrome

Couvelard A.
Hammel P.
Komminoth P.
Mete O.

Pacak K.
Perren A.
Stratakis C. A.

Definition

Von Hippel–Lindau syndrome (VHL) is an autosomal dominant cancer syndrome caused by germline *VHL* mutations leading to the development of various tumours, including retinal and CNS haemangioblastomas, renal cell carcinomas (RCCs) and renal cysts, phaeochromocytomas and paragangliomas, pancreatic serous cystadenomas and neuroendocrine tumours (NETs), and endolymphatic sac tumours (ELSTs).

Incidence and prevalence

The incidence of VHL is estimated at approximately 1 case per 36 000 live births {2282}.

Age distribution and penetrance

VHL has > 90% penetrance in patients aged ≥ 65 years {1712,2282}.

Diagnostic criteria

In patients with a family history of VHL, the clinical diagnosis requires only one major manifestation of the VHL tumour spectrum. In the absence of a family history, the clinical diagnosis requires at least two major manifestations, including one haemangioblastoma {2282}. De novo mutations occur in 20% of patients. *VHL* gene testing has facilitated the early diagnosis of VHL and allows for the diagnosis of atypical cases, because mutations are identified in > 95% of the patients {1712}.

Specific tumours and lesions

See Table 7.05.

CNS haemangioblastomas

Clinical features

Haemangioblastomas are a cardinal feature of VHL, occurring in 80% of patients {2901}; their sporadic counterparts account for only 1–2% of all intracranial neoplasms. They are frequently (i.e. in about 25% of cases) localized in the cerebellum, main stem, and dorsal spinal cord, whereas supratentorial lesions are rare (accounting for about 2.9% of cases) {2926}. VHL-associated haemangiomas

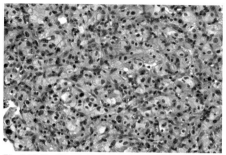

Fig. 7.23 Von Hippel–Lindau syndrome (VHL). Cerebellar haemangioblastoma in VHL showing a pseudoepithelial pattern.

are often multiple; occur in younger patients than do sporadic haemangiomas; and are associated with neurological deficits, increased intracranial pressure, or ataxia.

Pathology

Haemangioblastomas present as well-circumscribed, highly vascularized nodules, often in the wall of a large cyst. The tumours have a non-neoplastic component composed of abundant mature vascular structures with a rich capillary network, and a neoplastic component consisting of large vacuolated (so-called clear) lipid-containing stromal cells that harbour the *VHL* gene deletion {2903}. These histological features vary considerably, dependent on tumour size. Small

tumours can be nearly obscured by abundant reactive angiogenesis, a pattern that is frequently referred to as reticular or mesenchymal. Larger tumours may contain prominent epithelioid clusters of tumour cells, and are referred to as cellular or epithelioid {1098}.

The stromal cells are immunonegative for vascular markers such as CD31, cytokeratins, and EMA (which is important in the differential diagnosis with metastatic RCC). The HIF-regulated gene products VEGF and CAIX are highly expressed {1604}. The tumours are strongly positive for vimentin; are variably positive for S100; and may exhibit (focal) positivity for inhibin, GFAP, CD56 (also called NCAM), and neuron-specific enolase. NFP and synaptophysin are typically negative {267}. The Ki-67 proliferation index is usually < 1%.

Prognosis, prognostic factors, and treatment

Surgical excision is the treatment of choice. Multicentric tumours, and particularly brain stem and spinal tumours, are difficult to treat and cause substantial morbidity. Antiangiogenic inhibitors of growth factors such as VEGF or PDGF, and inhibitors of the numerous steps in the pathway of VHL, such as cyclin-dependent kinase blockers, are all potential

Table 7.05 Main manifestations of von Hippel–Lindau syndrome in the various organs affected

Affected organ(s)	Tumours or lesions
CNS	Haemangioblastomas
Retinas	Haemangioblastomas
Adrenal glands and paraganglia	Phaeochromocytomas, paragangliomas, and haemangioblastomas [a]
Kidneys	Renal cell carcinomas, renal cysts, and haemangioblastomas [a]
Pancreas	Neuroendocrine tumours, serous cystic neoplasms
Endolymphatic sac	Endolymphatic sac tumours
Epididymis	Epididymal papillary cystadenomas
Broad ligament and mesosalpinx	Cystadenomas of the broad ligament and mesosalpinx
Others [a] (lungs, liver, gallbladder, ampulla, common bile duct, peripheral nerves)	Haemangioblastomas, cysts, and neuroendocrine tumours

[a] Very rarely described cases.

therapeutic agents, but experience is limited {1841}.

Non-CNS haemangioblastomas

Retinal haemangioblastoma
Clinical features
As many as 85% of individuals with known VHL develop retinal haemangioblastoma {491}, which is also known as retinal angioma and angiomatosis retinae. It is the most common and earliest presentation of VHL and is found in gene carriers aged in their mid-20s {444}.

Pathology
The lesions are often multiple and bilateral, and vary in size and shape {1062}. Histologically, they are identical to CNS haemangioblastomas. Vacuolated or foamy stromal cells are interposed between variously sized vascular channels. The tumours lack endothelial cells, and some show glial cell proliferation.

Prognosis, prognostic factors, and treatment
At the age of 50 years, the estimated cumulative risk of visual loss is 35% among gene carriers and 55% among patients with retinal haemangiomas {2957}. Treatment (in particular, for preventing blindness) includes photocoagulation, cryotherapy, radiation, photodynamic therapy, and combinations of these modalities {444,1062}. Rarely, surgical excision is necessary.

Peripheral haemangioblastomas
Occasionally, haemangioblastomas identical to those seen in the CNS are found in peripheral nerves (e.g. the spinal nerve roots, cauda equina, and sciatic nerve) {2184,2678} or in extraneural tissues (e.g. the adrenal glands, liver, lungs, and kidneys) {639,703,2021,2318}.

Renal lesions
Clear cell renal cell carcinoma
Clinical features
As many as 40% of patients with VHL develop multicentric and bilateral clear cell RCC (ccRCC), and > 70% develop renal cysts {1705,1714}. The average age of patients with ccRCC and VHL is 37 years, and there is an equal sex distribution, in contrast with the average patient age of 61 years and male predominance of sporadic ccRCC {2130}.

Pathology
Grossly and histologically, VHL-associated RCCs resemble the classic clear cell type (ccRCC). They often contain cystic areas and are typically of low nuclear grade. In addition to a large tumour, multiple minute tumours are present. On microscopic examination, macroscopically normal-appearing parenchyma may be found to contain microfoci of ccRCC {1677}. According to the underlying germline mutation, ccRCCs are part of the spectrum of VHL type 1 or type 2A, with *VHL* mutations leading to decreased HIF1A degradation. The vast majority of sporadic ccRCCs harbour somatic *VHL* inactivation, with a similar impact on microvessel density. Sporadic ccRCCs without *VHL* mutation seem to be more aggressive. Genetically, VHL-associated ccRCCs are more homogeneous than their sporadic counterparts and have fewer copy-number events as secondary events {227}.

Prognostic factors and treatment
ccRCC is the most frequent malignant neoplasm of patients with VHL, and therefore an important mortality factor. Tumour size > 3 cm is an independent prognostic factor for survival in patients with VHL {1508}. VHL-associated RCCs are of lower grade than are sporadic ccRCCs.

Renal cysts
Renal cysts are preneoplastic changes and might result from disturbed microtubule function. Loss of the *VHL* wildtype allele in individual renal tubular cells occurs as a first event; although these cells are morphologically normal, they overexpress CAIX, which is an important hypoxia-inducible factor (HIF) downstream target {1893}. Entire tubular surfaces, smooth microcysts, and atypical cysts with epithelial dysplasia are also characterized by CAIX overexpression. Histologically, single cells may already show a clear-cell phenotype {1727}. There is frequently single-cell involvement in the proximal tubule, as well as microcysts and dysplastic lesions in the distal tubule. Cysts rarely progress to RCC, although a cyst-dependent pathway has been described {894}.

Adrenal medulla
Phaeochromocytoma and paraganglioma
Clinical features
Approximately 30% of patients with VHL develop phaeochromocytomas/paragangliomas, at a mean patient age of 30 years {2924}. Phaeochromocytoma in patients with VHL has a typical noradrenergic phenotype, with production

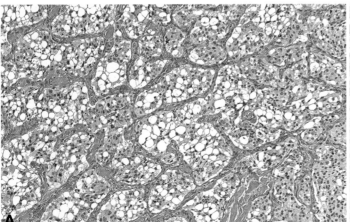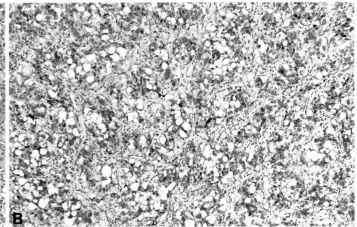

Fig. 7.24 Von Hippel–Lindau syndrome (VHL). VHL-related carotid body paraganglioma with clear-cell changes (**A**) and matching immunostaining for tyrosine hydroxylase (**B**).

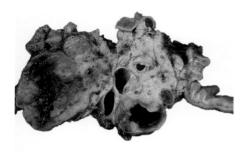

Fig. 7.25 Von Hippel–Lindau syndrome (VHL). Macroscopic view of the pancreas of a patient with VHL, containing several cysts and a large haemorrhagic neuroendocrine tumour.

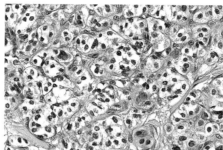

Fig. 7.26 Von Hippel–Lindau syndrome (VHL). Pancreatic neuroendocrine tumour in VHL, showing clear-cell features and nuclear atypia.

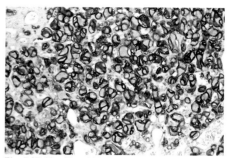

Fig. 7.27 Von Hippel–Lindau syndrome (VHL). Pancreatic neuroendocrine tumour in VHL, with the tumour cells expressing high levels of CAIX.

of norepinephrine and normetanephrine {749}. Rarely, the tumours can also produce dopamine and its metabolite 3-methoxytyramine {743}. In more than half of all patients with VHL, clinical signs and symptoms of catecholamine excess are minimal or absent, probably due to downregulation of adrenoceptors or because of the very small size of these tumours {749,1588,2924}. Patients with VHL with phaeochromocytomas/paragangliomas present with hypertension due to norepinephrine secretion, and less commonly, with palpations. Symptoms due to tumour size (VHL tumours are typically small) or metastatic disease are infrequent {1588}. Other common clinical presentations include sweating, nervousness, anxiety, and pallor.

Pathology
Half of the patients have a unilateral phaeochromocytoma, the other half have bilateral or multiple tumours. Occasionally, there are paragangliomas. The tumours typically show a thick vascular capsule, myxoid and hyalinized stroma, a rich vascular network intermixed with tumour cells containing variable clear and amphophilic cytoplasm, an absence of cytoplasmic hyaline globules, and a lack of atypia and mitoses {1424}. Unlike those associated with multiple endocrine neoplasia type 2, phaeochromocytomas associated with VHL lack medullary hyperplasia {423,1822,1829}. The clear-cell change is attributed to HIF-mediated lipid and glycogen accumulation in tumour cells {160,1937,2143,2525}. Consistent with their noradrenergic secretory phenotype, the tumours cells are mainly composed of norepinephrine-containing secretory granules with an eccentric electron-dense core {749}. Like those of other phaeochromocytomas/paragangliomas,

the tumour cells are positive for tyrosine hydroxylase, chromogranin A, and synaptophysin, but negative for keratins and transcription factors {1829,2077, 2090,2781}. Some paragangliomas may also express GATA3 {2590,2969}. Tyrosine hydroxylase distinguishes these tumours from pancreatic neuroendocrine neoplasms {423}. Strong membranous positivity for CAIX is also thought to be characteristic of VHL-associated phaeochromocytomas, but this finding requires further validation {2176}.

Prognosis, prognostic factors, and treatment
Because malignant behaviour cannot be predicted by any marker, malignancy is defined by the presence of metastasis {1829,2077,2090,2781}. Only 5% of the tumours present with metastasis, usually in association with a large phaeochromocytoma (> 5–6 cm in size) or with a paraganglioma {743,3098}. Complete

surgical resection is the treatment of choice.

Pancreatic lesions
Pancreatic neuroendocrine tumours
Clinical features
Pancreatic NETs (PanNETs) are observed in 11–17% of patients with VHL {266,1075,2282}. They are non-functioning (inactive). The mean patient age at diagnosis is 38 years (range: 16–68 years) {266,2282}.

Pathology
When present in patients with VHL, PanNETs are multiple in 50–56% of cases {1678,2151}. Grossly, they are well demarcated and are sometimes yellowish in colour due to lipid storage. They may contain fibrotic foci, probably reflecting the profibrogenic role of HIF {557,1141}. Histologically, they can have solid, trabecular, or glandular architecture, with several distinctive features: extreme

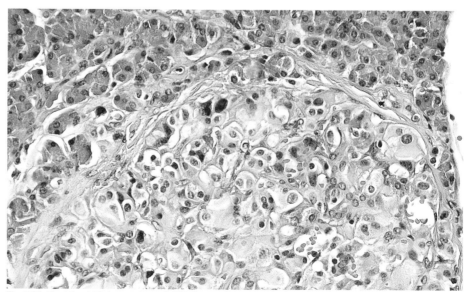

Fig. 7.28 Von Hippel–Lindau syndrome (VHL). Pancreatic neuroendocrine microadenoma in VHL, with cells showing a clear or eosinophilic cytoplasm.

hypervascularity {571}, nuclear atypia, and clear cells or multivacuolated lipid-rich cells. These changes are attributed to the activation of HIF, leading to a state of pseudohypoxia that results in lipid and glycogen accumulation with the tumour cells {1045}. In VHL-deficient PanNET cells, HIF is stabilized, with concomitant induction and expression of HIF-dependent targets, including VEGF, cyclin D1, and CAIX {2151,2624}. In about 70% of patients with VHL with resected PanNETs, the removed macrotumours are associated with microadenomatosis (i.e. the presence of several small tumours > 0.5 mm and < 5 mm) and abnormal islets that lack the normal qualitative and quantitative distribution of alpha, beta, delta, and PP cells and measure < 5 mm {1822,2151}. The microadenomas can be very small and seem to be less numerous (with 1–25 microadenomas per patient, mean: 7) {2151} than in multiple endocrine neoplasia type 1 {84}. Peliosis of islets and ductuloinsular complexes have also been described {423, 1822}; they are best detected with immunostaining for markers of the VHL/HIF pathway, especially CAIX {2151}. Precursor lesions often contain clear cells and nuclear atypia, and can be found within the ducts, contiguous to a pre-existing islet or mixed with acinar cells {2151}. The expression of molecules from the VHL/HIF pathway (especially HIF1A and CAIX) as a result of inactivation of the VHL gene provides strong evidence that these microscopic lesions are precursors to macrotumours. Clear-cell change can be identified in multiple endocrine neoplasia type 1 and sporadic NETs, but inhibin alpha expression in multifocal PanNETs should alert the diagnostician to the possibility of VHL-related pathogenesis {1045}.

Prognosis, prognostic factors, and treatment

Most PanNETs are slow-growing. In a retrospective study including 23 patients with VHL operated on for PanNETs, the median Ki-67 proliferation index was 3%, lymph node metastases were present in 43% of cases, and the long-term outcome was better than that seen with sporadic PanNETs. A parenchyma-sparing surgical strategy seems appropriate in patients with small PanNETs {633}.

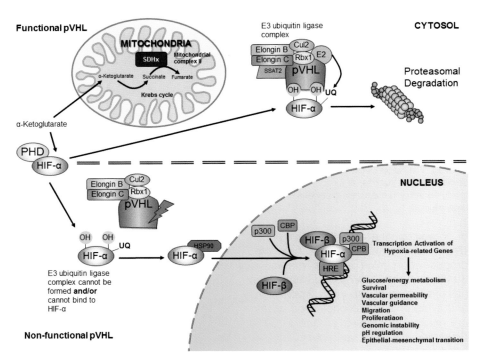

Fig. 7.29 Hypoxia-inducible factor signalling in von Hippel–Lindau syndrome. HIF1A / HIF-α is hydroxylated by PHDs for its recognition by the VHL protein (pVHL). pVHL, the *VHL* gene product, is the substrate recognition unit of the E3 ubiquitin (UQ) ligase complex known as the pVHL / elongin B / elongin C (VBC) complex, which targets HIF1A for proteasomal degradation in the presence of oxygen. The ubiquitination/degradation of HIF1A is promoted by the binding of SSAT2, which stabilizes the interaction of pVHL and elongin C. When mutations impairing or completely disrupting pVHL function occur, the activity of the VBC complex is compromised. HIF1A is no longer recognized by pVHL and is therefore not targeted for proteasomal degradation. It becomes stabilized, heterodimerizes with HIF1B, recruits coactivators, and binds to the core DNA sequence RCTCG at hypoxia-responsive elements (HREs) in target genes, where it activates their transcription. Adapted from Jochmanová I et al. {1265}.

Pancreatic cystic lesions

Pancreatic cystic lesions are frequent, occurring in as many as 91% of patients with VHL {1075,2151,2282}. They usually show the histopathological features of serous cystic neoplasms (microcystic and macrocystic serous cystadenomas). A literature review of reported data from 362 patients with VHL identified serous cystadenomas in 39 of the patients (11%) and simple cysts in 169 (47%) {460}. The lesions are usually multiple and are benign. Some are tiny (< 5 mm); others are solid or may include papillary areas, comparable to those described in VHL epididymis cystadenomas {1879,2151}. *VHL* deletions and prominent expression of HIF-signalling molecules are detected in all types of pancreatic cystic lesions in patients with VHL {1879,2151}.

Other lesions
Intestinal neuroendocrine tumours

NETs reported in patients with VHL include clear cell NETs of the ampulla and duodenum {1045,2577} and of the gallbladder and common bile duct {841, 1822}.

Endolymphatic sac tumours

In a recent study, the prevalence of ELSTs in patients with VHL was 3.6%, lower than the prevalence found in previous studies (11%) {181,1731}. ELST is bilateral in 30% of cases and can be the initial manifestation of the syndrome {181,1731}. VHL-associated ELSTs seem to be smaller (1.3 ± 1.1 cm, range: 0.2–5.2 cm) {1361}, less aggressive, and more fibrous than sporadic ELSTs {1971}. The mean patient age at diagnosis is 22 years (range: 12–50 years). The most common symptoms are audiovestibular, with progressive or sudden loss of hearing occurring in 84% of cases, tinnitus in 73%, and vertigo in 68% {1361,1731,1971}. No ELST genotype–phenotype correlations have been found {2190}.

ELST originates from the vestibular aqueduct endolymphatic epithelium and can grow to the cerebellopontine angle and/or the middle ear {993,2282}. Histologically, the tumour consists of papillary structures lined by a single row of cuboidal to columnar cells associated in some cases with cystic glandular structures lined by flattened cells and containing

Table 7.06 Genotype–phenotype correlations in von Hippel–Lindau syndrome (VHL)

VHL subtype	Haemangioblastoma	Renal cell carcinoma	Phaeochromocytoma
Type 1	+	+	–
Type 2A	+	–	+
Type 2B	+	+	+
Type 2C	–	–	+

eosinophilic colloid-like material. Some tumours show clear-cell areas, reminiscent of ccRCC. Vessels are numerous, and haemorrhage and haemosiderin deposits are frequent {993}. The tumour cells are positive for cytokeratin and EMA, and negative for CD31. They express HIF and its various downstream targets (e.g. CAIX, GLUT1, and VEGF). Numerous precursor structures can be found in tumour-free endolymphatic sacs and ducts of patients with VHL, consisting of multifocal small papillary and cystic structures and clusters of vacuolated clear cells, which also express HIF, CAIX, and GLUT1, with inactivation of the *VHL* wildtype allele {993}.

Epididymal papillary cystadenoma

Epididymal papillary cystadenomas occur in as many as 60% of males with VHL and are often bilateral. They arise from the epididymal duct and usually present as asymptomatic nodules in the region of the head of the epididymis. Large bilateral tumours can impair fertility. They are benign and do not usually require treatment.

Histologically, they are composed of papillary, tubular, and cystic structures lined by cuboidal to columnar clear glycogen-rich cells that give a positive periodic acid–Schiff (PAS) reaction. The cysts are often filled with a colloid-like secretion. CD31 immunostaining reveals extensive vascularization of the tumour stroma, in direct contact with overlying neoplastic epithelial cells {994}. Epididymal papillary cystadenomas arise secondary to inactivation of the wildtype copy of the *VHL* gene, followed by early and simultaneous activation of HIF, with upregulation of its

various downstream targets (e.g. CAIX, GLUT1, and VEGF). The tumours evolve from a variety of microscopic epithelial tumourlets confined to the efferent ductular system; these tumourlets are numerous and include complex epithelium, with clear-cell, cystic, and papillary changes {994}. Papillary tumours may also arise in the retroperitoneum and lung of patients with VHL {1397,2526}.

Cystadenoma of the broad ligament and mesosalpinx

These rare tumours occur in women with VHL. They are the counterparts of the more frequent epididymal cystadenomas in males, and are histologically similar. Their reported size was 3–6 cm (average: 4.5 cm) in a study of 5 cases, including 4 cases in patients with VHL {2016}. Macroscopically, these tumours have a fibrous capsule and are partly cystic and lobulated, with haemorrhagic foci and stellate fibrous scars {2016}. Histologically, they contain tubulopapillary structures (often hyalinized) containing haemosiderin and prominent subepithelial capillary networks, and are associated in some cases with clear cells arranged in a solid pattern with some tubular formation. The tumour cells are positive for CK7, vimentin, CAM5.2, PAX2, and CD10 {308,2016}.

Genetics

Gene structure and function

VHL is inherited in an autosomal dominant fashion. *VHL* is a tumour suppressor gene located on chromosome 3 (at 3p25.3). It comprises three exons and encodes two mRNA transcripts, which are 213 and 172 amino acids in length,

respectively (RefSeq ID: NM_000551). The *VHL* gene plays various roles, from targeting HIFA for degradation and suppression of aneuploidy to microtubule stabilization {895,1286}. The VHL protein is a critical part of a ubiquitin ligase protein complex that binds (via two hydroxylated prolines) to the alpha subunits of the HIF1 and HIF2 transcription factors and targets them for ubiquitination and proteasomal degradation {1307,1772}. Under normoxic conditions, the HIF1A subunits are rapidly degraded, but oxygen is an essential cofactor for the proline hydroxylase enzymes that must modify the HIF1A subunits for VHL protein binding to occur {1234,1236}. In hypoxia or when the VHL protein is absent or inactive, HIF1A and HIF2A are stabilized and activate the hypoxic gene response (e.g. VEGF, PDGFB, TGF-alpha, cyclin D1, etc.) {1287}.

Genotype–phenotype correlations
See Table 7.06.

Intrafamilial variation may be important, and interfamilial variation reflects genotype–phenotype correlations for phaeochromocytoma and RCC {1712}. VHL type 1 is characterized by retinal and CNS haemangioblastomas and by RCC, but not by phaeochromocytoma; the germline alterations are mainly deletions (30–40%), or missense substitutions and mutations that lead to synthesis of truncated proteins. VHL type 2 includes phaeochromocytoma. It is caused by germline missense mutations. Families with VHL type 2B have haemangioblastomas, renal cancers, and phaeochromocytomas; families with type 2A have a lower risk of renal cancer {1713}. VHL type 2C is caused by specific missense mutations, and patients only have phaeochromocytomas {1285}. Specific criteria have been recommended for referral to a medical team with expertise in VHL: ≥ 2 pancreatic serous cystic neoplasms, ≥ 2 PanNETs, or multiple pancreatic cysts plus any VHL-associated lesion {454}.

Familial paraganglioma–phaeochromocytoma syndromes caused by *SDHB*, *SDHC*, and *SDHD* mutations

Tischler A.S.
de Krijger R.R.
Gill A.
Matias-Guiu X.
Mete O.
Pacak K.
Stratakis C.A.

Definition
Familial paraganglioma–phaeochromocytoma syndromes are autosomal dominant tumour diseases caused by germline mutations in genes encoding subunits of succinate dehydrogenase (SDH).

Synonym
SDHx-related syndromes

Incidence and prevalence
Germline mutations in genes encoding SDH subunits are collectively the most common cause of hereditary paraganglioma–phaeochromocytoma {213,1968}. Together they account for the majority of familial groupings of these tumours {2124} and for almost 10% of apparently sporadic tumours that present with no familial or syndromic history {1968}. They also account for almost 30% of paediatric cases and 30–40% of tumours that metastasize {213,2124}. Mutations in *SDHB* are the most common (occurring in about 6–8% of all patients with phaeochromocytomas/paragangliomas), followed by mutations in *SDHD* (in 5–6%), *SDHC* (in 1–2%), and *SDHA* (in 1%) {599}. *SDHAF2* mutations are extremely rare {1497}. Regional variations attributable in part to founder mutations can alter the relative contributions of various genes {342,2124}.

Age distribution and penetrance
All of the paraganglioma syndrome types (PGL1–5) are autosomal dominant inherited disorders with highly variable penetrance that correlates to some degree with the driver gene. Approximately 75% of PGL1 carriers manifest disease by the age of 40 years. The penetrance of PGL2 is similarly high, but starting at a younger age. In contrast, only about 40% of patients with PGL4 manifest disease by the age of 40 years {213}. PGL3 and PGL5 have low penetrance, which has not been precisely calculated due to the relative rarity of these types {213,765}. PGL1 and PGL2 usually show a parent-of-origin effect: the mutation can be inherited from either parent, but disease usually manifests only following paternal transmission. This can lead to the skipping of generations in affected families, and must be considered when assessing family history. The pattern of inheritance for these two syndromes resembles maternal imprinting, but the mechanism remains unclear, although several possibilities have been proposed {184,1151}. Despite the overall correlation between genotype and penetrance, within an individual family or generation of a family, some carriers of a mutant allele may develop tumours and other carriers may not.

And there is no predictable sequence of development of phaeochromocytomas, paragangliomas, and other syndromically associated tumours {213}. Large-scale studies to precisely determine the age distribution and penetrance of SDH-deficient tumours are lacking.

Specific tumours and lesions
Hereditary paraganglioma syndromes show genotype–phenotype correlations associated with each of the susceptibility genes, as well as a degree of overlap with each other (Table 7.07) and with other diseases (see also the *Introduction* of Chapter 7, p. 242). The major paraganglioma syndromes are caused by mutations of *SDHB*, *SDHD*, and *SDHC*. At least 50% of *SDHB*-associated paragangliomas/phaeochromocytomas are extra-adrenal abdominal or thoracic paragangliomas, which are multifocal in 10–25% of cases; the rest are head and neck paragangliomas or phaeochromocytomas. In contrast, most *SDHD*-associated tumours are head and neck paragangliomas, which are multifocal in as many as 60% of cases {213}. *SDHC* is associated most often with solitary paragangliomas in the head and neck, with the thorax being the second most common site; phaeochromocytoma is extremely rare {765}.

Table 7.07 Tumour types associated with SDH-related syndromes

Tumour	PGL5/CSS (germline *SDHA* mutation)	PGL4/CSS (germline *SDHB* mutation)	PGL3/CSS (germline *SDHC* mutation)	PGL1/CSS (germline *SDHD* mutation)	PGL2/CSS (germline *SDHAF2* mutation)	Carney triad (*SDHC* promoter hypermethylation)
Phaeochromocytoma	+	+	+/–	+	+/–	–
Abdominal PGL	++	++++	+/–	+	+/–	+++
Head and neck PGL	+	++	++	+++	+	++
Thoracic PGL	+/–	++	+	++	+/–	+
SDH-deficient GIST	+++[a]	+	+	+	+/–	++++[a]
SDH-deficient RCC	+	+++	++	+/–	+/–	–
SDH-deficient PA	++	+	+	+	+/–	–
Pulmonary chondroma	–	–	–	–	–	++++

CSS, Carney–Stratakis syndrome (paraganglioma and gastrointestinal stromal tumour); GIST, gastrointestinal stromal tumour; NET, neuroendocrine tumour; PA, pituitary adenoma; PGL, paraganglioma; PGL1–5, paraganglioma syndrome types 1–5; RCC, renal cell carcinoma.
[a] 30% of SDH-deficient GISTs have been associated with *SDHA* mutations and 50% with Carney triad.

The presence or absence of biochemical function depends more on anatomical location than on the driver gene, with head and neck paragangliomas usually being hormonally silent {765}.

Other important tumours syndromically associated with SDH genes include gastrointestinal stromal tumours, renal cell carcinomas (RCCs), and pituitary adenomas.

SDH-deficient gastrointestinal stromal tumours have been associated with all SDH genes except *SDHAF2* {213}. Although they are rare overall, they define Carney–Stratakis syndrome (also called Carney–Stratakis dyad), which is the association of gastrointestinal stromal tumour with hereditary paragangliomas caused by any of the SDH genes. A counterpoint to the dyad is Carney triad, consisting of paraganglioma, gastrointestinal stromal tumour, and pulmonary chondroma. Although Carney triad is generally considered to be a non-hereditary disorder

caused by hypermethylation of the *SDHC* promoter, almost 10% of patients harbour germline variants in *SDHA*, *SDHB*, or *SDHD*, suggesting there might be a hereditary contribution to Carney triad in some cases {274}. SDH-deficient RCCs {2852} have been reported in as many as 14% of patients with *SDHB* mutations and 8% with *SDHD* mutations {213}. SDH-deficient pituitary adenomas {213, 663,2091} have been reported in association with mutations of *SDHA*, *SDHB*, and *SDHD* {213}. However, the syndromic significance of pituitary adenomas in individual patients can be difficult to ascertain because the tumours are also common both sporadically and in other syndromes {663}.

Diagnostic criteria
Because of the high prevalence of occult hereditary susceptibility, it is advisable that all patients with phaeochromocytomas or paragangliomas be

offered genetic testing where available {342,1587}. A targeted approach to testing currently predominates {1587} but is likely to be eventually replaced by global testing with next-generation sequencing technology {342,593}. Clinical guidelines for targeted testing are based mainly on tumour location, biochemical phenotype, family history, and syndromic associations {1587}. All patients with paragangliomas at any location and all patients with phaeochromocytomas that predominantly produce and/or secrete norepinephrine/normetanephrine and/or dopamine/3-methoxytyramine should be tested for SDH gene mutations {744,1587}.

SDH-related paragangliomas, particularly in the head and neck, often exhibit prominent vascularity and small cells with clear cytoplasm, but they cannot be reliably distinguished from tumours with other genetic backgrounds on the basis of morphology. However, immunohistochemistry for SDHB and SDHA proteins

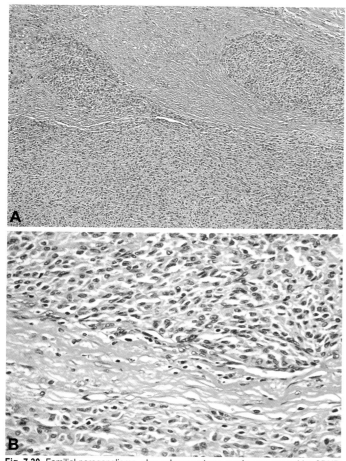

Fig. 7.30 Familial paraganglioma–phaeochromocytoma syndromes caused by *SDHB*, *SDHC*, and *SDHD* mutations. **A,B** SDH-deficient gastrointestinal stromal tumours showing multinodularity and epithelioid morphology.

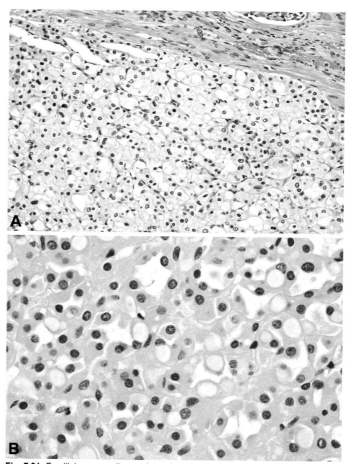

Fig. 7.31 Familial paraganglioma–phaeochromocytoma syndromes caused by *SDHB*, *SDHC*, and *SDHD* mutations. **A,B** SDH-deficient renal cell carcinomas showing cuboidal cells with flocculent and vacuolated cytoplasm arranged in a solid pattern, containing an entrapped non-neoplastic tubule (**A**).

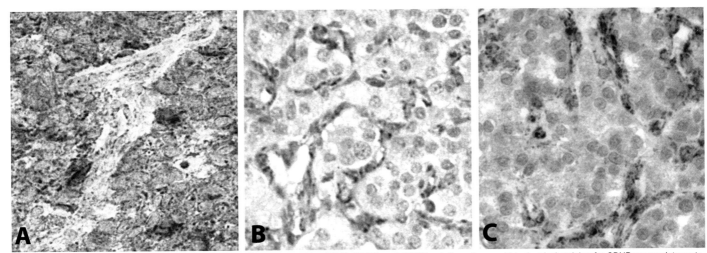

Fig. 7.32 Familial paraganglioma–phaeochromocytoma syndromes caused by *SDHB*, *SDHC*, and *SDHD* mutations. Immunohistochemical staining for SDHB: proper interpretation requires the presence of stained intratumoural endothelial cells as an intrinsic positive control. **A** Phaeochromocytoma with intact SDH (positive staining), defined by granular cytoplasmic staining of at least the same intensity in tumour cells as in endothelial cells. **B** SDH-deficient paraganglioma with completely negative tumour cells. **C** SDH-deficient paraganglioma with high background staining, which is interpreted as negative because the staining is weaker than in endothelial cells and is not granular.

is a useful diagnostic tool that can help to triage patients for genetic testing or serve as a surrogate marker when testing is not available. Immunoreactivity for SDHB is lost in SDH-deficient tumours caused by mutations of any of the SDH genes {601,2092,2849}, whereas immunoreactivity for SDHA is lost only with mutations of *SDHA* {1456}. The interobserver variability in the interpretation of SDH immunostaining is good, provided that guidelines are followed {2092}. Tumours with intact SDH show granular cytoplasmic staining corresponding to the distribution of mitochondria in both tumour cells and endothelial cells (which serve as essential intrinsic controls). In SDH-deficient tumours, the granular staining is lost in the tumour cells but persists in the endothelium.

SDH-deficient gastrointestinal stromal tumours and RCCs often exhibit distinctive histological features, which are particularly important to recognize if these tumours are the initial manifestation of hereditary disease. SDH-deficient gastrointestinal stromal tumours, whether caused by germline mutations or occurring in Carney triad {1071}, usually occur in children or young adults, are located in the stomach, and have epithelioid morphology. They are often multifocal and can show plexiform involvement of the muscularis propria {1840}. Distinctive features reported in SDH-deficient RCCs include cuboidal cells with indistinct borders and bubbly cytoplasm arranged in solid nests surrounding tubules or cystic

spaces. Vacuolated cytoplasmic inclusions that apparently correspond to giant mitochondria can also be present in SDH-deficient RCC {978}, whereas vacuoles that do not appear related to mitochondria have been reported as a feature of SDH-deficient pituitary adenoma {663}. Immunohistochemical staining for SDHB and SDHA has confirmed the presence of SDH deficiency in gastrointestinal stromal tumours {976}, RCCs {978}, and a subset of pituitary adenomas {663,2091,3020} in patients with phaeochromocytoma/paraganglioma, and in subsets of gastrointestinal stromal tumours and RCCs that arise de novo. It has been recommended that all RCCs exhibiting unusual morphology or arising in patients with a relevant family history be stained for SDHB {978}.

Genetics
Gene function
SDH is a mitochondrial enzyme that functions as the interface between the tricarboxylic acid cycle and the electron transport chain, in which it constitutes complex II. SDH converts succinate to fumarate, and in the process generates two electrons to be used for generating ATP (complex V) by oxidative phosphorylation.

The enzyme consists of four subunits encoded by separate genes: *SDHA*, *SDHB*, *SDHC*, and *SDHD*. The SDHA and SDHB subunits are located in the mitochondrial matrix. SDHC and SDHD anchor the complex to the inner mitochondrial

membrane, where the electron transport chain resides, and also provide the binding site for the electron acceptor ubiquinone. The succinate binding site and catalytic subunit of the SDH complex is SDHA, a flavoprotein that requires participation of its flavin moiety for the enzymatic reaction to take place {1133}. SDHB tunnels the electrons produced in the enzymatic reaction from the mitochondrial matrix to the electron transport chain (Fig. 7.33). An additional gene, *SDHAF2*, encodes a factor required for incorporation of flavin adenine dinucleotide into SDHA {1081}.

Germline mutations
Hereditary susceptibility to paragangliomas and syndromically associated tumours is conferred by autosomal dominant transmission of loss-of-function mutations in genes encoding any of the SDH subunits or in *SDHAF2*. Loss or inactivation of the wildtype allele together with other genetic changes is required for tumorigenesis, although the precise mechanism of tumorigenesis is still poorly understood. The second hit usually consists of a large deletion rather than a point mutation, probably encompassing tumour suppressor genes in addition to the wildtype SDH allele {184}. Due to the dual role of SDH, impaired catalytic function causes both accumulation of succinate and complete cessation of mitochondrial electron transport, resulting in the generation of reactive oxygen species. The initial driver of tumorigenesis is currently

believed to be succinate, which causes SDH-deficient tumours to express a pseudohypoxic signalling profile characterized by increased expression of hypoxia-sensitive transcription factors and their target genes. Non-hypoxic effects of succinate and reactive oxygen species have been posited to alter additional signalling pathways and to cause additional mutations {184}. A shared characteristic of all SDH-deficient phaeochromocytomas and paragangliomas is a methylator phenotype resulting in hypermethylation of histones and of the promoter regions of multiple genes {951,1595}. Another shared characteristic is destabilization of the SDH enzyme complex and selective degradation of subunits, providing the basis for immunohistochemical staining as an aid in the detection and differential diagnosis of SDH-deficient tumours {601, 2849} (see Diagnostic criteria).

The mechanistic basis of the genotype–phenotype correlations associated with various SDH gene mutations is unknown {429,1133}.

Prognosis and predictive factors

The prognosis of paragangliomas caused by SDH gene mutations depends on genotype, tumour location and size {2471}, and patient age at diagnosis {2471}. At least 30% of tumours with *SDHB* mutations metastasize, whereas metastases are less common with *SDHD* mutations and rare with *SDHC* mutations {863}. The likelihood of developing multiple tumours also depends on genotype, and is highest with mutations of *SDHB* {1970}. Among tumours with *SDHB* mutations, the highest risks of metastasis are associated with tumours > 5 cm and with tumours located in the abdomen {2471}.

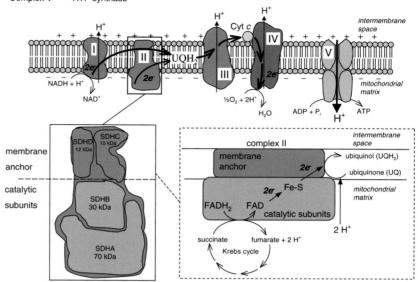

Integral membrane protein-complexes of the respiratory chain:
Complex I   NADH-ubiquinone reductase
Complex II   Succinate:ubiquinone reductase
Complex III   Ubiquinone-cytochrome C reductase
Complex IV   Cytochrome *c* oxidase
Complex V   ATP synthase

Fig. 7.33 Structure and functions of succinate dehydrogenase (SDH). SDH is the interface between the Krebs cycle and the mitochondrial electron transport chain, in which it constitutes complex II. Electrons generated in the normal conversion of succinate to fumarate are used to generate ATP by oxidative phosphorylation. Inactivating SDH gene mutations have the dual effect of causing succinate accumulation and blocking electron transport. Adapted from Müller et al {1926}.

Tumours in children or adolescents pose a particularly high risk {1384,1425}.

There is no cure other than complete surgical excision, which does not rule out the delayed presentation of metastatic disease. However, both primary and metastatic tumours often grow very slowly. Watchful waiting is therefore possible in some cases, and may be preferable to potentially harmful surgery or other interventions for tumours in some locations, particularly in the head, neck, and heart {307,1246,1549,1744}. In some cases, the prognosis may depend more on the behaviour of syndromically associated tumours (in particular gastrointestinal stromal tumours {399}) than on the paragangliomas themselves.

Molecular studies of SDH-related phaeochromocytomas and paragangliomas have suggested a few potential drug targets for treating metastases {429,441, 1247}, but there have been few clinical trials, with mixed results {429}. A low proportion of proliferating cells might reduce the effectiveness of some pharmacological agents {2194}.

Neurofibromatosis type 1

Perren A.
Pacak K.
Stratakis C. A.

Definition

Neurofibromatosis type 1 (NF1) is an autosomal dominant tumour syndrome caused by mutations in the *NF1* gene leading to multiple neurofibromas, café-au-lait spots, freckling of the axilla and/or groin, bone dysplasia, brain stem gliomas, phaeochromocytomas, duodenal neuroendocrine tumours (NETs), gastrointestinal stromal tumours, and malignant peripheral nerve sheath tumours (MPNSTs). NF1 is the most common inherited disease associated with neurofibromas (accounting for 90% of such cases), followed by neurofibromatosis type 2.

Synonyms

von Recklinghausen disease; peripheral neurofibromatosis

Incidence and prevalence

NF1 has an incidence of 1 case per 2500–3000 live births {2992}. In Finland, the prevalence is 1 case per 4400 population {2195}. The highest prevalence has been recorded in Israeli soldiers: 1 case per 1000 individuals (0.94 cases per 1000 men and 1.19 cases per 1000 women) {937}.

Age distribution and penetrance

Age distribution and penetrance vary depending on the presenting lesions, and are therefore reported in conjunction with the individual lesions below.

Table 7.08 Diagnostic criteria for neurofibromatosis type 1 (NF1): two or more must be present

1.	≥ 6 café-au-lait spots, the greatest diameter of which is > 5 mm in prepubertal patients and > 15 mm in postpubertal patients
2.	≥ 2 neurofibromas of any type, or ≥ 1 plexiform neurofibroma
3.	Axillary or inguinal freckling
4.	Optic glioma
5.	≥ 2 Lisch nodules
6.	A distinctive osseous lesion, such as sphenoid dysplasia or pseudoarthrosis
7.	A first-degree relative with NF1

Diagnostic criteria

The diagnostic criteria for NF1, established at the 1987 United States National Institutes of Health Consensus Development Conference on neurofibromatosis {1959}, are listed in Table 7.08. Clinicians should note a potential segmental involvement {1217}, which is only about one thirtieth as frequent as classic NF1. By 8 years of age, 97% of children with NF1 clinically fulfil the diagnostic criteria; by 20 years the rate is 100% {640}.

Specific tumours and lesions

Skin lesions
Penetrance and clinical features
Solitary café-au-lait spots are frequent, but are non-diagnostic of NF1. Clinically, only the presence of ≥ 6 lesions supports the diagnosis of NF1 {76}. Multiple neurofibromas are one of the most typical features in both children and adults. The clinical diagnosis of NF1 requires the presence of ≥ 2 neurofibromas or 1 plexiform neurofibroma {76}. Most of these tumours are benign, but they can invade local structures, especially nerves, resulting in specific clinical presentations. Malignancy is rare and associated with the occurrence of MPNSTs whose precursor lesions are plexiform neurofibromas. Most skin lesions appear during early childhood. Café-au-lait spots occur in > 95% of patients, and skin freckling in about 50% of patients {1268}. Neurofibromas, although very pathognomonic of NF1, affect only 40–60% of patients {897, 1789}.

Pathology
Café-au-lait spots are histologically characterized by basal hyperpigmentation with or without suprabasal melanosis. A minor melanocytic hyperplasia may be observed. Macromelanosomes (2–6 μm) have been reported as morphological markers of childhood neurofibromatosis; however, these pigmented cytoplasmic bodies are also found in lentigo simplex, dysplastic naevi, and the café-au-lait spots of McCune–Albright syndrome.

Neurofibromas are benignly behaving tumours of Schwann cells or their precursor cells, expressing S100. All neurofibroma variants (reviewed in {2315}) can be seen in patients with NF1. Localized cutaneous neurofibromas can affect the dermis or subcutis, and show no site predilection. The tumours are unencapsulated, round, and composed of a mixture of bland neoplastic Schwann cells and perineural cells, axons, and fibroblasts accompanied by fibrous matrix. Diffuse cutaneous and subcutaneous neurofibroma is much less common and is characterized by a plaque-like tumour, usually in the head and neck region. Pseudomeissnerian corpuscles are frequent. Only 10% are associated with NF1. Malignant change is infrequent. Plexiform neurofibromas occur almost exclusively in patients with NF1. Involvement of branching nerves results in worm-like so-called plexiform tangles. Many plexiform neurofibromas are present at birth or may continue to appear until adolescence. They occur in

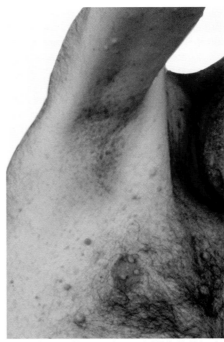

Fig. 7.34 Neurofibromatosis type 1 (NF1). Multiple pigmented spots and neurofibromas along with characteristic axillary freckling in a patient with NF1.

about 30% of patients with NF1. Plexiform neurofibromas are precursor lesions to MPNST; their risk of progression is 2–5%. About 50% of MPNSTs arise in patients with NF1. MPNSTs show a wide range of histological appearances. Cutaneous MPNSTs, which are very rare, display fascicles of alternating cellularity, whorls, palisades, or rosette-like arrangements. MPNSTs with rhabdomyosarcomatous and heterologous epithelial elements (malignant triton tumours) are particularly strongly associated with NF1 {2774}. All deep-seated sarcomas with a clear association to a nerve and without a clear line of differentiation should be considered MPNSTs {2315}, and all unclear sarcomas in patients with NF1 should be considered MPNSTs until proven otherwise. About 50% of MPNSTs express S100 weakly, and a minority show perineurial differentiation. The lifetime risk of patients with NF1 for developing MPNST is 8–13% {804}; early detection and resection are essential.

Duodenal neuroendocrine tumours
Penetrance and clinical features
Duodenal somatostatin-producing NETs usually occur at or in the ampulla of Vater. They are the second most common duodenal NETs, and 30% are associated with NF1. Duodenal gangliocytic paragangliomas may coexist, but are present in < 5% of patients {2273,2643}. These tumours usually present with signs and symptoms related to the localization of the tumour, including abdominal pain, anaemia, melaena, jaundice, and weight loss. A somatostatinoma syndrome seems to be uncommon {929,1036} or even non-existent. Most patients presenting with NF1-related duodenal NETs are aged 40–50 years {2273}.

Pathology
The lesions are solitary and often polypoid, with a mean diameter of 2 cm, and typically affect the major papilla and/or the ampulla. Advanced lesions infiltrate the sphincter of Oddi, duodenal wall, and/or pancreatic head and are then associated with lymph node metastases. Occasionally, the duodenal NET is combined with a gastrointestinal stromal tumour {929,2386} or an adenoma or adenocarcinoma {667}. The histological growth pattern is typically tubular and glandular, with psammoma bodies in the lumina in two thirds of cases. The psammoma

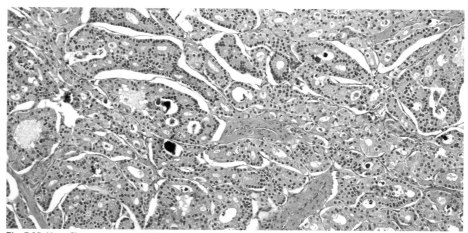
Fig. 7.35 Neurofibromatosis type 1 (NF1). Ampullary duodenal neuroendocrine tumour in NF1 showing typically glandular architecture and psammoma bodies.

bodies are composed of calcium apatite crystals {48}. Immunohistochemically, all duodenal NETs express synaptophysin, chromogranin A, and somatostatin.

Phaeochromocytoma
Age distribution, penetrance, and clinical features
Phaeochromocytomas usually occur during the fourth or fifth decade of life {747}, and < 5% are associated with NF1 {180,1198,2134,2923}. They are typically located in the adrenal glands {180}; extra-adrenal localization is rare {745}. About 10% of the patients have multiple tumours. NF1-related phaeochromocytomas present with classic symptoms and signs related to the excess release of epinephrine and metanephrine, and include hypertension, palpitations, sweating, nervousness, anxiety, and pallor {1588}. Metastases develop in < 5% of cases.

Pathology
Histologically, NF1-associated phaeochromocytomas do not differ from sporadic phaeochromocytomas, except that they are more frequently of the composite type {1379}. Their resemblance to sporadic phaeochromocytomas might be related to the fact that 20% of the sporadic lesions harbour somatic NF1 mutations {2975}. NF1 phaeochromocytomas lack the high microvessel density typical of von Hippel–Lindau syndrome–associated phaeochromocytomas.

CNS lesions
Although CNS lesions are not required for the establishment of a clinical diagnosis of NF1, they are very important because

they may lead to serious clinical consequences. CNS lesions include grade I pilocytic astrocytoma and optic, brain stem, and malignant gliomas. Optic gliomas develop almost exclusively in children, usually prior to the age of 7 years, with a median patient age at presentation of 4 years {261,1630}. Optic gliomas are the most common brain tumours and occur in 20% of patients; in some patients, optic gliomas cause loss of vision and various visual abnormalities (e. g. strabismus, colour vision changes, and proptosis). Brain stem gliomas are usually benign. They are found in as many as 4% of patients, and typically present in patients aged about 10 years; {1887,2187,2838}. In adult patients, the incidence of malignant gliomas is higher than in the general population {1057,1759}.

Pathology
About 15% of patients with NF1 develop brain tumours {714}; pilocytic astrocytomas are most frequent, whereas diffuse astrocytoma, gliomatosis, and pleomorphic xanthoastrocytoma are rare. Unidentified bright objects on MRI are a frequent abnormality in the brain stem of patients with NF1 {1887}. They are often multiple and bilateral, and are thought to constitute sites of vacuolar change {683}. Many of the low-grade gliomas (e.g. clinically indolent optic pilocytic astrocytoma) in patients with NF1 are not biopsied; therefore, little is known about specific histological features. Genetically, NF1-associated pilocytic astrocytomas show NF1 inactivation rather than the BRAF activation found in sporadic tumours.

Bone lesions

The most common bone lesions are skeletal dysplasias such as sphenoid wing, orbital bone, and long bone dysplasias. Ciliary bone cysts and giant cell granulomas are rare {76}. Fibrosarcomas, malignant fibrous histiocytomas, and primary neurogenic sarcomas are very rare but can lead to metastatic disease {712}.

Pathology

The bone lesions of patients with NF1 do not show specific histomorphological features.

Genetics

When the genetic testing performed includes various methods to test for splicing defects, deletions, both large chromosomal and smaller gene rearrangements, and other mutations, *NF1* gene abnormalities are currently found in > 90% of patients with the clinical diagnosis of NF1 {1816}. The disease is inherited as an autosomal dominant trait, and prenatal testing is now routinely available for known carriers. However, about half of all cases occur due to new (de novo) mutations, often due to paternal mosaicism.

The *NF1* gene codes for a protein called neurofibromin {852}, which is a RAS GTPase-activating protein; therefore, NF1 is part of a group of human diseases that are collectively known as RASopathies {2249}. The *NF1* gene is large, spanning > 350 kb of DNA on chromosome 17q11.2, which codes for at least 56 exons. Neurofibromin has multiple domains that interact with and regulate multiple signalling pathways in addition to RAS signalling, such as protein kinase A {2751}. Neurofibromin acts as a tumour

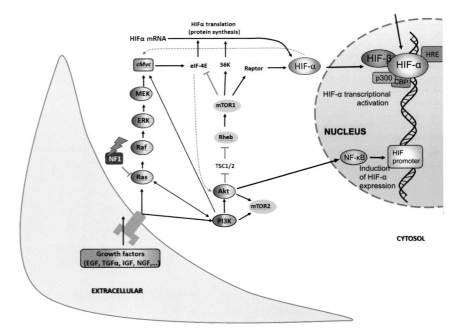

Fig. 7.36 In a normal cell, NF1 constrains RAS activity. Loss of NF1 expression (e.g. due to inactivating mutations in the *NF1* gene) leads to upregulation of the RAS/MAPK signalling pathway. RAS activation results in the activation of downstream pathways: MAPK, PI3K, and mTOR. These pathways are involved in proliferation, differentiation, survival, migration, and angiogenesis, and they increase HIF1A signalling in many cancers. ERK, a component of the RAS/MAPK pathway, directly phosphorylates HIF1A and the transcription factor SP1, thereby inducing transcription of VEGF, a key regulator of angiogenesis. MAPKs also promote nuclear accumulation of HIF1A. Another downstream target of PI3K is NF-kappaB, and cross-talk between the HIFA pathways and NF-kappaB signalling has been postulated. Overexpression of NF-kappaB subunits induces HIF1A mRNA expression and transcription. Adapted from I Jochmanová et al. {1265}.

suppressor gene; its inactivation due to mutations leads to increased signalling by the RAS oncogenes {2249}.

Although patients with larger deletions of the gene and surrounding genomic material have more severe phenotypes, there is little genotype–phenotype correlation among patients with classic NF1 and *NF1* mutations (other than chromosomal deletions). This may be due to genetic modifiers at other chromosomal loci {2145}.

Prognosis and predictive factors

Patients with NF1 should receive care in multidisciplinary clinics where they can receive all services they need, which may include preventive therapies such as surgeries {852}. There is wide variability of outcomes, depending on tumour burden.

Carney complex

Kirschner L. S.
Lloyd R. V.
Stratakis C. A.

Definition

Carney complex is an autosomal dominant tumour syndrome caused by *PRKAR1A* mutations, leading to spotty skin pigmentation, myxomatosis, endocrine overactivity, and schwannomas {398, 402}. The associated endocrine disorders include functioning tumours of the adrenal and pituitary glands and generally non-functioning tumours of the thyroid, testes, and ovaries. Rarely, tumours occur in the liver and pancreas.

Synonyms

LAMB syndrome (lentigines, atrial myxomas, mucocutaneous myxomas, and blue naevi); NAME syndrome (naevi, atrial myxomas, myxoid neurofibromas, and ephelides)

Incidence and prevalence

Carney complex is rare. The largest registry, maintained through joint efforts of the United States National Institutes of Health (NIH) and the European Network for the Study of Adrenal Tumours (ENSAT), includes > 400 cases. This registry provided the basis for the largest published patient series (353 patients) {232}. Of these patients, 258 (73%) were classified as having Carney complex type 1, with a detectable mutation in *PRKAR1A*, and 240 patients (68%) were from families with ≥ 2 affected members, whereas 32% had no identifiable family history. There was a female predominance among affected individuals; the female-to-male ratio was almost 2:1, with 221 women (63% of the cohort) versus 132 men (37%). Many additional patients have been reported in small numbers from other groups around the world, bringing the total number of cases described to > 750.

Age distribution and penetrance

Patients with Carney complex typically manifest pigmentation early in life, usually before puberty. In families known to carry mutations, this is often the earliest physical manifestation, although pigmentation can vary. However, because pigmentation (so-called birthmarks) is also common in the general population, the pigmentation occurring in de novo cases of Carney complex typically does not raise medical concern until other manifestations develop. Although pigmentation in patients with Carney complex does not resolve, it may become less prominent as patients age.

The course of Carney complex varies, but subtle manifestations are common beginning in the teenage years; these may include any of the endocrine manifestations (e. g. Cushing syndrome and growth hormone excess) or myxomatosis. The median patient age at detection is about 20 years, although cases have been identified in patients as young as 2 years and as late as in the fifth decade of life. In most cases, the disease has as indolent course; patients may first experience a few subtle manifestations and then accumulate additional lesions as they age.

Diagnostic criteria

The diagnostic criteria for Carney complex, initially described in the early 2000s {2657}, include typical skin pigmentation (lentiginosis or multiple blue or epithelioid blue naevi), myxomas (cardiac, cutaneous, mucosal, or breast), specific endocrine tumours (primary pigmented nodular adrenocortical disease, acromegaly, large cell calcifying Sertoli cell tumours, thyroid cancer, or multiple thyroid nodules), and any of a number of other rare tumours such as pigmented melanotic schwannoma, osteochondromyxoma, and multiple breast adenomas. Any patient with two of these diagnoses meets the clinical criteria for Carney complex. Patients can also be diagnosed with Carney complex if they fulfil any one of the major criteria and have an affected family member, or if they fulfil one major criterion in the context of either an inactivating mutation in *PRKAR1A* or an activating mutation or increased copy number of one of the protein kinase A (PKA) catalytic subunit genes (*PRKACA* and *PRKACB*) {560}.

Specific tumours and lesions

Skin pigmentation
Lentiginosis

Lentigines are pigmented cutaneous macules with various appearances, including localized hyperpigmentation of the basal epidermis. There may be increased melanocytes. Other lesions may show coarse melanin granules in the epidermis. Hyperplasia of the epidermis with prominent rete pegs may also be present.

Other pigmented naevi

Pigmented or blue naevi are seen on the extremities and trunk, and less commonly on the head and neck. They are darkly pigmented, domed, and usually < 1 cm. Microscopically, they are poorly circumscribed, located in the dermis, and contain two types of melanocytes: one type is heavily pigmented, globular, and fusiform and the other is lightly pigmented, polygonal, and spindled {401}.

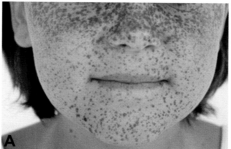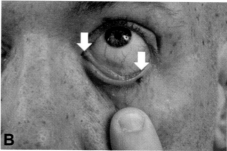

Fig. 7.37 Pigmentation in Carney complex. **A** Facial lentigines in a patient with unusually extensive involvement. **B** Carney complex pigmentation in the canthus and eyelid. Most patients have involvement of unusual sites.

The melanocytes are usually located along the dermal collagen bundle.

Myxomas
Cardiac myxomas
Cardiac myxomas in Carney complex are usually multifocal and are found in the atria as well as the left and right ventricles. They range in size from 0.3 to > 5 cm {1723}. The gross and microscopic appearances of cardiac myxomas in Carney complex and in isolated cases are similar. Histologically, they are hypocellular lesions with scattered polygonal and spindle cells in pools of ground substances.

Extracardiac myxomas
Myxomas can also occur in other sites, including the skin, external auditory canal, eyelid, mucocutaneous locations, and breast. Histologically, they show scattered polygonal, stellate, and spindle cells in pools of ground substances. Capillaries are usually prominent. Cutaneous lesions, when in contact with the overlying epidermis, may induce epidermal proliferation into the dermis, which becomes incorporated into the myxoma.

Endocrine tumours
Primary pigmented nodular adrenocortical disease
The adrenal glands contain small black or brown cortical nodules ranging from < 1 mm to 4 mm in diameter. Some of the micronodules may extend to the immediate pericapsular adipose tissue, and this should not be considered evidence of low-grade malignancy. Some of the nodules are present at the corticomedullary junction, but they do not usually extend into the medulla. Microscopically, the nodules are composed of enlarged globular cortical cells with granular eosinophilic cytoplasm that often contains lipochrome pigment. The surrounding uninvolved adrenal cortex may show signs of atrophy, and myelolipomatous changes may be present in the cortex. Immunohistochemical staining is usually positive for inhibin alpha, melan-A, and synaptophysin {404,2530}.

Pituitary tumours
Patients may present with acromegaly-associated tumours or with symptoms due to mixed somatotroph and lactotroph tumours. Abnormalities in the anterior pituitary range from macroadenomas to hyperplasia of cells producing growth hormone and prolactin (mammosomatotrophs). In one series, mammosomatotroph hyperplasia was present in 5 of 8 cases, in proximity to the adenoma tissue {1503,2078}. Adenomas usually show a diffuse pattern of growth, with round and polygonal cells containing round or oval nuclei. Immunohistochemical analysis of the tumours usually shows growth hormone, prolactin, or a combination of the two hormones. Ultrastructural examination of the adenomas shows large tightly packed cells with complex interdigitations. The cells usually have abundant rough endoplasmic reticulum and conspicuous Golgi complexes. Dense-core secretory granules of 200–250 nm in diameter are present.

Thyroid nodules and carcinomas
Thyroid abnormalities are not uncommon in Carney complex {2656}. They range from follicular hyperplasia and/or cystic changes to carcinomas. Benign follicular lesions or adenomas have been reported. The carcinomas may include papillary and follicular types. In many cases of Carney complex, only fine-needle aspiration biopsy was done, so the exact pathological findings in the nodules have not been clearly defined {2656}. Increased PRKAR1A expression has recently been reported in association with aggressive and undifferentiated thyroid tumours {854}, although other reports indicate that decreased PRKAR1A is seen in advanced thyroid tumours {2407}.

Gonadal tumours
Large cell calcifying Sertoli cell tumour and ovarian cystadenoma or cystadenocarcinoma
Large cell calcifying Sertoli cell tumour occurs in a small proportion of male patients with Carney complex. The tumours can be very large and replace the entire testis or can be microscopic foci within the testis {2208}. Large cell calcifying Sertoli cell tumours are usually bilateral and calcified. Microscopic examination shows patterns varying from solid to trabecular. An intratubular or in situ component may be present. The tumour cells are large, with abundant eosinophilic cytoplasm. Mitotic figures are uncommon. Distinctly laminated calcospherites are a common finding. Leydig cell tumours and adrenal cortical rest tumours may also be seen {402}.

The ovarian lesions in Carney complex range from ovarian cysts to serous cystadenomas and rare malignant tumours, including endometrioid cystadenocarcinomas and mucinous adenocarcinomas {2658}.

Peripheral nervous system
Pigmented melanotic schwannoma
Psammomatous melanotic schwannoma is one of the rare peripheral nerve sheath tumours that is associated with Carney complex. Some of these tumours may be malignant, with recurrences or metastases {398,407}. The tumours affect the posterior spinal nerve roots, alimentary tract (especially the oesophagus and stomach), bone, and skin. Most of the tumours are symptomatic. They have a black, brown, or blue appearance; are usually encapsulated; and are solid or

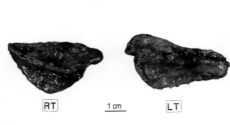
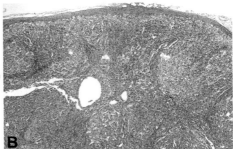
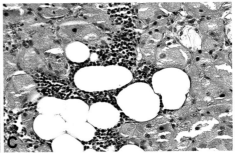

A **B** **C**

Fig. 7.38 Primary pigmented nodular adrenocortical disease (PPNAD) in Carney complex. **A** Adrenal glands showing multiple pigmented nodules measuring 1–4 mm. **B** Histological section of PPNAD showing multiple nodules. **C** Adrenal gland with a myelolipomatous focus and pigmentation of cortical cells.

spongy. Microscopic examination shows a well-circumscribed but incompletely encapsulated tumour with spindle and epithelioid cells, melanin, psammoma bodies, and adipose tissue. The spindle cells are arranged in interlacing fascicles and show whorling and occasionally nuclear palisading. Immunostaining is usually positive for S100 protein and vimentin, whereas staining for GFAP, actin, and keratin is negative. Ultrastructural examination usually reveals cells with elongated processes, continuous basal lamina, and melanosomes, as well as premelanosomes and intercellular long-spacing collagen.

Other tumours

Osteochondromyxomas are rare in Carney complex. They tend to appear early in life, and can exhibit either a blastic or lytic appearance {400}. They often exhibit a polymorphic histology, including areas of polygonal, stellate, or bipolar cells. Immature osteoid is present, with increased numbers of osteoclasts, indicating rapid bone remodelling. Areas of hyaline fibrosis may also be observed.

Rarely, tumours can also occur in the liver (hepatocellular carcinoma) and pancreas (acinar cell carcinoma) {945,952}.

Genetics

Most patients with Carney complex have inactivating mutations in *PRKAR1A*. The bulk of these are null mutations, including nonsense mutations, splice-site mutations, and micro- and macrodeletions, leading to nonsense-mediated mRNA decay and complete suppression of protein production {1393,1394}. Missense mutations have also been reported; in such cases, the protein is also non-functional {560}.

It is unclear whether loss of the normal allele is required for tumour formation. Analysis by FISH suggests that loss of heterozygosity is common in tumours {1763}, although tumour analysis at the protein level has detected residual

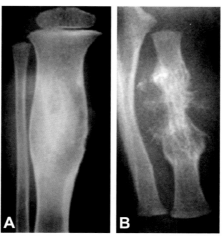

Fig. 7.39 Osteochondromyxoma. **A** Radiographical appearance of osteochondromyxoma showing a blastic lesion. **B** Radiographical appearance of osteochondromyxoma showing a lytic lesion.

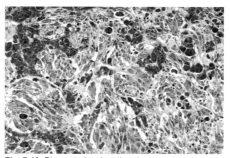

Fig. 7.40 Pigmented melanotic schwannoma.

PRKAR1A. However, it is unclear whether that protein was isolated from the tumour cells themselves or from the surrounding stroma. Comparative data from mouse models of *Prkar1a* mutations suggest that complete loss is necessary for the phenotype {3067}, although mouse models may not faithfully represent human tumorigenesis.

PRKAR1A itself is a protein that has been known for many years; it is the type 1A regulatory subunit of the cAMP-dependent PKA. cAMP/PKA signalling is essential for hormone secretion in many endocrine tissues, including those affected in Carney complex. It has been demonstrated that loss of PRKAR1A results in

increased PKA activity, leading to the tumour phenotype {1393}. The identification of the targets of PKA phosphorylation that are required for tumorigenesis is an area of active research.

Because disease-associated mutations result in complete loss of function, there is generally a poor correlation between phenotype and genotype. It has been suggested that specific mutations may be associated with specific features, but the small numbers of patients with each mutation (other than the two common mutations) make it difficult to distinguish variations associated with specific mutations from specific phenotypes within families due to other genetic and/or environmental factors.

The other genetic mutations associated with Carney complex and primary pigmented nodular adrenocortical disease (as noted above) are all associated with increases in PKA signalling. Mutations in *PDE8B* and *PDE11A* cause decreased phosphodiesterase activity and thereby increase cAMP and downstream PKA signalling. In the rare patients with additional copies of the PKA catalytic subunit (*PRKACA*), a different mechanism leads to similarly increased downstream signalling and a similar phenotype.

Prognosis and predictive factors

Most of the tumours associated with Carney complex are benign and slow-growing. Exceptions are the schwannomas, which can behave more aggressively, although not nearly as aggressively as melanomas, with which they can be confused due to their striking melanotic pigmentation. The other tumour type that can cause catastrophic acute consequences in Carney complex is cardiac myxoma, although this is a feature of cardiac myxomas in general, and is not due to malignancy per se. In families and/or patients with multiple cardiac myxomas, complications from open heart surgery may also lead to a reduction in overall lifespan.

McCune–Albright syndrome

Mete O.
Boyce A. M.
Stratakis C. A.
Weinstein L. S.

Definition
McCune–Albright syndrome (MAS) is a tumour disorder caused by somatic activating *GNAS* mutations resulting in mosaic disease with wide clinical variability and a broad spectrum of lesions, including fibrous dysplasia (FD); café-au-lait spots; and various endocrinopathies leading to hyperfunctioning syndromes such as gonadotropin-independent precocious puberty, hyperthyroidism, growth hormone (GH) excess or mixed GH and prolactin excess, Cushing syndrome, and FGF23-mediated hypophosphataemia.

Synonyms
Albright syndrome; fibrous dysplasia (polyostotic and monostotic); Mazabraud syndrome

Incidence and prevalence
MAS/FD with multisystem involvement is rare. There are no reliable data establishing disease prevalence; however, estimates range between 1 case per 1 million and 1 case per 100 000 population {303}. In contrast, FD (particularly as monostotic disease) is relatively common; it has been estimated to account for as many as 7% of all benign bone tumours {303}.

Age distribution and penetrance
The clinical spectrum of MAS/FD is broad, ranging from asymptomatic findings to neonatal lethality. The phenotype reflects the distribution of *GNAS* mutations and the role of G$_s$-alpha in mutation-bearing tissues. Penetrance is high and primarily determined by the number and location of mutant cells {1082}. Café-au-lait spots are usually apparent at or shortly after birth {546}. FD lesions manifest during the first few years of life and expand during childhood {1095}. Most clinically significant bone lesions are detectable by the age of 10 years, with few appearing in patients aged > 15 years {1095}. Endocrinopathies are generally apparent before the age of 5 years, with the exception of FGF23-mediated hypophosphataemia, which may wax and wane {301,546}.

Diagnostic criteria
MAS is clinically diagnosed in individuals fulfilling two or more of the following criteria: (1) café-au-lait spots with characteristic features, including irregular borders and distribution showing an association with (i. e. respecting) the midline of the body; (2) polyostotic or monostotic FD, which is usually diagnosed based on its characteristic ground-glass (occasionally sclerotic) radiographical appearance – however, biopsy and mutation testing may be beneficial for lesions with a non-classic appearance and isolated monostotic disease; (3) any of the following endocrinopathies: gonadotropin-independent precocious puberty, testicular lesions with or without precocious puberty, thyroid lesions with or without non-autoimmune hyperthyroidism, GH excess or mixed GH and prolactin excess, FD-associated renal phosphate wasting with or without hypophosphataemia, and neonatal Cushing syndrome.

The presence of any feature of MAS should prompt evaluation for additional manifestations. In individuals whose only finding is monostotic FD, the identification of a *GNAS* mutation is required to establish the diagnosis. The association of polyostotic FD and intramuscular myxomas is categorized as Mazabraud syndrome.

Specific tumours and lesions

Endocrine manifestations
Precocious puberty
Clinical features
The most common endocrine manifestation in girls is gonadotropin-independent precocious puberty {216,716,1753,2396}. Precocious puberty in MAS is isosexual, due to peripheral estrogen and/or testosterone production {216,1753,2088,2951}.

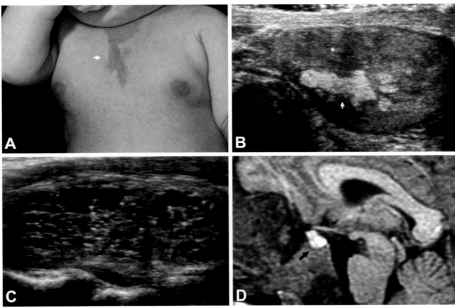

Fig. 7.41 McCune–Albright syndrome. **A** Photograph of a 1-year-old girl showing a characteristic café-au-lait spot (arrow), with irregular borders and location respecting the midline of the body. Note the presence of breast budding due to precocious puberty. **B** Testicular ultrasonography from a 48-year-old man with macroorchidism and a history of precocious puberty, showing discrete hyperechoic lesions (arrow) and surrounding heterogeneity (asterisk). **C** Thyroid ultrasonography from a 7-year-old girl with hyperthyroidism, showing a diffusely heterogeneous appearance and multiple hypoechoic lesions. **D** Contrast-enhanced sagittal MRI from a 30-year-old woman with growth hormone excess, showing a multinodular pituitary macroadenoma (arrow). Also apparent is extensive, heterogeneous-appearing fibrous dysplasia in the skull base (asterisk).

One series revealed that the prevalence of gonadal involvement is equal between the sexes; however, precocious puberty is more frequent in girls (accounting for ~80% of cases) than in boys (accounting for ~20%) {302,1753,2951}. In girls, precocity presents with episodic vaginal bleeding and breast budding, coinciding with the development of single or multiple estrogen-producing ovarian cysts. Between cysts, symptoms are generally absent. Affected boys develop enlarged testes with or without excess testosterone production {2951}. Ultrasonography is useful to screen gonads in MAS. Ovarian cysts may be either present or absent due to the episodic nature of their development. Testicular microlithiasis, hyperechoic lesions, hypoechoic lesions, heterogeneity, and focal calcifications can be identified in most boys irrespective of precocity {302,642}.

Pathology
Follicular cysts lined by granulosa cells are frequently identified in girls with MAS-related precocity {609,1753}. A single case of borderline ovarian serous tumour {490} and another of virilizing sclerosing stromal tumour have been reported in MAS {296}. Testicular enlargement results from maturation and growth of seminiferous tubules. In a recent study, orchiectomy specimens revealed large foci of Leydig cell hyperplasia indistinguishable from Leydig cell tumours {302}. Sertoli cell proliferations (including Sertoli cell intraepithelial neoplasia), bilateral testicular germ cell tumours (including embryonal carcinoma), and testicular adrenal rests have also been reported {302,716}.

Hyperthyroidism
Clinical features
Hyperthyroidism is the second most common endocrine manifestation in MAS {546,1752}. A comprehensive literature review identified subclinical or clinical hyperthyroidism in as many as 77% of patients with MAS-related goitre {433, 546,1752}. However, approximately 30% of patients with hyperthyroidism did not have clinically detectable goitre or thyroiditis {1752}; this absence of thyroiditis suggests that microscopic clonal follicular epithelial proliferations with *GNAS* mutations lead to thyroid hormone secretion. Abnormal ultrasound findings have been reported in 54% of patients {546,1752}. Even in the absence of hyperthyroidism,

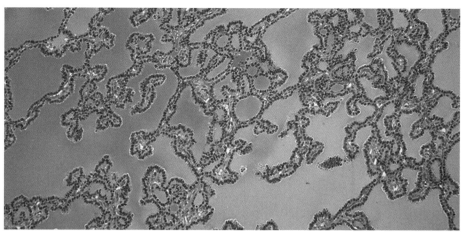

Fig. 7.42 McCune–Albright syndrome (MAS). Functioning thyroid nodules in MAS can show intrafollicular centripetal papillary growth, called follicular adenoma with papillary growth. Terms such as "papillary hyperplasia" and "nodular hyperplasia" should not be used.

affected patients have a higher triiodothyronine-to-thyroxine ratio, which is partially explained by cAMP-induced 5'-deiodinase activity {433,1752}.

Pathology
In a 1997 review of MAS-related thyroid abnormalities {1752}, multiple thyroid nodules were interpreted as multinodular hyperplasia, papillary hyperplasia, or goitre; solitary nodules were interpreted as follicular adenoma {1752}. Like nonsyndromic functioning thyroid nodules (which are typically associated with either *TSHR* or *GNAS* activating clonal mutations {1931,2084,2185}), the solitary or multiple functioning nodules that occur in MAS appear warm or hot on scan {2534} and can cause subclinical or clinical hyperthyroidism. Regardless of size, such nodules are called follicular adenomas with papillary growth (or papillary adenomas), and are histologically characterized by benign follicular epithelial proliferations with intrafollicular centripetal papillary projections {102,1821}. Rare cases of inflammatory thyroiditis and thyroid carcinomas have been described {545,1752}.

Growth hormone and prolactin excess
Clinical features
The diagnosis of MAS-related pituitary disease is often challenging, and it is frequently delayed as a result {2395}. MAS-related acromegaly is always associated with FD of the skull base {2395}. Most patients with MAS-related acromegaly have a normal height, which may be attributable to FD, precocity, and/or hyperthyroidism {2395}. Synchronous hyperprolactinaemia occurs in about 80% of

patients {2395}. Diffuse pituitary enlargement, microadenoma, macroadenoma, and multifocal microadenoma have been reported {2395,2902}. Despite the presence of biochemical acromegaly, MRI fails to detect lesions in some cases {36, 2395,2902}.

Pathology
MAS-related pituitary disease is heterogeneous and typically involves a subset of PIT1-lineage adenohypophyseal cells, including mammosomatotrophs and somatotrophs {1011,1822,2395, 2902}. Some patients present with mammosomatotroph or somatotroph hyperplasia; others develop mammosomatotroph or somatotroph adenomas {1011, 1467,2395,2902}. Although findings of the non-tumorous anterior pituitary were largely unavailable in some reports; evidence suggests a hyperplasia-to-neoplasia progression sequence and multicentric microadenomas in extended resection specimens {1822,2902}. Given the heterogeneous nature of MAS-related pituitary disease, total hypophysectomy is required for surgical cure {457,702, 2384,2902}.

Adrenal Cushing syndrome
Clinical features
Adrenal involvement manifests in the first year of life {337,2396}, and affects 1.7–7.5% of patients {38,337,1689,2296}. Weight gain with decreasing growth velocity is characteristic of Cushing syndrome in childhood {707}; however, neonates may develop failure to thrive {337}. Spontaneous resolution has been described in some neonates {1390}.

Pathology

The hallmark of MAS-related Cushing syndrome is bilateral nodular hyperplasia, which also encompasses presentations with bilateral primary bimorphic adrenocortical disease {409,707,2396, 2654}. Although primary bimorphic adrenocortical disease is not specific to MAS, it is histologically characterized by diffuse nodular hyperplasia juxtaposed with areas of atrophic cortex, resulting in a bimorphic appearance {409}. Hyperplastic foci are distinguished by strong inhibin alpha and synaptophysin expression, whereas the thin atrophic cortex reveals strong CD56 expression and lack of zona reticularis {409}. Rare examples of bilateral adenomas have also been described in MAS {409}.

Renal phosphate wasting
Clinical features
Renal phosphate wasting is common, and may be associated with hypophosphataemia and osteomalacia/rickets {544,1216A,1422}.

Pathology
The underlying mechanism relates to proximal tubulopathy mediated by the phosphaturic factor FGF23, which is released from FD tissue {1422,2292,2396}. FGF23 production is related to overall FD burden, and hypophosphataemia is typically seen in patients with significant skeletal disease {544}.

Non-endocrine or rare manifestations
Café-au-lait spots and FD are characteristic non-endocrine manifestations of MAS. Rare manifestations include oral pigmentation {2169}, gastrointestinal polyps {3087}, breast cancer {1200,2715}, hepatobiliary and pancreatic neoplasms {943,2122}, hepatobiliary dysfunction {569}, cardiac disease {569,2528,2855}, and platelet dysfunction {133}, along with hyperplasia of thymus {569,2855}, spleen {569,2855}, and pancreatic islets {569,2855}.

Genetics
GNAS chromosomal location and gene structure
MAS/FD results from postzygotic somatic activating (gain-of-function) mutations in G_s-alpha, one of several transcripts encoded by GNAS at 20q13.2-q13.3 {2964}. GNAS is a complex locus with

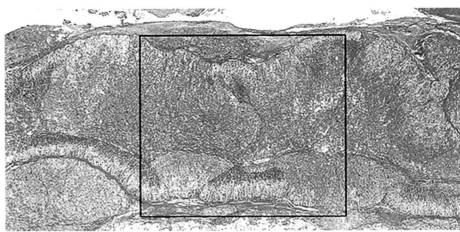

Fig. 7.43 McCune–Albright syndrome. Primary bimorphic adrenocortical disease is characterized by diffuse nodular hyperplasia. The boxed area shows a variegated appearance due to alternating areas of compact cell hyperplasia interspersed with areas of cortical atrophy.

an imprinted expression pattern. Multiple gene products, including maternal, paternal, and biallelic-expressed transcripts, are derived from four promoters and 5' exons that splice onto a common set of downstream exons (exons 2–13) {2964}. Somatic GNAS mutations in MAS/FD occur at one of two residues: Arg201 (accounting for > 95% of the mutations) {1689} and Gln227 (accounting for < 5%) {1207}.

Gene expression and function
The major product of GNAS is G_s-alpha, which is generated by the most downstream promoter (exon 1). G_s-alpha is the ubiquitously expressed heterotrimeric G-protein alpha subunit, which couples seven-transmembrane receptors to the cAMP-generating enzyme adenylyl cyclase and is required for the intracellular cAMP response to hormones and other extracellular signals. The GNAS variants at Arg201 and Gln227 disrupt G_s-alpha's intrinsic GTPase activity, causing constitutive activation and abnormal cAMP signalling {1543}.

Genotype–phenotype correlations
There are no known genotype–phenotype correlations. Clinical presentation and disease severity are likely determined by the degree of mosaicism and the location and extent of affected tissues.

Genetic counselling
MAS/FD results from activating mutations that are always somatic. This disorder is virtually never inherited, presumably due to the fact that germline mutations are likely lethal {1082}. Counselling should emphasize that, although no pregnancy is at zero risk, the risk of recurrence appears to be no higher than that in the general population.

Prognosis and predictive factors
The prognosis for individuals with MAS varies, depending on disease location and severity. Endocrinopathies persist throughout childhood and adulthood, with the exception of FGF23-mediated hypophosphataemia, which may worsen during periods of rapid linear growth and ameliorate in adulthood when FD disease activity wanes. Endocrinopathies can generally be controlled with pharmacotherapies {301}.

Optimizing the treatment of endocrinopathies may improve outcomes in FD. Untreated GH excess is associated with expansion of craniofacial FD, resulting in macrocephaly and vision loss {304}. Hypophosphataemia increases fractures and bone pain {1583}.

GNAS mutations in MAS/FD are weakly oncogenic, and affected tissues likely carry a small increased risk of malignant transformation. FD rarely undergoes sarcomatous degeneration {2361, 2726}, and additional cancers (as summarized above) have been reported. Radiotherapy and uncontrolled GH excess may increase the risk of malignant transformation.

Familial non-medullary thyroid cancer

LiVolsi V.
Eng C.
Foulkes W. D.
Nosé V.
Schmid K. W.

Several entities are categorized as familial thyroid cancers of follicular cells, including follicular, oncocytic, papillary, and anaplastic carcinomas. The syndromes associated with these follicular neoplasms include Cowden syndrome and other syndromes caused by *PTEN* mutations, familial adenomatous polyposis, and the less well understood familial differentiated carcinoma (usually papillary thyroid carcinoma) without other organ involvement.

Cowden syndrome and PTEN-related lesions

Definition
Cowden syndrome is an autosomal dominant disorder characterized by multiple hamartomas involving multiple tissues. There is a high risk of breast, thyroid, endometrial, renal, and colon cancers {770}, and the skin tumour trichilemmoma is pathognomonic. Cowden syndrome is caused by germline mutations in *PTEN* or other genes (i.e. SDH genes, *PIK3CA*, *AKT1*, *KLLN*, or *SEC23B*) {1711, 1978} (see *Follicular thyroid carcinoma*, p. 92). Follicular thyroid carcinomas are overrepresented in individuals with Cowden syndrome carrying germline *PTEN* mutations.

Synonyms
PTEN hamartoma tumour syndrome; Bannayan–Riley–Ruvalcaba syndrome; Proteus syndrome; Proteus-like syndrome

Incidence and prevalence
Cowden syndrome is the most common syndrome associated with familial non-medullary thyroid cancer. The annual incidence of Cowden syndrome is about 1 case per 200 000 population {770,818}. Estimates of the frequency of de novo *PTEN* mutations range from 10% to 48% {1818}. Individuals with germline *PTEN* mutations have a 35% lifetime risk of thyroid cancer {2712}.
The diagnosis of Cowden syndrome is made only when a *PTEN* pathogenic

variant is identified. Cases are missed due to the complexity of the clinical criteria; many manifestations of Cowden syndrome are common, and only about half of the patients have a family history {354}. Because Cowden syndrome confers a considerable risk for cancer, its recognition is important, so that cancer screening and genetic counselling can be initiated.

Age distribution and penetrance
Affected individuals usually present by their late 20s. The lifetime risk of developing breast cancer is 85%, and it occurs at a younger patient age than do sporadic lesions {660}. The lifetime risk of thyroid cancer (usually follicular and rarely papillary, but never medullary) is approximately 35%.

Clinical features
The clinical presentations can vary, even among members of the same family. Clinical criteria for Cowden syndrome {282, 1002} have been delineated by the National Comprehensive Cancer Network (NCCN) {249} (Table 7.09). Affected individuals usually have macrocephaly, dermal trichilemmomas, and papillomatous papules. The classic pathognomonic criterion of Cowden syndrome is trichilemmomas. Cowden syndrome is difficult to recognize due to its diverse clinical features, including various carcinomas {2712}.

Macroscopy
Thyroid tumours can occur anywhere in the gland and are often multifocal. Carcinomas, adenomas, and hyperplastic nodules may coexist. Hyperplastic nodules present grossly as multiple, firm, yellowish-tan, well-circumscribed nodules.

Microscopy
The thyroid lesions in patients with Cowden syndrome affect the follicular cells: multinodular goitre, multiple adenomatous nodules (occurring in 75% of cases), follicular adenoma (in 25%), follicular carcinoma (45%), and papillary

carcinoma (60%) {1563}. In addition, there is lymphocytic thyroiditis and C-cell hyperplasia (each occurring in 55% of cases), but medullary thyroid carcinoma is not part of Cowden syndrome {214,982, 1563,2057,2207,2527,2586}. Follicular carcinoma is a major diagnostic criterion for Cowden syndrome, and benign follicular nodules are minor criteria {1563}. The follicular and papillary (including follicular-variant papillary) lesions show histology identical to that of their sporadic counterparts (see *Papillary thyroid carcinoma*, p. 81, and *Follicular thyroid carcinoma*, p. 92). There is a tendency for the follicular proliferations to show oncocytic cytology. Multiple nodules both benign and malignant within the thyroid gland (especially in a young patient) should raise the suspicion of Cowden syndrome {365}. The constellation of histological

Table 7.09 Major and minor diagnostic criteria for Cowden syndrome and their frequency of occurrence

Major criteria	
Breast carcinoma	85%
Mucocutaneous lesions	
Trichilemmomas	
Keratoses	
Oral mucosal papillomas	
Cutaneous papules	
Pigmentation of penis	
Endometrial carcinoma	32%
Non-medullary thyroid carcinoma	35%
Macrocephaly	95%
Gastrointestinal hamartomas	
Lhermitte–Duclos disease	
Minor criteria	
Mental retardation	
Autism	
Fibrocystic breast disease	
Nodular thyroid hyperplasia	50–67%
Thyroid adenomas	
Lipomas	
Renal cell carcinoma	28%
Uterine fibroids	

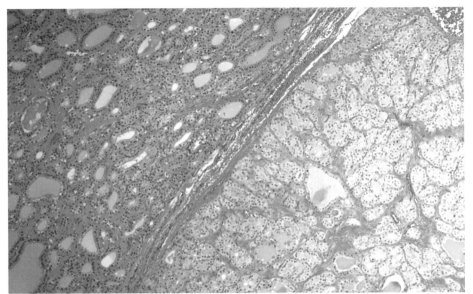
Fig. 7.44 Cowden syndrome. Adenomatous thyroid nodule in a patient with known *PTEN* mutation.

findings in thyroidectomy specimens from Cowden syndrome is unusual, but non-specific {1563,2207}. Most carcinomas arise in a background of multiple adenomatous nodules {365,2207}. Immunohistochemistry for PTEN shows loss of expression in the follicular cells {157, 2207}. There is no correlation between specific *PTEN* mutations and pathological findings {2207}.

Genetic profile
Cowden syndrome is an autosomal dominant inherited cancer syndrome associated with follicular thyroid carcinoma, papillary thyroid carcinoma (PTC), and the follicular variant of PTC. It is caused by germline mutations in several genes, most importantly the tumour suppressor gene *PTEN*; 10–44% of cases are due to a de novo mutation. Overexpression of PTEN results in phosphatase-dependent cell-cycle arrest at the G1 phase and/or apoptosis, depending on the cell type.

Genetic susceptibility
Cases with mutation of an SDH gene or of both *PTEN* and an SDH gene show predominant PTC histology, whereas cases with germline *PTEN* mutation are more likely to be follicular thyroid carcinoma or the follicular variant of PTC {1975,1978}.

Prognosis and predictive factors
The prognosis of the carcinomas occurring in Cowden syndrome depends on the stage and subtype of the lesion (see the *Prognosis and predictive factors*

sections of *Papillary thyroid carcinoma*, p. 91, and *Follicular thyroid carcinoma*, p. 95). Adenomas and adenomatous nodules are benign.

Familial adenomatous polyposis and APC-related lesions

Definition
Familial adenomatous polyposis (FAP) is an autosomal dominant disorder characterized by multiple colorectal adenomatous polyps and a high risk of cancers (colorectal, thyroid, and others). The responsible gene is *APC*. Some patients develop distinctive thyroid neoplasms. FAP is diagnosed in individuals with either ≥ 100 colorectal adenomatous polyps or < 100 adenomatous polyps and a relative with FAP.

Synonyms
APC-associated polyposis conditions include FAP, Gardner syndrome (FAP, desmoid tumours, and osteomas), and Turcot syndrome (FAP and medulloblastoma).

Incidence and prevalence
The prevalence is 3 cases per 100 000 population.

Etiology
There is one predisposition gene for FAP: *APC* on 5q22. The finding of a germline *APC* mutation establishes the molecular diagnosis of FAP, or more broadly, an *APC*-associated polyposis condition {1249}.

Clinical features
In FAP, extracolonic tumours include small intestinal carcinoma (in the duodenum and ampulla of Vater), hepatoblastoma, and desmoids. There is a female predominance {437,438,1599}.

Localization
Thyroid tumours in FAP have specific histology. They can occur anywhere in the gland and are frequently multiple {506, 1579,2794}.

Macroscopy
Grossly, the thyroid tumours can range from < 1 cm to > 8 cm. They are fleshy, white to tan, and firm.

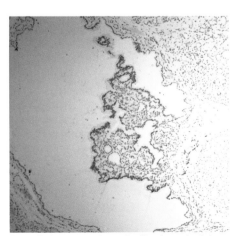

Fig. 7.45 Cowden syndrome. Adenomatous nodule with loss of PTEN expression in follicular cells and expression in endothelial cells.

Fig. 7.46 Cowden syndrome. Papillary hyperplastic focus immunostained for PTEN. Loss of expression in follicular cells.

Microscopy

FAP is associated with the cribriform-morular variant of papillary thyroid carcinoma, which occurs in 1–12% of FAP cases {1248,1249,2640}. The thyroid tumours are often circumscribed or partly encapsulated, with foci of invasion. Tumour patterns include solid, trabecular, spindled, and cribriform; some areas contain papillae and follicles that are devoid of colloid (imparting a lacy pattern to the lesion). The tumour cells can be columnar or cuboidal; spindle cell areas can transition to whorls or squamoid morules. The nuclei are stratified, crowded, and often round to oval with rare grooves or pseudoinclusions, some with prominent nucleoli. Clear, biotin-rich, eosinophilic nuclear inclusions have been described {369,1491}.

Immunophenotype

Immunohistochemistry shows positive nuclear reaction for TTF1 and a weak and very focal presence of thyroglobulin (often negative). Beta-catenin staining shows cytoplasmic and nuclear positivity in cases associated with FAP, reflecting the molecular changes that occur in the syndrome (i.e. permanent activation of the WNT pathway, with aberrant nuclear expression of beta-catenin).

Tumours of identical morphology can occur as sporadic lesions without background FAP {364,2670}. These tend to occur in older patients, and are unifocal {2196}. However, genetic testing is required whenever a cribriform-morular tumour is found, because some mutations in the APC gene may be associated with delayed manifestations in older individuals.

Genetic profile

APC is a tumour suppressor gene with multiple functions: cell migration, differentiation, proliferation, genetic stability, and apoptosis {1958}. The APC protein is linked to an array of cellular processes {1967}; its negative regulation of the WNT/beta-catenin pathway links APC to intestinal stem cell regulation {2480}. Mutations in APC are associated with a number of related syndromes (Gardner syndrome, Turcot syndrome, hereditary desmoid disease, and attenuated FAP), all subsumed under the term "familial adenomatous polyposis" {872}. Nearly all mutations in APC that cause FAP result in a truncated protein, but these proteins may be expressed and can retain some functions {2469}. Some associations between the position of the APC mutation and the occurrence of differentiated thyroid carcinoma (the cribriform-morular variant) in FAP have been reported {437}. In sporadic cases, germline mutations in PIK3CA have been reported {1507}.

Genetic susceptibility

There is only one susceptibility gene for FAP, but there are > 825 pathogenic germline mutations. Germline APC mutations confer a > 99% penetrance by the age of 40 years. In individuals with FAP and thyroid cancer, most germline APC mutations have been found to be 5' to codon 1220, occurring 5' to the APC mutation cluster region (codons 1286–1513) {437,1249,2820}.

Prognosis and predictive factors

The prognosis of the cribriform-morular variant of papillary thyroid carcinoma is good, with most patients cured by surgery. Rare cases of aggressive behaviour have been documented {369}.

Non-syndromic familial thyroid cancer

Definition

"Familial non-medullary thyroid cancer", or better "non-syndromic familial thyroid cancer", is a catch-all term for a group of heterogeneous disorders including familial non-medullary thyroid carcinomas, mainly papillary thyroid carcinoma (PTC). Although efforts to identify susceptibility genes have been underway for more than 15 years, these efforts are hampered by the complexity and heterogeneity of the entities' etiology. Families have also been described in which multiple members have multinodular goitre (familial multinodular goitre).

Synonym

Familial papillary thyroid carcinoma

Clinical features

The major clue to the diagnosis of non-syndromic familial thyroid cancer is a strong family history of thyroid nodules and cancers. Apart from family history, the clinical and radiological findings are identical to those of sporadic PTCs (see *Papillary thyroid carcinoma*, p. 81). In some patients known to have a strong family history, screening for thyroid nodules with atypical characteristics by ultrasound or other imaging techniques may allow for early detection and treatment.

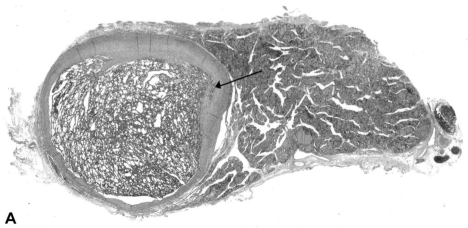

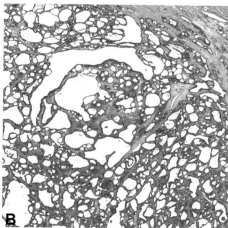

Fig. 7.47 Familial adenomatous polyposis. Cribriform-morular variant of papillary thyroid carcinoma. **A** Encapsulated tumour with focus of capsular invasion (arrow). **B** Higher-power view shows the so-called lace-like pattern.

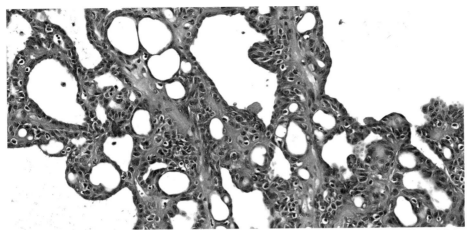
Fig. 7.48 Familial adenomatous polyposis. The cribriform-morular variant of papillary thyroid carcinoma. Empty follicles lined by elongated nuclei that are not cleared.

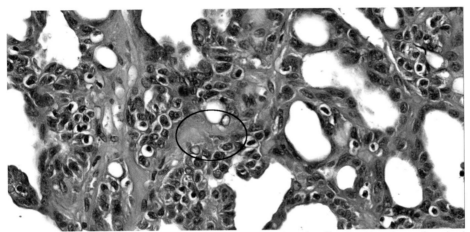
Fig. 7.49 Familial adenomatous polyposis. The cribriform-morular variant of papillary thyroid carcinoma. Occasional cleared nuclei (e.g. circled) are present.

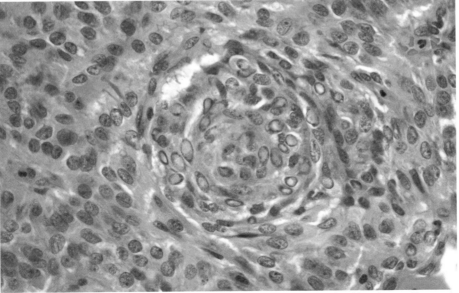
Fig. 7.50 Familial adenomatous polyposis. The cribriform-morular variant of papillary thyroid carcinoma with a morule in the background of spindle cells. Note the nuclear staining.

Localization

These tumours have no specific site predilection within the thyroid. They can occur anywhere within the lobes or isthmus of the gland.

Microscopy

Various patterns and subtypes of PTC or papillary thyroid microcarcinoma may be seen, which are not known to differ from those seen in sporadic tumours.

Genetics

Although efforts to identify susceptibility genes have been underway for more than 15 years, these efforts are hampered by the complexity and heterogeneity of the entities' etiology. There appear to be multiple private (i.e. found only in a single population) predisposition alleles for non-syndromic PTC (e.g. *SRRM2*) {2796}. Predisposition alleles for familial non-medullary thyroid cancer, such as the recently reported *HABP2* {927}, are common polymorphisms {928,2625, 2797,2815}. The genetic basis for familial multinodular goitre is unclear, but several groups have identified *DICER1* mutations in families with familial multinodular goitre with or without associated PTCs {611,700, 1609}.

Prognosis and predictive factors

The prognosis for these thyroid tumours, chiefly PTCs, is similar to that of sporadic PTCs of similar stage and subtype. Although the frequency of multifocal tumours may be increased in familial cases, there is no evidence that this adversely affects outcomes. In patients known to have a strong family history of PTC, screening may lead to detection of small, early lesions. Prompt treatment may produce excellent prognostic results in these cases. A possible exception is that familial papillary microcarcinoma syndrome may have a poor prognosis, despite the small size of the tumours {378,1692}; histologically, some of these lesions have shown vascular invasion, a very unusual finding in sporadic microcarcinomas.

Werner syndrome and Carney complex

Definition

Werner syndrome (WS) is an autosomal recessive progerioid disorder characterized by premature ageing and cancer predisposition. Individuals develop normally until their 20s, when loss and greying of hair, type 2 diabetes, cataracts, and osteoporosis develop {2061}. A single gene, WRN (also called RECQL2), on 8p12 is associated with WS {3079}. Carney complex is characterized by skin pigmentary abnormalities, myxomas, endocrine tumours or overactivity, and schwannomas. Primary pigmented nodular adrenocortical disease, causing Cushing syndrome, is the most common endocrine lesion in Carney complex, occurring in approximately 25% of patients. As many as 75% of individuals with germline mutations in PRKAR1A are found to have Carney complex.

Synonyms

Carney complex: LAMB syndrome (lentigines, atrial myxomas, mucocutaneous myxomas, and blue naevi); NAME syndrome (naevi, atrial myxomas, myxoid neurofibromas, and ephelides)

Incidence and prevalence

The incidence of WS has been roughly estimated to be 1 case per 100 000 population in Japan and 1 case per 1–10 million population outside of Japan. Of note is the clustering of WS in Sardinia, Italy. Data from academic centres and registries indicate the existence of about 400 unrelated Carney complex probands globally {2659}.

Clinical features

The diagnosis of WS is considered in individuals with four cardinal signs {2061, 3079}: bilateral cataracts (present in 99% of cases), premature thinning and greying of scalp hair (in 100%), typical skin pathology (96%), and short stature (95%). All four of these signs are found in 90% of WS cases. Approximately 45% of individuals with WS have neoplasms, including follicular thyroid carcinomas. The classic clinical features of Carney complex are lentiginosis (spotty pigmentation), endocrine overactivity, and cardiac myxomas. A definitive diagnosis of Carney complex requires two or more of the phenotypes in the diagnostic criteria listed on p.269 to be present {1754}.

Localization

Thyroid tumours and nodules can develop anywhere within the thyroid.

Macroscopy

No specific features distinguish these tumours from their sporadic counterparts.

Microscopy

The thyroid tumours in WS are almost all of follicular origin, and include follicular, papillary, and even anaplastic carcinomas. In one series of Japanese patients, anaplastic carcinoma accounted for 13% of the thyroid cancers {1223}. In Carney complex, most of the thyroid tumours are follicular adenomas {2659}, but both follicular and papillary carcinomas have been observed.

Genetics

WS is an autosomal recessive disorder characterized by germline homozygous or compound heterozygous mutations in WRN (also called RECQL2) {3079}. To date, no other predisposition genes have been found. However, individuals with rare atypical WS cases or paediatric-onset progeria (Hutchinson–Gilford progeria syndrome, which is an autosomal dominant disorder) carry germline mutations in LMNA. WRN has a transcript of 5765 bp and consists of 35 exons. It encodes a multifunctional nuclear protein of 1432 amino acids that is a member of the RecQ family of DNA helicases, which means it preferentially unwinds DNA structures. ATP-dependent WRN activities can be modified by interactions with other proteins, such as p53, RPA, and the KU complex. Biochemical and cell biological studies suggest that the WRN protein is involved in DNA repair, recombination, replication, and transcription, as well as in combined functions such as DNA repair during replication. More than 75 pathogenic WRN mutations have been identified; they are typically truncating, with a few missense. In the Japanese population, the c.3139-1G>C splicing mutation, which is a founder mutation resulting in exon 26 skipping, accounts for 60% of WS cases {2435}. In the Sardinian population of Italy, another founder mutation, c.2089-3024A>G, inserts a new exon between exons 18 and 19 {1748}. The founder mutations in these two populations probably account for the elevated frequencies of WS in the populations.

Prognosis and predictive factors

There are no known prognostic factors that differ from those of sporadic lesions.

DICER1 syndrome

Foulkes W. D.
Kovacs K.

Definition

DICER1 syndrome is an autosomal dominant pleiotropic tumour syndrome caused by germline DICER1 mutations that usually lead to tumours and dysplasias with onset in childhood, adolescence, or early adulthood, including pleuropulmonary blastoma (PPB); cystic nephroma; and endocrine-related lesions such as multinodular goitre, ovarian Sertoli–Leydig cell tumour, gynandroblastoma, juvenile granulosa cell tumour, and pituitary blastoma (associated with infantile-onset Cushing disease).

Synonym

Pleuropulmonary blastoma familial tumour and dysplasia syndrome

Incidence and prevalence

The precise incidence is unknown, but DICER1 syndrome is rare. In the Exome Aggregation Consortium (ExAC) dataset (http://exac.broadinstitute.org/), only 6 loss-of-function DICER1 mutations have been found in the > 60 000 individuals sequenced. An estimated 50 cases of PPB are diagnosed annually in the USA, and about 70% are associated with germline DICER1 mutations {320}. Assuming about 10% of mutation carriers develop PPB by the age of 6 years, and given the estimate of about 3.9 million live births per year in the USA, the annual

incidence of DICER1 mutations may be approximately 9 cases per 100 000 live births. The prevalence of mutations must be substantially higher, given that many carriers go unidentified and most associated conditions are non-lethal.

Age distribution and penetrance

Nearly all PPBs present by the age of 6 years {874,1817,2204}. Another frequent phenotype is cystic nephroma (a benign, multiloculated cystic renal dysplasia), with > 90% of cases occurring by the age of 4 years {276}. Ovarian sex cord–stromal tumours, most commonly Sertoli–Leydig cell tumours, have been reported in patients aged 2–45 years, but most occur in patients aged 10–25 years {874}. Nodular thyroid hyperplasia, often progressing to clinically evident multinodular goitre, generally develops in childhood and adolescence, but can remain occult and not clinically evident for decades {2298}. The very rare pituitary blastoma occurs by the age of 24 months {626}. Other conditions associated with DICER1 mutations (see below) are generally too rare for reliable estimates. The penetrance of DICER1 mutations is uncertain because the most common manifestations may be occult changes in lung, kidney, and thyroid that are detectable only with systematic detailed imaging of carriers. However, it is likely that > 50% of female DICER1 mutation carriers develop multinodular goitre in their lifetime {1351}.

Diagnostic criteria

There are no established diagnostic criteria for DICER1 syndrome (other than a deleterious germline mutation in DICER1). Some tumours are either so rare or so characteristic that any affected individual is likely to carry a germline DICER1 mutation {874}, including PPB, cystic nephroma {129,276}, nasal chondromesenchymal hamartoma {2646}, ciliary body medulloepithelioma {129,628, 2206}, pituitary blastoma, embryonal rhabdomyosarcoma of the cervix {624, 873}, and anaplastic sarcoma of the

kidney {701,1351}. Pituitary blastoma appears to be pathognomonic of DICER1 mutation {626}, and Sertoli–Leydig cell tumour and multinodular goitre in an individual or kindred are very highly suggestive of germline mutation {2298}. In contrast, pineoblastoma is only moderately suggestive of mutation {625}.

Specific tumours and lesions

DICER1 syndrome features a number of highly characteristic tumour and tumour-like conditions that generally arise in childhood or young adulthood {874}. The most important endocrine manifestations are nodular thyroid hyperplasia (which can result in multinodular goitre {2247} or more rarely differentiated thyroid carcinoma {627,2364}) and ovarian sex cord–stromal tumours (in particular Sertoli–Leydig cell tumour). Ovarian Sertoli cell tumours, gynandroblastoma, and juvenile granulosa cell tumours (often at the single-case level) have also been reported {2482}. These tumours can produce symptoms via hormone secretion. Pituitary blastoma appears to be pathognomonic of germline DICER1 mutation and is associated with infantile-onset Cushing disease {626}. The list of other associated conditions (some of which are discussed above) includes PPB, cystic nephroma {129} (very occasionally leading to anaplastic sarcoma of the

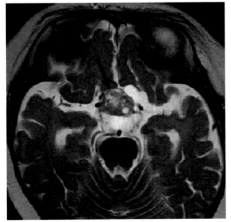

Fig. 7.51 DICER1 syndrome. T2-weighted axial MRI showing a pituitary tumour (arrow).

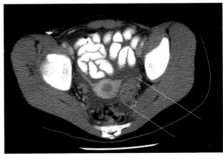

Fig. 7.52 DICER1 syndrome. Sertoli–Leydig cell tumour. CT performed after administration of intravenous and oral contrast demonstrates a left ovarian mass (white lines) measuring 2.6 × 3.9 cm. The endometrium is thickened (the uterus is shown centrally, left of the ovarian mass), and there is free fluid in the pelvis, although these findings may also occur physiologically in a postpubescent patient.

kidney), embryonal rhabdomyosarcoma of the cervix, nasal chondromesenchymal hamartoma, and ciliary body medulloepithelioma {874}, as well as a variety of rare to very rare intracranial tumours such as pineoblastoma {625}, primitive neuroectodermal tumours at other sites {1485}, and cerebral sarcoma {2205}. More common paediatric tumours, such as Wilms tumour, are also associated, but few such cases have been reported {1398, 2081,2237,2582A,3014}. One seminoma was reported in a carrier of a variant of unknown significance in *DICER1* syndrome {2582A}. The co-occurrence of an ovarian Sertoli–Leydig cell tumour with a thyroid carcinoma is highly suggestive of *DICER1* syndrome {725}.

Genetics

The chromosomal location is 14q32.13. The 27 exons of *DICER1* encode a protein of 1922 amino acids, comprising several structurally distinct domains with diverse functions. These domains contain highly evolutionarily conserved amino acids. The known domains (from N-terminus to C-terminus) are the DExD/H-box helicase domain, the transactivation response RNA-binding protein-binding domain, the helicase conserved C-terminal domain, a domain of unknown function known as DUF283, the platform and PAZ domains, the connector helix, the RNase IIIa and IIIb domains, and the double-stranded RNA-binding domain {874}. The RNase III domains are discussed further below. DICER1 has several known functions, but the most intensively investigated relates to maturation of microRNAs from precursor molecules. DICER1 acts as a molecular ruler, measuring and then cutting hairpin precursors into mature 5p and 3p forms {3100}. Germline mutations typically result in protein truncation and likely affect global processing, whereas second somatic missense mutations in the metal ion–binding RNase IIIa and IIIb domains occur in most tumours studied to date, and result in reduced 3p and 5p microRNAs, respectively {874}. Rare individuals carry germline or mosaic mutations of the critical metal ion–binding domains, and the resulting phenotypes are more severe than those associated with protein truncating mutations, in terms of

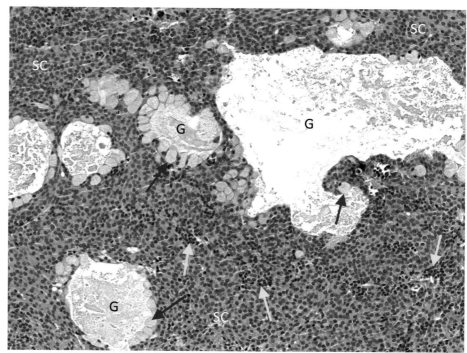

Fig. 7.53 *DICER1* syndrome. Pituitary blastoma composed of large secretory cells (SC) with scattered clusters of small, more primitive cells (yellow arrows). There are also some glands (G) lined by mucous cells (blue arrows).

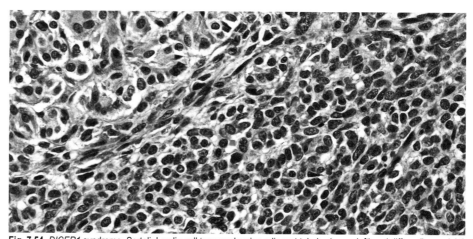

Fig. 7.54 *DICER1* syndrome. Sertoli–Leydig cell tumour showing adjacent tubular (upper left) and diffuse (lower right) architectural patterns.

both patient age at onset and the number of organs involved {628}. It is likely that these RNase III mutations have oncogenic properties {320,2942}.

Prognosis and predictive factors

There are no data to suggest that the presence of a germline *DICER1* mutation influences the prognosis associated with *DICER1*-related tumours as compared with that of their sporadic counterparts.

In general, the outcome following a diagnosis of ovarian sex cord–stromal tumour, cystic nephroma, embryonal rhabdomyosarcoma of the cervix, multinodular goitre, differentiated thyroid carcinoma, nasal chondromesenchymal hamartoma, or ciliary body medulloepithelioma is favourable, whereas cystic-solid and solid PPB, pituitary blastoma, and anaplastic sarcoma of the kidney may have survival rates as low as 50% {626,1817,2907}.

Glucagon cell hyperplasia and neoplasia

Sipos B.
Hammel P.
Klöppel G.

Definition

Glucagon cell hyperplasia and neoplasia (GCHN) is an inherited autosomal recessive disorder caused by germline *GCGR* mutations that lead to the development of islet glucagon cell hyperplasia and glucagon cell microtumours and macrotumours. The disorder is unrelated to multiple endocrine neoplasia type 1 and von Hippel–Lindau syndrome.

Synonyms

Glucagon cell adenomatosis; Mahvash disease/syndrome

Incidence and prevalence

GCHN is an extremely rare disease, with only about 10 cases reported to date.

Age distribution and penetrance

Males and females seem to be equally affected. Patient age ranges from 25 to 68 years.

Diagnostic criteria

Patients present with non-specific symptoms such as abdominal pain, altered bowel habits, fatigue, diabetes, and acute pancreatitis. When measured, serum glucagon levels are found to be elevated. One patient had a severe lethal glucagonoma syndrome {2066}. Other patients had no glucagonoma syndrome despite high serum glucagon levels. Abdominal imaging may reveal multiple small and single large pancreatic tumours that are also detectable by super spatial resolution scintigraphy {1130, 2580,3081}.

Macroscopy

Macroscopically, the pancreas can be normal-sized or enlarged. On the cut surface, there are multiple whitish-yellow nodules ranging in diameter from a few millimetres to 8 cm {1130,2580,3081}.

Microscopy

Throughout all of the pancreatic tissue, there are normal-sized and hypertrophic islets randomly distributed between microadenomas and in some cases also single macrotumours. Large tumours may undergo cystic transformation and focal calcification. The tumour cells are monomorphic and exhibit round to

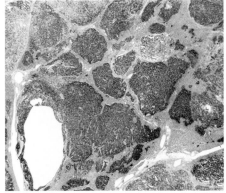

Fig. 7.56 Glucagon cell hyperplasia and neoplasia. Synaptophysin staining highlights multiple neuroendocrine tumours, one with a cystic change. In between the tumours are hyperplastic and normal islets.

oval nuclei. The mitotic activity is very low. There has been one reported case with micrometastases in regional lymph nodes {1130,2580}.

Both the microadenomas and the macrotumours are almost exclusively composed of cells that are immunopositive for glucagon. In the hypertrophic islets, glucagon-positive cells outnumber insulin cells and also somatostatin and PP cells. In one case, a few microadenomas stained for pancreatic polypeptide. All endocrine cells express SSTR2A. The Ki-67 proliferation index is very low (< 1%) {1130,2580,3081}.

Genetics

About 50% of the examined patients with GCHN showed germline mutations of the *GCGR* gene, located on chromosome 17q25 {1130,1846,2580,3081}. GCHN harbours either homozygous *GCGR* mutations or at least two heterozygous mutations leading to premature stop codons or probably deficient protein expression. Lack of glucagon signalling in the liver probably causes a disturbance in a presumed feedback mechanism between the liver and the glucagon cells, which in turn leads to glucagon cell hyperplasia and elevated glucagon levels. Findings in one index patient and his parents indicate that GCHN with *GCGR* mutations has an autosomal recessive inheritance

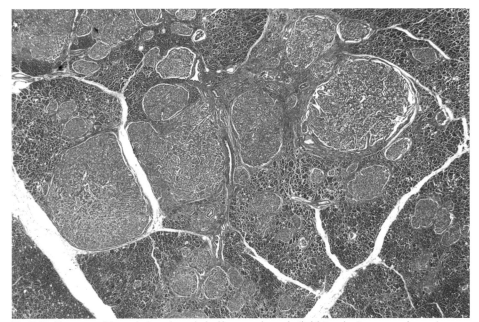

Fig. 7.55 Glucagon cell hyperplasia and neoplasia. Numerous hyperplastic islets, microtumours, and macrotumours are intermixed with normal islets.

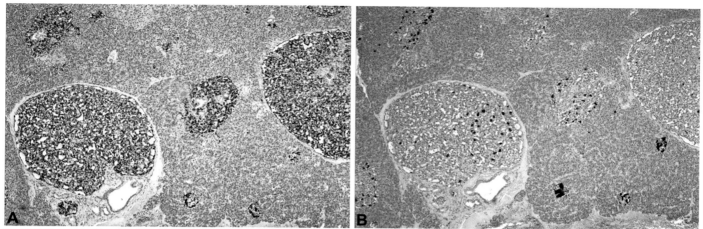

Fig. 7.57 Glucagon cell hyperplasia and neoplasia. **A** Glucagon is expressed predominantly in tumours, as well as in hyperplastic islets. **B** Insulin expression gradually becomes reduced or lost as the diameters of microtumours increase.

pattern {2580}. In patients without *GCGR* mutations the disease mechanisms are unclear {34,2580}. No alterations in *MEN1* or *VHL* were identified. GCHN with *GCGR* mutations seems to have a more advanced phenotype in terms of the number of hypertrophic islets and microadenomas and the occurrence of macrotumours. Lymph node metastases were found in one patient with wildtype *GCGR* {2580}.

Prognosis and predictive factors

In all but one reported case, GCHN has followed a benign clinical course. No recurrence of the disease has been noted in patients who underwent partial pancreatectomy {2580}; however, follow-up of such patients is mandatory, because the tumours can metastasize. One patient died of glucagonoma syndrome that caused severe migratory necrotizing erythema and sepsis {2066}.

Contributors

Dr Ihab ABDULKADER NALLIB
Department of Pathology
University Clinical Hospital
University of Santiago de Compostela
Travesía da Choupana, s/n
15706 Santiago de Compostela
SPAIN
Tel. +34 981 950 854
Fax +34 981 950 889
ihab.abdulkader.nallib@sergas.es

Dr N. Volkan ADSAY*
Department of Anatomic Pathology
Emory University
1364 Clifton Road Northeast, Room H-180B
Atlanta GA 30322
USA
Tel. +1 404 712 4179
Fax +1 404 727 2519
volkan.adsay@emory.edu

Dr Abir AL GHUZLAN
Histopathology Unit
Translational Research Laboratory
Institut Gustave Roussy
39 B Rue Camille Desmoulins
94805 Villejuif
FRANCE
Tel. +33 1 42 11 44 61
Fax +33 1 42 11 52 63
abir.alghuzlan@gustaveroussy.fr

Dr Jorge ALBORES SAAVEDRA
Department of Pathology
Médica Sur Clinic and Foundation
Puente de Piedra 150, Toriello Guerra,
Tlalpan
14050 Mexico City
MEXICO
Tel. +52 1 55 5424 7227
Fax +52 1 55 5424 7227
dralboresjorge@gmail.com

Dr Martin ANLAUF
Institute of Pathology and Cytology
St. Vincenz Krankenhaus
Auf dem Schafsberg
65549 Limburg
GERMANY
Tel. +49 6431 939 6314
Fax +49 6431 23304
anlauf@patho-limburg.de;
anlauf@patho-uegp.de

Dr Andrew ARNOLD
Center for Molecular Medicine
University of Connecticut School of Medicine
263 Farmington Avenue
Farmington CA 06030-3101
USA
Tel. +1 860 679 7640
Fax +1 860 679 7639
aarnold@uchc.edu

Dr Sofia ASIOLI
Department of Biomedical and Neuromotor
Sciences (DIBINEM)
Surgical Pathology Section
University of Bologna Hospital, Via Altura 3
40126 Bologna
ITALY
Tel. +39 51 622 5006
Fax +39 51 622 5759
sofia.asioli@gmail.com; sofia.asioli3@unibo.it

Dr Sébastien AUBERT
Institut de Pathologie
Pôle de Biologie Pathologie Génétique,
CHRU
Avenue Oscar Lambret
59037 Lille Cedex
FRANCE
Tel. +33 3 20 44 49 85
sebastien.aubert@chru-lille.fr;
sebastien.aubert@inserm.fr

Dr Zubair W. BALOCH
Dept of Pathology and Laboratory Medicine
Hospital of the University of Pennsylvania
Perelman School of Medicine
3400 Spruce Street, 6 Founders, Room 6.043
Philadelphia PA 19104-4283
USA
Tel. +1 215 662 3209
Fax +1 215 349 8994
baloch@mail.med.upenn.edu

Dr Armando BARTOLAZZI
Department of Pathology
Sant'Andrea Hospital
Via di Grottarossa 1035
00189 Roma
ITALY
Tel. +39 347 8666 854;
      +39 06 33 775 321
Fax +39 06 33 775 032
armando.bartolazzi@ki.se

Dr Fulvio BASOLO
Department of Pathology
University of Pisa
Via Roma 57
56021 Pisa
ITALY
Tel. +39 5099 2892
Fax +39 5099 2481
fulvio.basolo@med.unipi.it

Dr Gazanfer BELGE
Center for Human Genetics and
Genetic Counseling
University of Bremen
Leobener Str. ZHG
28359 Bremen
GERMANY
Tel. +49 421 218 61570
Fax +49 421 218 61505
belge@uni-bremen.de

Dr John P. BILEZIKIAN
Department of Medicine
Columbia University
Presbyterian Hospital
622 West 168th Street, Room 8W-864
New York NY 10032
USA
Tel. +1 212 305 6238
Fax +1 212 305 6486
jpb2@columbia.edu; boneboss@aol.com

Dr Tetiana BOGDANOVA
Institute of Endocrinology and Metabolism
69 Vyshgorodskaya Street
04114 Kiev
UKRAINE
Tel. +380 50 381 7401;
      +380 44 248 6901
tutla@mail.ru

Dr Fred T. BOSMAN*
Department of Pathology
University of Lausanne Medical Center
25 Rue du Bugnon
1011 Lausanne
SWITZERLAND
Tel. +41 21 731 10 30
Fax +41 21 314 72 05
fred.bosman@chuv.ch

* Indicates participation in the Working Group Meeting on the WHO Classification of Tumours of Endocrine Organs that was held in Lyon, France, 26–28 April 2016.
# Indicates disclosure of interests.

Dr Alison M. BOYCE
Skeletal Clinical Studies Unit
Craniofacial and Skeletal Diseases Branch
NIDCR, National Institutes of Health
30 Convent Drive, Room 228, MSC 4320
Bethesda MD 20892
USA
Tel. +1 301 443 2700
Fax +1 301 480 9962
boyceam@nidcr.nih.gov

Dr Jerome S. BURKE#
Department of Pathology
Alta Bates Summit Medical Center
2450 Ashby Avenue
Berkeley CA 94705
USA
Tel. +1 510 204 1642
Fax +1 510 549 2671
burkej@sutterhealth.org

Dr José Manuel CAMESELLE TEIJEIRO
Department of Anatomic Pathology
University Clinical Hospital
University of Santiago de Compostela
Travesía da Choupana, s/n
15706 Santiago de Compostela
SPAIN
Tel. +34 981 950 858
Fax +34 981 950 889
josemanuel.cameselle@usc.es

Dr Carlo CAPELLA
Dept of Surgical and Morphological Sciences
University of Insubria
Via O. Rossi 9
21100 Varese
ITALY
Tel. +39 332 270 601
Fax +39 332 270 600
carlo.capella@uninsubria.it

Dr Maria Luisa CARCANGIU*
Department of Anatomical Pathology
Fondazione IRCCS
Istituto Nazionale dei Tumori
Via Giacomo Venezian 1
20133 Milano
ITALY
Tel. +39 348 019 7903
Fax +39 022 390 2877
marialuisa.carcangiu@istitutotumori.mi.it

Dr John K.C. CHAN*
Department of Pathology
Queen Elizabeth Hospital
Gascoigne Road, Kowloon
Hong Kong SAR
CHINA
Tel. +852 3506 6830
Fax +832 2385 2455
jkcchan@ha.org.hk

Dr Herbert CHEN
Department of Surgery
University of Alabama at Birmingham
1808 7th Avenue South
Suite 502
Birmingham AL 35233
USA
Tel. +1 205 934 3333
herbchen@uab.edu

Dr Liang CHENG
Department of Pathology
Indiana University School of Medicine
350 West 11th Street, Room 4010
Indianapolis IN 46202-4108
USA
Tel. +1 317 491 6442
Fax +1 317 491 6419
lcheng@iupui.edu; liang_cheng@yahoo.com

Dr Rebecca D. CHERNOCK
Department of Pathology & Immunology
Washington University School of Medicine
660 South Euclid Avenue, Campus Box 8118
St Louis MO 63110
USA
rchernock@path.wustl.edu

Dr Wah CHEUK
Department of Pathology
Queen Elizabeth Hospital
Gascoigne Road, Kowloon
Hong Kong SAR
CHINA
Tel. +852 3506 5739
Fax +852 2385 2455
cheuk_wah@hotmail.com

Dr John C. CHEVILLE
Dept of Laboratory Medicine and Pathology
Mayo Clinic
200 First Street Southwest
Rochester MN 55905
USA
Tel. +1 507 284 3867
Fax +1 507 284 1599
cheville.john@mayo.edu

Dr George P. CHROUSOS
Biomedical Research Foundation,
Academy of Athens
4 Soranou Ephessiou Street
Athens 115 27
GREECE
Tel. +30 21 0 659 7546
Fax +30 21 0 659 7545
chrousog@mail.nih.gov;
chrousge@med.uoa.gr; chrousos@gmail.com

Dr Khoon Leong CHUAH
Department of Pathology
Tan Tock Seng Hospital
11 Jalan Tan Tock Seng
Singapore 308433
SINGAPORE
gzzckl@singnet.com.sg

Dr Stefan COSTINEAN
Department of Pathology
University of Nebraska Medical Center
S 42nd Street & Emile Street
Omaha NE 68198
USA
Tel. +1 402 559 6106
stefan.costinean@unmc.edu;
scostinean@yahoo.de

Dr Anne COUVELARD#
Department of Pathology
Bichat Hospital, AP-HP
46 Rue Henri Huchard
75877 Paris Cedex 18
FRANCE
Tel. +33 1 40 25 80 12
Fax +33 1 40 25 80 00
anne.couvelard@aphp.fr

Dr Ronald R. de KRIJGER*
Department of Pathology
Josephine Nefkens Institute, Room Be222
Erasmus MC, University Medical Center
3000 CA Rotterdam PO Box 2040
THE NETHERLANDS
Tel. +31 10 408 7901
Fax +31 10 408 9487
r.dekrijger@erasmusmc.nl,
r.dekrijger@rdgg.nl

Dr Gonzague de PINIEUX
Service d'Anatomie et
Cytologie Pathologiques
Trousseau Hospital
CHRU de Tours
Avenue de la République
37044 Tours
FRANCE
Tel. +33 2 34 38 94 17
gonzague.dubouexic@univ-tours.fr

Dr Ronald A. DeLELLIS
Dept of Pathology and Laboratory Medicine
Alpert Medical School, Brown University
Rhode Island Hospital
593 Eddy Street
Providence RI 02903
USA
Tel. +1 401 444 4483
ronald_delellis@brown.edu;
ron.delellis@gmail.com; rdelellis@lifespan.org

Dr Karl Michael DERWAHL
St. Hedwig Hospital Berlin
Große Hamburger Str. 5-11
10115 Berlin
GERMANY
m.burkard@alexianer.de;
k.derwahl@alexianer.de

Dr David M. DORFMAN
Department of Hematology
Brigham and Women's Hospital and
Harvard Medical School
75 Francis Street
Boston MA 02215
USA
Tel. +1 617 732 7518
Fax +1 617 731 4872
ddorfman@partners.org

Dr Rossella ELISEI#
Endocrine Unit
Dept of Clinical and Experimental Medicine
University of Pisa
Via Paradisa 2
56124 Pisa
ITALY
rossella.elisei@med.unipi.it

Dr Adel K. EL-NAGGAR*
University of Texas
MD Anderson Cancer Center
1515 Holcombe Boulevard, Unit 085
Houston TX 77030
USA
Tel. +1 713 792 3109
Fax +1 713 745 1105
anaggar@mdanderson.org

Dr Catarina ELOY
Department of Pathology
IPATIMUP / Porto Medical School
Rua Júlio Amaral de Carvalho, 45
4200-135 Porto
PORTUGAL
Tel. +351 225 570 700
Fax +351 225 570 799
celoy@ipatimup.pt;
catarinaeloy@hotmail.com

Dr Charis ENG
Genomic Medicine Institute
Cleveland Clinic Main Campus
Mail Code: NE50
9500 Euclid Avenue
Cleveland OH 44195
USA
Tel. +1 216 636 1768
engc@ccf.org

Dr Jonathan I. EPSTEIN
Department of Pathology
Johns Hopkins Medical Institutions
Weinberg Building, Room 2242
401 North Broadway
Baltimore MD 21231-2410
USA
Tel. +1 410 955 5043
Fax +1 443 287 3818
jepstein@jhmi.edu

Dr Lori A. ERICKSON
Dept of Laboratory Medicine and Pathology
Mayo Clinic
200 First Street Southwest
Rochester MN 55905
USA
erickson.lori@mayo.edu

Dr Vincenzo EUSEBI
Department of Pathology
University of Bologna
Ospedale Bellaria, Via Altura 3
40139 Bologna
ITALY
vincenzo.eusebi@unibo.it

Dr Harry L. EVANS
Division of Anatomic Pathology
Department of Surgical Pathology
University of Texas
MD Anderson Cancer Center
1515 Holcombe Boulevard, Box 0085
Houston TX 77030
USA
hevans@mdanderson.org

Dr Fabio FACCHETTI
Department of Pathology
University of Brescia – Spedali Civili Brescia
Piazzale Spedali Civili, 1
25123 Brescia
ITALY
Tel. +39 30 3995 426
Fax +39 30 3995 377
fabio.facchetti@unibs.it

Dr Guido FADDA
Department of Anatomic Pathology
Università Cattolica
Largo Francesco Vito 1
00168 Roma
ITALY
Tel. +39 06 3015 4433
guido.fadda@unicatt.it

Dr James A. FAGIN#
Department of Endocrinology
Memorial Sloan Kettering Cancer Center
1275 York Avenue
New York NY 10065
USA
faginj@mskcc.org

Dr William C. FAQUIN
Department of Pathology
Massachusetts General Hospital
55 Fruit Street, Warren 219
Boston MA 02114
USA
Tel. +1 617 573 3957
wfaquin@partners.org

Dr Giovanni FELLEGARA#
Department of Pathology
Centro Diagnostico Italiano
Via Simone Saint Bon 20
20147 Milano
ITALY
Tel. +39 02 4831 7788
giovanni.fellegara@cdi.it

Dr Judith A. FERRY
Department of Pathology
Massachusetts General Hospital
55 Fruit Street
Boston MA 02114
USA
Tel. +1 617 726 4826
Fax +1 617 726 9312
jferry@partners.org

Dr Cyril FISHER
Department of Histopathology
Royal Marsden Hospital
203 Fulham Road
London SW3 6JJ
UNITED KINGDOM
Tel. +44 780 82631
Fax +44 780 82578
cyrilfisher@gmail.com

Dr William D. FOULKES
Department of Human Genetics
McGill University
1001 Boulevard Décarie
Montreal QC H4A 3J1
CANADA
Tel. +1 514 451 1227
Fax +1 514 412 4296
william.foulkes@mcgill.ca

Dr Kaarle O. FRANSSILA
Department of Pathology
University of Helsinki
PO Box 21
00014 Helsinki
FINLAND
Tel. +358 40 551 7035
kaarle.franssila@kolumbus.fi

Dr Larissa V. FURTADO
Department of Pathology
University of Chicago Medicine
5841 South Maryland Avenue
Room N-305, MC 1089
Chicago IL 60637
USA
Tel. +1 773 702 2980
Fax +1 773 834 3449
larissa.furtado@hsc.utah.edu

Dr Kim R. GEISINGER
Department of Pathology
University of Mississippi Medical Center
2500 North State Street
Jackson MS 39216
USA
Tel. +1 601 984 1530
Fax +1 601 984 1531
krgeisin@yahoo.com

Dr Ronald A. GHOSSEIN
Department of Pathology
Memorial Sloan Kettering Cancer Center
1275 York Avenue
New York NY 10021
USA
ghossein@mskcc.org;
ghosseir@mskcc.org

Dr Anthony GILL*
Department of Anatomical Pathology
Royal North Shore Hospital
Reserve Road
NSW 2065 St Leonards
AUSTRALIA
Tel. +61 2 9926 4399
Fax +61 2 9926 4084
affgill@med.usyd.edu.au

Dr Thomas J. GIORDANO*#
Department of Pathology
University of Michigan Health System
1500 East Medical Center Drive
Ann Arbor MI 48109
USA
Tel. +1 734 615 4470
Fax +1 734 763 4851
giordano@umich.edu

Dr Dario GIUFFRIDA
Division of Medical Oncology
Istituto Oncologico del Mediterraneo
Via Penninazzo 7
95037 Viagrande CT
ITALY
Tel. +39 957 895 000
Fax +39 957 901 400
giuffridadario@alice.it

Dr Ashley GROSSMAN*#
Oxford Centre for Diabetes, Endocrinology &
Metabolism
University of Oxford
Churchill Hospital, Headington
Oxford OX3 7LE
UNITED KINGDOM
Tel. +44 1865 857 308
Fax +44 1865 857 311
ashley.grossman@ocdem.ox.ac.uk

Dr Philip Ian HAIGH
Department of Surgery
Kaiser Permanente Los Angeles
Medical Center
4760 West Sunset Boulevard
Los Angeles CA 90027
USA
Tel. +1 323 783 5674
Fax +1 323 783 8747
philip.i.haigh@kp.org

Dr Pascal HAMMEL#
Department of Digestive Oncology
Hôpital Beaujon
Assistance Publique
Hôpitaux de Paris, AP-HP
100 Boulevard du Général Leclerc
92110 Clichy
FRANCE
Tel. +33 1 40 87 56 14
pascal.hammel@bjn.aphp.fr

Dr Ian D. HAY
Division of Endocrinology, Diabetes,
Metabolism, and Nutrition
Mayo Clinic
200 First Street Southwest
Rochester MN 55905
USA
Tel. +1 507 266 3769
Fax +1 507 284 5745
hay.ian@mayo.edu

Dr Geoffrey N. HENDY
Department of Experimental Therapeutics
and Metabolism, Research Institute of McGill
University Health Centre, Room EM1.3226
RI-MUHC Glen Site, 1001 Boulevard Décarie
Montreal QC H4A 3J1
CANADA
Tel. +1 514 934 1934 ext. 35165
Fax +1 514 933 8784
geoffrey.hendy@mcgill.ca

Dr Ralph H. HRUBAN
Department of Pathology
Johns Hopkins University School of Medicine
600 North Wolfe Street, Carnegie 415
Baltimore MD 21287-6417
USA
Tel. +1 410 955 9790
Fax +1 410 955 0394
rhruban@jhmi.edu

Dr Jennifer L. HUNT
Department of Pathology
University of Arkansas for Medical Sciences
4301 West Markham Street, Mail Slot 517
Little Rock AR 72205
USA
Tel. +1 501 686 5170
Fax +1 501 296 1184
jlhunt@uams.edu; jhunt2@uams.edu

Dr Elaine S. JAFFE
Laboratory of Pathology, Center for Cancer
Research, National Cancer Institute
Building 10, Room 3S 235
10 Center Drive, MSC-1500
Bethesda MD 20892-1500
USA
Tel. +1 301 480 8040
Fax +1 301 480 8089
ejaffe@mail.nih.gov

Dr Pierre-Alexandre JUST
Pathology Department
AP-HP, Hôpitaux Universitaires Paris-Centre
Université Paris Descartes, Hôpital Cochin
27 Rue du Faubourg Saint-Jacques
75679 Paris
FRANCE
Tel. +33 1 58 41 14 62
pierre-alexandre.just@cch.aphp.fr

Dr Kennichi KAKUDO*
Department of Pathology
Nara Hospital
Kindai University Faculty of Medicine
1248-1 Otoda-cho
Ikoma-shi, Nara-ken 630-0293
JAPAN
Tel. +81 743 77 0880 (090 9709 8632)
Fax +81 743 77 0890
kakudo@thyroid.jp

Dr Klaus KASERER
Labor Kaserer & Salzer OG
Fachärzte für Pathologie
Reisnerstr. 5, Stiege 3, TOP II
1030 Wien
AUSTRIA
Tel. +43 1 712 58 04
Fax +43 1 714 01 56
office@labor-kaserer.at;
kaserer@labor-kaserer.at

Dr Ryohei KATOH
Department of Pathology
University of Yamanashi
1110 Shimokato
Chuo-shi, Yamanashi-ken 409-3898
JAPAN
Tel. +81 55 273 9529
Fax +81 55 273 9534
rkatoh@yamanashi.ac.jp

Dr Akira KAWASHIMA
Department of Radiology
Mayo Clinic
13400 East Shea Boulevard
Scottsdale AZ 85259
USA
Tel. +1 480 342 0898
Fax +1 480 301 4303
kawashima.akira@mayo.edu

Dr Electron KEBEBEW
Endocrine Oncology Branch
National Institutes of Health
Building 10, Hatfield CRC, Room 4-5952
Bethesda MD 20892
USA
Tel. +1 301 496 5049
Fax +1 301 402 1788
kebebewe@mail.nih.gov

Dr Na Rae KIM
Department of Pathology
Gachon University Gil Medical Center
21 Namdong-daero,
774 Beon-gil, Namdong-gu
Incheon 21565
REPUBLIC OF KOREA
Tel. +82 32 460 3073
Fax +82 32 460 2394
clara_nrk@gilhospital.com

Dr Noriko KIMURA*
Dept of Clinical Research, Pathology Division
National Hospital Organization
Hakodate Hospital
18-16 Kawahara-cho
Hakodate-shi Hokkaido 041-8512
JAPAN
Tel. +81 138 51 6281
Fax +81 138 30 1020
kimura-path@hnh.hosp.go.jp

Dr Lawrence S. KIRSCHNER#
Dept of Internal Medicine - Endocrinology
Ohio State University College of Medicine
579 McCampbell Hall
1581 Dodd Drive
Columbus OH 43210
USA
Tel. +1 614 685 9170
Fax +1 614 293 5264
lawrence.kirschner@osumc.edu

Dr David S. KLIMSTRA*#
Department of Pathology
Memorial Sloan Kettering Cancer Center
1275 York Avenue
New York NY 10065
USA
Tel. +1 212 639 8410
Fax +1 212 772 8521
klimstrd@mskcc.org

Dr Günter KLÖPPEL*#
Department of Pathology
Technical University Munich
Ismaninger Str. 22
81675 Munich
GERMANY
Tel. +49 894 140 4161
Fax +49 894 140 4865
guenter.kloeppel@alumni.uni-kiel.de;
guenter.kloeppel@tum.de

Dr Christian A. KOCH
University of Mississippi Medical Center
2500 North State Street
Jackson MS 39216
USA
Tel. +1 601 815 2005
ckoch@umc.edu

Dr Paul KOMMINOTH*
Institute of Pathology
Stadtspital Triemli
Birmensdorferstrasse 497
8063 Zurich
SWITZERLAND
Tel. +41 44 416 53 00
Fax +41 44 416 53 99
paul.komminoth@triemli.zuerich.ch

Dr Tetsuo KONDO
Department of Pathology
University of Yamanashi
1110 Shimokato
Chuo-shi, Yamanashi-ken 409-3898
JAPAN
Tel. +81 55 273 9529
Fax +81 55 273 9534
ktetsuo@yamanashi.ac.jp

Dr George KONTOGEORGOS*
Department of Pathology
G. Gennimatas Athens General Hospital
KOFKA Building, 1st floor
154 Messogion Avenue
Athens 115 27
GREECE
Tel. +30 21 0 778 4302
Fax +30 21 0 770 5980
gkonto@med.uoa.gr

Dr Márta KORBONITS#
Department of Endocrinology
Barts and The London School of
Medicine and Dentistry
Queen Mary University of London
Charterhouse Square
London EC1M 6BQ
UNITED KINGDOM
m.korbonits@qmul.ac.uk

Dr Kalman KOVACS
Dept of Laboratory Medicine and
Pathobiology
St. Michael's Hospital
30 Bond Street
Toronto ON M5B 1W8
CANADA
Tel. +1 416 864 5858
Fax +1 416 864 5648
kovacsk@smh.toronto.on.ca

Dr Stefano LA ROSA*
Service of Clinical Pathology
Lausanne University Hospital
Institute of Pathology
25, rue du Bugnon
1011 Lausanne
SWITZERLAND
Tel. +41 21 314 71 62
Fax +41 21 314 72 05
stefano.larosa@chuv.ch

Dr Ernest LACK
Joint Pathology Center
606 Stephen Sitter Avenue
Building 606
Silver Spring MD 20910
USA
Tel. +1 301 295 5652
Fax +1 301 295 5675
ernest.lack.ctr@mail.mil

Dr Alfred King Yin LAM
Department of Pathology
Griffith University School of Medicine
Gold Coast Campus
QLD 4222 Gold Coast
AUSTRALIA
Tel. +61 7 5678 0718
Fax +61 7 5687 6797
a.lam@griffith.edu.au

Dr Janez LAMOVEC
Department of Pathology
Institute of Oncology
Zaloška Cesta 2
1000 Ljubljana
SLOVENIA
jlamovec@onko-i.si

Dr Catharina LARSSON
Department of Oncology-Pathology
Karolinska Institutet
Karolinska University Hospital-
Solna R8:04
171 76 Stockholm
SWEDEN
Tel. +46 8 517 739 30
catharina.larsson@ki.se

Dr Sigurd F. LAX
Department of Pathology
Landeskrankenhaus Graz Süd-West,
Standort West
Göstinger Str. 22
8020 Graz
AUSTRIA
Tel. +43 316 5466 5502
Fax +43 316 5466 5504
sigurd.lax@kages.at

Dr Virginia LiVOLSI*#
Dept of Pathology and Laboratory Medicine
University of Pennsylvania Medical Center
3400 Spruce Street, Founders 6-040
Philadelphia PA 19104
USA
Tel. +1 215 662 6544
Fax +1 215 662 7042
linus@mail.med.upenn.edu

Dr Ricardo V. LLOYD*
Dept of Pathology and Laboratory Medicine
University of Wisconsin
School of Medicine and Public Health
600 Highland Avenue
Madison WI 53792-8550
USA
Tel. +1 608 265 4377
Fax +1 608 265 6215
rvlloyd@wisc.edu

Dr M. Beatriz S. LOPES*
Department of Pathology (Neuropathology)
University of Virginia Health System
1215 Lee Street, Box 800214 – HSC
Charlottesville VA 22908-0214
USA
Tel. +1 434 924 9175
Fax +1 434 924 9177
msl2e@virginia.edu

Dr Xavier MATIAS-GUIU
Department of Pathology
Hospital Universitari Arnau de Vilanova
Av. Alcalde Rovira Roure, 80
25198 Lleida
SPAIN
Tel. +34 973 705 340
fjmatiasguiu.lleida.ics@gencat.cat

Dr Akira MATSUNO
Department of Neurosurgery
Teikyo University School of Medicine
2-11-1 Kaga, Itabashi-ku
Tokyo 173-8605
JAPAN
Tel. +81 3 3964 1211
Fax +81 3 5375 1716
akirakun@med.teikyo-u.ac.jp

Dr L. Jeffrey MEDEIROS
Department of Hematopathology
University of Texas
MD Anderson Cancer Center
1515 Holcombe Boulevard
Houston TX 77030
USA
Tel. +1 713 745 2535
Fax +1 713 792 7273
ljmedeiros@mdanderson.org

Dr Maria J. MERINO
Laboratory of Pathology
Center for Cancer Research,
National Cancer Institute
Building 10, Room 2B 44
10 Center Drive
Bethesda MD 20892
USA
Tel. +1 301 496 3326
mjmerino@mail.nih.gov

Dr Ozgur METE
Department of Pathology
University Health Network
200 Elizabeth Street
Toronto ON M5G 2C4
CANADA
Tel. +1 416 340 3004
Fax +1 416 340 5517
ozgur.mete2@uhn.ca

Dr Jeffrey F. MOLEY
Department of Surgery
Washington University School of Medicine
660 South Euclid Avenue, Campus Box 8109
St Louis MO 63110
USA
Tel. +1 314 747 0064
Fax +1 314 747 1310
moleyj@wustl.edu

Dr Kathleen T. MONTONE
Dept of Pathology and Laboratory Medicine
Division of Surgical Pathology
Perelman School of Medicine
University of Pennsylvania
3400 Spruce Street, Founders 6-039
Philadelphia PA 19104
USA
kmontone@upenn.edu;
kathleen.montone@uphs.upenn.edu

Dr Hans MORREAU
Leiden University Medical Center
Albinusdreef 2, PO Box 9600, LI-Q
2300 RC Leiden
THE NETHERLANDS
Tel. +31 71 526 6630
j.morreau@lumc.nl

Dr Lois MULLIGAN
Dept of Pathology and Molecular Medicine
Queen's University
Botterell Hall, Room 315A
10 Stuart Street
Kingston ON K7L 3N6
CANADA
Tel. +1 613 533 6000 ext. 77475
Fax +1 613 533 6830
mulligal@queensu.ca

Dr Yuri E. NIKIFOROV*
Division of Molecular Genomic Pathology
University of Pittsburgh School of Medicine
Clinical Lab Building, 8th Floor, Room 8031
3477 Euler Way
Pittsburgh PA 15213
USA
Tel. +1 412 802 6083
Fax +1 412 802 6799
nikiforovye@upmc.edu

Dr Hiroshi NISHIOKA
Dept of Hypothalamic and Pituitary Surgery
Toranomon Hospital
2-2-2 Toranomon, Minato-ku
Tokyo 105-0001
JAPAN
Tel. +81 3 3588 1111
Fax +81 3 3582 7068
nishioka@tokyo-med.ac.jp

Dr Daisuke NONAKA
Department of Pathology
Christie NHS Foundation Trust
Wilmslow Road
Manchester M20 4BX
UNITED KINGDOM
Tel. +44 161 446 3277
Fax +44 161 446 3300
dnonaka@msn.com;
daisuke.nonaka@christie.nhs.uk

Dr Vania NOSÉ
Department of Pathology
Massachusetts General Hospital
55 Fruit Street, Warren 214
Boston MA 02114-2696
USA
Tel. +1 617 643 7201
vnose@mgh.harvard.edu

Dr Kjell ÖBERG
Department of Medical Sciences,
Endocrine Oncology
Uppsala University
Akademiska sjukhuset ing 40 5 tr
751 85 Uppsala
SWEDEN
Tel. +46 18 611 4917
Fax +46 70 425 0688
kjell.oberg@medsci.uu.se

Dr Hiroko OHGAKI*
Section of Molecular Pathology
International Agency for Research on Cancer
150 Cours Albert Thomas
69372 Lyon Cedex 08
FRANCE
Tel. +33 4 72 73 85 34
Fax +33 4 72 73 86 98
ohgaki@iarc.fr

Dr Nobuyuki OHIKE
Division of Pathology
Showa University Fujigaoka Hospital
1-30 Fujigaoka, Aoba-ku
Yokohama-shi, Kanagawa-ken 227-8501
JAPAN
Tel. +81 45 971 1151
Fax +81 45 972 6242
ohike@med.showa-u.ac.jp

Dr Josep ORIOLA
Sección de Genética Molecular
Centro de Diagnóstico Biomédico – CDB
Hospital Clinic
Carrer de Villarroel, 170
08036 Barcelona
SPAIN
Tel. +34 932 275 400
joriola@clinic.ub.es

Dr Robert Y. OSAMURA*
International University of Health and Welfare
(IUHW).Tokai University School of Medicine,
Department of Diagnostic Pathology
Nippon Kokan Hospital (NKK)
1-2-1 Kokan St. Kawasaki-ku
Kawasaki-city, Kanagawa
JAPAN
Tel. +81 44 333 5591
Fax +81 44 333 5599
osamura@iuhw.ac.jp

Dr Karel PACAK
Section on Medical Neuroendocrinology
National Institutes of Health
Building 10, Room 1-3140
10 Center Drive
Bethesda MD 20892
USA
Tel. +1 301 402 4592
karel@mail.nih.gov

Dr Thomas G. PAPATHOMAS
Department of Pathology
King's College Hospital NHS Foundation Trust
Denmark Hill
London SE5 9RS
UNITED KINGDOM
thomaspapathomas@nhs.net

Dr Mauro PAPOTTI*#
Department of Oncology
University of Turin
Via Santena 7
10126 Turin
ITALY
Tel. +39 011 633 4623
Fax +39 011 663 5267
mauro.papotti@unito.it

Dr Ralf PASCHKE
Division of Endocrinology and Metabolism,
Provincial Endocrine Tumour Team,
Richmond Road Diagnosis and Treatment
Centre (RRDTC)
1820 Richmond RD SW, Calgary AB T2T5C7
CANADA
Tel. +1 403 955 8969
Fax +1 403 955 8248
ralf.paschke@ucalgary.ca

Dr Natalia S. PELLEGATA
Institute of Pathology
Helmholtz Zentrum München
Deutsches Forschungszentrum für
Gesundheit und Umwelt (GmbH)
Ingolstädter Landstr. 1
85764 Neuherberg
GERMANY
Tel. +49 89 3187 2633
natalia.pellegata@helmholtz-muenchen.de

Dr Aurel PERREN
Institute of Pathology
University of Bern
Murtenstrasse 31
3010 Bern
SWITZERLAND
Tel. +41 31 632 32 22
Fax +41 31 632 49 95
aurel.perren@pathology.unibe.ch

Dr Simonetta PIANA
Pathology Unit
Arcispedale Santa Maria Nuova - IRCCS
Viale Risorgimento 80
42124 Reggio Emilia
ITALY
Tel. +39 522 295 919
Fax +39 522 296 954
piana.simonetta@asmn.re.it

Dr António E. PINTO
Department of Anatomical Pathology
Instituto Português de Oncologia de Lisboa,
Francisco Gentil
Rua Professor Lima Basto
Lisbon
PORTUGAL
aepinto@ipolisboa.min-saude.pt

Dr Manju L. PRASAD
Department of Pathology
Yale School of Medicine
200 South Frontage Road, PO Box 208070
New Haven CT 06520
USA
Tel. +1 203 785 4862
Fax +1 203 737 2922
manju.prasad@yale.edu

Dr Gregory W. RANDOLPH
Thyroid and Parathyroid Endocrine Surgery
Department of Otolaryngology
Massachusetts Eye and Ear Infirmary
243 Charles Street
Boston MA 02114
USA
Tel. +1 617 966 3707
Fax +1 617 573 3914
gregory.randolph@meei.harvard.edu

Dr Alberto RIGHI
Department of Pathology
Rizzoli Institute
Via di Barbiano 1/10
40136 Bologna
ITALY
Tel. +39 51 636 662
Fax +39 51 636 6592
alberto.righi@ior.it

Dr Guido RINDI#
Institute of Anatomic Pathology
Catholic University
Policlinico Agostino Gemelli
Largo Agostino Gemelli 8
00168 Roma
ITALY
Tel. +39 06 3015 5883
Fax +39 06 3015 7008
guido.rindi@unicatt.it

Dr Federico RONCAROLI
Department of Cellular Pathology
Division of Neuroscience and Experimental
Psychology
Salford Royal Hospital NHS Foundation Trust
Stott Lane
Salford – M6 8HD
UNITED KINGDOM
Tel. +44 161 206 2329
federico.roncaroli@manchester.ac.uk

Dr Juan ROSAI*#
Centro Diagnostico Italiano
Via Simone Saint Bon 20
20147 Milano
ITALY
Tel. +39 02 4831 7649
Fax +39 02 4831 7650
juan.rosai@cdi.it; rosai@cdi.it

Dr Fabio ROTONDO
Department of Laboratory Medicine
Division of Pathology
St. Michael's Hospital
30 Bond Street
Toronto ON M5B 1W8
CANADA
Tel. +1 416 864 6060 ext. 77216
Fax +1 416 864 5648
rotondof@smh.ca

Dr Brian ROUS*
National Cancer Registration Service,
Eastern Office
Victoria House, Capital Park
Fulbourn, Cambridge CB21 5XA
UNITED KINGDOM
Tel. +44 122 321 3625
Fax +44 122 321 3571
brian.rous@phe.gov.uk

Dr Aleš RYŠKA
Fingerland Department of Pathology
Charles University Faculty of Medicine
Faculty Hospital
500 05 Hradec Kralove
CZECH REPUBLIC
Tel. +420 495 833 748
Fax +420 495 832 004
ryskaa@lfhk.cuni.cz; ryskaale@fnhk.cz;
ryskaale@gmail.com

Dr Peter SADOW
Pathology Service
Massachusetts General Hospital
55 Fruit Street, Warren 219
Boston MA 02114
USA
Tel. +1 617 573 3157
Fax +1 617 573 3389
psadow@partners.org;
psadaw@mgh.harvard.edu

Dr Hironobu R. SASANO
Department of Pathology
Tohoku University School of Medicine
2-1 Seiryou-machi, Aoba-ku
Sendai-shi, Miyagi-ken 980-8575
JAPAN
Tel. +81 22 717 8050
Fax +81 22 273 5976
hsasano@patholo2.med.tohoku.ac.jp

Dr Aldo SCARPA
Department of Pathology
University and Hospital Trust of Verona
Policlinico GB Rossi
Piazzale Ludovico Antonio Scuro 10
37134 Verona
ITALY
Tel. +39 045 812 4043
Fax +39 045 812 7432
aldo.scarpa@univr.it

Dr Kurt W. SCHMID
Institute of Pathology and Neuropathology
University Hospital Essen
University Duisburg-Essen
Hufelandstr. 55
45147 Essen
GERMANY
Tel. +49 2 01 7 23 28 90
Fax +49 2 01 7 23 59 26
kw.schmid@uk-essen.de

Dr Arthur B. SCHNEIDER#
Section of Endocrinology
University of Illinois at Chicago
1819 West Polk Street (M/C 640)
Chicago IL 60612
USA
Tel. +1 312 996 6060
Fax +1 312 413 0437
abschnei@uic.edu

Dr Jean-Yves SCOAZEC
Department of Pathology
Gustave Roussy
114 Rue Édouard-Vaillant
94805 Villejuif
FRANCE
Tel. +33 1 42 11 44 11
Fax +33 1 42 11 52 80
jy.scoazec@gmail.com;
jean-yves.scoazec@gustaveroussy.fr

Dr Hiroyuki SHIMADA
Dept of Pathology and Laboratory Medicine
Children's Hospital Los Angeles
4650 Sunset Boulevard, MS 43
Los Angeles CA 90027
USA
Tel. +1 323 361 5813
Fax +1 323 361 8005
hshimada@chla.usc.edu

Dr Michio SHIMIZU
Diagnostic Pathology Center
Hakujikai Memorial Hospital
5-11-1 Shikahama, Adachi-ku
Tokyo 123-0864
JAPAN
Tel. +81 3 3899 1311
Fax +81 3 3855 2851
shimizu@hakujikai.org

Dr Bence SIPOS
Department of Pathology and Neuropathology
University Hospital Tübingen
Liebermeisterstr. 8
72076 Tübingen
GERMANY
Tel. +49 7071 298 0215
Fax +49 7071 292 991
bence.sipos@med.uni-tuebingen.de

Dr Robert SMALLRIDGE#
Mayo Clinic
4500 San Pablo Road
Jacksonville FL 322224
USA
Tel. +1 904 953 2392
smallridge.robert@mayo.edu

Dr Paula SOARES
IPATIMUP – Cancer Biology
Rua Júlio Amaral de Carvalho, 45
4200-135 Porto
PORTUGAL
Tel. +351 225 570 700
Fax +351 225 570 799
psoares@ipatimup.pt

Dr Manuel SOBRINHO SIMÕES*
Department of Pathology
Porto Medical Faculty / IPATIMUP
Rua Júlio Amaral de Carvalho, 45
4200-135 Porto
PORTUGAL
Tel. +351 225 570 700
Fax +351 225 570 799
ssimoes@ipatimup.pt

Dr Ernst J.M. SPEEL
Department of Pathology
Maastricht University Medical Center
P. Debyelaan 25
PO Box 5800
6229 HX Maastricht
THE NETHERLANDS
Tel. +31 43 387 4614
Fax +31 43 387 6613

Dr Constantine A. STRATAKIS
Eunice Kennedy Shriver National Institute
of Child Health and Human Development
Building 31, Room 2A46 MSC2425
Bethesda MD 20892
USA
Tel. +1 301 594 5984
Fax +1 301 480 6480
stratakc@mail.nih.gov; nichdsd@mail.nih.gov;
stratakc@cc1.nichd.nih.gov

Dr Iwao SUGITANI
Department of Endocrine Surgery
Nippon Medical School
Graduate School of Medicine
1-1-5 Sendagi, Bunkyo-ku
Tokyo 113-8603
JAPAN
Tel. +81 3 5814 6219
Fax +81 3 5685 0985
isugitani@nms.ac.jp

Dr Luis V. SYRO
Department of Neurosurgery
Hospital Pablo Tobón Uribe and
Clinica Medellín
Carrera 65 B # 30 – 95. Cons 220
Medellín 050030
COLOMBIA
Tel. +57 4 444 6152 Ext 7220
lvsyro@une.net.co

Dr Giovanni TALLINI*
Scuola di Medicina e Chirurgia
Anatomia Patologica, Università di Bologna
Ospedale Bellaria, Via Altura 3
40139 Bologna
ITALY
Tel. +39 51 622 5757
Fax +39 51 622 5759
giovanni.tallini@ausl.bo.it;
giovanni.tallini@unibo.it

Dr Lester D.R. THOMPSON
Department of Pathology, Southern California
Permanente Medical Group
Woodland Hills Medical Center
5601 De Soto Avenue
Woodland Hills CA 91365
USA
Tel. +1 818 719 2613
Fax +1 818 719 2309
lester.d.thompson@kp.org

Dr Tarik TIHAN
Neuropathology Division
University of California, San Francisco
505 Parnassus Avenue, Room M551
San Francisco CA 94143-0102
USA
Tel. +1 415 476 5236
Fax +1 415 476 7963
tarik.tihan@ucsf.edu

Dr Arthur S. TISCHLER*
Department of Pathology and Laboratory
Medicine
Tufts MedicalCenter
800 Washington Street, Box 802
Boston MA 02111
USA
Tel. +1 617 636 1038
Fax +1 617 636 8302
atischler@tuftsmedicalcenter.org

Dr Frédérique TISSIER
Service d'Anatomie Pathologique 1
Hôpital Universitaire de la Pitié-Salpêtrière
AP-HP, Université Pierre-et-Marie-Curie
83 Boulevard de l'Hôpital
75651 Paris Cedex 13
FRANCE
Tel. +33 1 42 17 77 89
Fax +33 1 42 17 77 77
frederique.tissier@psl.aphp.fr

Dr Jacqueline TROUILLAS*
Unité INSERM 1028: Laboratoire d'Histologie
et Embryologie Moleculaires
Faculté de Medecine Lyon Est
Rue Guillaume Paradin
69372 Lyon Cedex 8
FRANCE
Tel. +33 4 78 77 86 54
Fax +33 4 78 77 86 52
jacqueline.trouillas@univ-lyon1.fr

Dr William Y.W. TSANG
Department of Pathology
Queen Elizabeth Hospital
Gascoigne Road, Kowloon
Hong Kong SAR
CHINA
Tel. +852 3506 8888
tsangyw@ha.org.hk; wywtsang@gmail.com

Dr R. Michael TUTTLE
Endocrinology Service
Memorial Sloan Kettering Cancer Center
1275 York Avenue
New York NY 10021
USA
Tel. +1 646 888 2716
Fax +1 646 888 2700
tuttlem@mskcc.org

Dr Philippe VIELH
Département de Pathologie
Laboratoire National de Santé
1 Rue Louis Rech
L – 3555 Dudelange
LUXEMBOURG
Tel. +352 2810 0346
Fax +352 2810 0342
philippe.vielh@lns.etat.lu

Dr Marco VOLANTE#
Department of Oncology
University of Turin
San Luigi Hospital
Regione Gonzole 10
10043 Orbassano TO
ITALY
Tel. +39 011 670 5464
Fax +39 011 902 6753
marco.volante@unito.it

Dr Steven G. WAGUESPACK
Endocrine Neoplasia & Hormonal Disorders
University of Texas
MD Anderson Cancer Center
1400 Pressler Street, Unit 1461, FCT12.5030
Houston TX 77030-3722
USA
Tel. +1 713 792 2841
Fax +1 713 794 4065
swagues@mdanderson.org

Dr Paul E. WAKELY, Jr
Department of Pathology
Ohio State University Wexner Medical Center
405 Doan Hall
410 West 10th Avenue
Columbus OH 43210
USA
Tel. +1 614 293 9232
Fax +1 614 293 7626
paul.wakely@osumc.edu

Dr Lee S. WEINSTEIN
Metabolic Diseases Branch, National Institute
of Diabetes and Digestive and Kidney
Diseases, National Institutes of Health
10 Center Drive, Building 10, Room 8C101
Bethesda MD 20814
USA
Tel. +1 301 402 2923
Fax +1 301 402 0374
leew@mail.nih.gov

Dr Lawrence M. WEISS
Clarient Pathology Services, Inc.
31 Columbia
Aliso Viejo CA 92656
USA
Tel. +1 626 227 6438
weiss11111@gmail.com

Dr Bruce M. WENIG
Department of Pathology
Moffitt Cancer Center
12902 Magnolia Drive
Tampa, FL 33612
USA
Tel. +1 813 745 2213
Fax +1 813 745 8479
bruce.wenig@moffitt.org

Dr William H. WESTRA
Head and Neck Pathology Laboratory
Johns Hopkins School of Medicine
Weinberg Building, Room 2242
401 North Broadway
Baltimore MD 21231
USA
Tel. +1 410 614 3964
Fax +1 410 955 0115
wwestra@jhmi.edu

Dr Mark R. WICK
Department of Pathology
University of Virginia Health System
PO Box 800214
1215 Lee Street
Charlottesville VA 22908-0214
USA
mrw9c@virginia.edu; mrwick1@usa.net

Dr Michelle D. WILLIAMS*
Department of Pathology
MD Anderson Cancer Center
University of Texas
1515 Holcombe Boulevard, Unit 085
Houston TX 77030
USA
Tel. +1 713 794 1765
Fax +1 713 563 1848
mdwillia@mdanderson.org

Dr Christian WITTEKIND
University Hospital Leipzig
Pathology Institute
Liebigstr. 26
04103 Leipzig
GERMANY
Tel. +49 341 971 5000
Fax +49 341 971 5009
christian.wittekind@medizin.uni-leipzig.de

Dr Andrew WOTHERSPOON
Department of Histopathology
Royal Marsden Hospital
Fulham Road
London SW3 6JJ
UNITED KINGDOM
andrew.wotherspoon@rmh.nhs.uk

Dr Shozo YAMADA#
Dept of Hypothalamic and Pituitary Surgery
Toranomon Hospital
2-2-2 Toranomon, Minato-ku
Tokyo 105-0001
JAPAN
Tel. +81 3 3588 1111
Fax +81 3 3582 7068
syamadays11@hotmail.com

Dr William F. YOUNG, Jr
Division of Endocrinology, Diabetes,
Metabolism, and Nutrition
Mayo Clinic
200 First Street Southwest
Rochester MN 55905
USA
Tel. +1 507 284 2511
Fax +1 507 284 2191
wyoung@mayo.edu

Dr Giuseppe ZAMBONI
Department of Pathology, University of Verona
Sacro Cuore Don Calabria Hospital
Via Don A. Sempreboni 5
37024 Negrar VR
ITALY
Tel. +39 045 6013 415
Fax +39 045 6013 921
giuseppe.zamboni@univr.it;
giuseppe.zamboni@sacrocuore.it

Declaration of interests

Dr **Burke** reports being a partner in Pathology Services Incorporated in Berkeley CA, USA.

Dr **Couvelard** reports receiving personal consulting fees from Ipsen and research support and travel support from Novartis.

Dr **Elisei** reports receiving personal consulting fees from Bayer, AstraZeneca, Exelixis, Genzyme, and Eisai and personal speaking fees from Bayer, Genzyme, Eisai, and Exelixis. Dr Elisei reports receiving travel support from Bayer and Genzyme.

Dr **Fagin** reports having been on an advisory panel for Quest Diagnostics.

Dr **Fellegara** reports having received personal consulting fees from Veracyte.

Dr **Giordano** reports being on a clinical advisory board for PDI/Interpace Diagnostics. Dr Giordano reports having been on a clinical advisory board for, and having received research support and personal honoraria from, Asuragen. Dr Giordano reports holding intellectual property rights for the gene expression profile of papillary thyroid carcinoma, patented by the University of Michigan.

Dr **Grossman** reports receiving personal speaking fees from, and being on advisory boards for, Ipsen, Novartis, HRA Pharma, and Shire.

Dr **Hammel** reports receiving personal consulting fees from Celgene and having received personal consulting fees from AstraZeneca. Dr Hammel reports receiving travel support from Merck Serono and research support from Erytech.

Dr **Kirschner** reports holding a patent for the gene that causes Carney complex.

Dr **Klimstra** reports having received personal consulting fees from Wren Laboratories and personal speaking fees from Novartis.

Dr **Klöppel** reports receiving personal speaking fees from Novartis and Ipsen.

Dr **Korbonits** reports receiving research support and personal speaking fees from Pfizer.

Dr **LiVolsi** reports receiving personal consulting fees from Veracyte.

Dr **Papotti** reports being on an advisory board for Eli Lilly and having been on advisory boards for Clovis Oncology and Boehringer Ingelheim. Dr Papotti reports having received research support from Novartis.

Dr **Rindi** reports receiving personal speaking fees from Ipsen and having received personal speaking fees from Novartis. Dr Rindi reports having received personal consulting fees from AAA SA, Bracco Imaging, and Ipsen.

Dr **Rosai** reports receiving personal consulting fees from Veracyte.

Dr **Schneider** reports having received personal consulting fees from Kirkland & Ellis LLP.

Dr **Smallridge** reports that the Mayo Clinic receives non-financial research support, through the National Cancer Institute (NCI) cooperative group Alliance, from Daiichi Sankyo.

Dr **Volante** reports that the Department of Oncology at the University of Turin receives research support from Novartis. Dr Volante reports receiving personal speaking fees from Novartis and Teijin Pharma.

Dr **Yamada** reports receiving personal honoraria from Pfizer, Eli Lilly Japan, and Novartis.

IARC/WHO Committee for the International Classification of Diseases for Oncology (ICD-O)

Dr Freddie BRAY
Section of Cancer Surveillance
International Agency for Research on Cancer
150 Cours Albert Thomas
69372 Lyon Cedex 08
FRANCE
Tel. +33 4 72 73 84 53
Fax +33 4 72 73 86 96
brayf@iarc.fr

Mrs April FRITZ
A. Fritz and Associates, LLC
21361 Crestview Road
Reno NV 89521
USA
Tel. +1 775 636 7243
Fax +1 888 891 3012
april@afritz.org

Dr Robert JAKOB
Data Standards and Informatics
Information, Evidence and Research
World Health Organization (WHO)
20 Avenue Appia
1211 Geneva 27
SWITZERLAND
Tel. +41 22 791 58 77
Fax +41 22 791 48 94
jakobr@who.int

Dr Paul KLEIHUES
Faculty of Medicine
University of Zurich
Pestalozzistrasse 5
8032 Zurich
SWITZERLAND
Tel. +41 44 362 21 10
Fax +41 44 251 06 65
kleihues@pathol.uzh.ch

Dr Günter KLÖPPEL
Department of Pathology
Technical University Munich
Ismaninger Str. 22
81675 Munich
GERMANY
Tel. +49 894 140 4161
Fax +49 894 140 4865
guenter.kloeppel@alumni.uni-kiel.de;
guenter.kloeppel@tum.de

Dr Ricardo V. LLOYD
Dept of Pathology and Laboratory Medicine
University of Wisconsin
School of Medicine and Public Health
600 Highland Avenue
Madison WI 53792-8550
USA
Tel. +1 608 265 4377
Fax +1 608 265 6215
rvlloyd@wisc.edu

Dr Hiroko OHGAKI
Section of Molecular Pathology
International Agency for Research on Cancer
150 Cours Albert Thomas
69372 Lyon Cedex 08
FRANCE
Tel. +33 4 72 73 85 34
Fax +33 4 72 73 86 98
ohgaki@iarc.fr

Dr Marion PIÑEROS
Section of Cancer Surveillance
International Agency for Research on Cancer
150 Cours Albert Thomas
69372 Lyon Cedex 08
FRANCE
Tel. +33 4 72 73 84 18
Fax +33 4 72 73 86 96
pinerosm@iarc.fr

Dr Brian ROUS
National Cancer Registration Service,
Eastern Office
Victoria House, Capital Park
Fulbourn, Cambridge CB21 5XA
UNITED KINGDOM
Tel. +44 122 321 3625
Fax +44 122 321 3571
brian.rous@phe.gov.uk

Dr Leslie H. SOBIN
Frederick National Laboratory for
Cancer Research, Cancer Human Biobank
National Cancer Institute
6110 Executive Boulevard, Suite 250
Rockville MD 20852
USA
Tel. +1 301 443 7947
Fax +1 301 402 9325
leslie.sobin@nih.gov

Sources of figures and tables

Sources of figures

1.01	Osamura RY
1.02	Osamura RY
1.03 A–C	Osamura RY
1.04 A–C	Osamura RY
1.05 A–C	Osamura RY
1.06	Osamura RY
1.07	Osamura RY
1.08	Osamura RY
1.09	Modified from Pituitary, Pit-1 positive alpha-subunit positive nonfunctioning human pituitary adenomas: a dedifferentiated GH cell lineage? 1: 1999, pp. 269–271, RY Osamura, S Tahara, K Komatsubara, Y Itoh, H Kajiwara, R Kurotani, N Sanno, A Teramoto. With permission of Springer.
1.10 A,B	Yamada S
1.11 A–C	Mete O
1.12 A–D	Mete O
1.13 A–C	Mete O
1.14 A,B	Grossman A
1.15 A,B	Mete O
1.16 A	Nosé V
1.16 B,C	Mete O
1.17 A–C	Reprinted with permission from Mete O, Asa SL (2012). Clinicopathological correlations in pituitary adenomas. Brain Pathol. 22:443–53.
1.18 A,B	Nosé V
1.19 A,B	Nosé V
1.20	Osamura RY
1.21 A–C	Osamura RY
1.22 A,B	Yamada S
1.23 A,B	Mete O
1.24 A–C	Mete O
1.25 A,B	Mete O
1.26 A–C	Mete O
1.27	Reprinted by permission from Macmillan Publishers Ltd: Nat Genet. Reincke M, Sbiera S, Hayakawa A, Theodoropoulou M, Osswald A, Beuschlein F, et al. Mutations in the deubiquitinase gene USP8 cause Cushing's disease. 2015; 47(1):31–8. Copyright 2017.
1.28 A,B	Yamada S
1.29	Yamada S
1.30 A–C	Yamada S
1.31 A–D	Yamada S
1.32	Nishioka H
1.33	Nishioka H
1.34 A,B	Mete O
1.35 A	Erickson LA
1.35 B	Osamura RY
1.36	Erickson LA
1.37 A–C	Kontogeorgos G
1.38 A–C	Reprinted with permission

	from Erickson D, Scheithauer BW, Atkinson J, Horvath E, Kovacs K, Lloyd RV, Young WF Jr (2009). Silent subtype 3 pituitary adenoma: a clinicopathologic analysis of the Mayo Clinic experience. Clin Endocrinol (Oxf.) 71(1):92–9.
1.39	Faustini-Fustini M Pituitary Unit IRCCS Institute of Neurological Science of Bologna Bologna, Italy
1.40 A–C	Roncaroli F
1.41 A–C	Roncaroli F
1.42 A–C	Henry K Imperial College London Charing Cross Hospital Campus Department of Histopathology London, United Kingdom; and 23rd Congress of the European Society of Pathology, Helsinki 2011, with permission.
1.43 A,B	Roncaroli F
1.44	Kovacs K
1.45	Kovacs K
1.46	Tihan T
1.47	Kleihues P {1674} University of Zurich, Switzerland
1.48 A–C	Tihan T
1.48 D	Lopes MBS
1.48 E	Nishioka H
1.49	Nishioka H
1.50	Tihan T
1.51	Tihan T
1.52 A,B	Osamura RY
1.53 A,B	Osamura RY
1.54 A–E	Osamura RY
1.55	Kovacs K
1.56	Kovacs K
1.57	Lopes MBS
1.58	Lopes MBS
1.59	Chen L Dept. of Pathology Xuanwu Hospital Beijing, China
1.60 A,B	Roncaroli F
1.61 A–C	Yamada S
1.62 A	Lopes MBS
1.62 B,C	Mete O
1.63 A	Mete O
1.63 B	Lopes MBS
1.64	Lopes MBS
1.65 A	Tihan T
1.65 B	Lopes MBS
1.66	Lopes MBS
1.67 A–D	Lopes MBS
1.68 A–C	Lopes MBS
1.69 A–C	Lopes MBS
1.70	Osamura RY
1.71 A,B	Osamura RY
1.72 A	Tihan T
1.72 B,C	Lopes MBS

1.72 D	Tihan T
1.73 A,B	Osamura RY
1.74 A–C	Osamura RY
2.01	Derwahl KM
2.02	Nikiforov YE
2.03 A,B	Nikiforov YE
2.04 A–C	Nikiforov YE
2.05 A,B	Nikiforov YE
2.06	Nikiforov YE
2.07	Nikiforov YE
2.08	Nikiforov YE
2.09 A–C	Nikiforov YE
2.10	Nikiforov YE
2.11	Baloch ZW
2.12	Nikiforov YE
2.13 A	Carney JA
2.13 B,C	Volante M
2.14 A,B	Papotti M
2.15 A,B	Volante M
2.16 A,B	Tallini G
2.17 A,B	Tallini G
2.18	Fish S Dept. of Medicine Endocrinology Service Memorial Sloan Kettering Cancer Center New York NY, USA
2.19	Kakudo K
2.20	Williams MD
2.21 A–C	Nikiforov YE
2.22 A,B	Nikiforov YE
2.23 A–C	Nikiforov YE
2.24	Rosai J
2.25	Rosai J
2.26 A–D	Baloch ZW
2.27	Rosai J
2.28	Rosai J
2.29 A,B	Rosai J
2.30	Rosai J
2.31	Rosai J
2.32	Reprinted with permission from Rosai J, DeLellis RA, Carcangiu ML, Frable J, Tallini G (2015). Tumors of the thyroid and parathyroid glands. In: AFIP atlas of tumor pathology. Series 4, Fascicle 21. Washington DC: American Registry of Pathology Press.
2.33	Rosai J
2.34	Rosai J
2.35	Rosai J
2.36	Rosai J
2.37	Wenig BM
2.38	Rosai J
2.39 A,B	Baloch ZW
2.40 A,B	Baloch ZW
2.41	Baloch ZW
2.42 A,B	Baloch ZW
2.43 A	See above, 2.32
2.43 B	Piana S
2.44 A,B	Rosai J
2.45	Lloyd RV

2.46	Rosai J
2.47 A,B	Rosai J
2.48	Reprinted from Cell, Vol. 159, Issue 3, Cancer Genome Atlas Research Network, Integrated genomic characterization of papillary thyroid carcinoma, 2014:676–90, Copyright (2017), with permission from Elsevier.
2.49	See above, 2.48
2.50	Eloy C
2.51 A,B	Baloch ZW
2.52 A,B	Sadow P
2.53	Bartolazzi A
2.54	Bartolazzi A
2.55	Baloch ZW
2.56	Tallini G
2.57	Tallini G
2.58 A–D	Tallini G
2.59	Tallini G
2.60	Matias-Guiu X
2.61	Tallini G
2.62 A–C	Tallini G
2.62 D	Aubert S
2.63	Reprinted with permission from Volante M, Collini P, Nikiforov YE, et al. (2007). Poorly differentiated thyroid carcinoma: the Turin proposal for the use of uniform diagnostic criteria and an algorithmic diagnostic approach. Am J Surg Pathol. 31(8):1256–64.
2.64 A	Chernock RD
2.64 B	Aubert S
2.64 C	Chernock RD
2.65	El-Naggar AK
2.66	El-Naggar AK
2.67 A	Baloch ZW
2.67 B	Faquin WC
2.68 A–D	Williams MD
2.68 E	Tallini G
2.68 F	Williams MD
2.69	El-Naggar AK
2.70	Lam AKY
2.71	Carcangiu ML
2.72	Lam AKY
2.73 A	Matias-Guiu X
2.73 B	See above, 2.32
2.74 A	Baloch ZW
2.74 B	Baloch ZW
2.75	DeLellis RA
2.76	DeLellis RA
2.77	DeLellis RA
2.78	DeLellis RA
2.79	DeLellis RA
2.80	DeLellis RA
2.81 A,B	Al Ghuzlan A
2.82	Erickson LA
2.83	Erickson LA
2.84	Erickson LA
2.85	DeLellis RA
2.86	Erickson LA
2.87	DeLellis RA
2.88	Eusebi V
2.89	Tallini G
2.90	DeLellis RA
2.91 A–C	DeLellis RA
2.92	DeLellis RA
2.93	Volante M
2.94	Volante M
2.95 A,B	Volante M
2.96 A,B	Shimizu M

2.97 A–D	Volante M
2.98 A–C	Giordano TJ
2.99	This figure was published in Wenig B (2016). Atlas of head and neck pathology, 3rd ed. Figure 28-86, p. 1398. Copyright Elsevier (2017).
2.100	Cameselle Teijeiro JM
2.101	Cameselle Teijeiro JM
2.102	Cameselle Teijeiro JM
2.103	Cameselle Teijeiro JM
2.104	Wenig BM
2.105	Albores Saavedra J
2.106	Albores Saavedra J
2.107	Albores Saavedra J
2.108	Albores Saavedra J
2.109	Sobrinho Simões M
2.110	Cameselle Teijeiro JM
2.111	Cameselle Teijeiro JM
2.112	Chan JKC
2.113	Chan JKC
2.114 A–B	Chan JKC
2.115 A–D	Chan JKC
2.116	Kakudo K
2.117	Kakudo K
2.118	Kakudo K
2.119	Kakudo K
2.120	Kakudo K
2.121	Kakudo K
2.122	Kakudo K
2.123	Matias-Guiu X
2.124	Thompson LDR
2.125	Thompson LDR
2.126	Thompson LDR
2.127	Thompson LDR
2.128	Thompson LDR
2.129	Volante M
2.130	Wick MR
2.131 A,B	Wick MR
2.132 A,B	Wick MR
2.133 A	Ryška A
2.133 B,C	Wick MR
2.134 A–C	Wick MR
2.135 A,B	Wick MR
2.136	Thompson LDR
2.137	Thompson LDR
2.138	Thompson LDR
2.139	Thompson LDR
2.140	Thompson LDR
2.141	Thompson LDR
2.142	Thompson LDR
2.143	Reprinted with permission from Rodriguez I, Ayala E, Caballero C, De Miguel C, Matias-Guiu X, Cubilla AL, et al. (2001). Solitary fibrous tumor of the thyroid gland: report of seven cases. Am J Surg Pathol. 25(11):1424–8.
2.144	Cameselle Teijeiro JM
2.145	Cameselle Teijeiro JM
2.146	Cameselle Teijeiro JM
2.147	Cameselle Teijeiro JM
2.148 A	Thompson LDR
2.148 B	Chan JKC
2.149	Chan JKC
2.150	Chan JKC
2.151	Chan JKC
2.152 A,B	Thompson LDR
2.153	Chan JKC
2.154	Chan JKC
2.155	Chan JKC
2.156	Chan JKC

2.157 A–C	Chan JKC
2.158 A,B	Chan JKC
2.159	Thompson LDR
2.160	Thompson LDR
2.161	Thompson LDR
2.162 A–D	Thompson LDR
2.163 A,B	Fadda G
2.164 A,B	Fadda G
2.165 A,B	Sadow P
2.166	Fadda G
2.167	Fadda G
3.01 A,B	DeLellis RA
3.02 A,B	DeLellis RA
3.03 A,B	DeLellis RA
3.04 A,B	DeLellis RA
3.05 A,B	DeLellis RA
3.06 A,B	DeLellis RA
3.07 A	Gill A
3.07 B,C	DeLellis RA
3.08	DeLellis RA
3.09 A	Höög A Dept of pathology Karolinska University Hospital, Stockholm Dept of pathology Linköping University Hospital, Linköping, Sweden
3.09 B	DeLellis RA
3.10 A	Haigh PI
3.10 B	DeLellis RA
3.11 A	Sadow P
3.11 B	Erickson LA
3.12	See above, 2.32
3.13 A,B	DeLellis RA
3.14 A,B	DeLellis RA
3.15 A	DeLellis RA
3.15 B	Erickson LA
3.16 A	DeLellis RA
3.16 B	Erickson LA
3.17	DeLellis RA
3.18 A	DeLellis RA
3.18 B	Gill A
3.19	Erickson LA
3.20	Erickson LA
4.01 A–C	Kawashima A
4.02 A–D	Giordano TJ
4.03 A–C	Giordano TJ
4.04 A,B	Giordano TJ
4.05	Reprinted by permission from Macmillan Publishers Ltd: Assié G, Jouinot A, Bertherat J (2014). The 'omics' of adrenocortical tumours for personalized medicine. Nature Reviews Endocrinology 10(4):215–28. Copyright (2014).
4.06	Reprinted from Zheng S, Cherniack AD, Dewal N, et al. (2016). Comprehensive pan-genomic characterization of adrenocortical carcinoma. Cancer Cell 29(5):723–36. Copyright (2017). With permission from Elsevier.
4.07 A,B	Young WF
4.08 A	Sasano HR
4.08 B,C	Tischler AS
4.09 A,B	Giordano TJ
4.10 A,B	Thompson LDR
4.11	Reprinted from Monticone S, Else T, Mulatero P, Williams TA,

Rainey WE (2015). Understanding primary aldosteronism: impact of next generation sequencing and expression profiling. Mol Cell Endocrinol. 399:311–20. Copyright 2017. With permission from Elsevier.

4.12A   Reprinted from Cheng JY, Gill AJ, Kumar SK (2015). Granulosa cell tumour of the adrenal. Pathology. 47(5):487–9. Copyright (2015). With permission from Elsevier.

4.12B   Thompson LDR

4.13   Yokoyama H
Dr Hiroshi Yokoyama's Urology Clinic
Fukuoka, Japan

4.14   Thompson LDR
4.15A   Sasano HR
4.15B   Sasano HR
4.16   Thompson LDR
4.17   Thompson LDR
4.18A   Thompson LDR
4.18B   Fisher C
4.19A   Lam AKY
4.19B   Lack E
4.20   Lack E
4.21   Weiss LM
4.22   Lam AKY
4.23A   Lack E
4.23B   Sasano HR

5.01A,B   Kawashima A
5.02   Kawashima A
5.03A   Lam AKY
5.03B   Tischler AS
5.03C   Reprinted with permission from Page DL, DeLellis RA, Hough AJ Jr (1985). Tumors of the adrenal. In: AFIP atlas of tumor pathology. Series 2, Fascicle 23. Washington DC: Armed Forces Institute of Pathology.
5.04A   Tischler AS
5.04B   Thompson LDR
5.05A,B   Tischler AS
5.06A,B   Tischler AS
5.07A,B   Tischler AS
5.08A   Tischler AS
5.08B,C   Lack E
5.09A–C   Tischler AS
5.10A,B   Tischler AS
5.11A,B   Tischler AS
5.12A–C   Lack EE
5.13A   Lack EE
5.13B   Tischler AS
5.14   Pacak K
5.15A,B   Shiga K
Department of Head & Neck Surgery
Iwate Medical University School of medicine
Morioka, Japan
5.16   Kimura N
5.17A–D   Kimura N
5.18A–D   Kimura N
5.19A–C   Imamura H
Division of Pediatrics Department of Reproductive and Developmental Medicine
University of Miyazaki
Miyazaki, Japan

5.20   See above, 5.19A–C
5.21A–F   Kimura N
5.22A   Reprinted with permission from Hirano K, Amano A, Kimura N, et al. (2011) A surgical repair case of cardiac paraganglioma invading the left atrium. Shinzo;43:803-810.
5.22B,C   Kimura N
5.23A–C   Nichikawa T
Yokohama Rosai Hospital
Yokohama, Japan
5.24A–D   Kijima H
Department of Pathology and Bioscience
Hirosaki University School of Medicine
Hirosaki, Japan
5.25A–D   Kimura N
5.26A–F   Shimada H
5.27A–C   Shimada H
5.28A,B   Shimada H
5.29A–C   Shimada H
5.30A,B   Tischler AS
5.31A–D   Tischler AS
5.32A–D   Tischler AS
5.33A–C   Tischler AS

6.01A   Klöppel G
6.01B   Klimstra DS
6.02A,B   Adsay NV
6.03A,B   Klöppel G
6.04A–D   Klimstra DS
6.05A,B   Klimstra DS
6.06   Klimstra DS
6.07A,B   Klimstra DS
6.08   Klimstra DS
6.09   Klimstra DS
6.10   Klimstra DS
6.11   Klimstra DS
6.12   Klimstra DS
6.13   Klimstra DS
6.14   Klimstra DS
6.15   Klöppel G
6.16   Klöppel G
6.17   Klimstra DS
6.18   Rindi G
6.19   Wild D
Department of Radiology & Nuclear Medicine
University Hospital of Basel
Basel, Switzerland
6.20   Missiaglia E, Dalai I, Barbi S, Beghelli S, Falconi M, della Peruta M, et al. (2010). Pancreatic endocrine tumors: expression profiling evidences a role for AKT-mTOR pathway. J Clin Oncol. 28(2):245–55. Reprinted with permission. © (2010) American Society of Clinical Oncology. All rights reserved.
6.21   Klöppel G
6.22   Perren A
6.23   Perren A
6.24   Perren A
6.25   Klöppel G
6.26   Klöppel G
6.27   Klöppel G
6.28   Couvelard A
6.29   Couvelard A
6.30   Couvelard A
6.31A–C   Couvelard A, Hentic O (2015).

Glucagonoma. In: La Rosa S, Sessa F, editors. Pancreatic neuroendocrine neoplasms: practical approach to diagnosis, classification, and therapy. Cham: Springer International Publishing AG; pp. 81–8. With permission of Springer.

6.32A   Dominioni L
General and Thoracic Surgery
University of Insubria
Varese, Italy
6.32B   La Rosa S
6.33A–C   La Rosa S
6.34   Klöppel G
6.35   Rindi G
6.36   Rindi G
6.37A–C   Öberg K
6.38   Capella C
6.39   Capella C
6.40   Hruban RH
6.41A,B   Hruban RH
6.42A,B   Osamura RY
6.43   Adsay NV
6.44   Adsay NV
6.45   Klöppel G
6.46   Klöppel G
6.47   Adsay NV
6.48   Klöppel G
6.49   Klöppel G
6.50A,B   Ohike N
6.51A–C   Ohike N
6.52A,B   Klöppel G

7.01   Komminoth P
7.02   Komminoth P
7.03   Gan HW, Bulwer C, Jeelani O, Levine MA, Korbonits M, Spoudeas HA (2015). Treatment-resistant pediatric giant prolactinoma and multiple endocrine neoplasia type 1. Int J Pediatr Endocrinol. 2015(1):15. Reprinted with permission of BioMed Central.
7.04   Komminoth P
7.05   Komminoth P
7.06   Klöppel G
7.07   Komminoth P
7.08   Komminoth P
7.09   Komminoth P
7.10   Komminoth P
7.11   Image reprinted with permission from Thomas N. Darling, MD, PhD, Uniformed Services University of the Health Sciences, published by Medscape Drugs & Diseases (http://emedicine.medscape.com/), 2016, available from: http://emedicine.medscape.com/article/1093723-overview.
7.12A–C   Mete O
7.13   Mete O
7.14   Mete O
7.15   Waguespack SG
7.16   Waguespack SG
7.17   Adapted by permission from Macmillan Publishers Ltd: Waguespack SG, Rich TA, Perrier ND, Jimenez C, Cote GJ (2011). Management of medullary thyroid carcinoma and

MEN2 syndromes in childhood. Nature Reviews Endocrinology 7(10):596–607. Copyright (2011).

7.18	Pellegata NS
7.19	Gill A
7.20	Gill A
7.21	Gill A
7.22	Dray M
	Histology Department
	Waikato Hospital
	Hamilton, New Zealand
7.23	Couvelard A
7.24 A,B	Mete O
7.25	Couvelard A
7.26	Couvelard A
7.27	Couvelard A
7.28	Couvelard A
7.29	Adapted from Jochmanová I, Yang C, Zhuang Z, Pacak K. Hypoxia-inducible factor signaling in pheochromocytoma: turning the rudder in the right direction. J Natl Cancer Inst. 2013 Sep 4;105(17):1270-83. By permission of Oxford University Press.
7.30 A,B	Gill A
7.31A,B	Gill A
7.32 A–C	Tischler AS
7.33	Müller U, Troidl C, Niemann S (2005). SDHC mutations in hereditary paraganglioma/pheochromocytoma. Fam Cancer. 4:9–12. With permission of Springer.
7.34	Pacak K
7.35	Klimstra DS
7.36	See above, 7.29
7.37A,B	Stratakis CA
7.38 A	Lloyd RV
7.38 B	Komminoth P
7.38 C	Lloyd RV
7.39 A,B	Carney JA, Boccon-Gibod L, Jarka DE, Tanaka Y, Swee RG, Unni KK, et al. (2001). Osteochondromyxoma of bone: a congenital tumor associated with lentigines and other unusual disorders. Am J Surg Pathol. 25(2):164–76.
7.40	Woodruff JM (deceased)
7.41 A–D	Boyce AM
7.42	Mete O
7.43	Carney JA, Young WF, Stratakis CA (2011). Primary bimorphic adrenocortical disease: cause of hypercortisolism in McCune-Albright syndrome. Am J Surg Pathol. 35(9):1311–26.
7.44	Nosé V
7.45	Nosé V
7.46	Nosé V
7.47A,B	LiVolsi V
7.48	LiVolsi V
7.49	LiVolsi V
7.50	Nosé V
7.51	Foulkes WD
7.52	Foulkes WD
7.53	Foulkes WD
7.54	Foulkes WD
7.55	Klöppel G
7.56	Klöppel G
7.57A,B	Klöppel G

Sources of figures on front cover

Top left	Young WF
Top centre	DeLellis RA
Top right	Komminoth P
Middle left	Osamura RY
Middle centre	Klöppel G
Middle right	Chan JKC
Bottom left	Reprinted by permission from Macmillan Publishers Ltd: Nat Genet. Reincke M, Sbiera S, Hayakawa A, Theodoropoulou M, Osswald A, Beuschlein F, et al. Mutations in the deubiquitinase gene USP8 cause Cushing's disease. 2015;47(1):31–8. Copyright 2017.
Bottom centre	Shimada H
Bottom right	Reprinted from Monticone S, Else T, Mulatero P, Williams TA, Rainey WE (2015). Understanding primary aldosteronism: impact of next generation sequencing and expression profiling. Mol Cell Endocrinol. 399:311–20. Copyright 2017. With permission from Elsevier.

Sources of tables

1.04	Montone KT (2015). The differential diagnosis of sinonasal/nasopharyngeal neuroendocrine/neuroectodermally derived tumors. Archives of Pathology & Laboratory Medicine 139(12):1498–507. ©2015 College of American Pathologists.
1.05	Lopes MBS
1.06	Lopes MBS
2.01	Modified with permission from Rosai J, DeLellis RA, Carcangiu ML, Frable J, Tallini G (2015). Tumors of the thyroid and parathyroid glands. In: AFIP atlas of tumor pathology. Series 4, Fascicle 21. Washington DC: American Registry of Pathology Press.
2.02	Williams MD
2.03	Tallini G
2.04	Tallini G
2.05	Adapted with permission from: Nikiforov YE, Seethala RR, Tallini G, Baloch ZW, Basolo F, Thompson LD, et al. (2016) Nomenclature Revision for Encapsulated Follicular Variant of Papillary Thyroid Carcinoma: A Paradigm Shift to Reduce Overtreatment of Indolent Tumors. JAMA Oncol. 2:1023-9.
2.06	Soares P
2.07	LiVolsi V
2.08	Tallini G
2.09	Tallini G
2.10	Tallini G
2.11	Cameselle Tejeiro JM
2.12	Kakudo K
2.13	Thompson LDR
4.01	Adapted with permission from: DeLellis RA, Lloyd RV, Heitz PU, Eng C. (eds) (2004) WHO Classification of Tumours. Pathology and Genetics of Endocrine Organs. 3rd ed. Lyon, IARCPress.
4.02	Giordano TJ
4.03	Modified with permission from Else T, Kim AC, Sabolch A, Raymond VM, Kandathil A, Caoili EM, et al. (2014). Adrenocortical carcinoma. Endocr Rev 35(2):282–326.
4.04	Giordano TJ
4.05	Cheng L
5.03	Adapted from Kleihues P, Cavenee WK, editors (2000). World Health Organization classification of tumours. Pathology and genetics of tumours of the nervous system. 3rd ed. Lyon: IARCPress.
5.04	Shimada H
5.05	Shimada H
5.06	Cohn SL, Pearson AD, London WB, Monclair T, Ambros PF, Brodeur GM, et al. (2009). The International Neuroblastoma Risk Group (INRG) classification system: an INRG Task Force report. J Clin Oncol. 27(2):289–97. Reprinted with permission. ©2009 American Society of Clinical Oncology. All rights reserved.
6.02	Komminoth P
6.03	Klimstra DS
6.04	Klimstra DS
7.01	Klöppel G
7.02	Komminoth P
7.03	DeLellis RA
7.04	Pellegata NS
7.05	Couvelard A
7.06	Hammel P
7.07	Perren A
7.08	Perren A
7.09	LiVolsi V

TNM Classification

Brierley JD, Gospodarowicz MK, Wittekind Ch, editors (2017). TNM Classification of Malignant Tumours. 8th ed. John Wiley & Sons. A help desk for specific questions about TNM classification is available at http://www.uicc.org/resources/tnm/helpdesk.

AJCC Staging

Amin MB, Edge S, Greene F, et al. Editors. (2017) AJCC Cancer Staging Manual. 8th ed. New York: Springer. Used with permission of the American Joint Committee on Cancer (AJCC), Chicago, Illinois.

References

1. Abele TA, Yetkin ZF, Raisanen JM, et al. (2012). Non-pituitary origin sellar tumours mimicking pituitary macroadenomas. Clin Radiol. 67:821–7. PMID:22749386
1A. Abdulkader M, Abdulla K, Rakha E, et al. (2006). Routine elastic staining assists detection of vascular invasion in colorectal cancer. Histopathology. 49:487–92. PMID: 17064294
2. Abi-Raad R, Virk RK, Dinauer CA, et al. (2015). C-Cell Neoplasia in Asymptomatic Carriers of RET Mutation in Extracellular Cysteine-Rich and Intracellular Tyrosine Kinase Domain. Hum Pathol. 46:1121–8. PMID:26033033
3. Abraham DT, Low TH, Messina M, et al. (2011). Medullary thyroid carcinoma: long-term outcomes of surgical treatment. Ann Surg Oncol. 18:219–25. PMID:20878247
4. Acharya S, Sarafoglou K, LaQuaglia M, et al. (2003). Thyroid neoplasms after therapeutic radiation for malignancies during childhood or adolescence. Cancer. 97:2397–403. PMID:12733137
5. Adamson AR, Grahame-Smith DG, Bogomoletz V, et al. (1971). Malignant argentaffinoma with carcinoid syndrome and hypoglycaemia. Br Med J. 3:93–4. PMID:5314568
6. Adeniran AJ, Zhu Z, Gandhi M, et al. (2006). Correlation between genetic alterations and microscopic features, clinical manifestations, and prognostic characteristics of thyroid papillary carcinomas. Am J Surg Pathol. 30:216–22. PMID:16434896
7. Adsay NV, Andea A, Basturk O, et al. (2004). Secondary tumors of the pancreas: an analysis of a surgical and autopsy database and review of the literature. Virchows Arch. 444:527–35. PMID:15057558
8. Afkhami M, Karunamurthy A, Chiosea S, et al. (2016). Histopathologic and Clinical Characterization of Thyroid Tumors Carrying the BRAF(K601E) Mutation. Thyroid. 26:242–7. PMID:26422023
9. Aflorei ED, Korbonits M (2014). Epidemiology and etiopathogenesis of pituitary adenomas. J Neurooncol. 117:379–94. PMID:24481996
10. Afrogheh AH, Meserve E, Sadow PM, et al. (2016). Molecular characterization of an endometrial endometrioid adenocarcinoma metastatic to a thyroid Hürthle cell adenoma showing cancerization of follicles. Endocr Pathol. 27:213–9. PMID:26687112
11. Afroz N, Khan N, Hassan J, et al. (2011). Role of imprint cytology in the intraoperative diagnosis of pituitary adenomas. Diagn Cytopathol. 39:138–40. PMID:21254464
12. Agaimy A, Erlenbach-Wünsch K, Konukiewitz B, et al. (2013). ISL1 expression is not restricted to pancreatic well-differentiated neuroendocrine neoplasms, but is also commonly found in well and poorly differentiated neuroendocrine neoplasms of extrapancreatic origin. Mod Pathol. 26:995–1003. PMID:23503646
13. Agarwal A, Mehrotra PK, Jain M, et al. (2010). Size of the tumor and pheochromocytoma of the adrenal gland scaled score (PASS): can they predict malignancy? World J Surg. 34:3022–8. PMID:20703467
14. Agarwal SK (2013). Multiple endocrine neoplasia type 1. Front Horm Res. 41:1–15. PMID:23652667
15. Agarwal SK, Mateo CM, Marx SJ (2009). Rare germline mutations in cyclin-dependent kinase inhibitor genes in multiple endocrine neoplasia type 1 and related states. J Clin Endocrinol Metab. 94:1826–34. PMID:19141585
16. Agarwal SK, Ozawa A, Mateo CM, et al. (2009). The MEN1 gene and pituitary tumours. Horm Res. 71 Suppl 2:131–8. PMID:19407509
17. Agha A, Carpenter R, Bhattacharya S, et al. (2007). Parathyroid carcinoma in multiple endocrine neoplasia type 1 (MEN1) syndrome: two case reports of an unrecognised entity. J Endocrinol Invest. 30:145–9. PMID:17392605
18. Agustsson TT, Baldvinsdottir T, Jonasson JG, et al. (2015). The epidemiology of pituitary adenomas in Iceland, 1955–2012: a nationwide population-based study. Eur J Endocrinol. 173:655–64. PMID:26423473
19. Ahmad K, Fayos JV (1978). Pituitary fibrosarcoma secondary to radiation therapy. Cancer. 42:107–10. PMID:667787
20. Ahuja AT, Chan ES, Allen PW, et al. (1998). Carcinoma showing thymiclike differentiation (CASTLE tumor). AJNR Am J Neuroradiol. 19:1225–8. PMID:9726458
21. AIRTUM Working Group (2013). Italian cancer figures, report 2013: Multiple tumours. Epidemiol Prev. 37(4–5 Suppl 1):1–152. PMID:24259384
22. AIRTUM Working Group; CCM; AIEOP Working Group (2013). Italian cancer figures, report 2012: Cancer in children and adolescents. Epidemiol Prev. 37(1 Suppl 1):1–225. PMID:23585445
23. Aitken RE, Bartley PC, Bryant SJ, et al. (1975). The effect of multiphasic biochemical screening on the diagnosis of primary hyperparathyroidism. Aust N Z J Med. 5:224–6. PMID:1057934
24. Akahani S, Nangia-Makker P, Inohara H, et al. (1997). Galectin-3: a novel antiapoptotic molecule with a functional BH1 (NWGR) domain of Bcl-2 family. Cancer Res. 57:5272–6. PMID:9393748
25. Akaishi J, Sugino K, Kameyama K, et al. (2015). Clinicopathologic features and outcomes in patients with diffuse sclerosing variant of papillary thyroid carcinoma. World J Surg. 39:1728–35. PMID:25743484
26. Åkerström T, Crona J, Delgado Verdugo A, et al. (2012). Comprehensive re-sequencing of adrenal aldosterone producing lesions reveal three somatic mutations near the KCNJ5 potassium channel selectivity filter. PLoS One. 7:e41926. PMID:22848660
27. Akishima-Fukasawa Y, Yoshihara A, Ishikawa Y, et al. (2011). Malignant adrenal rest tumor of the retroperitoneum producing adrenocortical steroids. Endocr Pathol. 22:112–7. PMID:21374072
28. Akiyama T, Shida T, Yoshitomi H, et al. (2016). Expression of Sex Determining Region Y-Box 2 and Pancreatic and Duodenal Homeobox 1 in Pancreatic Neuroendocrine Tumors. Pancreas. 45:522–7. PMID:26491904
29. Akslen LA, LiVolsi VA (2000). Prognostic significance of histologic grading compared with subclassification of papillary thyroid carcinoma. Cancer. 88:1902–8. PMID:10760768
30. Al-Bahri S, Tariq A, Lowentritt B, et al. (2014). Giant bilateral adrenal myelolipoma with congenital adrenal hyperplasia. Case Rep Surg. 2014:728198. PMID:25140269
31. Al-Dahmani K, Mohammad S, Imran F, et al. (2016). Sellar Masses: An Epidemiological Study. Can J Neurol Sci. 43:291–7. PMID:26522017
32. Al-Ghamdi S, Fageeh N, Dewan M (2000). Malignant schwannoma of the thyroid gland. Otolaryngol Head Neck Surg. 122:143–4. PMID:10629502
33. Al-Mefty O, Holoubi A, Rifai A, et al. (1985). Microsurgical removal of suprasellar meningiomas. Neurosurgery. 16:364–72. PMID:3982616
34. Al-Sarireh B, Haidermota M, Verbeke C, et al. (2013). Glucagon cell adenomatosis without glucagon receptor mutation. Pancreas. 42:360–2. PMID:23407487
35. Alahmadi H, Lee D, Wilson JR, et al. (2012). Clinical features of silent corticotroph adenomas. Acta Neurochir (Wien). 154:1493–8. PMID:22619024
36. Alband N, Korbonits M (2014). Familial pituitary tumors. Handb Clin Neurol. 124:339–60. PMID:25248598
37. Albany C, Jain A, Ulbright TM, et al. (2011). Lung cancer, thyroid cancer or both: An unusual case presentation. J Thorac Dis. 3:271–3. PMID:22263102
38. Albers N, Jörgens S, Deiss D, et al. (2002). McCune-Albright syndrome–the German experience. J Pediatr Endocrinol Metab. 15 Suppl 3:897–901. PMID:12199348
39. Albert S (2013). Primary Burkitt lymphoma of the thyroid. Ear Nose Throat J. 92:E1–2. PMID:24366706
40. Albores-Saavedra J (1989). C-cell hyperplasia. Am J Surg Pathol. 13:987–9. PMID:2802014
41. Albores-Saavedra J, Gould E, Vardaman C, et al. (1991). The macrofollicular variant of papillary thyroid carcinoma: a study of 17 cases. Hum Pathol. 22:1195–205. PMID:1748427
42. Albores-Saavedra J, Gu X, Luna MA (2003). Clear cells and thyroid transcription factor I reactivity in sclerosing mucoepidermoid carcinoma of the thyroid gland. Ann Diagn Pathol. 7:348–53. PMID:15018117
43. Albores-Saavedra J, Housini I, Vuitch F, et al. (1997). Macrofollicular variant of papillary thyroid carcinoma with minor insular component. Cancer. 80:1110–6. PMID:9305712
44. Albores-Saavedra J, LiVolsi VA, Williams ED (1985). Medullary carcinoma. Semin Diagn Pathol. 2:137–46. PMID:3843691
45. Albores-Saavedra J, Monforte H, Nadji M, et al. (1988). C-cell hyperplasia in thyroid tissue adjacent to follicular cell tumors. Hum Pathol. 19:795–9. PMID:2900208
46. Albores-Saavedra J, Sharma S (2001). Poorly differentiated follicular thyroid carcinoma with rhabdoid phenotype: a clinicopathologic, immunohistochemical and electron microscopic study of two cases. Mod Pathol. 14:98–104. PMID:11235911
47. Albores-Saavedra JA, Krueger JE (2001). C-cell hyperplasia and medullary thyroid microcarcinoma. Endocr Pathol. 12:365–77. PMID:11914470
48. Albrecht S, Gardiner GW, Kovacs K, et al. (1989). Duodenal somatostatinoma with psammoma bodies. Arch Pathol Lab Med. 113:517–20. PMID:2565711
49. Albuquerque FC, Weiss MH, Kovacs K, et al. (1999). A functioning composite 'corticotroph' pituitary adenoma with interspersed adrenocortical cells. Pituitary. 1:279–84. PMID:11081209
50. Alevizaki M, Papageorgiou G, Rentziou G, et al. (2009). Increasing prevalence of papillary thyroid carcinoma in recent years in Greece: the majority are incidental. Thyroid. 19:749–54. PMID:19534620
51. Alevizaki M, Saltiki K (2015). Primary Hyperparathyroidism in MEN2 Syndromes. Recent Results Cancer Res. 204:179–86. PMID:26494389
52. Alexander VR, Manjaly JG, Pepper CM, et al. (2015). Head and neck teratomas in children–A series of 23 cases at Great Ormond Street Hospital. Int J Pediatr Otorhinolaryngol. 79:2008–14. PMID:26611341
53. Alexandraki KI, Grossman AB (2010). The ectopic ACTH syndrome. Rev Endocr Metab Disord. 11:117–26. PMID:20544290
54. Alexandraki KI, Munayem Khan M, Chahal HS, et al. (2012). Oncogene-induced senescence in pituitary adenomas and carcinomas. Hormones (Athens). 11:297–307. PMID:22908062
55. Alexandrescu S, Brown RE, Tandon N, et al. (2012). Neuron precursor features of spindle cell oncocytoma of adenohypophysis. Ann Clin Lab Sci. 42:123–9. PMID:22585606
56. Ali A, Serra S, Asa SL, et al. (2006). The predictive value of CK19 and CD99 in pancreatic endocrine tumors. Am J Surg Pathol. 30:1588–94. PMID:17122516
57. Allen CE, Ladisch S, McClain KL (2015). How I treat Langerhans cell histiocytosis. Blood. 126:26–35. PMID:25827831
58. Allolio B, Fassnacht M (2006). Clinical review: Adrenocortical carcinoma: clinical update. J Clin Endocrinol Metab. 91:2027–37. PMID:16551738
59. Altenähr E, Arps H, Montz R, et al. (1979). Quantitative ultrastructural and radioimmunologic assessment of parathyroid gland activity in primary hyperparathyroidism. Lab Invest. 41:303–12. PMID:491543
60. Altenähr E, Saeger W (1973). Light and electron microscopy of parathyroid carcinoma. Report of three cases. Virchows Arch A Pathol Pathol Anat. 360:107–22. PMID:4200384
61. Altinay S, Ozen A, Namal E, et al. (2014). Electron microscopic analysis of an angiosarcoma of the thyroid from a non-Alpine endemic goiter region: A case report and brief review of the literature. Oncol Lett. 8:2117–21. PMID:25289092
62. Alves Filho W, Mahmoud RR, Ramos DM, et al. (2014). Malignant solitary fibrous tumor of the thyroid: a case-report and review of the literature. Arq Bras Endocrinol Metabol. 58:402–6. PMID:24936737
63. Alves P, Soares P, Fonseca E, et al. (1999). Papillary Thyroid Carcinoma Overexpresses Fully and Underglycosylated Mucins Together with Native and Sialylated Simple Mucin Antigens and Histo-Blood Group Antigens. Endocr Pathol. 10:315–24. PMID:12114768
64. Alwaheeb S, Rambaldini G, Boerner S, et al. (2006). Worrisome histologic alterations following fine-needle aspiration of the parathyroid. J Clin Pathol. 59:1094–6. PMID:17021134
65. Alzouebi M, Goepel JR, Horsman JM, et al. (2012). Primary thyroid lymphoma: the 40 year experience of a UK lymphoma treatment centre. Int J Oncol. 40:2075–80. PMID:22367111
66. Amacher AM, Goyal B, Lewis JS Jr, et al. (2015). Prevalence of a hobnail pattern in papillary, poorly differentiated, and anaplastic thyroid carcinoma: a possible manifestation of high-grade transformation. Am J Surg Pathol. 39:260–5. PMID:25321328
67. Amal B, El Fatemi H, Souaf I, et al. (2013).

A rare primary tumor of the thyroid gland: report a new case of leiomyosarcoma and literature review. Diagn Pathol. 8:36. PMID:23445571
68. Amar L, Baudin E, Burnichon N, et al. (2007). Succinate dehydrogenase B gene mutations predict survival in patients with malignant pheochromocytomas or paragangliomas. J Clin Endocrinol Metab. 92:3822–8. PMID:17652212
69. Amar L, Bertherat J, Baudin E, et al. (2005). Genetic testing in pheochromocytoma or functional paraganglioma. J Clin Oncol. 23:8812–8. PMID:16314641
70. Amato B, Bianco T, Compagna R, et al. (2014). Surgical resection of carotid body paragangliomas: 10 years of experience. Am J Surg. 207:293–8. PMID:24119888
71. Ambros PF, Ambros IM, Brodeur GM, et al. (2009). International consensus for neuroblastoma molecular diagnostics: report from the International Neuroblastoma Risk Group (INRG) Biology Committee. Br J Cancer. 100:1471–82. PMID:19401703
72. Amiel J, Laudier B, Attié-Bitach T, et al. (2003). Polyalanine expansion and frameshift mutations of the paired-like homeobox gene PHOX2B in congenital central hypoventilation syndrome. Nat Genet. 33:459–61. PMID:12640453
72A. Amin MB, Edge S, Greene F, et al. Editors. (2017) AJCC Cancer Staging Manual. 8th ed. New York: Springer.
73. An J, Oh YL, Shin JH, et al. (2010). Primary schwannoma of the thyroid gland: a case report. Acta Cytol. 54(5 Suppl):857–62. PMID:21053556
74. Anand VK, Osborne CM, Harkey HL 3rd (1993). Infiltrative clival pituitary adenoma of ectopic origin. Otolaryngol Head Neck Surg. 108:178–83. PMID:8441545
75. Andersen GS, Toftdahl DB, Lund JO, et al. (1988). The incidence rate of phaeochromocytoma and Conn's syndrome in Denmark, 1977–1981. J Hum Hypertens. 2:187–9. PMID:3236322
76. Anderson JL, Gutmann DH (2015). Neurofibromatosis type 1. Handb Clin Neurol. 132:75–86. PMID:26564071
77. Ando M, Nakanishi Y, Asai M, et al. (2008). Mucoepidermoid carcinoma of the thyroid gland showing marked ciliation suggestive of its pathogenesis. Pathol Int. 58:741–4. PMID:18844942
78. Andrews GA, Kniseley RM (1956). Transformation of thyroidal carcinoma to clear-cell type. Am J Clin Pathol. 26:1427–38. PMID:13394549
79. Andrion A, Mazzucco G, Torchio B (1992). FNA cytology of thyroid neurilemmoma (schwannoma). Diagn Cytopathol. 8:311–2. PMID:1606890
80. Anlauf M, Bauersfeld J, Raffel A, et al. (2009). Insulinomatosis: a multicentric insulinoma disease that frequently causes early recurrent hyperinsulinemic hypoglycemia. Am J Surg Pathol. 33:339–46. PMID:19011561
81. Anlauf M, Enosawa T, Henopp T, et al. (2008). Primary lymph node gastrinoma or occult duodenal microgastrinoma with lymph node metastases in a MEN1 patient: the need for a systematic search for the primary tumor. Am J Surg Pathol. 32:1101–5. PMID:18520436
82. Anlauf M, Garbrecht N, Bauersfeld J, et al. (2007). Hereditary neuroendocrine tumors of the gastroenteropancreatic system. Virchows Arch. 451 Suppl 1:S29–38. PMID:17684762
83. Anlauf M, Perren A, Meyer CL, et al. (2005). Precursor lesions in patients with multiple endocrine neoplasia type 1-associated duodenal gastrinomas. Gastroenterology. 128:1187–98. PMID:15887103
84. Anlauf M, Schlenger R, Perren A, et al. (2006). Microadenomatosis of the endocrine pancreas in patients with and without the multiple endocrine neoplasia type 1 syndrome. Am J Surg Pathol. 30:560–74. PMID:16699310
85. Annamalai AK, Dean AF, Kandasamy N, et al. (2012). Temozolomide responsiveness in aggressive corticotroph tumours: a case report and review of the literature. Pituitary. 15:276–87. PMID:22076588
86. Ansell SM, Grant CS, Habermann TM (1999). Primary thyroid lymphoma. Semin Oncol. 26:316–23. PMID:10375088
87. Aquilina K, Boop FA (2011). Nonneoplastic enlargement of the pituitary gland in children. J Neurosurg Pediatr. 7:510–5. PMID:21529191
88. Arezzo A, Patetta R, Ceppa P, et al. (1998). Mucoepidermoid carcinoma of the thyroid gland arising from a papillary epithelial neoplasm. Am Surg. 64:307–11. PMID:9544139
89. Arita K, Uozumi T, Kuwabara S, et al. (1991). A case of pituitary adenoma producing both growth hormone (GH) and adrenocorticotropic hormone (ACTH). Endocrinol Jpn. 38:271–8. PMID:1665412
90. Armand R, Cappola AR, Horenstein RB, et al. (2004). Adrenal cortical adenoma with excess black pigment deposition, combined with myelolipoma and clinical Cushing's syndrome. Int J Surg Pathol. 12:57–61. PMID:14765276
91. Arola J, Salmenkivi K, Liu J, et al. (2000). p53 and Ki67 in adrenocortical tumors. Endocr Res. 26:861–5. PMID:11196463
92. Aron M, Kapila K, Verma K (2005). Neural tumours of the neck presenting as thyroid nodules: a report of three cases. Cytopathology. 16:206–9. PMID:16048507
93. Arora N, Scognamiglio T, Lubitz CC, et al. (2009). Identification of borderline thyroid tumors by gene expression array analysis. Cancer. 115:5421–31. PMID:19658182
94. Asa SL (2011). Tumors of the pituitary gland. In: AFIP atlas of tumor pathology. Series 4, Fascicle 15. Washington DC: American Registry of Pathology Press.
95. Asa SL (2004). My approach to oncocytic tumours of the thyroid. J Clin Pathol. 57:225–32. PMID:14990587
96. Asa SL, Dardick I, Van Nostrand AW, et al. (1988). Primary thyroid thymoma: a distinct clinicopathologic entity. Hum Pathol. 19:1463–7. PMID:3056830
97. Asa SL, Digiovanni R, Jiang J, et al. (2007). A growth hormone receptor mutation impairs growth hormone autofeedback signaling in pituitary tumors. Cancer Res. 67:7505–11. PMID:17671221
98. Asa SL, Ezzat S (2002). The pathogenesis of pituitary tumours. Nat Rev Cancer. 2:836–49. PMID:12415254
99. Asa SL, Ezzat S (2009). The pathogenesis of pituitary tumors. Annu Rev Pathol. 4:97–126. PMID:19400692
100. Asa SL, Ezzat S (2014). Genomic approaches to problems in pituitary neoplasia. Endocr Pathol. 25:209–13. PMID:24272682
101. Asa SL, Kovacs K, Horvath E, et al. (1984). Sellar glomangioma. Ultrastruct Pathol. 7:49–54. PMID:6097000
102. Asa SL, Mete O (2013). Thyroid neoplasms of follicular cell derivation: a simplified approach. Semin Diagn Pathol. 30:178–85. PMID:24144287
103. Asa SL, Scheithauer BW, Bilbao JM, et al. (1984). A case for hypothalamic acromegaly: a clinicopathological study of six patients with hypothalamic gangliocytomas producing growth hormone-releasing factor. J Clin Endocrinol Metab. 58:796–803. PMID:6423659
104. Asare EA, Sturgeon C, Winchester DJ, et al. (2015). Parathyroid Carcinoma: An Update on Treatment Outcomes and Prognostic Factors from the National Cancer Data Base (NCDB). Ann Surg Oncol. 22:3990–5. PMID:26077914
105. Asgharian B, Turner ML, Gibril F, et al. (2004). Cutaneous tumors in patients with multiple endocrine neoplasm type 1 (MEN1) and gastrinomas: prospective study of frequency and development of criteria with high sensitivity and specificity for MEN1. J Clin Endocrinol Metab. 89:5328–36. PMID:15531478
106. Asioli S, Erickson LA, Righi A, et al. (2010). Poorly differentiated carcinoma of the thyroid: validation of the Turin proposal and analysis of IMP3 expression. Mod Pathol. 23:1269–78. PMID:20562850
107. Asioli S, Erickson LA, Righi A, et al. (2013). Papillary thyroid carcinoma with hobnail features: histopathologic criteria to predict aggressive behavior. Hum Pathol. 44:320–8. PMID:23036367
108. Asioli S, Erickson LA, Sebo TJ, et al. (2010). Papillary thyroid carcinoma with prominent hobnail features: a new aggressive variant of moderately differentiated papillary carcinoma. A clinicopathologic, immunohistochemical, and molecular study of eight cases. Am J Surg Pathol. 34:44–52. PMID:19956062
109. Asioli S, Maletta F, Pagni F, et al. (2014). Cytomorphologic and molecular features of hobnail variant of papillary thyroid carcinoma: case series and literature review. Diagn Cytopathol. 42:78–84. PMID:23913779
110. Asioli S, Righi A, Volante M, et al. (2014). Cell size as a prognostic factor in oncocytic poorly differentiated carcinomas of the thyroid. Hum Pathol. 45:1489–95. PMID:24745614
111. Assié G, Jouinot A, Bertherat J (2014). The 'omics' of adrenocortical tumours for personalized medicine. Nat Rev Endocrinol. 10:215–28. PMID:24492180
112. Assié G, Letouzé E, Fassnacht M, et al. (2014). Integrated genomic characterization of adrenocortical carcinoma. Nat Genet. 46:607–12. PMID:24747642
113. Asteria C, Anagni M, Fugazzola L, et al. (2002). MEN1 gene mutations are a rare event in patients with sporadic neuroendocrine tumors. Eur J Intern Med. 13:319–23. PMID:12144911
114. Asteria C, Anagni M, Persani L, et al. (2001). Loss of heterozygosity of the MEN1 gene in a large series of TSH-secreting pituitary adenomas. J Endocrinol Invest. 24:796–801. PMID:11765049
115. Astrom K, Cohen JE, Willett-Brozick JE, et al. (2003). Altitude is a phenotypic modifier in hereditary paraganglioma type 1: evidence for an oxygen-sensing defect. Hum Genet. 113:228–37. PMID:12811540
116. Attiyeh EF, London WB, Mossé YP, et al. (2005). Chromosome 1p and 11q deletions and outcome in neuroblastoma. N Engl J Med. 353:2243–53. PMID:16306521
117. Aubertine CL, Flieder DB (2004). Primary paraganglioma of the lung. Ann Diagn Pathol. 8:237–41. PMID:15290677
118. Avetisian IL, Petrova GV (1996). Latent thyroid pathology in residents of Kiev, Ukraine. J Environ Pathol Toxicol Oncol. 15:239–43. PMID:9216814
119. Awad SS, Miskulin J, Thompson N (2003). Parathyroid adenomas versus four-gland hyperplasia as the cause of primary hyperparathyroidism in patients with prolonged lithium therapy. World J Surg. 27:486–8. PMID:12658498
120. Aylwin SJ, Bodi I, Beaney R (2016). Pronounced response of papillary craniopharyngioma to treatment with vemurafenib, a BRAF inhibitor. Pituitary. 19:544–6. PMID:26115708
121. Azizan EA, Murthy M, Stowasser M, et al. (2012). Somatic mutations affecting the selectivity filter of KCNJ5 are frequent in 2 large unselected collections of adrenal aldosteronomas. Hypertension. 59:587–91. PMID:22252394
122. Azizan EA, Poulsen H, Tuluc P, et al. (2013). Somatic mutations in ATP1A1 and CACNA1D underlie a common subtype of adrenal hypertension. Nat Genet. 45:1055–60. PMID:23913004
123. Babouk NL (2004). Solitary fibrous tumor of the thyroid gland. Saudi Med J. 25:805–7. PMID:15195217
124. Bacon CM, Diss TC, Ye H, et al. (2009). Follicular lymphoma of the thyroid gland. Am J Surg Pathol. 33:22–34. PMID:18830125
125. Badalian-Very G, Vergilio JA, Degar BA, et al. (2010). Recurrent BRAF mutations in Langerhans cell histiocytosis. Blood. 116:1919–23. PMID:20519626
126. Badawi RA, Scott-Coombes D (2002). Ancient schwannoma masquerading as a thyroid mass. Eur J Surg Oncol. 28:88–90. PMID:11869021
127. Bae KT, Fuangtharnthip P, Prasad SR, et al. (2003). Adrenal masses: CT characterization with histogram analysis method. Radiology. 228:735–42. PMID:12954893
128. Baguet JP, Hammer L, Mazzuco TL, et al. (2004). Circumstances of discovery of phaeochromocytoma: a retrospective study of 41 consecutive patients. Eur J Endocrinol. 150:681–6. PMID:15132724
129. Bahubeshi A, Bal N, Rio Frio T, et al. (2010). Germline DICER1 mutations and familial cystic nephroma. J Med Genet. 47:863–6. PMID:21036787
130. Bai S, Baloch ZW, Samulski TD, et al. (2015). Poorly differentiated oncocytic (hürthle cell) follicular carcinoma: an institutional experience. Endocr Pathol. 26:164–9. PMID:25898815
131. Bai S, LiVolsi VA, Fraker DL, et al. (2012). Water-clear parathyroid adenoma: report of two cases and literature review. Endocr Pathol. 23:196–200. PMID:22638654
132. Baisakh MR, Mohapatra N, Adhikary SD, et al. (2014). Malignant peripheral nerve sheath tumor of adrenal gland with heterologus osseous differentiation in a case of Von Recklinghausen's disease. Indian J Pathol Microbiol. 57:130–2. PMID:24739852
133. Bajpai A, Greenway A, Zacharin M (2008). Platelet dysfunction and increased bleeding tendency in McCune-Albright syndrome. J Pediatr. 153:287–9. PMID:18639732
134. Bakuła-Zalewska E, Cameron R, Gałczyński JP, et al. (2015). Hyaline matrix in hyalinizing trabecular tumor: Findings in fine-needle aspiration smears. Diagn Cytopathol. 43:710–3. PMID:25352467
135. Balci S, Saglam A, Oruckaptan H, et al. (2015). Pituitary adenoma with gangliocytic component: report of 5 cases with focus on immunoprofile of gangliocytic component. Pituitary. 18:23–30. PMID:24430434
136. Bale GF (1950). Teratoma of the neck in the region of the thyroid gland; a review of the literature and report of 4 cases. Am J Pathol. 26:565–79. PMID:15419285
137. Balili I, Sullivan S, Mckeever P, et al. (2014). Pituitary carcinoma with endolymphatic sac metastasis. Pituitary. 17:210–3. PMID:23645293
138. Ballav C, Naziat A, Mihai R, et al. (2012). Mini-review: pheochromocytomas causing the ectopic ACTH syndrome. Endocrine. 42:69–73. PMID:22396144
139. Baloch Z, LiVolsi VA, Tondon R (2013). Aggressive variants of follicular cell derived thyroid carcinoma; the so called 'real thyroid carcinomas'. J Clin Pathol. 66:733–43. PMID:23626010
140. Baloch ZW, Abraham S, Roberts S, et al. (1999). Differential expression of cytokeratins in follicular variant of papillary carcinoma: an immunohistochemical study and its diagnostic utility. Hum Pathol. 30:1166–71. PMID:10534163
141. Baloch ZW, Fleisher S, LiVolsi VA, et al. (2002). Diagnosis of "follicular neoplasm": a gray zone in thyroid fine-needle aspiration cytology. Diagn Cytopathol. 26:41–4. PMID:11782086
142. Baloch ZW, LiVolsi VA (1998). Fine-Needle

Aspiration Cytology of Papillary Hürthle Cell Carcinoma with Lymphocytic Stroma "Warthin-Like Tumor" of the Thyroid. Endocr Pathol. 9:317–23. PMID:12114779
143. Baloch ZW, LiVolsi VA (1999). Tumor-to-tumor metastasis to follicular variant of papillary carcinoma of thyroid. Arch Pathol Lab Med. 123:703–6. PMID:10420227
144. Baloch ZW, LiVolsi VA (2002). Etiology and significance of the optically clear nucleus. Endocr Pathol. 13:289–99. PMID:12665647
145. Baloch ZW, LiVolsi VA (2014). Follicular-patterned afflictions of the thyroid gland: reappraisal of the most discussed entity in endocrine pathology. Endocr Pathol. 25:12–20. PMID:24464744
146. Baloch ZW, LiVolsi VA (2015). C-Cells and their Associated Lesions and Conditions: A Pathologists Perspective. Turk Patoloji Derg. 31 Suppl 1:60–79. PMID:26177318
147. Baloch ZW, Solomon AC, LiVolsi VA (2000). Primary mucoepidermoid carcinoma and sclerosing mucoepidermoid carcinoma with eosinophilia of the thyroid gland: a report of nine cases. Mod Pathol. 13:802–7. PMID:10912941
148. Balogun JA, Monsalves E, Juraschka K, et al. (2015). Null cell adenomas of the pituitary gland: an institutional review of their clinical imaging and behavioral characteristics. Endocr Pathol. 26:63–70. PMID:25403448
149. Bando H, Sano T, Ohshima T, et al. (1992). Differences in pathological findings and growth hormone responses in patients with growth hormone-producing pituitary adenoma. Endocrinol Jpn. 39:355–63. PMID:1446651
150. Banerjee SS, Eyden BP, Wells S, et al. (1992). Pseudoangiosarcomatous carcinoma: a clinicopathological study of seven cases. Histopathology. 21:13–23. PMID:1634198
151. Banerjee SS, Harris M (2000). Morphological and immunophenotypic variations in malignant melanoma. Histopathology. 36:387–402. PMID:10792480
152. Bansal M, Gandhi M, Ferris RL, et al. (2013). Molecular and histopathologic characteristics of multifocal papillary thyroid carcinoma. Am J Surg Pathol. 37:1586–91. PMID:23797723
153. Barbosa SL, Rodien P, Leboulleux S, et al. (2005). Ectopic adrenocorticotropic hormone-syndrome in medullary carcinoma of the thyroid: a retrospective analysis and review of the literature. Thyroid. 15:618–23. PMID:16029131
154. Barghorn A, Komminoth P, Bachmann D, et al. (2001). Deletion at 3p25.3–p23 is frequently encountered in endocrine pancreatic tumours and is associated with metastatic progression. J Pathol. 194:451–8. PMID:11523053
155. Barghorn A, Speel EJ, Farspour B, et al. (2001). Putative tumor suppressor loci at 6q22 and 6q23-q24 are involved in the malignant progression of sporadic endocrine pancreatic tumors. Am J Pathol. 158:1903–11. PMID:11395364
156. Barker EV, Cervigne NK, Reis PP, et al. (2009). microRNA evaluation of unknown primary lesions in the head and neck. Mol Cancer. 8:127. PMID:20028561
157. Barletta JA, Bellizzi AM, Hornick JL (2011). Immunohistochemical staining of thyroidectomy specimens for PTEN can aid in the identification of patients with Cowden syndrome. Am J Surg Pathol. 35:1505–11. PMID:21921783
158. Barman S, Mandal KC, Mukhopadhyay M (2014). Adrenal myelolipoma: An incidental and rare benign tumor in children. J Indian Assoc Pediatr Surg. 19:236–8. PMID:25336809
159. Barnes L (2009). Metastases to the head and neck: an overview. Head Neck Pathol. 3:217–24. PMID:20596975
160. Barontini M, Dahia PL (2010). VHL disease. Best Pract Res Clin Endocrinol Metab. 24:401–13. PMID:20833332
161. Barreau O, Assié G, Wilmot-Roussel H, et al. (2013). Identification of a CpG island methylator phenotype in adrenocortical carcinomas. J Clin Endocrinol Metab. 98:E174–84. PMID:23093492
162. Barreau O, de Reynies A, Wilmot-Roussel H, et al. (2012). Clinical and pathophysiological implications of chromosomal alterations in adrenocortical tumors: an integrated genomic approach. J Clin Endocrinol Metab. 97:E301–11. PMID:22112813
163. Bartolazzi A, Gasbarri A, Papotti M, et al. (2001). Application of an immunodiagnostic method for improving preoperative diagnosis of nodular thyroid lesions. Lancet. 357:1644–50. PMID:11425367
164. Bartsch DK, Albers MB, Lopez CL, et al. (2016). Bronchopulmonary Neuroendocrine Neoplasms and Their Precursor Lesions in Multiple Endocrine Neoplasia Type 1. Neuroendocrinology. 103:240–7. PMID:26113081
165. Bartsch DK, Slater EP, Albers M, et al. (2014). Higher risk of aggressive pancreatic neuroendocrine tumors in MEN1 patients with MEN1 mutations affecting the CHES1 interacting MENIN domain. J Clin Endocrinol Metab. 99:E2387–91. PMID:25210877
166. Barzon L, Pasquali C, Grigoletto C, et al. (2001). Multiple endocrine neoplasia type 1 and adrenal lesions. J Urol. 166:24–7. PMID:11435815
167. Barzon L, Sonino N, Fallo F, et al. (2003). Prevalence and natural history of adrenal incidentalomas. Eur J Endocrinol. 149:273–85. PMID:14514341
168. Baskin HJ, Cobin RH, Duick DS, et al. (2002). American Association of Clinical Endocrinologists medical guidelines for clinical practice for the evaluation and treatment of hyperthyroidism and hypothyroidism. Endocr Pract. 8:457–69. PMID:15260011
169. Basolo F, Giannini R, Monaco C, et al. (2002). Potent mitogenicity of the RET/PTC3 oncogene correlates with its prevalence in tall-cell variant of papillary thyroid carcinoma. Am J Pathol. 160:247–54. PMID:11786418
170. Basolo F, Torregrossa L, Giannini R, et al. (2010). Correlation between the BRAF V600E mutation and tumor invasiveness in papillary thyroid carcinomas smaller than 20 millimeters: analysis of 1060 cases. J Clin Endocrinol Metab. 95:4197–205. PMID:20631031
171. Bassett JH, Forbes SA, Pannett AA, et al. (1998). Characterization of mutations in patients with multiple endocrine neoplasia type 1. Am J Hum Genet. 62:232–44. PMID:9463336
172. Bassiouni H, Asgari S, Stolke D (2006). Tuberculum sellae meningiomas: functional outcome in a consecutive series treated microsurgically. Surg Neurol. 66:37–44, discussion 44–5. PMID:16793435
173. Basturk O, Tang L, Hruban RH, et al. (2014). Poorly differentiated neuroendocrine carcinomas of the pancreas: a clinicopathologic analysis of 44 cases. Am J Surg Pathol. 38:437–47. PMID:24503751
174. Basturk O, Yang Z, Tang LH, et al. (2015). The high-grade (WHO G3) pancreatic neuroendocrine tumor category is morphologically and biologically heterogenous and includes both well differentiated and poorly differentiated neoplasms. Am J Surg Pathol. 39:683–90. PMID:25723112
175. Bates AS, Farrell WE, Bicknell EJ, et al. (1997). Allelic deletion in pituitary adenomas reflects aggressive biological activity and has potential value as a prognostic marker. J Clin Endocrinol Metab. 82:818–24. PMID:9062489
176. Batsakis JG, Littler ER, Oberman HA (1964). Teratomas of the neck. A clinicopathologic appraisal. Arch Otolaryngol. 79:619–24. PMID:14135081
177. Baudin E, Bidart JM, Rougier P, et al. (1999). Screening for multiple endocrine neoplasia type 1 and hormonal production in apparently sporadic neuroendocrine tumors. J Clin Endocrinol Metab. 84:69–75. PMID:9920064
178. Baudin E, Do Cao C, Cailleux AF, et al. (2003). Positive predictive value of serum thyroglobulin levels, measured during the first year of follow-up after thyroid hormone withdrawal, in thyroid cancer patients. J Clin Endocrinol Metab. 88:1107–11. PMID:12629092
179. Bauer AJ, Terrell R, Doniparthi NK, et al. (2002). Vascular endothelial growth factor monoclonal antibody inhibits growth of anaplastic thyroid cancer xenografts in nude mice. Thyroid. 12:953–61. PMID:12490072
180. Bausch B, Koschker AC, Fassnacht M, et al. (2006). Comprehensive mutation scanning of NF1 in apparently sporadic cases of pheochromocytoma. J Clin Endocrinol Metab. 91:3478–81. PMID:16787982
181. Bausch B, Wellner U, Peyre M, et al. (ELST) Consortium (2016). Characterization of endolymphatic sac tumors and von Hippel-Lindau disease in the International Endolymphatic Sac Tumor Registry. Head Neck. 38 Suppl 1:E673–9. PMID:25867206
182. Bayley JP, Kunst HP, Cascon A, et al. (2010). SDHAF2 mutations in familial and sporadic paraganglioma and phaeochromocytoma. Lancet Oncol. 11:366–72. PMID:20071235
183. Bayraktar F, Kebapcilar L, Kocdor MA, et al. (2006). Cushing's syndrome due to ectopic CRH secretion by adrenal pheochromocytoma accompanied by renal infarction. Exp Clin Endocrinol Diabetes. 114:444–7. PMID:17039427
184. Baysal BE, Maher ER (2015). 15 YEARS OF PARAGANGLIOMA: Genetics and mechanism of pheochromocytoma-paraganglioma syndromes characterized by germline SDHB and SDHD mutations. Endocr Relat Cancer. 22:T71–82. PMID:26113606
185. Baysal BE, Willett-Brozick JE, Lawrence EC, et al. (2002). Prevalence of SDHB, SDHC, and SDHD germline mutations in clinic patients with head and neck paragangliomas. J Med Genet. 39:178–83. PMID:11897817
186. Beard CM, Sheps SG, Kurland LT, et al. (1983). Occurrence of pheochromocytoma in Rochester, Minnesota, 1950 through 1979. Mayo Clin Proc. 58:802–4. PMID:6645626
187. Beasley MB, Lantuejoul S, Abbondanzo S, et al. (2003). The P16/cyclin D1/Rb pathway in neuroendocrine tumors of the lung. Hum Pathol. 34:136–42. PMID:12612881
188. Beauchesne P, Trouillas J, Barral F, et al. (1995). Gonadotropic pituitary carcinoma: case report. Neurosurgery. 37:810–5, discussion 815–6. PMID:8559312
189. Beck-Peccoz P, Lania A, Beckers A, et al. (2013). 2013 European thyroid association guidelines for the diagnosis and treatment of thyrotropin-secreting pituitary tumors. Eur Thyroid J. 2:76–82. PMID:24783044
190. Beck-Peccoz P, Persani L (2002). Medical management of thyrotropin-secreting pituitary adenomas. Pituitary. 5:83–8. PMID:12675505
191. Beck-Peccoz P, Persani L, Lania A (2000). Thyrotropin-secreting pituitary adenomas. In: De Groot LJ, Beck-Peccoz P, Chrousos G, et al., editors. Endotext. South Dartmouth: MDText.com, Inc. PMID:25905212
192. Beck-Peccoz P, Persani L, Mannavola D, et al. (2009). Pituitary tumours: TSH-secreting adenomas. Best Pract Res Clin Endocrinol Metab. 23:597–606. PMID:19945025
193. Beckers A, Aaltonen LA, Daly AF, et al. (2013). Familial isolated pituitary adenomas (FIPA) and the pituitary adenoma predisposition due to mutations in the aryl hydrocarbon receptor interacting protein (AIP) gene. Endocr Rev. 34:239–77. PMID:23371967
194. Beckers A, Abs R, Willems PJ, et al. (1992). Aldosterone-secreting adrenal adenoma as part of multiple endocrine neoplasia type 1 (MEN1): loss of heterozygosity for polymorphic chromosome 11 deoxyribonucleic acid markers, including the MEN1 locus. J Clin Endocrinol Metab. 75:564–70. PMID:1639957
195. Beckers A, Daly AF (2007). The clinical, pathological, and genetic features of familial isolated pituitary adenomas. Eur J Endocrinol. 157:371–82. PMID:17893250
196. Beckers A, Lodish MB, Trivellin G, et al. (2015). X-linked acrogigantism syndrome: clinical profile and therapeutic responses. Endocr Relat Cancer. 22:353–67. PMID:25712922
197. Beckers A, Van Peer G, Carter DR, et al. (2015). MYCN-driven regulatory mechanisms controlling LIN28B in neuroblastoma. Cancer Lett. 366:123–32. PMID:26123663
198. Beer TW (1992). Malignant thyroid haemangioendothelioma in a non-endemic goitrous region, with immunohistochemical evidence of a vascular origin. Histopathology. 20:539–41. PMID:1607156
199. Beerman H, Rigaud C, Bogomoletz WV, et al. (1990). Melanin production in black medullary thyroid carcinoma (MTC). Histopathology. 16:227–33. PMID:2332208
200. Bégu-Le Corroller A, Valéro R, Moutardier V, et al. (2008). Aggressive multimodal therapy of sporadic malignant insulinoma can improve survival: a retrospective 35-year study of 12 patients. Diabetes Metab. 34(4 Pt 1):343–8. PMID:18556231
201. Beilan JA, Lawton A, Hajdenberg J, et al. (2013). Pheochromocytoma of the urinary bladder: a systematic review of the contemporary literature. BMC Urol. 13:22. PMID:23627260
202. Bejarano PA, Nikiforov YE, Swenson ES, et al. (2000). Thyroid transcription factor-1, thyroglobulin, cytokeratin 7, and cytokeratin 20 in thyroid neoplasms. Appl Immunohistochem Mol Morphol. 8:189–94. PMID:10981870
203. Belfiore A, La Rosa GL, Padova G, et al. (1987). The frequency of cold thyroid nodules and thyroid malignancies in patients from an iodine-deficient area. Cancer. 60:3096–102. PMID:3677033
204. Belfiore A, Sava L, Runello F, et al. (1983). Solitary autonomously functioning thyroid nodules and iodine deficiency. J Clin Endocrinol Metab. 56:283–7. PMID:6822638
205. Belge G, Rippe V, Meiboom M, et al. (2001). Delineation of a 150-kb breakpoint cluster in benign thyroid tumors with 19q13.4 aberrations. Cytogenet Cell Genet. 93:48–51. PMID:11474178
206. Belge G, Roque L, Soares J, et al. (1998). Cytogenetic investigations of 340 thyroid hyperplasias and adenomas revealing correlations between cytogenetic findings and histology. Cancer Genet Cytogenet. 101:42–8. PMID:9460499
207. Bellevicine C, Cozzolino I, Malapelle U, et al. (2012). Cytological and molecular features of papillary thyroid carcinoma with prominent hobnail features: a case report. Acta Cytol. 56:560–4. PMID:23075900
208. Bellevicine C, Vigliar E, Malapelle U, et al. (2015). Lung adenocarcinoma and its thyroid metastasis characterized on fine-needle aspirates by cytomorphology, immunocytochemistry, and next-generation sequencing. Diagn Cytopathol. 43:585–9. PMID:25900221
209. Bellingham GA, Dhir AK, Luke PP (2008). Case report: retroperitoneoscopic pheochromocytoma removal in an adult with Eisenmenger's syndrome. Can J Anaesth. 55:295–301. PMID:18451118
210. Bengtsson D, Schrøder HD, Andersen M, et al. (2015). Long-term outcome and MGMT as a predictive marker in 24 patients with atypical pituitary adenomas and pituitary carcinomas given treatment with temozolomide.

J Clin Endocrinol Metab. 100:1689–98. PMID:25646794

211. Benites Filho PR, Sakamoto D, Machuca TN, et al. (2005). Granular cell tumor of the neurohypophysis: report of a case with unusual age presentation. Virchows Arch. 447:649–52. PMID:16133355

212. Benito M, Asa SL, Livolsi VA, et al. (2005). Gonadotroph tumor associated with multiple endocrine neoplasia type 1. J Clin Endocrinol Metab. 90:570–4. PMID:15522929

213. Benn DE, Robinson BG, Clifton-Bligh RJ (2015). 15 YEARS OF PARAGANGLIOMA: Clinical manifestations of paraganglioma syndromes types 1-5. Endocr Relat Cancer. 22:T91–103. PMID:26273102

214. Bennett KL, Mester J, Eng C (2010). Germline epigenetic regulation of KILLIN in Cowden and Cowden-like syndrome. JAMA. 304:2724–31. PMID:21177507

215. Bentwich I, Avniel A, Karov Y, et al. (2005). Identification of hundreds of conserved and nonconserved human microRNAs. Nat Genet. 37:766–70. PMID:15965474

216. Bercaw-Pratt JL, Moorjani TP, Santos XM, et al. (2012). Diagnosis and management of precocious puberty in atypical presentations of McCune-Albright syndrome: a case series review. J Pediatr Adolesc Gynecol. 25:e9–13. PMID:22051789

217. Berezin M, Shimon I, Hadani M (1995). Prolactinoma in 53 men: clinical characteristics and modes of treatment (male prolactinoma). J Endocrinol Invest. 18:436–41. PMID:7594238

218. Berezowski K, Grimes MM, Gal A, et al. (1996). CD5 immunoreactivity of epithelial cells in thymic carcinoma and CASTLE using paraffin-embedded tissue. Am J Clin Pathol. 106:483–6. PMID:8853036

219. Berger G, Trouillas J, Bloch B, et al. (1984). Multihormonal carcinoid tumor of the pancreas. Secreting growth hormone-releasing factor as a cause of acromegaly. Cancer. 54:2097–108. PMID:6435852

220. Bergero N, De Pompa R, Sacerdote C, et al. (2005). Galectin-3 expression in parathyroid carcinoma: immunohistochemical study of 26 cases. Hum Pathol. 36:908–14. PMID:16112008

221. Bergholm U, Adami HO, Bergström R, et al. (1989). Clinical characteristics in sporadic and familial medullary thyroid carcinoma. A nationwide study of 249 patients in Sweden from 1959 through 1981. Cancer. 63:1196–204. PMID:2563669

222. Berho M, Suster S (1997). The oncocytic variant of papillary carcinoma of the thyroid: a clinicopathologic study of 15 cases. Hum Pathol. 28:47–53. PMID:9013831

223. Berkmann S, Tolnay M, Hänggi D, et al. (2010). Sarcoma of the sella after radiotherapy for pituitary adenoma. Acta Neurochir (Wien). 152:1725–35. PMID:20512596

224. Berna MJ, Annibale B, Marignani M, et al. (2008). A prospective study of gastric carcinoids and enterochromaffin-like cell changes in multiple endocrine neoplasia type 1 and Zollinger-Ellison syndrome: identification of risk factors. J Clin Endocrinol Metab. 93:1582–91. PMID:18270260

225. Bernini GP, Moretti A, Mannelli M, et al. (2005). Unique association of non-functioning pheochromocytoma, ganglioneuroma, adrenal cortical adenoma, hepatic and vertebral hemangiomas in a patient with a new intronic variant in the VHL gene. J Endocrinol Invest. 28:1032–7. PMID:16483185

226. Bernstein J, Virk RK, Hui P, et al. (2013). Tall cell variant of papillary thyroid microcarcinoma: clinicopathologic features with BRAF(V600E) mutational analysis. Thyroid. 23:1525–31. PMID:23682579

227. Beroukhim R, Brunet JP, Di Napoli A, et al. (2009). Patterns of gene expression and copy-number alterations in von-hippel lindau disease-associated and sporadic clear cell carcinoma of the kidney. Cancer Res. 69:4674–81. PMID:19470766

228. Berres ML, Allen CE, Merad M (2013). Pathological consequence of misguided dendritic cell differentiation in histiocytic diseases. Adv Immunol. 120:127–61. PMID:24070383

229. Berruti A, Fassnacht M, Haak H, et al. (2014). Prognostic role of overt hypercortisolism in completely operated patients with adrenocortical cancer. Eur Urol. 65:832–8. PMID:24268504

230. Berry CL, Keeling J, Hilton C (1969). Teratomata in infancy and childhood: a review of 91 cases. J Pathol. 98:241–52. PMID:5358276

231. Bertherat J (2012). Adrenocortical cancer in Carney complex: a paradigm of endocrine tumor progression or an association of genetic predisposing factors? J Clin Endocrinol Metab. 97:387–90. PMID:22312093

232. Bertherat J, Horvath A, Groussin L, et al. (2009). Mutations in regulatory subunit type 1A of cyclic adenosine 5´-monophosphate-dependent protein kinase (PRKAR1A): phenotype analysis in 353 patients and 80 different genotypes. J Clin Endocrinol Metab. 94:2085–91. PMID:19293268

233. Bertoin F, Letouzé E, Grignani P, et al. (2015). Genome-wide paternal uniparental disomy as a cause of Beckwith-Wiedemann syndrome associated with recurrent virilizing adrenocortical tumors. Horm Metab Res. 47:497–503. PMID:25365508

234. Besic N, Hocevar M, Zgajnar J, et al. (2005). Prognostic factors in anaplastic carcinoma of the thyroid-a multivariate survival analysis of 188 patients. Langenbecks Arch Surg. 390:203–8. PMID:15599758

235. Beskid M, Lorenc R, Rościszewska A (1971). C-cell thyroid adenoma in man. J Pathol. 103:1–4. PMID:4327780

236. Besson A, Dowdy SF, Roberts JM (2008). CDK inhibitors: cell cycle regulators and beyond. Dev Cell. 14:159–69. PMID:18267085

237. Betônico CC, Rodrigues R, Mendonça SC, et al. (2004). Primary hypothyroidism mimicking pituitary macroadenoma. Arq Bras Endocrinol Metabol. 48:423–6. [Portuguese] PMID:15640908

238. Beuschlein F, Boulkroun S, Osswald A, et al. (2013). Somatic mutations in ATP1A1 and ATP2B3 lead to aldosterone-producing adenomas and secondary hypertension. Nat Genet. 45:440–4, e1–2. PMID:23416519

239. Beuschlein F, Fassnacht M, Assié G, et al. (2014). Constitutive activation of PKA catalytic subunit in adrenal Cushing's syndrome. N Engl J Med. 370:1019–28. PMID:24571724

240. Beuschlein F, Strasburger CJ, Siegerstetter V, et al. (2000). Acromegaly caused by secretion of growth hormone by a non-Hodgkin's lymphoma. N Engl J Med. 342:1871–6. PMID:10861322

241. Beuschlein F, Weigel J, Saeger W, et al. (2015). Major prognostic role of Ki67 in localized adrenocortical carcinoma after complete resection. J Clin Endocrinol Metab. 100:841–9. PMID:25559399

242. Bezerra JE, Latronico AC (2014). MicroRNA era: the importance for diagnosis and prognosis of adrenocortical tumors. Biomed Res Int. 2014:381917. PMID:25050346

243. Bhandarkar ND, Chan J, Strome M (2005). A rare case of mucoepidermoid carcinoma of the thyroid. Am J Otolaryngol. 26:138–41. PMID:15742270

244. Bhatnagar P, Bhatnagar A, Kishan S, et al. (2004). Unusual widespread metastatic presentation of mixed medullary-follicular thyroid carcinoma. Clin Nucl Med. 29:303–5. PMID:15069329

245. Bhatoe HS, Kotwal N, Badwal S (2007). Clival pituitary adenoma with acromegaly: case report and review of literature. Skull Base. 17:265–8. PMID:18174927

246. Bhayana S, Booth GL, Asa SL, et al. (2005). The implication of somatotroph adenoma phenotype to somatostatin analog responsiveness in acromegaly. J Clin Endocrinol Metab. 90:6290–5. PMID:16118335

247. Biankin SA, Cachia AR (1999). Leiomyoma of the thyroid gland. Pathology. 31:64–6. PMID:10212928

248. Bielle F, Fréneaux P, Jeanne-Pasquier C, et al. (2012). PHOX2B immunolabeling: a novel tool for the diagnosis of undifferentiated neuroblastomas among childhood small round blue-cell tumors. Am J Surg Pathol. 36:1141–9. PMID:22790854

249. Biesecker LG, Happle R, Mulliken JB, et al. (1999). Proteus syndrome: diagnostic criteria, differential diagnosis, and patient evaluation. Am J Med Genet. 84:389–95. PMID:10360391

250. Bilbao JM, Horvath E, Kovacs K, et al. (1978). Intrasellar paraganglioma associated with hypopituitarism. Arch Pathol Lab Med. 102:95–8. PMID:341846

251. Bilginer B, Türk CC, Narin F, et al. (2015). Enigmatic entity in childhood: clival chordoma from a tertiary center's perspective. Acta Neurochir (Wien). 157:1587–93. PMID:26223909

252. Bilimoria KY, Bentrem DJ, Merkow RP, et al. (2007). Application of the pancreatic adenocarcinoma staging system to pancreatic neuroendocrine tumors. J Am Coll Surg. 205:558–63. PMID:17903729

253. Bilodeau S, Vallette-Kasic S, Gauthier Y, et al. (2006). Role of Brg1 and HDAC2 in GR trans-repression of the pituitary POMC gene and misexpression in Cushing disease. Genes Dev. 20:2871–86. PMID:17043312

254. Bisceglia M, Carosi I, Scillitani A, et al. (2009). Cystic lymphangioma-like adenomatoid tumor of the adrenal gland: Case presentation and review of the literature. Adv Anat Pathol. 16:424–32. PMID:19851133

255. Bisceglia M, Galliani C, Giannatempo G, et al. (2011). Solitary fibrous tumor of the central nervous system: a 15-year literature survey of 220 cases (August 1996–July 2011). Adv Anat Pathol. 18:356–92. PMID:21841406

256. Bisceglia M, Ludovico O, Di Mattia A, et al. (2004). Adrenocortical oncocytic tumors: report of 10 cases and review of the literature. Int J Surg Pathol. 12:231–43. PMID:15306935

257. Bishop JA, Sharma R, Westra WH (2011). PAX8 immunostaining of anaplastic thyroid carcinoma: a reliable means of discerning thyroid origin for undifferentiated tumors of the head and neck. Hum Pathol. 42:1873–7. PMID:21663937

258. Bishop JA, Wu G, Tufano RP, et al. (2012). Histological patterns of locoregional recurrence in Hürthle cell carcinoma of the thyroid gland. Thyroid. 22:690–4. PMID:22524498

259. Bisi H, Fernandes VS, de Camargo RY, et al. (1989). The prevalence of unsuspected thyroid pathology in 300 sequential autopsies, with special reference to the incidental carcinoma. Cancer. 64:1888–93. PMID:2676140

260. Bismar TA, Basturk O, Gerald WL, et al. (2004). Desmoplastic small cell tumor in the pancreas. Am J Surg Pathol. 28:808–12. PMID:15166674

261. Bizzarri C, Bottaro G (2015). Endocrine implications of neurofibromatosis 1 in childhood. Horm Res Paediatr. 83:232–41. PMID:25659607

262. Bjornsson J, Scheithauer BW, Okazaki H, et al. (1985). Intracranial germ cell tumors: pathobiological and immunohistochemical aspects of 70 cases. J Neuropathol Exp Neurol. 44:32–46. PMID:4038412

263. Black BK (1954). Carcinoma of the parathyroid. Ann Surg. 139:355–63. PMID:13149082

264. Black WC, Haff RC (1970). The surgical pathology of parathyroid chief cell hyperplasia. Am J Clin Pathol. 53:565–79. PMID:5444463

265. Blank A, Schmitt AM, Korpershoek E, et al. (2010). SDHB loss predicts malignancy in pheochromocytomas / sympathethic paragangliomas, but not through hypoxia signalling. Endocr Relat Cancer. 17:919–28. PMID:20702724

266. Blansfield JA, Choyke L, Morita SY, et al. (2007). Clinical, genetic and radiographic analysis of 108 patients with von Hippel-Lindau disease (VHL) manifested by pancreatic neuroendocrine neoplasms (PNETs). Surgery. 142:814–8, discussion 818.e1–2. PMID:18063061

267. Bleistein M, Geiger K, Franz K, et al. (2000). Transthyretin and transferrin in hemangioblastoma stromal cells. Pathol Res Pract. 196:675–81. PMID:11087054

268. Boari N, Losa M, Mortini P, et al. (2006). Intrasellar paraganglioma: a case report and review of the literature. Acta Neurochir (Wien). 148:1311–4, discussion 1314. PMID:17039304

269. Böcker W, Schröder S, Dralle H (1988). Minimal thyroid neoplasia. Recent Results Cancer Res. 106:131–8. PMID:3285408

270. Boecher-Schwarz HG, Fries G, Bornemann A, et al. (1992). Suprasellar granular cell tumor. Neurosurgery. 31:751–4, discussion 754. PMID:1407463

271. Boedeker CC, Hensen EF, Neumann HP, et al. (2014). Genetics of hereditary head and neck paragangliomas. Head Neck. 36:907–16. PMID:23913591

272. Boehm BO, Rosinger S, Belyi D, et al. (2011). The parathyroid as a target for radiation damage. N Engl J Med. 365:676–8. PMID:21848480

273. Bohórquez CL, González-Cámpora R, Loscertales MC, et al. (2003). Solitary fibrous tumor of the thyroid with capsular invasion. Pathol Res Pract. 199:687–90. PMID:14666971

274. Boikos SA, Xekouki P, Fumagalli E, et al. (2016). Carney triad can be (rarely) associated with germline succinate dehydrogenase defects. Eur J Hum Genet. 24:569–73. PMID:26173966

275. Boltze C, Roessner A, Landt O, et al. (2002). Homozygous proline at codon 72 of p53 as a potential risk factor favoring the development of undifferentiated thyroid carcinoma. Int J Oncol. 21:1151–4. PMID:12370767

276. Boman F, Hill DA, Williams GM, et al. (2006). Familial association of pleuropulmonary blastoma with cystic nephroma and other renal tumors: a report from the International Pleuropulmonary Blastoma Registry. J Pediatr. 149:850–4. PMID:17137906

277. Bondeson L, Bondeson AG (1996). Cytologic features in fine-needle aspirates from a sclerosing mucoepidermoid thyroid carcinoma with eosinophilia. Diagn Cytopathol. 15:301–5. PMID:8982585

278. Bondeson L, Bondeson AG, Thompson NW (1991). Papillary carcinoma of the thyroid with mucoepidermoid features. Am J Clin Pathol. 95:175–9. PMID:1992608

279. Bondeson L, Sandelin K, Grimelius L (1993). Histopathological variables and DNA cytometry in parathyroid carcinoma. Am J Surg Pathol. 17:820–9. PMID:8338192

280. Bongiovanni M, Bloom L, Krane JF, et al. (2009). Cytomorphologic features of poorly differentiated thyroid carcinoma: a multi-institutional analysis of 40 cases. Cancer. 117:185–94. PMID:19365842

281. Bongiovanni M, Piana S, Frattini M, et al. (2013). CDX2 expression in columnar variant of papillary thyroid carcinoma. Thyroid. 23:1498–9. PMID:23734674

282. Bonneau D, Longy M (2000). Mutations of the human PTEN gene. Hum Mutat. 16:109–22. PMID:10923032

283. Bonnet S, Gaujoux S, Launay P, et al. (2011). Wnt/β-catenin pathway activation in adrenocortical adenomas is frequently due to somatic CTNNB1-activating mutations, which are associated with larger and nonsecreting tumors: a study in cortisol-secreting and -nonsecreting tumors. J Clin Endocrinol Metab. 96:E419–26. PMID:21084400

284. Bonora E, Porcelli AM, Gasparre G, et al. (2006). Defective oxidative phosphorylation in thyroid oncocytic carcinoma is associated with pathogenic mitochondrial DNA mutations affecting complexes I and III. Cancer Res. 66:6087–96. PMID:16778181

285. Boos LA, Dettmer M, Schmitt A, et al. (2013). Diagnostic and prognostic implications of the PAX8-PPARγ translocation in thyroid carcinomas-a TMA-based study of 226 cases. Histopathology. 63:234–41. PMID:23738683

286. Boos S, Meyer E, Wimmer B, et al. (1991). Malignant triton tumor of the thyroid gland. Radiat Med. 9:159–61. PMID:1961942

287. Bordi C, Corleto VD, Azzoni C, et al. (2001). The antral mucosa as a new site for endocrine tumors in multiple endocrine neoplasia type 1 and Zollinger-Ellison syndromes. J Clin Endocrinol Metab. 86:2236–42. PMID:11344233

288. Borges MT, Lillehei KO, Kleinschmidt-DeMasters BK (2011). Spindle cell oncocytoma with late recurrence and unique neuroimaging characteristics due to recurrent subclinical intratumoral bleeding. J Neurooncol. 101:145–54. PMID:20495848

289. Borota OC, Scheithauer BW, Fougner SL, et al. (2009). Spindle cell oncocytoma of the adenohypophysis: report of a case with marked cellular atypia and recurrence despite adjuvant treatment. Clin Neuropathol. 28:91–5. PMID:19353839

290. Borson-Chazot F, Garby L, Raverot G, et al. (2012). Acromegaly induced by ectopic secretion of GHRH: a review 30 years after GHRH discovery. Ann Endocrinol (Paris). 73:497–502. PMID:23122576

291. Bosisio FM, Bickel JT (2013). "Glomeruloid" follicular thyroid adenoma. Int J Surg Pathol. 21:376. PMID:23637255

292. Bosse KR, Diskin SJ, Cole KA, et al. (2012). Common variation at BARD1 results in the expression of an oncogenic isoform that influences neuroblastoma susceptibility and oncogenicity. Cancer Res. 72:2068–78. PMID:22350409

293. Boulkroun S, Beuschlein F, Rossi GP, et al. (2012). Prevalence, clinical, and molecular correlates of KCNJ5 mutations in primary aldosteronism. Hypertension. 59:592–8. PMID:22275527

294. Boulkroun S, Samson-Couterie B, Dzib JF, et al. (2010). Adrenal cortex remodeling and functional zona glomerulosa hyperplasia in primary aldosteronism. Hypertension. 56:885–92. PMID:20937967

295. Bourgois B, Boman F, Nelken B, et al. (2004). Intractable diarrhoea revealing a neuroblastoma hypersecreting the vasoactive intestinal peptide. Arch Pediatr. 11:340–3. [French] PMID:15051093

296. Boussaïd K, Meduri G, Maiza JC, et al. (2013). Virilizing sclerosing-stromal tumor of the ovary in a young woman with McCune Albright syndrome: clinical, pathological, and immunohistochemical studies. J Clin Endocrinol Metab. 98:E314–20. PMID:23365131

297. Bovio S, Cataldi A, Reimondo G, et al. (2006). Prevalence of adrenal incidentaloma in a contemporary computerized tomography series. J Endocrinol Invest. 29:298–302. PMID:16699294

298. Bowker CM, Whittaker RS (1992). Malignant teratoma of the thyroid: case report and literature review of thyroid teratoma in adults. Histopathology. 21:81–3. PMID:1634206

299. Bown N, Cotterill S, Lastowska M, et al. (1999). Gain of chromosome arm 17q and adverse outcome in patients with neuroblastoma. N Engl J Med. 340:1954–61. PMID:10379019

300. Boyar Cetinkaya R, Aagnes B, Thiis-Evensen E, et al. (2017). Trends in incidence of neuroendocrine neoplasms in Norway: a report of 16,075 cases from 1993 through 2010. Neuroendocrinology. 104:1–10. PMID:26562558

301. Boyce AM, Bhattacharyya N, Collins MT (2013). Fibrous dysplasia and fibroblast growth factor-23 regulation. Curr Osteoporos Rep. 11:65–71. PMID:23532406

302. Boyce AM, Chong WH, Shawker TH, et al. (2012). Characterization and management of testicular pathology in McCune-Albright syndrome. J Clin Endocrinol Metab. 97:E1782–90. PMID:22745241

303. Boyce AM, Collins MT (1993). Fibrous dysplasia/McCune-Albright syndrome. In: Pagon RA, Adam MP, Ardinger HH, et al., editors. GeneReviews®. Seattle: University of Washington, Seattle. PMID:25719192

304. Boyce AM, Glover M, Kelly MH, et al. (2013). Optic neuropathy in McCune-Albright syndrome: effects of early diagnosis and treatment of growth hormone excess. J Clin Endocrinol Metab. 98:E126–34. PMID:23093488

305. Boyle NH, Ogg CS, Hartley RB, et al. (1999). Parathyroid carcinoma secondary to prolonged hyperplasia in chronic renal failure and in coeliac disease. Eur J Surg Oncol. 25:100–3. PMID:10188867

306. Bradley KJ, Hobbs MR, Buley ID, et al. (2005). Uterine tumours are a phenotypic manifestation of the hyperparathyroidism-jaw tumour syndrome. J Intern Med. 257:18–26. PMID:15606373

307. Bradshaw JW, Jansen JC (2005). Management of vagal paraganglioma: is operative resection really the best option? Surgery. 137:225–8. PMID:15674205

308. Brady A, Nayar A, Cross P, et al. (2012). A detailed immunohistochemical analysis of 2 cases of papillary cystadenoma of the broad ligament: an extremely rare neoplasm characteristic of patients with von hippel-lindau disease. Int J Gynecol Pathol. 31:133–40. PMID:22317868

309. Brady S, Lechan RM, Schwaitzberg SD, et al. (1997). Composite pheochromocytoma/ganglioneuroma of the adrenal gland associated with multiple endocrine neoplasia 2A: case report with immunohistochemical analysis. Am J Surg Pathol. 21:102–8. PMID:8990146

310. Abrams HL, Spiro R, Goldstein N (1950). Metastases in carcinoma; analysis of 1000 autopsied cases. Cancer. 3:74–85. PMID:15405683

311. Branch CL Jr, Laws ER Jr (1987). Metastatic tumors of the sella turcica masquerading as primary pituitary tumors. J Clin Endocrinol Metab. 65:469–74. PMID:3624409

312. Brandi ML, Gagel RF, Angeli A, et al. (2001). Guidelines for diagnosis and therapy of MEN type 1 and type 2. J Clin Endocrinol Metab. 86:5658–71. PMID:11739416

313. Brastianos PK, Shankar GM, Gill CM, et al. (2015). Dramatic Response of BRAF V600E Mutant Papillary Craniopharyngioma to Targeted Therapy. J Natl Cancer Inst. 108:108. PMID:26498373

314. Brastianos PK, Taylor-Weiner A, Manley PE, et al. (2014). Exome sequencing identifies BRAF mutations in papillary craniopharyngiomas. Nat Genet. 46:161–5. PMID:24413733

315. Brat DJ, Scheithauer BW, Eberhart CG, et al. (2001). Extraventricular neurocytomas: pathologic features and clinical outcome. Am J Surg Pathol. 25:1252–60. PMID:11688459

316. Brat DJ, Scheithauer BW, Staugaitis SM, et al. (2000). Pituicytoma: a distinctive low-grade glioma of the neurohypophysis. Am J Surg Pathol. 24:362–8. PMID:10716149

317. Brauckhoff M, Machens A, Hess S, et al. (2008). Premonitory symptoms preceding metastatic medullary thyroid cancer in MEN 2B: An exploratory analysis. Surgery. 144:1044–50, discussion 1050–3. PMID:19041016

318. Brauckhoff M, Machens A, Lorenz K, et al. (2014). Surgical curability of medullary thyroid cancer in multiple endocrine neoplasia 2B: a changing perspective. Ann Surg. 259:800–6. PMID:23979292

319. Brennan P (2015). Breast cancer risk in MEN1 – a cancer genetics perspective. Clin Endocrinol (Oxf). 82:327–229. PMID:25279812

320. Brenneman M, Field A, Yang J, et al. (2015). Temporal order of RNase IIIb and loss-of-function mutations during development determines phenotype in DICER1 syndrome: a unique variant of the two-hit tumor suppression model. F1000Res. 4:214. PMID:26925222

321. Bricaire L, Odou MF, Cardot-Bauters C, et al. (2013). Frequent large germline HRPT2 deletions in a French National cohort of patients with primary hyperparathyroidism. J Clin Endocrinol Metab. 98:E403–8. PMID:23293331

322. Bridenstine M, Kerr JM, Lillehei KO, et al. (2013). Cushing's disease due to mixed pituitary adenoma-gangliocytoma of the posterior pituitary gland presenting with Aspergillus sp. sinus infection. Clin Neuropathol. 32:377–83. PMID:23611590

323. Brierley JD, Gospodarowicz MK, Wittekind C, editors (2016). TNM Classification of Malignant Tumours. 8th ed. John Wiley & Sons.

324. Brierley J, Tsang R, Simpson WJ, et al. (1996). Medullary thyroid cancer: analyses of survival and prognostic factors and the role of radiation therapy in local control. Thyroid. 6:305–10. PMID:8875751

325. Brignardello E, Gallo M, Baldi I, et al. (2007). Anaplastic thyroid carcinoma: clinical outcome of 30 consecutive patients referred to a single institution in the past 5 years. Eur J Endocrinol. 156:425–30. PMID:17389456

326. Brito JP, Asi N, Bancos I, et al. (2015). Testing for germline mutations in sporadic pheochromocytoma/paraganglioma: a systematic review. Clin Endocrinol (Oxf). 82:338–45. PMID:24954084

327. Brochier S, Galland F, Kujas M, et al. (2010). Factors predicting relapse of nonfunctioning pituitary macroadenomas after neurosurgery: a study of 142 patients. Eur J Endocrinol. 163:193–200. PMID:20460423

328. Brodeur GM, Hogarty MD, Moose YP, et al. (2011). Neuroblastoma. In: Pizzo PA, Poplack DG, editors. Principles and practice of pediatric oncology. Philadelphia: Lippincott Williams & Wilkins; pp. 886–922.

329. Brodeur GM, Nakagawara A, Yamashiro DJ, et al. (1997). Expression of TrkA, TrkB and TrkC in human neuroblastomas. J Neurooncol. 31:49–55. PMID:9049830

330. Brodeur GM, Pritchard J, Berthold F, et al. (1993). Revisions of the international criteria for neuroblastoma diagnosis, staging, and response to treatment. J Clin Oncol. 11:1466–77. PMID:8336186

331. Brodeur GM, Seeger RC, Barrett A, et al. (1988). International criteria for diagnosis, staging, and response to treatment in patients with neuroblastoma. J Clin Oncol. 6:1874–81. PMID:3199170

332. Brodeur GM, Seeger RC, Schwab M, et al. (1984). Amplification of N-myc in untreated human neuroblastomas correlates with advanced disease stage. Science. 224:1121–4. PMID:6719137

333. Bronner MP, Clevenger CV, Edmonds PR, et al. (1988). Flow cytometric analysis of DNA content in Hürthle cell adenomas and carcinomas of the thyroid. Am J Clin Pathol. 89:764–9. PMID:3369368

334. Broughan TA, Leslie JD, Soto JM, et al. (1986). Pancreatic islet cell tumors. Surgery. 99:671–8. PMID:2424108

335. Brown K, Kristopaitis T, Yong S, et al. (1998). Cystic glucagonoma: A rare variant of an uncommon neuroendocrine pancreas tumor. J Gastrointest Surg. 2:533–6. PMID:10457311

336. Brown NA, Furtado LV, Betz BL, et al. (2014). High prevalence of somatic MAP2K1 mutations in BRAF V600E-negative Langerhans cell histiocytosis. Blood. 124:1655–8. PMID:24982505

337. Brown RJ, Kelly MH, Collins MT (2010). Cushing syndrome in the McCune-Albright syndrome. J Clin Endocrinol Metab. 95:1508–15. PMID:20157193

338. Brown RL, Wollman R, Weiss RE (2007). Transformation of a pituitary macroadenoma into to a corticotropin-secreting carcinoma over 16 years. Endocr Pract. 13:463–71. PMID:17872347

339. Brown S, O'Neill C, Suliburk J, et al. (2011). Parathyroid carcinoma: increasing incidence and changing presentation. ANZ J Surg. 81:528–32. PMID:22295377

340. Brunnemann RB, Ro JY, Ordonez NG, et al. (1999). Extrapleural solitary fibrous tumor: a clinicopathologic study of 24 cases. Mod Pathol. 12:1034–42. PMID:10574600

341. Buch H, El-Hadd T, Bicknell J, et al. (2002). Pituitary tumours are multiclonal from the outset: evidence from a case with dural metastases. Clin Endocrinol (Oxf). 56:817–22. PMID:12072054

342. Buffet A, Venisse A, Nau V, et al. (2012). A decade (2001–2010) of genetic testing for pheochromocytoma and paraganglioma. Horm Metab Res. 44:359–66. PMID:22517557

343. Buley ID, Gatter KC, Heryet A, et al. (1987). Expression of intermediate filament proteins in normal and diseased thyroid glands. J Clin Pathol. 40:136–42. PMID:3546391

344. Bullock M, Ren Y, O'Neill C, et al. (2016). TERT promoter mutations are a major indicator of recurrence and death due to papillary thyroid carcinomas. Clin Endocrinol (Oxf). 85:283–90. PMID:26667986

345. Bülow B, Jansson S, Juhlin C, et al. (2006). Adrenal incidentaloma – follow-up results from a Swedish prospective study. Eur J Endocrinol. 154:419–23. PMID:16498055

346. Burgess JR, Harle RA, Tucker P, et al. (1996). Adrenal lesions in a large kindred with multiple endocrine neoplasia type 1. Arch Surg. 131:699–702. PMID:8678766

347. Burlacu MC, Tichomirowa M, Daly A, et al. (2009). Familial pituitary adenomas. Presse Med. 38:112–6. [French] PMID:18990538

348. Burnichon N, Buffet A, Parfait B, et al. (2012). Somatic NF1 inactivation is a frequent event in sporadic pheochromocytoma. Hum Mol Genet. 21:5397–405. PMID:22962301

349. Burnichon N, Cascón A, Schiavi F, et al. (2012). MAX mutations cause hereditary and sporadic pheochromocytoma and paraganglioma. Clin Cancer Res. 18:2828–37. PMID:22452945

350. Burnichon N, Rohmer V, Amar L, et al. (2009). The succinate dehydrogenase genetic testing in a large prospective series of patients with paragangliomas. J Clin Endocrinol Metab. 94:2817–27. PMID:19454582

351. Burnichon N, Vescovo L, Amar L, et al. (2011). Integrative genomic analysis reveals somatic mutations in pheochromocytoma and paraganglioma. Hum Mol Genet. 20:3974–85. PMID:21784903

352. Busam KJ, Iversen K, Coplan KA, et al. (1998). Immunoreactivity for A103, an antibody to melan-A (Mart-1), in adrenocortical and other steroid tumors. Am J Surg Pathol. 22:57–63. PMID:9422316

353. Bush ZM, Longtine JA, Cunningham T, et al. (2010). Temozolomide treatment for aggressive pituitary tumors: correlation of clinical outcome with O(6)-methylguanine methyltransferase (MGMT) promoter methylation and expression. J Clin Endocrinol Metab. 95:E280–90. PMID:20668043

354. Butler MG, Dasouki MJ, Zhou XP, et al. (2005). Subset of individuals with autism spectrum disorders and extreme macrocephaly associated with germline PTEN tumour suppressor gene mutations. J Med Genet. 42:318–21. PMID:15805158

355. Cabanne F, Gérard-Marchant R, Heimann R, et al. (1974). Malignant tumors of the thyroid gland. Problems of histopathologic diagnosis. Apropos of 692 lesions collected by the thyroid cancer Cooperative Group of the O.E.R.T.C. Ann Anat Pathol (Paris). 19:129–48. [French] PMID:4480015

356. Cady B, Rossi R (1988). An expanded view of risk-group definition in differentiated thyroid carcinoma. Surgery. 104:947–53. PMID:3194846

357. Caillou B, Talbot M, Weyemi U, et al. (2011). Tumor-associated macrophages (TAMs) form an interconnected cellular supportive network in anaplastic thyroid carcinoma. PLoS One. 6:e22567. PMID:21811634

358. Calebiro D, Di Dalmazi G, Bathon K, et al. (2015). cAMP signaling in cortisol-producing adrenal adenoma. Eur J Endocrinol. 173:M99–106. PMID:26139209

359. Calender A, Giraud S, Porchet N, et al. (1998). Clinicogenetic study of MEN1: recent physiopathological data and clinical applications (GENEM). Ann Endocrinol (Paris). 59:444–51. [French] PMID:10189986

359A. Callender GG, Udelsman R. (2014). Surgery for primary hyperparathyroidism. Cancer. 120(23):3602–16. PMID: 25042934

360. Calò PG, Maxia S, Lai ML, et al. (2010). Sclerosing mucoepidermoid thyroid carcinoma requiring cervical reconstruction: a case report and review of the literature. Am Surg. 76:918–9. PMID:20726436

361. Calzolari F, Sartori PV, Talarico C, et al. (2008). Surgical treatment of intrathyroid metastases: preliminary results of a multicentric study. Anticancer Res. 28 5B:2885–8. PMID:19031929

362. Camacho P, Gordon D, Chiefari E, et al. (2000). A Phe 486 thyrotropin receptor mutation in an autonomously functioning follicular carcinoma that was causing hyperthyroidism. Thyroid. 10:1009–12. PMID:11128715

363. Cambiaso P, Amodio D, Procaccini E, et al. (2015). Pituicytoma and Cushing's Disease in a 7-Year-Old Girl: A Mere Coincidence? Pediatrics. 136:e1632–6. PMID:26553184

364. Cameselle-Teijeiro J, Chan JK (1999). Cribriform-morular variant of papillary carcinoma: a distinctive variant representing the sporadic counterpart of familial adenomatous polyposis-associated thyroid carcinoma? Mod Pathol. 12:400–11. PMID:10229505

365. Cameselle-Teijeiro J, Fachal C, Cabezas-Agrícola JM, et al. (2015). Thyroid Pathology Findings in Cowden Syndrome: A Clue for the Diagnosis of the PTEN Hamartoma Tumor Syndrome. Am J Clin Pathol. 144:322–8. PMID:26185318

366. Cameselle-Teijeiro J, Febles-Pérez C, Sobrinho-Simões M (1995). Papillary and mucoepidermoid carcinoma of the thyroid with anaplastic transformation: a case report with histologic and immunohistochemical findings that support a provocative histogenetic hypothesis. Pathol Res Pract. 191:1214–21. PMID:8927569

367. Cameselle-Teijeiro J, Febles-Pérez C, Sobrinho-Simões M (1997). Cytologic features of fine needle aspirates of papillary and mucoepidermoid carcinoma of the thyroid with anaplastic transformation. A case report. Acta Cytol. 41(4 Suppl):1356–60. PMID:9990275

368. Cameselle-Teijeiro J, Manuel Lopes J, Villanueva JP, et al. (2003). Lipomatous haemangiopericytoma (adipocytic variant of solitary fibrous tumour) of the thyroid. Histopathology. 43:406–8. PMID:14511266

369. Cameselle-Teijeiro J, Menasce LP, Yap BK, et al. (2009). Cribriform-morular variant of papillary thyroid carcinoma: molecular characterization of a case with neuroendocrine differentiation and aggressive behavior. Am J Clin Pathol. 131:134–42. PMID:19095577

370. Cameselle-Teijeiro J, Pardal F, Eloy C, et al. (2008). Follicular thyroid carcinoma with an unusual glomeruloid pattern of growth. Hum Pathol. 39:1540–7. PMID:18602667

371. Cameselle-Teijeiro J, Preto A, Soares P, et al. (2005). A stem cell role for thyroid solid cell nests. Hum Pathol. 36:590–1. PMID:15948129

372. Cameselle-Teijeiro J, Sobrinho-Simões M (1999). Cytomorphologic features of mucoepidermoid carcinoma of the thyroid. Am J Clin Pathol. 111:134–6. PMID:9894464

373. Cameselle-Teijeiro J, Varela-Duran J, Fonseca E, et al. (1994). Solitary fibrous tumor of the thyroid. Am J Clin Pathol. 101:535–8. PMID:8160648

374. Canaff L, Vanbellinghen JF, Kanazawa I, et al. (2012). Menin missense mutants encoded by the MEN1 gene that are targeted to the proteasome: restoration of expression and activity by CHIP siRNA. J Clin Endocrinol Metab. 97:E282–91. PMID:22090276

375. Cancer Genome Atlas Research Network (2014). Integrated genomic characterization of papillary thyroid carcinoma. Cell. 159:676–90. PMID:25417114

376. Cao D, Li L, Liu L, et al. (2014). Solitary extramedullary plasmacytoma of the adrenal gland: a rare case report with review of the literature. Int J Clin Exp Pathol. 7:9072–5. PMID:25674290

377. Cao D, Liu A, Wang F, et al. (2011). RNA-binding protein LIN28 is a marker for primary extragonadal germ cell tumors: an immunohistochemical study of 131 cases. Mod Pathol. 24:288–96. PMID:21057460

378. Cao J, Chen C, Chen C, et al. (2016). Clinicopathological features and prognosis of familial papillary thyroid carcinoma–a large-scale, matched, case-control study. Clin Endocrinol (Oxf). 84:598–606. PMID:26191611

379. Cao Y, Gao Z, Li L, et al. (2013). Whole exome sequencing of insulinoma reveals recurrent T372R mutations in YY1. Nat Commun. 4:2810. PMID:24326773

380. Cao Y, He M, Gao Z, et al. (2014). Activating hotspot L205R mutation in PRKACA and adrenal Cushing's syndrome. Science. 344:913–7. PMID:24700472

381. Caoili EM, Korobkin M, Francis IR, et al. (2002). Adrenal masses: characterization with combined unenhanced and delayed enhanced CT. Radiology. 222:629–33. PMID:11867777

382. Capasso M, Diskin SJ, Totaro F, et al. (2013). Replication of GWAS-identified neuroblastoma risk loci strengthens the role of BARD1 and affirms the cumulative effect of genetic variations on disease susceptibility. Carcinogenesis. 34:605–11. PMID:23222812

383. Capatina C, Ntali G, Karavitaki N, et al. (2013). The management of head-and-neck paragangliomas. Endocr Relat Cancer. 20:R291–305. PMID:23921204

384. Capella C, Bordi C, Monga G, et al. (1978). Multiple endocrine cell types in thyroid medullary carcinoma. Evidence for calcitonin, somatostatin, ACTH, 5HT and small granule cells. Virchows Arch A Pathol Anat Histol. 377:111–28. PMID:205037

385. Capella C, Polak JM, Buffa R, et al. (1983). Morphologic patterns and diagnostic criteria of VIP-producing endocrine tumors. A histologic, histochemical, ultrastructural, and biochemical study of 32 cases. Cancer. 52:1860–74. PMID:6627205

386. Capella C, Riva C, Leutner M, et al. (1995). Pituitary lesions in multiple endocrine neoplasia syndrome (MENS) type 1. Pathol Res Pract. 191:345–7. PMID:7479350

387. Caplin ME, Pavel M, Ćwikła JB, et al. (2014). Lanreotide in metastatic enteropancreatic neuroendocrine tumors. N Engl J Med. 371:224–33. PMID:25014687

388. Cappabianca P, Cirillo S, Alfieri A, et al. (1999). Pituitary macroadenoma and diaphragma sellae meningioma: differential diagnosis on MRI. Neuroradiology. 41:22–6. PMID:9987763

389. Cappelli C, Tironi A, Marchetti GP, et al. (2008). Aggressive thyroid carcinoma showing thymic-like differentiation (CASTLE): case report and review of the literature. Endocr J. 55:685–90. PMID:18560200

390. Carcangiu ML, Bianchi S (1989). Diffuse sclerosing variant of papillary thyroid carcinoma. Clinicopathologic study of 15 cases. Am J Surg Pathol. 13:1041–9. PMID:2490923

391. Carcangiu ML, Bianchi S, Savino D, et al. (1991). Follicular Hürthle cell tumors of the thyroid gland. Cancer. 68:1944–53. PMID:1913544

392. Carcangiu ML, Sibley RK, Rosai J (1985). Clear cell change in primary thyroid tumors. A study of 38 cases. Am J Surg Pathol. 9:705–22. PMID:4061729

393. Carcangiu ML, Zampi G, Pupi A, et al. (1985). Papillary carcinoma of the thyroid. A clinicopathologic study of 241 cases treated at the University of Florence, Italy. Cancer. 55:805–28. PMID:3967175

394. Carcangiu ML, Zampi G, Rosai J (1984). Poorly differentiated ("insular") thyroid carcinoma. A reinterpretation of Langhans' "wuchernde Struma". Am J Surg Pathol. 8:655–68. PMID:6476195

395. Carcangiu ML, Zampi G, Rosai J (1985). Papillary thyroid carcinoma: a study of its many morphologic expressions and clinical correlates. Pathol Annu. 20:1–44. PMID:3887295

396. Carda C, Ferrer J, Vilanova M, et al. (2005). Anaplastic carcinoma of the thyroid with rhabdomyosarcomatous differentiation: a report of two cases. Virchows Arch. 446:46–51. PMID:15517365

397. Carén H, Kryh H, Nethander M, et al. (2010). High-risk neuroblastoma tumors with 11q-deletion display a poor prognostic, chromosome instability phenotype with later onset. Proc Natl Acad Sci U S A. 107:4323–8. PMID:20145112

398. Carney JA (1990). Psammomatous melanotic schwannoma. A distinctive, heritable tumor with special associations, including cardiac myxoma and the Cushing syndrome. Am J Surg Pathol. 14:206–22. PMID:2305928

399. Carney JA (2013). Carney triad. Front Horm Res. 41:92–110. PMID:23652673

400. Carney JA, Boccon-Gibod L, Jarka DE, et al. (2001). Osteochondromyxoma of bone: a congenital tumor associated with lentigines and other unusual disorders. Am J Surg Pathol. 25:164–76. PMID:11176065

401. Carney JA, Ferreiro JA (1996). The epithelioid blue nevus. A multicentric familial tumor with important associations, including cardiac myxoma and psammomatous melanotic schwannoma. Am J Surg Pathol. 20:259–72. PMID:8772778

402. Carney JA, Gordon H, Carpenter PC, et al. (1985). The complex of myxomas, spotty pigmentation, and endocrine overactivity. Medicine (Baltimore). 64:270–83. PMID:4010501

403. Carney JA, Hirokawa M, Lloyd RV, et al. (2008). Hyalinizing trabecular tumors of the thyroid gland are almost all benign. Am J Surg Pathol. 32:1877–89. PMID:18813121

404. Carney JA, Libé R, Bertherat J, et al. (2014). Primary pigmented nodular adrenocortical disease: the original 4 cases revisited after 30 years for follow-up, new investigations, and molecular genetic findings. Am J Surg Pathol. 38:1266–73. PMID:24805858

405. Carney JA, Sizemore GW, Hayles AB (1978). Multiple endocrine neoplasia, type 2b. Pathobiol Annu. 8:105–53. PMID:364372

406. Carney JA, Sizemore GW, Tyce GM (1975). Bilateral adrenal medullary hyperplasia in multiple endocrine neoplasia, type 2: the precursor of bilateral pheochromocytoma. Mayo Clin Proc. 50:3–10. PMID:1110583

407. Carney JA, Stratakis CA (1998). Epithelioid blue nevus and psammomatous melanotic schwannoma: the unusual pigmented skin tumors of the Carney complex. Semin Diagn Pathol. 15:216–24. PMID:9711672

408. Carney JA, Stratakis CA, Young WF Jr (2013). Adrenal cortical adenoma: the fourth component of the Carney triad and an association with subclinical Cushing syndrome. Am J Surg Pathol. 37:1140–9. PMID:23681078

409. Carney JA, Young WF, Stratakis CA (2011). Primary bimorphic adrenocortical disease: cause of hypercortisolism in McCune-Albright syndrome. Am J Surg Pathol. 35:1311–26. PMID:21836496

410. Caron NR, Sturgeon C, Clark OH (2004). Persistent and recurrent hyperparathyroidism. Curr Treat Options Oncol. 5:335–45. PMID:15233910

411. Carpi A, Sagripanti A, Nicolini A, et al. (1998). Large needle aspiration biopsy for reducing the rate of inadequate cytology on fine needle aspiration specimens from palpable thyroid nodules. Biomed Pharmacother. 52:303–7. PMID:9809173

412. Carpten JD, Robbins CM, Villablanca A, et al. (2002). HRPT2, encoding parafibromin, is mutated in hyperparathyroidism-jaw tumor syndrome. Nat Genet. 32:676–80. PMID:12434154

413. Carrasco CA, Rojas-Z D, Chiorino R, et al. (2012). Primary pituitary lymphoma in immunocompetent patient: diagnostic problems and prolonged follow-up. Pituitary. 15:93–6. PMID:20146099

414. Carroll PV, Jenkins PJ (2016). Acromegaly. In: De Groot LJ, Chrousos G, Dungan K, et al., editors. Endotext. South Dartmouth: MDText.com, Inc. PMID:25905322

415. Carstens PH, Cressman FK Jr (1989). Malignant oncocytic carcinoid of the pancreas. Ultrastruct Pathol. 13:69–75. PMID:2919439

416. Cascón A, Comino-Méndez I, Currás-Freixes M, et al. (2015). Whole-exome sequencing identifies MDH2 as a new familial paraganglioma gene. J Natl Cancer Inst. 107:107. PMID:25766404

417. Cascón A, Huarte-Mendicoa CV, Javier Leandro-García L, et al. (2011). Detection of the first gross CDC73 germline deletion in an HPT-JT syndrome family. Genes Chromosomes Cancer. 50:922–9. PMID:21837707

418. Casey MB, Lohse CM, Lloyd RV (2003). Distinction between papillary thyroid hyperplasia and papillary thyroid carcinoma by immunohistochemical staining for cytokeratin 19, galectin-3, and HBME-1. Endocr Pathol. 14:55–60. PMID:12746563

419. Casey MB, Sebo TJ, Carney JA (2004). Hyalinizing trabecular adenoma of the thyroid gland identification through MIB-1 staining of fine-needle aspiration biopsy smears. Am J Clin Pathol. 122:506–10. PMID:15487446

420. Casey MB, Sebo TJ, Carney JA (2004). Hyalinizing trabecular adenoma of the thyroid gland: cytologic features in 29 cases. Am J Surg Pathol. 28:859–67. PMID:15223954

421. Casey R, Garrahy A, Tuthill A, et al. (2014). Universal genetic screening uncovers a novel presentation of an SDHAF2 mutation. J Clin Endocrinol Metab. 99:E1392–6. PMID:24712571

422. Cassarino DS, Auerbach A, Rushing EJ (2003). Widely invasive solitary fibrous tumor of the sphenoid sinus, cavernous sinus, and pituitary fossa. Ann Diagn Pathol. 7:169–73. PMID:12808569

423. Cassol C, Mete O (2015). Endocrine manifestations of von Hippel-Lindau disease. Arch Pathol Lab Med. 139:263–8. PMID:25611110

424. Castelblanco E, Gallel P, Ros S, et al. (2012). Thyroid paraganglioma. Report of 3 cases and description of an immunohistochemical profile useful in the differential diagnosis with medullary thyroid carcinoma, based on complementary DNA array results. Hum Pathol. 43:1103–12. PMID:22209341

425. Castleman B, Roth SI (1978). Tumors of the parathyroid gland. In: AFIP atlas of tumor pathology. Series 2, Fascicle 14. Washington DC: Armed Forces Institute of Pathology; pp. 74–9.

426. Castinetti F, Dufour H, Gaillard S, et al. (2015). Non-functioning pituitary adenoma: when and how to operate? What pathologic criteria for typing? Ann Endocrinol (Paris). 76:220–7. PMID:26070464

427. Castinetti F, Kroiss A, Kumar R, et al. (2015). 15 YEARS OF PARAGANGLIOMA: Imaging and imaging-based treatment of pheochromocytoma and paraganglioma. Endocr Relat Cancer. 22:T135–45. PMID:26045470

428. Castro P, Rebocho AP, Soares RJ, et al. (2006). PAX8-PPARgamma rearrangement is frequently detected in the follicular variant of papillary thyroid carcinoma. J Clin Endocrinol Metab. 91:213–20. PMID:16219715

429. Castro-Vega LJ, Lepoutre-Lussey C, Gimenez-Roqueplo AP, et al. (2016). Rethinking pheochromocytomas and paragangliomas from a genomic perspective. Oncogene. 35:1080–9. PMID:26028031

430. Castro-Vega LJ, Letouzé E, Burnichon N, et al. (2015). Multi-omics analysis defines core genomic alterations in pheochromocytomas and paragangliomas. Nat Commun. 6:6044. PMID:25625332

431. Cavaco BM, Barros L, Pannett AA, et al. (2001). The hyperparathyroidism-jaw tumour syndrome in a Portuguese kindred. QJM. 94:213–22. PMID:11294964

432. Ceccato F, Lombardi G, Manara R, et al. (2015). Temozolomide and pasireotide treatment for aggressive pituitary adenoma: expertise at a tertiary care center. J Neurooncol. 122:189–96. PMID:25555563

433. Celi FS, Coppotelli G, Chidakel A, et al. (2008). The role of type 1 and type 2 5'-deiodinase in the pathophysiology of the 3,5,3'-triiodothyronine toxicosis of McCune-Albright syndrome. J Clin Endocrinol Metab. 93:2383–9. PMID:18349068

434. Cerecer-Gil NY, Figuera LE, Llamas FJ, et al. (2010). Mutation of SDHB is a cause of hypoxia-related high-altitude paraganglioma. Clin Cancer Res. 16:4148–54. PMID:20592014

435. Cetani F, Pardi E, Borsari S, et al. (2004). Genetic analyses of the HRPT2 gene in primary hyperparathyroidism: germline and somatic mutations in familial and sporadic parathyroid tumors. J Clin Endocrinol Metab. 89:5583–91. PMID:15531515

436. Cetani F, Pardi E, Viacava P, et al. (2004). A reappraisal of the Rb1 gene abnormalities in the diagnosis of parathyroid cancer. Clin Endocrinol (Oxf). 60:99–106. PMID:14678295

437. Cetta F, Montalto G, Gori M, et al. (2000). Germline mutations of the APC gene in patients with familial adenomatous polyposis-associated thyroid carcinoma: results from a European cooperative study. J Clin Endocrinol Metab. 85:286–92. PMID:10634400

438. Cetta F, Ugolini G, Barellini L, et al. (2011). FAP associated cribriform morular variant of PTC: striking female prevalence and indolent course. Endocr J. 58:817–8. PMID:21878742

439. Ch'ng ES, Hoshida Y, Iizuka N, et al. (2007). Composite malignant pheochromocytoma with malignant peripheral nerve sheath tumour: a case with 28 years of tumour-bearing history. Histopathology. 51:420–2. PMID:17727489

440. Chabre O, Libé R, Assie G, et al. (2013). Serum miR-483-5p and miR-195 are predictive of recurrence risk in adrenocortical cancer patients. Endocr Relat Cancer. 20:579–94. PMID:23756429

441. Chae YC, Angelin A, Lisanti S, et al. (2013). Landscape of the mitochondrial Hsp90 metabolome in tumours. Nat Commun. 4:2139. PMID:23842546

442. Chakraborti S, Mahadevan A, Govindan A, et al. (2013). Pituicytoma: report of three cases with review of literature. Pathol Res Pract. 209:52–8. PMID:23237862

443. Chakraborty R, Hampton OA, Shen X, et al. (2014). Mutually exclusive recurrent somatic mutations in MAP2K1 and BRAF support a central role for ERK activation in LCH pathogenesis. Blood. 124:3007–15. PMID:25202140

444. Chan CC, Collins AB, Chew EY (2007). Molecular pathology of eyes with von Hippel-Lindau (VHL) Disease: a review. Retina. 27:1–7. PMID:17218907

445. Chan J (2002). Strict criteria should be applied in the diagnosis of encapsulated follicular variant of papillary thyroid carcinoma. Am J Clin Pathol. 117:16–8. PMID:11791591

446. Chan JK, Albores-Saavedra J, Battifora H, et al. (1991). Sclerosing mucoepidermoid thyroid carcinoma with eosinophilia. A distinctive low-grade malignancy arising from the metaplastic follicles of Hashimoto's thyroiditis. Am J Surg Pathol. 15:438–48. PMID:2035738

447. Chan JK, Carcangiu ML, Rosai J (1991). Papillary carcinoma of thyroid with exuberant nodular fasciitis-like stroma. Report of three cases. Am J Clin Pathol. 95:309–14. PMID:1996541

448. Chan JK, Rosai J (1991). Tumors of the neck showing thymic or related branchial pouch differentiation: a unifying concept. Hum Pathol. 22:349–67. PMID:2050369

449. Chan JK, Saw D (1986). The grooved nucleus. A useful diagnostic criterion of papillary carcinoma of the thyroid. Am J Surg Pathol. 10:672–9. PMID:3766846

450. Chan JK, Tsang WY (1995). Endocrine malignancies that may mimic benign lesions. Semin Diagn Pathol. 12:45–63. PMID:7770674

451. Chan JK, Tse CC (1988). Mucin production in metastatic papillary carcinoma of the thyroid. Hum Pathol. 19:195–200. PMID:3277907

452. Chan JK, Tsui MS, Tse CH (1987). Diffuse sclerosing variant of papillary carcinoma of the thyroid: a histological and immunohistochemical study of three cases. Histopathology. 11:191–201. PMID:2437003

453. Chan YF, Ma L, Boey JH, et al. (1986). Angiosarcoma of the thyroid. An immunohistochemical and ultrastructural study of a case in a Chinese patient. Cancer. 57:2381–8. PMID:3084061

454. Chan-Smutko G, Iliopoulos O (2010). Familial renal cell cancers and pheochromocytomas. In: Chung DC, Haber DA, editors. Principles of clinical cancer genetics: A handbook from the Massachusetts General Hospital. New York: Springer; pp. 109–28.

455. Chandrasekharappa SC, Guru SC, Manickam P, et al. (1997). Positional cloning of the gene for multiple endocrine neoplasia-type 1. Science. 276:404–7. PMID:9103196

456. Chang KC, Chen PI, Huang ZH, et al. (2002). Adrenal myelolipoma with translocation (3;21)(q25;p11). Cancer Genet Cytogenet. 134:77–80. PMID:11996801

457. Chanson P, Dib A, Visot A, et al. (1994). McCune-Albright syndrome and acromegaly: clinical studies and responses to treatment in five cases. Eur J Endocrinol. 131:229–34. PMID:7921205

458. Chapman DB, Lippert D, Geer CP, et al. (2010). Clinical, histopathologic, and radiographic indicators of malignancy in head and neck paragangliomas. Otolaryngol Head Neck Surg. 143:531–7. PMID:20869564

459. Chara L, Rodríguez B, Holgado E, et al. (2011). An unusual metastatic renal cell carcinoma with maintained complete response to sunitinib treatment. Case Rep Oncol. 4:583–6. PMID:22220154

460. Charlesworth M, Verbeke CS, Falk GA, et al. (2012). Pancreatic lesions in von Hippel-Lindau disease? A systematic review and meta-synthesis of the literature. J Gastrointest Surg. 16:1422–8. PMID:22370733

461. Chatzellis E, Alexandraki KI, Androulakis II, et al. (2015). Aggressive pituitary tumors. Neuroendocrinology. 101:87–104. PMID:25571935

462. Chaudhary RK, Barnes EL, Myers EN (1994). Squamous cell carcinoma arising in Hashimoto's thyroiditis. Head Neck. 16:582–5. PMID:7822183

463. Chaudhry NS, Ahmad F, Blieden C, et al. (2013). Suprasellar and sellar paraganglioma presenting as a nonfunctioning pituitary macroadenoma. J Clin Neurosci. 20:1615–8. PMID:23876285

464. Chem KT, Rosai J (1977). Follicular variant of thyroid papillary carcinoma: a clinicopathologic study of six cases. Am J Surg Pathol. 1:123–30. PMID:602974

465. Chen BB, Yeh CC, Chang TC, et al. (2005). Computed tomography diagnosis of primary thyroid teratoma. J Formos Med Assoc. 104:514–7. PMID:16091830

466. Chen C, Yang Y, Jin L, et al. (2013). Primary thyroid T-lymphoblastic lymphoma: a case report and review of the literature. Int J Clin Exp Pathol. 7:443–50. PMID:24427370

467. Chen CH, Boag AH, Beiko DT, et al. (2009). Composite paraganglioma-ganglioneuroma of the urinary bladder: a rare neoplasm causing hemodynamic crisis at tumour resection. Can Urol Assoc J. 3:E45–8. PMID:19829717

468. Chen H, Nicol TL, Udelsman R (1999). Clinically significant, isolated metastatic disease to the thyroid gland. World J Surg. 23:177–80, discussion 181. PMID:9880428

469. Chen H, Nicol TL, Zeiger MA, et al. (1998). Hürthle cell neoplasms of the thyroid: are there factors predictive of malignancy? Ann Surg. 227:542–6. PMID:9563543

470. Chen H, Sippel RS, O'Dorisio MS, et al. (NANETS) (2010). The North American Neuroendocrine Tumor Society consensus guideline for the diagnosis and management of neuroendocrine tumors: pheochromocytoma, paraganglioma, and medullary thyroid cancer. Pancreas. 39:775–83. PMID:20664475

471. Chen JH, Faquin WC, Lloyd RV, et al. (2011). Clinicopathological and molecular characterization of nine cases of columnar cell variant of papillary thyroid carcinoma. Mod Pathol. 24:739–49. PMID:21358618

472. Chen W, Wang J, Wang E, et al. (2010). Detection of clonal lymphoid receptor gene rearrangements in langerhans cell histiocytosis. Am J Surg Pathol. 34:1049–57. PMID:20551822

473. Chen Y, Takita J, Choi YL, et al. (2008). Oncogenic mutations of ALK kinase in neuroblastoma. Nature. 455:971–4. PMID:18923524

474. Chen YT, Kitabayashi N, Zhou XK, et al. (2008). MicroRNA analysis as a potential diagnostic tool for papillary thyroid carcinoma. Mod Pathol. 21:1139–46. PMID:18587330

475. Cheng JY, Gill AJ, Kumar SK (2015). Granulosa cell tumour of the adrenal. Pathology. 47:487–9. PMID:26126046

476. Chentli F, Belhimer F, Kessaci F, et al. (2012). Congenital craniopharyngioma: a case report and literature review. J Pediatr Endocrinol Metab. 25:1181–3. PMID:23329768

477. Chéreau N, Buffet C, Trésallet C, et al. (2016). Recurrence of papillary thyroid carcinoma with lateral cervical node metastases: Predictive factors and operative management. Surgery. 159:755–62. PMID:26435440

478. Chesnokova V, Zonis S, Wawrowsky K, et al. (2012). Clusterin and FOXL2 act concordantly to regulate pituitary gonadotroph adenoma growth. Mol Endocrinol. 26:2092–103. PMID:23051594

479. Chetty R (2011). Thyroid follicular adenoma composed of lipid-rich cells. Endocr Pathol. 22:31–4. PMID:21165779

480. Chetty R, Clark SP, Dowling JP (1993). Leiomyosarcoma of the thyroid: immunohistochemical and ultrastructural study. Pathology. 25:203–5. PMID:8367205

481. Chetty R, Clark SP, Pitson GA (1993). Primary small cell carcinoma of the pancreas. Pathology. 25:240–2. PMID:8265240

482. Chetty R, Clark SP, Taylor DA (1993). Pigmented pheochromocytomas of the adrenal medulla. Hum Pathol. 24:420–3. PMID:8491482

483. Chetty R, Goetsch S, Nayler S, et al. (1998). Spindle epithelial tumour with thymus-like element (SETTLE): the predominantly monophasic variant. Histopathology. 33:71–4. PMID:9726052

484. Chetty R, Pillay P, Jaichand V (1998). Cytokeratin expression in adrenal phaeochromocytomas and extra-adrenal paragangliomas. J Clin Pathol. 51:477–8. PMID:9771451

485. Cheuk W, Jacobson AA, Chan JK (2000). Spindle epithelial tumor with thymus-like differentiation (SETTLE): a distinctive malignant thyroid neoplasm with significant metastatic potential. Mod Pathol. 13:1150–5. PMID:11048811

486. Cheung CC, Boerner SL, MacMillan CM, et al. (2000). Hyalinizing trabecular tumor of the thyroid: a variant of papillary carcinoma proved by molecular genetics. Am J Surg Pathol. 24:1622–6. PMID:11117782

487. Cheung NK, Dyer MA (2013). Neuroblastoma: developmental biology, cancer genomics and immunotherapy. Nat Rev Cancer. 13:397–411. PMID:23702928

488. Cheung NK, Zhang J, Lu C, et al. (2012). Association of age at diagnosis and genetic mutations in patients with neuroblastoma. JAMA. 307:1062–71. PMID:22416102

489. Cheunsuchon P, Zhou Y, Zhang X, et al. (2011). Silencing of the imprinted DLK1-MEG3 locus in human clinically nonfunctioning pituitary adenomas. Am J Pathol. 179:2120–30. PMID:21871428

490. Chevalier N, Paris F, Fontana S, et al. (2015). Postpubertal Persistent Hyperestrogenemia in McCune-Albright Syndrome: Unilateral Oophorectomy Improved Fertility but Detected an Unexpected Borderline Epithelial Ovarian Tumor. J Pediatr Adolesc Gynecol. 28:e169–72. PMID:26321108

491. Chew EY (2005). Ocular manifestations of von Hippel-Lindau disease: clinical and genetic investigations. Trans Am Ophthalmol Soc. 103:495–511. PMID:17057815

492. Chia WK, Sharifah NA, Reena RM, et al. (2010). Fluorescence in situ hybridization analysis using PAX8- and PPARG-specific probes reveals the presence of PAX8-PPARG translocation and 3p25 aneusomy in follicular thyroid neoplasms. Cancer Genet Cytogenet. 196:7–13. PMID:19963130

493. Chiang MF, Brock M, Patt S (1990). Pituitary metastases. Neurochirurgia (Stuttg). 33:127–31. PMID:2203980

494. Chikani V, Lambie D, Russell A (2013). Pituitary metastases from papillary carcinoma of thyroid: a case report and literature review. Endocrinol Diabetes Metab Case Rep. 2013:130024. PMID:24616765

495. Chindris AM, Casler JD, Bernet VJ, et al. (2015). Clinical and molecular features of Hürthle cell carcinoma of the thyroid. J Clin Endocrinol Metab. 100:55–62. PMID:25259908

496. Chinezu L, Vasiljevic A, Jouanneau E, et al. (2014). Expression of somatostatin receptors, SSTR2A and SSTR5, in 108 endocrine pituitary tumors using immunohistochemical detection

with new specific monoclonal antibodies. Hum Pathol. 45:71–7. PMID:24182563
497. Chmielecki J, Crago AM, Rosenberg M, et al. (2013). Whole-exome sequencing identifies a recurrent NAB2-STAT6 fusion in solitary fibrous tumors. Nat Genet. 45:131–2. PMID:23313954
498. Chmielecki J, Hutchinson KE, Frampton GM, et al. (2014). Comprehensive genomic profiling of pancreatic acinar cell carcinomas identifies recurrent RAF fusions and frequent inactivation of DNA repair genes. Cancer Discov. 4:1398–405. PMID:25266736
499. Cho EY, Ahn GH (2001). Immunoexpression of inhibin alpha-subunit in adrenal neoplasms. Appl Immunohistochem Mol Morphol. 9:222–8. PMID:11556749
500. Cho JH, Park YH, Kim WS, et al. (2006). High incidence of mucosa-associated lymphoid tissue in primary thyroid lymphoma: a clinicopathologic study of 18 cases in the Korean population. Leuk Lymphoma. 47:2128–31. PMID:17071486
501. Choi GH, Yang MS, Yoon DH, et al. (2010). Pediatric cervical chordoma: report of two cases and a review of the current literature. Childs Nerv Syst. 26:835–40. PMID:20094721
502. Choi H, Kim S, Moon JH, et al. (2008). Multiple endocrine neoplasia type 1 with multiple leiomyomas linked to a novel mutation in the MEN1 gene. Yonsei Med J. 49:655–61. PMID:18729310
503. Choi M, Scholl UI, Yue P, et al. (2011). K+ channel mutations in adrenal aldosterone-producing adenomas and hereditary hypertension. Science. 331:768–72. PMID:21311022
504. Choi WJ, Baek JH, Ha EJ, et al. (2015). The ultrasonography features of hyalinizing trabecular tumor of the thyroid gland and the role of fine needle aspiration cytology and core needle biopsy in its diagnosis. Acta Radiol. 56:1113–8. PMID:25232186
505. Choi YM, Sung TY, Kim WG, et al. (2015). Clinical course and prognostic factors in patients with malignant pheochromocytoma and paraganglioma: A single institution experience. J Surg Oncol. 112:815–21. PMID:26464058
506. Chong Y, Shin JH, Oh YL, et al. (2013). Cribriform-morular variant of papillary thyroid carcinoma: ultrasonographic and clinical characteristics. Thyroid. 23:45–9. PMID:22892017
507. Chou A, Toon C, Pickett J, et al. (2013). von Hippel-Lindau syndrome. Front Horm Res. 41:30–49. PMID:23652669
508. Chow LS, Erickson LA, Abu-Lebdeh HS, et al. (2006). Parathyroid lipoadenomas: a rare cause of primary hyperparathyroidism. Endocr Pract. 12:131–6. PMID:16690459
509. Chow SM, Chan JK, Law SC, et al. (2003). Diffuse sclerosing variant of papillary thyroid carcinoma–clinical features and outcome. Eur J Surg Oncol. 29:446–9. PMID:12798749
510. Chow SM, Chan JK, Tse LL, et al. (2007). Carcinoma showing thymus-like element (CASTLE) of thyroid: combined modality treatment in 3 patients with locally advanced disease. Eur J Surg Oncol. 33:83–5. PMID:17085008
511. Chrisoulidou A, Mandanas S, Mitsakis P, et al. (2012). Parathyroid involvement in thyroid cancer: an unforeseen event. World J Surg Oncol. 10:121. PMID:22742583
512. Chrisoulidou A, Pazaitou-Panayiotou K, Georgiou E, et al. (2008). Ectopic Cushing's syndrome due to CRH secreting liver metastasis in a patient with medullary thyroid carcinoma. Hormones (Athens). 7:259–62. PMID:18694866
513. Christ E, Wild D, Forrer F, et al. (2009). Glucagon-like peptide-1 receptor imaging for localization of insulinomas. J Clin Endocrinol Metab. 94:4398–405. PMID:19820010
514. Christmas TJ, Chapple CR, Noble JG, et al. (1988). Hyperparathyroidism after neck irradiation. Br J Surg. 75:873–4. PMID:3179662
515. Chu PG, Lau SK, Weiss LM (2009). Keratin expression in endocrine organs and their neoplasms. Endocr Pathol. 20:1–10. PMID:19214802
516. Chung AY, Tran TB, Brumund KT, et al. (2012). Metastases to the thyroid: a review of the literature from the last decade. Thyroid. 22:258–68. PMID:22313412
517. Chung DC, Smith AP, Louis DN, et al. (1997). A novel pancreatic endocrine tumor suppressor gene locus on chromosome 3p with clinical prognostic implications. J Clin Invest. 100:404–10. PMID:9218518
518. Chung DH, Kim NR, Kim T, et al. (2015). Malignant glomus tumor of the thyroid gland where is heretofore an unreported organ: a case report and literature review. Endocr Pathol. 26:37–44. PMID:25544269
519. Chung J, Lee SK, Gong G, et al. (1999). Sclerosing Mucoepidermoid carcinoma with eosinophilia of the thyroid glands: a case report with clinical manifestation of recurrent neck mass. J Korean Med Sci. 14:338–41. PMID:10402181
520. Chung-Park M, Yang JT, McHenry CR, et al. (2003). Adenomatoid tumor of the adrenal gland with micronodular adrenal cortical hyperplasia. Hum Pathol. 34:818–21. PMID:14506647
521. Ciampi R, Knauf JA, Kerler R, et al. (2005). Oncogenic AKAP9-BRAF fusion is a novel mechanism of MAPK pathway activation in thyroid cancer. J Clin Invest. 115:94–101. PMID:15630448
522. Ciampi R, Mian C, Fugazzola L, et al. (2013). Evidence of a low prevalence of RAS mutations in a large medullary thyroid cancer series. Thyroid. 23:50–7. PMID:23240926
523. Cimino-Mathews A, Sharma R, Netto GJ (2011). Diagnostic use of PAX8, CAIX, TTF-1, and TGB in metastatic renal cell carcinoma of the thyroid. Am J Surg Pathol. 35:757–61. PMID:21451364
524. Cipriani NA, Nagar S, Kaplan SP, et al. (2015). Follicular Thyroid Carcinoma: How Have Histologic Diagnoses Changed in the Last Half-Century and What Are the Prognostic Implications? Thyroid. 25:1209–16. PMID:26440366
525. Cisco RM, Norton JA (2007). Surgery for gastrinoma. Adv Surg. 41:165–76. PMID:17972563
526. Cistaro A, Niccoli Asabella A, Coppolino P, et al. (2015). Diagnostic and prognostic value of ^{18}F-FDG PET/CT in comparison with morphological imaging in primary adrenal gland malignancies – a multicenter experience. Hell J Nucl Med. 18:97–102. PMID:26187207
527. Civantos F, Albores-Saavedra J, Nadji M, et al. (1984). Clear cell variant of thyroid carcinoma. Am J Surg Pathol. 8:187–92. PMID:6703194
528. Clain JB, Scherl S, Dos Reis L, et al. (2014). Extrathyroidal extension predicts extranodal extension in patients with positive lymph nodes: an important association that may affect clinical management. Thyroid. 24:951–7. PMID:24443878
529. Clark GR, Sciacovelli M, Gaude E, et al. (2014). Germline FH mutations presenting with pheochromocytoma. J Clin Endocrinol Metab. 99:E2046–50. PMID:25004247
530. Clayton EF, Ziober A, Yao Y, et al. (2013). Malignant tumors with clear cell morphology: a comparative immunohistochemical study with renal cell carcinoma antibody, Pax8, steroidogenic factor 1, and brachyury. Ann Diagn Pathol. 17:192–7. PMID:23218904
531. Clouston WM, Cannell GC, Fryar BG, et al. (1989). Virilizing adrenal adenoma in an adult with the Beckwith-Wiedemann syndrome: paradoxical response to dexamethasone. Clin Endocrinol (Oxf). 31:467–73. PMID:2534067
532. Cohen J, Gierlowski TC, Schneider AB (1990). A prospective study of hyperparathyroidism in individuals exposed to radiation in childhood. JAMA. 264:581–4. PMID:2366296
533. Cohen JB, Troxell M, Kong CS, et al. (2003). Ectopic intrathyroidal thymoma: a case report and review. Thyroid. 13:305–8. PMID:12729482
534. Cohen Y, Xing M, Mambo E, et al. (2003). BRAF mutation in papillary thyroid carcinoma. J Natl Cancer Inst. 95:625–7. PMID:12697856
535. Cohn KH, Silen W (1982). Lessons of parathyroid reoperations. Am J Surg. 144:511–7. PMID:7137458
536. Cohn SL, Pearson AD, London WB, et al. (2009). The International Neuroblastoma Risk Group (INRG) classification system: an INRG Task Force report. J Clin Oncol. 27:289–97. PMID:19047291
537. Coire CI, Horvath E, Kovacs K, et al. (1997). Cushing's Syndrome from an Ectopic Pituitary Adenoma with Peliosis: A Histological, Immunohistochemical, and Ultrastructural Study and Review of the Literature. Endocr Pathol. 8:65–74. PMID:12114673
538. Coiré CI, Horvath E, Kovacs K, et al. (1998). A composite silent corticotroph pituitary adenoma with interspersed adrenocortical cells: case report. Neurosurgery. 42:650–4. PMID:9527001
539. Coleman KD, Wright JA, Ghosh M, et al. (2009). Estradiol modulation of hepatocyte growth factor by stromal fibroblasts in the female reproductive tract. Fertil Steril. 92:1107–9. PMID:19423096
540. Coli A, Di Giorgio A, Castri F, et al. (2010). Sarcomatoid carcinoma of the adrenal gland: A case report and review of literature. Pathol Res Pract. 206:59–65. PMID:19369012
541. Collienne M, Timmesfeld N, Bergmann SR, et al. (2015). Adrenal incidentaloma and subclinical Cushing's syndrome: a longitudinal follow-up study by endoscopic ultrasound. Ultraschall Med. EPUB 2015. PMID:26529351
542. Collini P, Mattavelli F, Pellegrinelli A, et al. (2006). Papillary carcinoma of the thyroid gland of childhood and adolescence: Morphologic subtypes, biologic behavior and prognosis: a clinicopathologic study of 42 sporadic cases treated at a single institution during a 30-year period. Am J Surg Pathol. 30:1420–6. PMID:17063083
543. Collini P, Sampietro G, Rosai J, et al. (2003). Minimally invasive (encapsulated) follicular carcinoma of the thyroid gland is the low-risk counterpart of widely invasive follicular carcinoma but not of insular carcinoma. Virchows Arch. 442:71–6. PMID:12536317
544. Collins MT, Chebli C, Jones J, et al. (2001). Renal phosphate wasting in fibrous dysplasia of bone is part of a generalized renal tubular dysfunction similar to that seen in tumor-induced osteomalacia. J Bone Miner Res. 16:806–13. PMID:11341325
545. Collins MT, Sarlis NJ, Merino MJ, et al. (2003). Thyroid carcinoma in the McCune-Albright syndrome: contributory role of activating Gs alpha mutations. J Clin Endocrinol Metab. 88:4413–7. PMID:12970318
546. Collins MT, Singer FR, Eugster E (2012). McCune-Albright syndrome and the extraskeletal manifestations of fibrous dysplasia. Orphanet J Rare Dis. 7 Suppl 1:S4. PMID:22640971
547. Comino-Méndez I, de Cubas AA, Bernal C, et al. (2013). Tumoral EPAS1 (HIF2A) mutations explain sporadic pheochromocytoma and paraganglioma in the absence of erythrocytosis. Hum Mol Genet. 22:2169–76. PMID:23418310
548. Comstock JM, Willmore-Payne C, Holden JA, et al. (2009). Composite pheochromocytoma: a clinicopathologic and molecular comparison with ordinary pheochromocytoma and neuroblastoma. Am J Clin Pathol. 132:69–73. PMID:19864235
549. Cong H, Li T, Chen G, et al. (2015). Missed Initial Diagnosis of Malignant Struma Ovarii Containing Follicular Thyroid Carcinoma: Metastatic Pulmonary Recurrence 17 yr After Ovariectomy. Int J Gynecol Pathol. 34:445–9. PMID:26262453
550. Conzo G, Candela G, Tartaglia E, et al. (2014). Leiomyosarcoma of the thyroid gland: A case report and literature review. Oncol Lett. 7:1011–4. PMID:24944660
551. Cook AM, Vini L, Harmer C (1999). Squamous cell carcinoma of the thyroid: outcome of treatment in 16 patients. Eur J Surg Oncol. 25:606–9. PMID:10556008
552. Cook MN, Olshan AF, Guess HA, et al. (2004). Maternal medication use and neuroblastoma in offspring. Am J Epidemiol. 159:721–31. PMID:15051581
553. Cooper DS, Doherty GM, Haugen BR, et al. (2006). Management guidelines for patients with thyroid nodules and differentiated thyroid cancer. Thyroid. 16:109–42. PMID:16420177
554. Cooper O (2015). Silent corticotroph adenomas. Pituitary. 18:225–31. PMID:25534889
555. Corbetta S, Pizzocaro A, Peracchi M, et al. (1997). Multiple endocrine neoplasia type 1 in patients with recognized pituitary tumours of different types. Clin Endocrinol (Oxf). 47:507–12. PMID:9425388
556. Corbo V, Dalai I, Scardoni M, et al. (2010). MEN1 in pancreatic endocrine tumors: analysis of gene and protein status in 169 sporadic neoplasms reveals alterations in the vast majority of cases. Endocr Relat Cancer. 17:771–83. PMID:20566584
557. Corcos O, Couvelard A, Giraud S, et al. (2008). Endocrine pancreatic tumors in von Hippel-Lindau disease: clinical, histological, and genetic features. Pancreas. 37:85–93. PMID:18580449
558. Cornett WR, Sharma AK, Day TA, et al. (2007). Anaplastic thyroid carcinoma: an overview. Curr Oncol Rep. 9:152–8. PMID:17288883
559. Corrado S, Corsello SM, Maiorana A, et al. (2014). Papillary thyroid carcinoma with predominant spindle cell component: report of two rare cases and discussion on the differential diagnosis with other spindled thyroid neoplasm. Endocr Pathol. 25:307–14. PMID:24356783
560. Correa R, Salpea P, Stratakis CA (2015). Carney complex: an update. Eur J Endocrinol. 173:M85–97. PMID:26130139
561. Corrin B, Gilby ED, Jones NF, et al. (1973). Oat cell carcinoma of the pancreas with ectopic ACTH secretion. Cancer. 31:1523–7. PMID:4350960
562. Cortet-Rudelli C, Bonneville JF, Borson-Chazot F, et al. (2015). Post-surgical management of non-functioning pituitary adenoma. Ann Endocrinol (Paris). 76:228–38. PMID:26116412
563. Costa AM, Herrero A, Fresno MF, et al. (2008). BRAF mutation associated with other genetic events identifies a subset of aggressive papillary thyroid carcinoma. Clin Endocrinol (Oxf). 68:618–34. PMID:18070147
564. Costa-Guda J, Arnold A (2014). Genetic and epigenetic changes in sporadic endocrine tumors: parathyroid tumors. Mol Cell Endocrinol. 386:46–54. PMID:24035866
565. Costa-Guda J, Imanishi Y, Palanisamy N, et al. (2013). Allelic imbalance in sporadic parathyroid carcinoma and evidence for its de novo origins. Endocrine. 44:489–95. PMID:23435613
566. Costa-Guda J, Marinoni I, Molatore S, et al. (2011). Somatic mutation and germline sequence abnormalities in CDKN1B, encoding p27Kip1, in sporadic parathyroid adenomas. J Clin Endocrinol Metab. 96:E701–6. PMID:21289244
567. Costa-Guda J, Soong CP, Parekh VI, et al. (2013). Germline and somatic mutations

in cyclin-dependent kinase inhibitor genes CDKN1A, CDKN2B, and CDKN2C in sporadic parathyroid adenomas. Horm Cancer. 4:301–7. PMID:23715670
568. Costinean S, Balatti V, Bottoni A, et al. (2012). Primary intrathyroidal paraganglioma: histopathology and novel molecular alterations. Hum Pathol. 43:2371–5. PMID:23079201
569. Courtoy PJ (1991). Endocytosis 1990: from basic biology to health and disease. Second European Workshop on Endocytosis sponsored by the European Molecular Biology Organization and NATO, Paris, France October 1–5, 1990. New Biol. 3:243–52. PMID:1678967
570. Couvelard A, Hentic O (2015). Glucagonoma. In: La Rosa S, Sessa F, editors. Pancreatic neuroendocrine neoplasms: practical approach to diagnosis, classification, and therapy. Cham: Springer International Publishing AG; pp. 81–8.
571. Couvelard A, O'Toole D, Turley H, et al. (2005). Microvascular density and hypoxia-inducible factor pathway in pancreatic endocrine tumours: negative correlation of microvascular density and VEGF expression with tumour progression. Br J Cancer. 92:94–101. PMID:15558070
572. Covington MF, Chin SS, Osborn AG (2011). Pituicytoma, spindle cell oncocytoma, and granular cell tumor: clarification and meta-analysis of the world literature since 1893. AJNR Am J Neuroradiol. 32:2067–72. PMID:21960498
573. Cox TM, Fagan EA, Hillyard CJ, et al. (1979). Role of calcitonin in diarrhoea associated with medullary carcinoma of the thyroid. Gut. 20:629–33. PMID:226460
574. Coyle D, Friedmacher F, Puri P (2014). The association between Hirschsprung's disease and multiple endocrine neoplasia type 2a: a systematic review. Pediatr Surg Int. 30:751–6. PMID:24972642
575. Cozzolino I, Malapelle U, Carlomagno C, et al. (2010). Metastasis of colon cancer to the thyroid gland: a case diagnosed on fine-needle aspirate by a combined cytological, immunocytochemical, and molecular approach. Diagn Cytopathol. 38:932–5. PMID:20213843
576. Crabtree JS, Scacheri PC, Ward JM, et al. (2001). A mouse model of multiple endocrine neoplasia, type 1, develops multiple endocrine tumors. Proc Natl Acad Sci U S A. 98:1118–23. PMID:11158604
577. Craig JR, Hart WR (1979). Extragenital adenomatoid tumor: Evidence for the mesothelial theory of origin. Cancer. 43:1678–81. PMID:156063
578. Craver RD, Lipscomb JT, Suskind D, et al. (2001). Malignant teratoma of the thyroid with primitive neuroepithelial and mesenchymal sarcomatous components. Ann Diagn Pathol. 5:285–92. PMID:11598856
579. Cromer MK, Starker LF, Choi M, et al. (2012). Identification of somatic mutations in parathyroid tumors using whole-exome sequencing. J Clin Endocrinol Metab. 97:E1774–81. PMID:22740705
580. Crona J, Delgado Verdugo A, Maharjan R, et al. (2013). Somatic mutations in H-RAS in sporadic pheochromocytoma and paraganglioma identified by exome sequencing. J Clin Endocrinol Metab. 98:E1266–71. PMID:23640968
581. Crotty TB, Scheithauer BW, Young WF Jr, et al. (1995). Papillary craniopharyngioma: a clinicopathological study of 48 cases. J Neurosurg. 83:206–14. PMID:7616262
582. Crowley RK, Al-Derazi Y, Lynch K, et al. (2012). Acromegaly associated with gangliocytoma. Ir J Med Sci. 181:353–5. PMID:19789938
583. Cruz MC, Marques LP, Sambade C, et al. (1991). Primary mucinous carcinoma of the thyroid gland. Surg Pathol. 4:266–73.
584. Cryns VL, Thor A, Xu HJ, et al. (1994). Loss of the retinoblastoma tumor-suppressor gene in parathyroid carcinoma. N Engl J Med. 330:757–61. PMID:7906387
585. Cubilla AL, Hajdu SI (1975). Islet cell carcinoma of the pancreas. Arch Pathol. 99:204–7. PMID:163633
586. Cudennec YF, Trannoy P, Briche T, et al. (1992). Thyroid teratoma in adults. Rev Laryngol Otol Rhinol (Bord). 113:213–5. [French] PMID:1344539
587. Cugati G, Singh M, Symss NP, et al. (2012). Primary intrasellar schwannoma. J Clin Neurosci. 19:1584–5. PMID:22959445
588. Cunningham JT, Rodgers JT, Arlow DH, et al. (2007). mTOR controls mitochondrial oxidative function through a YY1-PGC-1alpha transcriptional complex. Nature. 450:736–40. PMID:18046414
589. Cunningham SC, Suh HS, Winter JM, et al. (2006). Retroperitoneal paraganglioma: single-institution experience and review of the literature. J Gastrointest Surg. 10:1156–63. PMID:16966036
590. Cuny T, Barlier A (2013). The significance of MEN1 mutations in pituitary carcinomas. Biomark Med. 7:567–9. PMID:23905891
591. Cuny T, Pertuit M, Sahnoun-Fathallah M, et al. (2013). Genetic analysis in young patients with sporadic pituitary macroadenomas: besides AIP don't forget MEN1 genetic analysis. Eur J Endocrinol. 168:533–41. PMID:23321498
592. Cupisti K, Wolf A, Raffel A, et al. (2007). Long-term clinical and biochemical follow-up in medullary thyroid carcinoma: a single institution's experience over 20 years. Ann Surg. 246:815–21. PMID:17968174
593. Currás-Freixes M, Inglada-Pérez L, Mancikova V, et al. (2015). Recommendations for somatic and germline genetic testing of single pheochromocytoma and paraganglioma based on findings from a series of 329 patients. J Med Genet. 52:647–56. PMID:26269449
594. Cusick JF, Ho KC, Hagen TC, et al. (1982). Granular-cell pituicytoma associated with multiple endocrine neoplasia type. J Neurosurg. 56:594–6. PMID:7062133
595. Cutlan RT, Greer JE, Wong FS, et al. (2000). Immunohistochemical characterization of thyroid gland angiomatoid tumors. Exp Mol Pathol. 69:159–64. PMID:11001864
595A. Därr R, Nambuba J, Del Rivero J, et al. (2016) Novel insights into the polycythemia-paraganglioma-somatostatinoma syndrome. Endocr Relat Cancer 23:899–908. PMID:27679736
596. d'Alessandro AF, Montenegro FL, Brandão LG, et al. (2012). Supernumerary parathyroid glands in hyperparathyroidism associated with multiple endocrine neoplasia type 1. Rev Assoc Med Bras (1992). 58:323–7. PMID:22735224
597. D'Angelo D, Palmieri D, Mussnich P, et al. (2012). Altered microRNA expression profile in human pituitary GH adenomas: down-regulation of miRNA targeting HMGA1, HMGA2, and E2F1. J Clin Endocrinol Metab. 97:E1128–38. PMID:22564666
598. D'Antonio A, Addesso M, De Dominicis G, et al. (2007). Mucinous carcinoma of thyroid gland. Report of a primary and a metastatic mucinous tumour from ovarian adenocarcinoma with immunohistochemical study and review of literature. Virchows Arch. 451:847–51. PMID:17704943
599. Dahia PL (2014). Pheochromocytoma and paraganglioma pathogenesis: learning from genetic heterogeneity. Nat Rev Cancer. 14:108–19. PMID:24442145
600. Dahia PL, Aguiar RC, Honegger J, et al. (1998). Mutation and expression analysis of the p27/kip1 gene in corticotrophin-secreting tumours. Oncogene. 16:69–76. PMID:9467944
601. Dahia PL, Ross KN, Wright ME, et al. (2005). A HIF1alpha regulatory loop links hypoxia and mitochondrial signals in pheochromocytomas. PLoS Genet. 1:72–80. PMID:16103922
602. Dall'Igna P, Virgone C, De Salvo GL, et al. (2014). Adrenocortical tumors in Italian children: analysis of clinical characteristics and P53 status. Data from the national registries. J Pediatr Surg. 49:1367–71. PMID:25148739
603. Daly AF, Beckers A (2008). Update on the treatment of pituitary adenomas: familial and genetic considerations. Acta Clin Belg. 63:418–24. PMID:19170361
604. Daly AF, Rixhon M, Adam C, et al. (2006). High prevalence of pituitary adenomas: a cross-sectional study in the province of Liege, Belgium. J Clin Endocrinol Metab. 91:4769–75. PMID:16968795
605. Daly AF, Tichomirowa MA, Beckers A (2009). Update on familial pituitary tumors: from multiple endocrine neoplasia type 1 to familial isolated pituitary adenoma. Horm Res. 71 Suppl 1:105–11. PMID:19153518
606. Damiani S, Filotico M, Eusebi V (1991). Carcinoma of the thyroid showing thymoma-like features. Virchows Arch A Pathol Anat Histopathol. 418:463–6. PMID:2035260
607. Damiani S, Fratamico F, Lapertosa G, et al. (1991). Alcian blue and epithelial membrane antigen are useful markers in differentiating benign from malignant papillae in thyroid lesions. Virchows Arch A Pathol Anat Histopathol. 419:131–5. PMID:1871955
608. Daniels GH (2011). Screening for medullary thyroid carcinoma with serum calcitonin measurements in patients with thyroid nodules in the United States and Canada. Thyroid. 21:1199–207. PMID:21936671
609. Danon M, Robboy SJ, Kim S, et al. (1975). Cushing syndrome, sexual precocity, and polyostotic fibrous dysplasia (Albright syndrome) in infancy. J Pediatr. 87(6 Pt 1):917–21. PMID:171361
610. Darling TN, Skarulis MC, Steinberg SM, et al. (1997). Multiple facial angiofibromas and collagenomas in patients with multiple endocrine neoplasia type 1. Arch Dermatol. 133:853–7. PMID:9236523
611. Darrat I, Bedoyan JK, Chen M, et al. (2013). Novel DICER1 mutation as cause of multinodular goiter in children. Head Neck. 35:E369–71. PMID:23728841
612. Das P, Haresh KP, Suri V, et al. (2010). Malignant hemangiopericytoma of pituitary fossa. Indian J Pathol Microbiol. 53:109–11. PMID:20090235
613. Das S, Kalyani R (2008). Sclerosing mucoepidermoid carcinoma with eosinophilia of the thyroid. Indian J Pathol Microbiol. 51:34–6. PMID:18417848
614. Dasgupta A, Teerthanath S, Jayakumar M, et al. (2014). Primary cavernous haemangioma of the thyroid – a case report. J Clin Diagn Res. 8:151–2. PMID:24701513
615. Davenport E, Lennard T (2014). Acute hypercortisolism: what can the surgeon offer? Clin Endocrinol (Oxf). 81:498–502. PMID:24802156
616. Davies L, Morris LG, Haymart M, et al. (2015). American Association Of Clinical Endocrinologists and American College Of Endocrinology disease state clinical review: the increasing incidence of thyroid cancer. Endocr Pract. 21:686–96. PMID:26135963
617. Davis DA, Medline NM (1970). Spironolactone (aldactone) bodies: concentric lamellar formations in the adrenal cortices of patients treated with spironolactone. Am J Clin Pathol. 54:22–32. PMID:5504616
618. Dawson J, Bloom SR, Cockel R (1983). A unique apudoma producing the glucagonoma and gastrinoma syndromes. Postgrad Med J. 59:315–6. PMID:6878103
619. Dayan CM, Daniels GH (1996). Chronic autoimmune thyroiditis. N Engl J Med. 335:99–107. PMID:8649497
620. de Angelis M, Cappabianca P (2014). Thyrotropin pituitary adenomas. World Neurosurg. 82:1026–7. PMID:24954258
621. De Crea C, Raffaelli M, Sessa L, et al. (2014). Actual incidence and clinical behaviour of follicular thyroid carcinoma: an institutional experience. ScientificWorldJournal. 2014:952095. PMID:24741369
622. de Cubas AA, Korpershoek E, Inglada-Pérez L, et al. (2015). DNA Methylation Profiling in Pheochromocytoma and Paraganglioma Reveals Diagnostic and Prognostic Markers. Clin Cancer Res. 21:3020–30. PMID:25825477
623. de Fraipont F, El Atifi M, Cherradi N, et al. (2005). Gene expression profiling of human adrenocortical tumors using complementary deoxyribonucleic Acid microarrays identifies several candidate genes as markers of malignancy. J Clin Endocrinol Metab. 90:1819–29. PMID:15613424
624. de Kock L, Boshari T, Martinelli F, et al. (2016). Adult-Onset Cervical Embryonal Rhabdomyosarcoma and DICER1 Mutations. J Low Genit Tract Dis. 20:e8–10. PMID:26461232
625. de Kock L, Sabbaghian N, Druker H, et al. (2014). Germ-line and somatic DICER1 mutations in pineoblastoma. Acta Neuropathol. 128:583–95. PMID:25022261
626. de Kock L, Sabbaghian N, Plourde F, et al. (2014). Pituitary blastoma: a pathognomonic feature of germ-line DICER1 mutations. Acta Neuropathol. 128:111–22. PMID:24839956
627. de Kock L, Sabbaghian N, Soglio DB, et al. (2014). Exploring the association Between DICER1 mutations and differentiated thyroid carcinoma. J Clin Endocrinol Metab. 99:E1072–7. PMID:24617712
628. de Kock L, Wang YC, Revil T, et al. (2016). High-sensitivity sequencing reveals multi-organ somatic mosaicism causing DICER1 syndrome. J Med Genet. 53:43–52. PMID:26475046
629. de Krijger RR, Papathomas TG (2012). Adrenocortical neoplasia: evolving concepts in tumorigenesis with an emphasis on adrenal cortical carcinoma variants. Virchows Arch. 460:9–18. PMID:22086150
630. de la Monte SM, Hutchins GM, Moore GW (1984). Endocrine organ metastases from breast carcinoma. Am J Pathol. 114:131–6. PMID:6140849
631. de Laat JM, Dekkers OM, Pieterman CR, et al. (2015). Long-Term Natural Course of Pituitary Tumors in Patients With MEN1: Results From the DutchMEN1 Study Group (DMSG). J Clin Endocrinol Metab. 100:3288–96. PMID:26126205
632. de Laat JM, Pieterman CR, van den Broek MF, et al. (2014). Natural course and survival of neuroendocrine tumors of thymus and lung in MEN1 patients. J Clin Endocrinol Metab. 99:3325–33. PMID:24915123
633. de Mestier L, Gaujoux S, Cros J, et al. (2015). Long-term Prognosis of Resected Pancreatic Neuroendocrine Tumors in von Hippel-Lindau Disease Is Favorable and Not Influenced by Small Tumors Left in Place. Ann Surg. 262:384–8. PMID:25185468
634. de Montpréville VT, Mussot S, Gharbi N, et al. (2005). Paraganglioma with ganglioneuromatous component located in the posterior mediastinum. Ann Diagn Pathol. 9:110–4. PMID:15806520
635. de Oliveira Andrade LJ, Santos França L, Santos França L, et al. (2010). Double pituitary prolactinoma. J Clin Endocrinol Metab. 95:4848–9. PMID:21051581
636. de Reyniès A, Assié G, Rickman DS, et al. (2009). Gene expression profiling reveals a new classification of adrenocortical tumors and identifies molecular predictors of malignancy and survival. J Clin Oncol. 27:1108–15. PMID:19139432
637. Siqueira PF, Mathez AL, Pedretti DB, et al. (2015). Pituitary metastasis of lung neuroendocrine carcinoma: case report and literature review. Arch Endocrinol Metab. 59:548–53. PMID:26677090
638. Dean PG, van Heerden JA, Farley DR, et al. (2000). Are patients with multiple endocrine neoplasia type I prone to premature death? World J Surg. 24:1437–41. PMID:11038219

639. Deb P, Pal S, Dutta V, et al. (2012). Adrenal haemangioblastoma presenting as phaeochromocytoma: a rare manifestation of extraneural hemangioblastoma. Endocr Pathol. 23:187–90. PMID:22544391
640. DeBella K, Szudek J, Friedman JM (2000). Use of the national institutes of health criteria for diagnosis of neurofibromatosis 1 in children. Pediatrics. 105(3 Pt 1):608–14. PMID:10699117
641. Decaussin M, Bernard MH, Adeleine P, et al. (2002). Thyroid carcinomas with distant metastases: a review of 111 cases with emphasis on the prognostic significance of an insular component. Am J Surg Pathol. 26:1007–15. PMID:12170087
642. Defilippi C, Chiappetta D, Marzari D, et al. (2006). Image diagnosis in McCune-Albright syndrome. J Pediatr Endocrinol Metab. 19 Suppl 2:561–70. PMID:16789618
643. DeGroot LJ, Kaplan EL, McCormick M, et al. (1990). Natural history, treatment, and course of papillary thyroid carcinoma. J Clin Endocrinol Metab. 71:414–24. PMID:2380337
644. Dehner LP, Hill DA (2009). Adrenal cortical neoplasms in children: why so many carcinomas and yet so many survivors? Pediatr Dev Pathol. 12:284–91. PMID:19326954
645. Dekker PB, Kuipers-Dijkshoorn N, Hogendoorn PC, et al. (2003). G2M arrest, blocked apoptosis, and low growth fraction may explain indolent behavior of head and neck paragangliomas. Hum Pathol. 34:690–8. PMID:12874765
646. del Pozo C, García-Pascual L, Balsells M, et al. (2011). Parathyroid carcinoma in multiple endocrine neoplasia type 1. Case report and review of the literature. Hormones (Athens). 10:326–31. PMID:22281890
647. Delattre JY, Castelain C, Davila L, et al. (1990). Metastasis to the pituitary stalk in a case of breast cancer. Rev Neurol (Paris). 146:455–6. [French] PMID:2204991
648. DeLellis RA (1993). Orphan Annie eye nuclei: a historical note. Am J Surg Pathol. 17:1067–8. PMID:8372945
649. DeLellis RA (2011). Parathyroid tumors and related disorders. Mod Pathol. 24 Suppl 2:S78–93. PMID:21455204
650. DeLellis RA, Lloyd RV, Heitz PU, et al., editors (2004). World Health Organization classification of tumours. Pathology and genetics of tumours of endocrine organs. 3rd ed. Lyon: IARCPress.
651. DeLellis RA, May L, Tashjian AH Jr, et al. (1978). C-cell granule heterogeneity in man. An ultrastructural immunocytochemical study. Lab Invest. 38:263–9. PMID:633851
652. DeLellis RA, Nunnemacher G, Wolfe HJ (1977). C-cell hyperplasia. An ultrastructural analysis. Lab Invest. 36:237–48. PMID:839736
653. DeLellis RA, Rule AH, Spiler I, et al. (1978). Calcitonin and carcinoembryonic antigen as tumor markers in medullary thyroid carcinoma. Am J Clin Pathol. 70:587–94. PMID:360824
654. DeLellis RA, Wolfe HJ, Gagel RF, et al. (1976). Adrenal medullary hyperplasia. A morphometric analysis in patients with familial medullary thyroid carcinoma. Am J Pathol. 83:177–96. PMID:1275056
655. Delemer B (2012). MEN1 and pituitary adenomas. Ann Endocrinol (Paris). 73:59–61. PMID:22542456
656. Delgrange E, Trouillas J, Maiter D, et al. (1997). Sex-related difference in the growth of prolactinomas: a clinical and proliferation marker study. J Clin Endocrinol Metab. 82:2102–7. PMID:9215279
657. Delgrange E, Vasiljevic A, Wierinckx A, et al. (2015). Expression of estrogen receptor alpha is associated with prolactin pituitary tumor prognosis and supports the sex-related difference in tumor growth. Eur J Endocrinol. 172:791–801. PMID:25792376
658. Delitala AP, Vidili G, Manca A, et al. (2014). A case of thyroid metastasis from pancreatic cancer: case report and literature review. BMC Endocr Disord. 14:6. PMID:24428866
659. Delle Fave G, Kwekkeboom DJ, Van Cutsem E, et al. (2012). ENETS Consensus Guidelines for the management of patients with gastroduodenal neoplasms. Neuroendocrinology. 95:74–87. PMID:22262004
660. Delnatte C, Sanlaville D, Mougenot JF, et al. (2006). Contiguous gene deletion within chromosome arm 10q is associated with juvenile polyposis of infancy, reflecting cooperation between the BMPR1A and PTEN tumor-suppressor genes. Am J Hum Genet. 78:1066–74. PMID:16685657
661. Delprat C, Aricò M (2014). Blood spotlight on Langerhans cell histiocytosis. Blood. 124:867–72. PMID:24894775
662. Demicco EG, Harms PW, Patel RM, et al. (2015). Extensive survey of STAT6 expression in a large series of mesenchymal tumors. Am J Clin Pathol. 143:672–82. PMID:25873501
663. Dénes J, Swords F, Rattenberry E, et al. (2015). Heterogeneous genetic background of the association of pheochromocytoma/paraganglioma and pituitary adenoma: results from a large patient cohort. J Clin Endocrinol Metab. 100:E531–41. PMID:25494863
664. Deng XR, Wang G, Kuang CJ, et al. (2005). Metastasis of leiomyosarcoma to the thyroid. Chin Med J (Engl). 118:174–6. PMID:15667806
665. Denzinger S, Burger M, Hartmann A, et al. (2007). Spontaneous rupture of a benign giant adrenal adenoma. APMIS. 115:381–4. PMID:17504308
666. Derringer GA, Thompson LD, Frommelt RA, et al. (2000). Malignant lymphoma of the thyroid gland: a clinicopathologic study of 108 cases. Am J Surg Pathol. 24:623–39. PMID:10800981
667. Deschamps L, Dokmak S, Guedj N, et al. (2010). Mixed endocrine somatostatinoma of the ampulla of vater associated with a neurofibromatosis type 1: a case report and review of the literature. JOP. 11:64–8. PMID:20065557
668. Deshmukh NS, Mangham DC, Warfield AT, et al. (2001). Solitary fibrous tumour of the thyroid gland. J Laryngol Otol. 115:940–2. PMID:11779319
669. Deshpande V, Fernandez-del Castillo C, Muzikansky A, et al. (2004). Cytokeratin 19 is a powerful predictor of survival in pancreatic endocrine tumors. Am J Surg Pathol. 28:1145–53. PMID:15316313
670. Dettmer M, Schmitt A, Steinert H, et al. (2011). Poorly differentiated thyroid carcinomas: how much poorly differentiated is needed? Am J Surg Pathol. 35:1866–72. PMID:21989341
671. Dettmer M, Schmitt A, Steinert H, et al. (2012). Poorly differentiated oncocytic thyroid carcinoma–diagnostic implications and outcome. Histopathology. 60:1045–51. PMID:22348590
672. Dettmer MS, Perren A, Moch H, et al. (2014). MicroRNA profile of poorly differentiated thyroid carcinomas: new diagnostic and prognostic insights. J Mol Endocrinol. 52:181–9. PMID:24443580
673. Dettmer MS, Schmitt A, Steinert H, et al. (2015). Tall cell papillary thyroid carcinoma: new diagnostic criteria and mutations in BRAF and TERT. Endocr Relat Cancer. 22:419–29. PMID:25870252
674. Dettori T, Frau DV, Lai ML, et al. (2003). Aneuploidy in oncocytic lesions of the thyroid gland: diffuse accumulation of mitochondria within the cell is associated with trisomy 7 and progressive numerical chromosomal alterations. Genes Chromosomes Cancer. 38:22–31. PMID:12874783
675. Di Dalmazi G, Kisker C, Calebiro D, et al. (2014). Novel somatic mutations in the catalytic subunit of the protein kinase A as a cause of adrenal Cushing's syndrome: a European multicentric study. J Clin Endocrinol Metab. 99:E2093–100. PMID:25057884
676. Di Ieva A, Rotondo F, Syro LV, et al. (2014). Aggressive pituitary adenomas–diagnosis and emerging treatments. Nat Rev Endocrinol. 10:423–35. PMID:24821329
677. Diaz-Arias AA, Bickel JT, Loy TS, et al. (1992). Follicular carcinoma with clear cell change arising in lingual thyroid. Oral Surg Oral Med Oral Pathol. 74:206–11. PMID:1508530
678. Diaz-Cano SJ, de Miguel M, Blanes A, et al. (2001). Germline RET 634 mutation positive MEN 2A-related C-cell hyperplasias have genetic features consistent with intraepithelial neoplasia. J Clin Endocrinol Metab. 86:3948–57. PMID:11502837
679. Diaz-Perez R, Quiroz H, Nishiyama RH (1976). Primary mucinous adenocarcinoma of thyroid gland. Cancer. 38:1323–5. PMID:182353
680. Dickersin GR, Vickery AL Jr, Smith SB (1980). Papillary carcinoma of the thyroid, oxyphil cell type, "clear cell" variant: a light- and electron-microscopic study. Am J Surg Pathol. 4:501–9. PMID:7435777
681. Diolaiti D, McFerrin L, Carroll PA, et al. (2015). Functional interactions among members of the MAX and MLX transcriptional network during oncogenesis. Biochim Biophys Acta. 1849:484–500. PMID:24857747
682. Diolombi ML, Khani F, Epstein JI (2016). Diagnostic dilemmas in enlarged and diffusely hemorrhagic adrenal glands. Hum Pathol. 53:63–72. PMID:27001431
683. DiPaolo DP, Zimmerman RA, Rorke LB, et al. (1995). Neurofibromatosis type 1: pathologic substrate of high-signal-intensity foci in the brain. Radiology. 195:721–4. PMID:7754001
684. Diskin SJ, Capasso M, Schnepp RW, et al. (2012). Common variation at 6q16 within HACE1 and LIN28B influences susceptibility to neuroblastoma. Nat Genet. 44:1126–30. PMID:22941191
685. Diskin SJ, Hou C, Glessner JT, et al. (2009). Copy number variation at 1q21.1 associated with neuroblastoma. Nature. 459:987–91. PMID:19536264
686. Djalilian HR, Linzie B, Maisel RH (2000). Malignant teratoma of the thyroid: review of literature and report of a case. Am J Otolaryngol. 21:112–5. PMID:10758996
687. Dobashi Y, Sugimura H, Sakamoto A, et al. (1994). Stepwise participation of p53 gene mutation during dedifferentiation of human thyroid carcinomas. Diagn Mol Pathol. 3:9–14. PMID:8162258
688. Doherty GM, Lairmore TC, DeBenedetti MK (2004). Multiple endocrine neoplasia type 1 parathyroid adenoma development over time. World J Surg. 28:1139–42. PMID:15490065
689. Doi M, Imai T, Shichiri M, et al. (2003). Octreotide-sensitive ectopic ACTH production by islet cell carcinoma with multiple liver metastases. Endocr J. 50:135–43. PMID:12803233
690. Dolecek TA, Propp JM, Stroup NE, et al. (2012). CBTRUS statistical report: primary brain and central nervous system tumors diagnosed in the United States in 2005–2009. Neuro Oncol. 14 Suppl 5:v1–49. PMID:23095881
691. Domingue ME, Marbaix E, Do Rego JL, et al. (2015). Infrasellar pituitary gangliocytoma causing Cushing's syndrome. Pituitary. 18:738–44. PMID:25183169
692. Dominguez-Malagon H, Delgado-Chavez R, Torres-Najera M, et al. (1989). Oxyphil and squamous variants of medullary thyroid carcinoma. Cancer. 63:1183–8. PMID:2917321
693. Dominguez-Malagon H, Guerrero-Medrano J, Suster S (1995). Ectopic poorly differentiated (insular) carcinoma of the thyroid. Report of a case presenting as an anterior mediastinal mass. Am J Clin Pathol. 104:408–12. PMID:7572790
694. Donangelo I, Araújo PB, Antenuzi D, et al. (2005). Tumor deletion mapping of chromosomal region 13q14 in 43 growth hormone secreting pituitary adenomas. Endocrine. 28:131–6. PMID:16388084
695. Dong W, Zhang H, Zhang P, et al. (2013). The changing incidence of thyroid carcinoma in Shenyang, China before and after universal salt iodization. Med Sci Monit. 19:49–53. PMID:23314590
696. Donghi R, Longoni A, Pilotti S, et al. (1993). Gene p53 mutations are restricted to poorly differentiated and undifferentiated carcinomas of the thyroid gland. J Clin Invest. 91:1753–60. PMID:8473515
697. Donovan DT, Levy ML, Furst EJ, et al. (1989). Familial cutaneous lichen amyloidosis in association with multiple endocrine neoplasia type 2A: a new variant. Henry Ford Hosp Med J. 37:147–50. PMID:2576950
698. Donow C, Pipeleers-Marichal M, Schröder S, et al. (1991). Surgical pathology of gastrinoma. Site, size, multicentricity, association with multiple endocrine neoplasia type 1, and malignancy. Cancer. 68:1329–34. PMID:1678681
699. Dorfman DM, Shahsafaei A, Miyauchi A (1998). Intrathyroidal epithelial thymoma (ITET)/carcinoma showing thymus-like differentiation (CASTLE) exhibits CD5 immunoreactivity: new evidence for thymic differentiation. Histopathology. 32:104–9. PMID:9543665
700. Doros L, Schultz KA, Stewart DR, et al. (1993). DICER1-related disorders. In: Pagon RA, Adam MP, Ardinger HH, et al., editors. GeneReviews®. Seattle: University of Washington, Seattle. PMID:24761742
701. Doros LA, Rossi CT, Yang J, et al. (2014). DICER1 mutations in childhood cystic nephroma and its relationship to DICER1-renal sarcoma. Mod Pathol. 27:1267–80. PMID:24481001
702. Dötsch J, Kiess W, Hänze J, et al. (1996). Gs alpha mutation at codon 201 in pituitary adenoma causing gigantism in a 6-year-old boy with McCune-Albright syndrome. J Clin Endocrinol Metab. 81:3839–42. PMID:8923825
703. Doyle LA, Fletcher CD (2014). Peripheral hemangioblastoma: clinicopathologic characterization in a series of 22 cases. Am J Surg Pathol. 38:119–27. PMID:24145646
704. Dreijerink KM, Derks JL, Cataldo I, et al. (2015). Genetics and Epigenetics of Pancreatic Neuroendocrine Tumors and Pulmonary Carcinoids. Front Horm Res. 44:115–38. PMID:26303708
705. Dreijerink KM, Valk GD (2015). Reply to: Breast cancer risk in MEN1–a cancer genetics perspective. Clin Endocrinol (Oxf). 83:141. PMID:25409873
706. Drelon C, Berthon A, Mathieu M, et al. (2016). EZH2 is overexpressed in adrenocortical carcinoma and is associated with disease progression. Hum Mol Genet. 25:2789–800. PMID:27149985
706A. Drougat L, Espiard S, Bertherat J (2015). Genetics of primary bilateral macronodular adrenal hyperplasia: a model for early diagnosis of Cushing's syndrome? Eur J Endocrinol. 173(4):M121–31. PMID:26264719
707. Duan K, Gomez Hernandez K, Mete O (2015). Clinicopathological correlates of adrenal Cushing's syndrome. J Clin Pathol. 68:175–86. PMID:25425660
708. Duan K, Gomez Hernandez K, Mete O (2015). Clinicopathological correlates of hyperparathyroidism. J Clin Pathol. 68:771–87. PMID:26163537
709. Duan K, Mete Ö (2015). Parathyroid Carcinoma: Diagnosis and Clinical Implications. Turk Patoloji Derg. 31 Suppl 1:80–97. PMID:26177319
710. Dubois S, Guyétant S, Menei P, et al. (2007). Relevance of Ki-67 and prognostic factors for recurrence/progression of gonadotropic

adenomas after first surgery. Eur J Endocrinol. 157:141–7. PMID:17656591

711. Dubois SG, London WB, Zhang Y, et al. (2008). Lung metastases in neuroblastoma at initial diagnosis: A report from the International Neuroblastoma Risk Group (INRG) project. Pediatr Blood Cancer. 51:589–92. PMID:18649370

712. Ducatman BS, Scheithauer BW, Dahlin DC (1983). Malignant bone tumors associated with neurofibromatosis. Mayo Clin Proc. 58:578–82. PMID:6310276

713. Ducatman BS, Scheithauer BW, Piepgras DG, et al. (1986). Malignant peripheral nerve sheath tumors. A clinicopathologic study of 120 cases. Cancer. 57:2006–21. PMID:3082508

714. Duffner PK, Cohen ME, Seidel FG, et al. (1989). The significance of MRI abnormalities in children with neurofibromatosis. Neurology. 39:373–8. PMID:2494565

715. Duh QY, Hybarger CP, Geist R, et al. (1987). Carcinoids associated with multiple endocrine neoplasia syndromes. Am J Surg. 154:142–8. PMID:2886072

716. Dumitrescu CE, Collins MT (2008). McCune-Albright syndrome. Orphanet J Rare Dis. 3:12. PMID:18489744

717. Dundr P, Dudorkinová D, Povýsil C, et al. (2003). Pigmented composite paraganglioma-ganglioneuroma of the urinary bladder. Pathol Res Pract. 199:765–9. PMID:14708645

718. Dupuy M, Bonneville F, Grunenwald S, et al. (2012). Primary sellar neuroblastoma. A new case and review of literature. Ann Endocrinol (Paris). 73:216–21. PMID:22497798

719. Duregon E, Fassina A, Volante M, et al. (2013). The reticulin algorithm for adrenocortical tumor diagnosis: a multicentric validation study on 245 unpublished cases. Am J Surg Pathol. 37:1433–40. PMID:23774167

720. Duregon E, Molinaro L, Volante M, et al. (2014). Comparative diagnostic and prognostic performances of the hematoxylin-eosin and phospho-histone H3 mitotic count and Ki-67 index in adrenocortical carcinoma. Mod Pathol. 27:1246–54. PMID:24434900

721. Duregon E, Rapa I, Votta A, et al. (2014). MicroRNA expression patterns in adrenocortical carcinoma variants and clinical pathologic correlations. Hum Pathol. 45:1555–62. PMID:24890943

722. Duregon E, Volante M, Bollito E, et al. (2015). Pitfalls in the diagnosis of adrenocortical tumors: a lesson from 300 consultation cases. Hum Pathol. 46:1799–807. PMID:26472162

723. Duregon E, Volante M, Cappia S, et al. (2011). Oncocytic adrenocortical tumors: diagnostic algorithm and mitochondrial DNA profile in 27 cases. Am J Surg Pathol. 35:1882–93. PMID:21989346

724. Duregon E, Volante M, Giorcelli J, et al. (2013). Diagnostic and prognostic role of steroidogenic factor 1 in adrenocortical carcinoma: a validation study focusing on clinical and pathologic correlates. Hum Pathol. 44:822–8. PMID:23158211

725. Durieux E, Descotes F, Mauduit C, et al. (2016). The co-occurrence of an ovarian Sertoli-Leydig cell tumor with a thyroid carcinoma is highly suggestive of a DICER1 syndrome. Virchows Arch. 468:631–6. PMID:26983701

726. Dvorakova S, Vaclavikova E, Sykorova V, et al. (2008). Somatic mutations in the RET proto-oncogene in sporadic medullary thyroid carcinomas. Mol Cell Endocrinol. 284:21–7. PMID:18282654

727. Dwight T, Mann K, Benn DE, et al. (2013). Familial SDHA mutation associated with pituitary adenoma and pheochromocytoma/paraganglioma. J Clin Endocrinol Metab. 98:E1103–8. PMID:23633203

728. Dwight T, Nelson AE, Theodosopoulos G, et al. (2002). Independent genetic events associated with the development of multiple parathyroid tumors in patients with primary hyperparathyroidism. Am J Pathol. 161:1299–306. PMID:12368203

729. Dwight T, Thoppe SR, Foukakis T, et al. (2003). Involvement of the PAX8/peroxisome proliferator-activated receptor gamma rearrangement in follicular thyroid tumors. J Clin Endocrinol Metab. 88:4440–5. PMID:12970322

730. Dworakowska D, Grossman AB (2012). The molecular pathogenesis of corticotroph tumours. Eur J Clin Invest. 42:665–76. PMID:22098190

731. Dyer EH, Civit T, Abecassis JP, et al. (1994). Functioning ectopic supradiaphragmatic pituitary adenomas. Neurosurgery. 34:529–32, discussion 532. PMID:7832831

732. Ebrahimi SA, Wang EH, Wu A, et al. (1999). Deletion of chromosome 1 predicts prognosis in pancreatic endocrine tumors. Cancer Res. 59:311–5. PMID:9927038

733. ECC 2015—Neuroendocrine Cancer (2015). SSA therapies—177Lu-DOTATATE is a better one in NETTER-1. Nat Rev Clin Oncol. 12:684.

734. Echevarría ME, Fangusaro J, Goldman S (2008). Pediatric central nervous system germ cell tumors: a review. Oncologist. 13:690–9. PMID:18586924

735. Eckert F, Schmid U, Gloor F, et al. (1986). Evidence of vascular differentiation in anaplastic tumours of the thyroid–an immunohistological study. Virchows Arch A Pathol Anat Histopathol. 410:203–15. PMID:3099463

736. Edge S, Byrd DR, Compton CC, et al., editors (2010). AJCC cancer staging manual. 7th ed. New York: Springer; pp. 87–96.

737. Edis AJ (1977). Surgical anatomy and technique of neck exploration for primary hyperparathyroidism. Surg Clin North Am. 57:495–504. PMID:867217

738. Egashira N, Takekoshi S, Takei M, et al. (2011). Expression of FOXL2 in human normal pituitaries and pituitary adenomas. Mod Pathol. 24:765–73. PMID:21478824

739. Ege B, Leventoğlu S (2013). Primary leiomyosarcoma of the thyroid. J Korean Surg Soc. 85:43–6. PMID:23833760

740. Egloff B (1983). The hemangioendothelioma of the thyroid. Virchows Arch A Pathol Anat Histopathol. 400:119–42. PMID:6412429

741. Eisenhofer G, Goldstein DS, Kopin IJ, et al. (2003). Pheochromocytoma: rediscovery as a catecholamine-metabolizing tumor. Endocr Pathol. 14:193–212. PMID:14586065

742. Eisenhofer G, Kopin IJ, Goldstein DS (2004). Catecholamine metabolism: a contemporary view with implications for physiology and medicine. Pharmacol Rev. 56:331–49. PMID:15317907

743. Eisenhofer G, Lenders JW, Siegert G, et al. (2012). Plasma methoxytyramine: a novel biomarker of metastatic pheochromocytoma and paraganglioma in relation to established risk factors of tumour size, location and SDHB mutation status. Eur J Cancer. 48:1739–49. PMID:22036874

744. Eisenhofer G, Lenders JW, Timmers H, et al. (2011). Measurements of plasma methoxytyramine, normetanephrine, and metanephrine as discriminators of different hereditary forms of pheochromocytoma. Clin Chem. 57:411–20. PMID:21262951

745. Eisenhofer G, Pacak K, Huynh TT, et al. (2010). Catecholamine metabolomic and secretory phenotypes in phaeochromocytoma. Endocr Relat Cancer. 18:97–111. PMID:21051559

746. Eisenhofer G, Peitzsch M (2014). Laboratory evaluation of pheochromocytoma and paraganglioma. Clin Chem. 60:1486–99. PMID:25332315

747. Eisenhofer G, Timmers HJ, Lenders JW, et al. (2011). Age at diagnosis of pheochromocytoma differs according to catecholamine phenotype and tumor location. J Clin Endocrinol Metab. 96:375–84. PMID:21147885

748. Eisenhofer G, Tischler AS, de Krijger RR (2012). Diagnostic tests and biomarkers for pheochromocytoma and extra-adrenal paraganglioma: from routine laboratory methods to disease stratification. Endocr Pathol. 23:4–14. PMID:22180288

749. Eisenhofer G, Walther MM, Huynh TT, et al. (2001). Pheochromocytomas in von Hippel-Lindau syndrome and multiple endocrine neoplasia type 2 display distinct biochemical and clinical phenotypes. J Clin Endocrinol Metab. 86:1999–2008. PMID:11344198

750. Ejerblad S, Grimelius L, Johansson H, et al. (1976). Studies on the non-adenomatous glands in patients with a solitary parathyroid adenoma. Ups J Med Sci. 81:31–6. PMID:1273998

751. El-Daly H, Rao P, Palazzo F, et al. (2010). A rare entity of an unusual site: adenomatoid tumour of the adrenal gland: a case report and review of the literature. Patholog Res Int. 2010:702472. PMID:21151721

752. El-Maqsoud NM, Tawfiek ER, Abdelmeged A, et al. (2016). The diagnostic utility of the triple markers Napsin A, TTF-1, and PAX8 in differentiating between primary and metastatic lung carcinomas. Tumour Biol. 37:3123–34. PMID:26427663

753. el-Naggar AK, Batsakis JG, Luna MA, et al. (1988). Hürthle cell tumors of the thyroid. A flow cytometric DNA analysis. Arch Otolaryngol Head Neck Surg. 114:520–1. PMID:3355687

754. el-Sahrigy D, Zhang XM, Elhosseiny A, et al. (2004). Signet-ring follicular adenoma of the thyroid diagnosed by fine needle aspiration. Report of a case with cytologic description. Acta Cytol. 48:87–90. PMID:14969188

755. Elder EE, Xu D, Höög A, et al. (2003). KI-67 AND hTERT expression can aid in the distinction between malignant and benign pheochromocytoma and paraganglioma. Mod Pathol. 16:246–55. PMID:12640105

756. Eldor R, Glaser B, Fraenkel M, et al. (2011). Glucagonoma and the glucagonoma syndrome – cumulative experience with an elusive endocrine tumour. Clin Endocrinol (Oxf). 74:593–8. PMID:21470282

756A. Elisei R, Bottici V, Luchetti F, et al. (2004). Impact of routine measurement of serum calcitonin on the diagnosis and outcome of medullary thyroid cancer: experience in 10,864 patients with nodular thyroid disorders. J Clin Endocrinol Metab. 89:163–8. PMID: 14715844

757. Elisei R, Cosci B, Romei C, et al. (2008). Prognostic significance of somatic RET oncogene mutations in sporadic medullary thyroid cancer: a 10-year follow-up study. J Clin Endocrinol Metab. 93:682–7. PMID:18073307

758. Elisei R, Schlumberger MJ, Müller SP, et al. (2013). Cabozantinib in progressive medullary thyroid cancer. J Clin Oncol. 31:3639–46. PMID:24002501

759. Elliott DD, Sellin R, Egger JF, et al. (2005). Langerhans cell histiocytosis presenting as a thyroid gland mass. Ann Diagn Pathol. 9:267–74. PMID:16198954

760. Elliott DD, Sherman SI, Busaidy NL, et al. (2008). Growth factor receptors expression in anaplastic thyroid carcinoma: potential markers for therapeutic stratification. Hum Pathol. 39:15–20. PMID:17949783

761. Eloy C, Oliveira M, Vieira J, et al. (2014). Carcinoma of the thyroid with ewing family tumor elements and favorable prognosis: report of a second case. Int J Surg Pathol. 22:260–5. PMID:23637256

762. Eloy C, Santos J, Soares P, et al. (2011). Intratumoural lymph vessel density is related to presence of lymph node metastases and separates encapsulated from infiltrative papillary thyroid carcinoma. Virchows Arch. 459:595–605. PMID:22081104

763. Eloy JA, Mortensen M, Gupta S, et al. (2007). Metastasis of uterine leiomyosarcoma to the thyroid gland: case report and review of the literature. Thyroid. 17:1295–7. PMID:17988195

764. Else T, Kim AC, Sabolch A, et al. (2014). Adrenocortical carcinoma. Endocr Rev. 35:282–326. PMID:24423978

765. Else T, Marvin ML, Everett JN, et al. (2014). The clinical phenotype of SDHC-associated hereditary paraganglioma syndrome (PGL3). J Clin Endocrinol Metab. 99:E1482–6. PMID:24758179

766. Elsheikh TM, Asa SL, Chan JK, et al. (2008). Interobserver and intraobserver variation among experts in the diagnosis of thyroid follicular lesions with borderline nuclear features of papillary carcinoma. Am J Clin Pathol. 130:736–44. PMID:18854266

767. Elston MS, Gill AJ, Conaglen JV, et al. (2008). Wnt pathway inhibitors are strongly down-regulated in pituitary tumors. Endocrinology. 149:1235–42. PMID:18079202

768. Elston MS, Meyer-Rochow GY, Conaglen HM, et al. (2015). Increased SSTR2A and SSTR3 expression in succinate dehydrogenase-deficient pheochromocytomas and paragangliomas. Hum Pathol. 46:390–6. PMID:25554089

769. Elston MS, Meyer-Rochow GY, Dray M, et al. (2015). Early Onset Primary Hyperparathyroidism Associated with a Novel Germline Mutation in CDKN1B. Case Rep Endocrinol. 2015:510985. PMID:26257968

770. Eng C (1993). PTEN hamartoma tumor syndrome. In: Pagon RA, Adam MP, Ardinger HH, et al., editors. GeneReviews®. Seattle: University of Washington, Seattle. PMID:20301661

771. Eng C (1996). Seminars in medicine of the Beth Israel Hospital, Boston. The RET proto-oncogene in multiple endocrine neoplasia type 2 and Hirschsprung's disease. N Engl J Med. 335:943–51. PMID:8782503

772. Eng C (1998). Genetics of Cowden syndrome: through the looking glass of oncology. Int J Oncol. 12:701–10. PMID:9472113

773. Eng C (2000). Multiple endocrine neoplasia type 2 and the practice of molecular medicine. Rev Endocr Metab Disord. 1:283–90. PMID:11706742

774. Eng C (2010). Mendelian genetics of rare–and not so rare–cancers. Ann N Y Acad Sci. 1214:70–82. PMID:20946573

775. Eng C, Clayton D, Schuffenecker I, et al. (1996). The relationship between specific RET proto-oncogene mutations and disease phenotype in multiple endocrine neoplasia type 2. International RET mutation consortium analysis. JAMA. 276:1575–9. PMID:8918855

776. Eng C, Mulligan LM, Healey CS, et al. (1996). Heterogeneous mutation of the RET proto-oncogene in subpopulations of medullary thyroid carcinoma. Cancer Res. 56:2167–70. PMID:8616867

777. Eng C, Smith DP, Mulligan LM, et al. (1994). Point mutation within the tyrosine kinase domain of the RET proto-oncogene in multiple endocrine neoplasia type 2B and related sporadic tumours. Hum Mol Genet. 3:237–41. PMID:7911697

778. Enriquez ML, Lal P, Ziober A, et al. (2012). The use of immunohistochemical expression of SF-1 and EMA in distinguishing adrenocortical tumors from renal neoplasms. Appl Immunohistochem Mol Morphol. 20:141–5. PMID:22553814

779. Erdem E, Angtuaco EC, Van Hemert R, et al. (2003). Comprehensive review of intracranial chordoma. Radiographics. 23:995–1009. PMID:12853676

780. Erhamamci S, Reyhan M, Kocer NE, et al. (2014). Simultaneous occurrence of medullary and differentiated thyroid carcinomas. Report of 4 cases and brief review of the literature. Hell J Nucl Med. 17:148–52. PMID:24997082

781. Erickson D, Kudva YC, Ebersold MJ, et al. (2001). Benign paragangliomas: clinical presentation and treatment outcomes in 236 patients. J Clin Endocrinol Metab. 86:5210–6. PMID:11701678

782. Erickson D, Scheithauer B, Atkinson J, et al. (2009). Silent subtype 3 pituitary adenoma: a clinicopathologic analysis of the Mayo Clinic experience. Clin Endocrinol (Oxf). 71:92–9. PMID:19170710

783. Erickson LA, Jalal SM, Goellner JR, et al. (2001). Analysis of Hürthle cell neoplasms of the thyroid by interphase fluorescence in situ hybridization. Am J Surg Pathol. 25:911–7. PMID:11420462

784. Erickson LA, Jin L, Goellner JR, et al. (2000). Pathologic features, proliferative activity, and cyclin D1 expression in Hürthle cell neoplasms of the thyroid. Mod Pathol. 13:186–92. PMID:10697277

785. Erickson LA, Jin L, Papotti M, et al. (2002). Oxyphil parathyroid carcinomas: a clinico-pathologic and immunohistochemical study of 10 cases. Am J Surg Pathol. 26:344–9. PMID:11859206

786. Erickson LA, Jin L, Wollan P, et al. (1999). Parathyroid hyperplasia, adenomas, and carcinomas: differential expression of p27Kip1 protein. Am J Surg Pathol. 23:288–95. PMID:10078919

787. Erickson LA, Vrana JA, Theis J, et al. (2015). Analysis of Amyloid in Medullary Thyroid Carcinoma by Mass Spectrometry-Based Proteomic Analysis. Endocr Pathol. 26:291–5. PMID:26304852

788. Eriksson B, Orlefors H, Oberg K, et al. (2005). Developments in PET for the detection of endocrine tumours. Best Pract Res Clin Endocrinol Metab. 19:311–24. PMID:15763703

789. Erkiliç S, Erkiliç A, Bayazit YA (2003). Primary leiomyoma of the thyroid gland. J Laryngol Otol. 117:832–4. PMID:14653931

790. Erlic Z, Hoffmann MM, Sullivan M, et al. (2010). Pathogenicity of DNA variants and double mutations in multiple endocrine neoplasia type 2 and von Hippel-Lindau syndrome. J Clin Endocrinol Metab. 95:308–13. PMID:19906784

791. Erovic BM, Harris L, Jamali M, et al. (2012). Biomarkers of parathyroid carcinoma. Endocr Pathol. 23:221–31. PMID:23001705

792. Esapa CT, Johnson SJ, Kendall-Taylor P, et al. (1999). Prevalence of Ras mutations in thyroid neoplasia. Clin Endocrinol (Oxf). 50:529–35. PMID:10468914

793. Espiard S, Bertherat J (2013). Carney complex. Front Horm Res. 41:50–62. PMID:23652670

794. Esposito F, Cappabianca P, Del Basso De Caro M, et al. (2004). Endoscopic endonasal transsphenoidal removal of an intra-suprasellar schwannoma mimicking a pituitary adenoma. Minim Invasive Neurosurg. 47:230–4. PMID:15346320

795. Esposito I, Segler A, Steiger K, et al. (2015). Pathology, genetics and precursors of human and experimental pancreatic neoplasms: An update. Pancreatology. 15:598–610. PMID:26365060

796. Essig GF Jr, Porter K, Schneider D, et al. (2013). Fine needle aspiration and medullary thyroid carcinoma: the risk of inadequate preoperative evaluation and initial surgery when relying upon FNAB cytology alone. Endocr Pract. 19:920–7. PMID:23757627

797. Esteves C, Neves C, Augusto L, et al. (2015). Pituitary incidentalomas: analysis of a neuroradiological cohort. Pituitary. 18:777–81. PMID:25800168

798. Estrella JS, Broaddus RR, Mathews A, et al. (2014). Progesterone receptor and PTEN expression predict survival in patients with low- and intermediate-grade pancreatic neuroendocrine tumors. Arch Pathol Lab Med. 138:1027–36. PMID:25076292

799. Eubanks PJ, Sawicki MP, Samara GJ, et al. (1997). Pancreatic endocrine tumors with loss of heterozygosity at the multiple endocrine neoplasia type I locus. Am J Surg. 173:518–20. PMID:9207166

800. Eugster E (2015). Gigantism. In: De Groot LJ, Beck-Peccoz P, Chrousos G, et al., editors. Endotext. South Dartmouth: MDText.com, Inc. PMID:25905378

801. Eusebi V, Carcangiu ML, Dina R, et al. (1990). Keratin-positive epithelioid angiosarcoma of thyroid. A report of four cases. Am J Surg Pathol. 14:737–47. PMID:1696070

802. Eusebi V, Damiani S, Riva C, et al. (1990). Calcitonin free oat-cell carcinoma of the thyroid gland. Virchows Arch A Pathol Anat Histopathol. 417:267–71. PMID:2166978

803. Evangelisti C, de Biase D, Kurelac I, et al. (2015). A mutation screening of oncogenes, tumor suppressor gene TP53 and nuclear encoded mitochondrial complex I genes in oncocytic thyroid tumors. BMC Cancer. 15:157. PMID:25880213

804. Evans DG, Baser ME, McGaughran J, et al. (2002). Malignant peripheral nerve sheath tumours in neurofibromatosis 1. J Med Genet. 39:311–4. PMID:12011145

805. Evans HL (1984). Follicular neoplasms of the thyroid. A study of 44 cases followed for a minimum of 10 years, with emphasis on differential diagnosis. Cancer. 54:535–40. PMID:6733684

806. Evans HL (1987). Encapsulated papillary neoplasms of the thyroid. A study of 14 cases followed for a minimum of 10 years. Am J Surg Pathol. 11:592–7. PMID:3618882

807. Evenepoel L, Papathomas TG, Krol N, et al. (2015). Toward an improved definition of the genetic and tumor spectrum associated with SDH germ-line mutations. Genet Med. 17:610–20. PMID:25394176

808. Eytan S, Kim KY, Bleich D, et al. (2015). Isolated double pituitary adenomas: A silent corticotroph adenoma and a microprolactinoma. J Clin Neurosci. 22:1676–8. PMID:26067545

809. Ezaki H, Ebihara S, Fujimoto Y, et al. (1992). Analysis of thyroid carcinoma based on material registered in Japan during 1977–1986 with special reference to predominance of papillary type. Cancer. 70:808–14. PMID:1643612

810. Ezzat S, Asa SL (2006). Mechanisms of disease: The pathogenesis of pituitary tumors. Nat Clin Pract Endocrinol Metab. 2:220–30. PMID:16932287

811. Ezzat S, Asa SL, Stefaneanu L, et al. (1994). Somatotroph hyperplasia without pituitary adenoma associated with a long standing growth hormone-releasing hormone-producing bronchial carcinoid. J Clin Endocrinol Metab. 78:555–60. PMID:8126126

812. Ezzat S, Ezrin C, Yamashita S, et al. (1993). Recurrent acromegaly resulting from ectopic growth hormone gene expression by a metastatic pancreatic tumor. Cancer. 71:66–70. PMID:8416728

813. Ezzat S, Horvath E, Harris AG, et al. (1994). Morphological effects of octreotide on growth hormone-producing pituitary adenomas. J Clin Endocrinol Metab. 79:113–8. PMID:8027215

814. Ezzat S, Kontogeorgos G, Redelmeier DA, et al. (1995). In vivo responsiveness of morphological variants of growth hormone-producing pituitary adenomas to octreotide. Eur J Endocrinol. 133:686–90. PMID:8548053

815. Ezzat S, Mader R, Fischer S, et al. (2006). An essential role for the hematopoietic transcription factor Ikaros in hypothalamic-pituitary-mediated somatic growth. Proc Natl Acad Sci U S A. 103:2214–9. PMID:16467156

816. Ezzat S, Yu S, Asa SL (2003). Ikaros isoforms in human pituitary tumors: distinct localization, histone acetylation, and activation of the 5' fibroblast growth factor receptor-4 promoter. Am J Pathol. 163:1177–84. PMID:12937159

817. Ezzat S, Zheng L, Winer D, et al. (2006). Targeting N-cadherin through fibroblast growth factor receptor-4: distinct pathogenetic and therapeutic implications. Mol Endocrinol. 20:2965–75. PMID:16857743

818. Fackenthal JD, Marsh DJ, Richardson AL, et al. (2001). Male breast cancer in Cowden syndrome patients with germline PTEN mutations. J Med Genet. 38:159–64. PMID:11238682

819. Fagin JA, Matsuo K, Karmakar A, et al. (1993). High prevalence of mutations of the p53 gene in poorly differentiated human thyroid carcinomas. J Clin Invest. 91:179–84. PMID:8423216

820. Fahlbusch R, Schott W (2002). Pterional surgery of meningiomas of the tuberculum sellae and planum sphenoidale: surgical results with special consideration of ophthalmological and endocrinological outcomes. J Neurosurg. 96:235–43. PMID:11838796

821. Falconi M, Bartsch DK, Eriksson B, et al. (2012). ENETS Consensus Guidelines for the management of patients with digestive neuroendocrine neoplasms of the digestive system: well-differentiated pancreatic non-functioning tumors. Neuroendocrinology. 95:120–34. PMID:22261872

821A. Falconi M, Eriksson B, Kaltsas G, et al. (2016) ENETS Consensus Guidelines update for the management of patients with functional pancreatic neuroendocrine tumors and non-functional pancreatic neuroendocrine tumors. Neuroendocrinology. 103:153–71. PMID:26742109

822. Famini P, Maya MM, Melmed S (2011). Pituitary magnetic resonance imaging for sellar and parasellar masses: ten-year experience in 2598 patients. J Clin Endocrinol Metab. 96:1633–41. PMID:21470998

823. Fan S, Jiang Y, Yao Y, et al. (2013). Pituitary ACTH-secreting adenoma in Addison's disease: a case report. Clin Neurol Neurosurg. 115:2543–6. PMID:24216004

824. Fang SH, Lal G (2011). Parathyroid cancer. Endocr Pract. 17 Suppl 1:36–43. PMID:21454239

825. Faquin WC, Wong LQ, Afrogheh AH, et al. (2016). Impact of reclassifying noninvasive follicular variant of papillary thyroid carcinoma on the risk of malignancy in The Bethesda System for Reporting Thyroid Cytopathology. Cancer Cytopathol. 124:181–7. PMID:26457584

826. Farhat NA, Faquin WC, Sadow PM (2013). Primary mucoepidermoid carcinoma of the thyroid gland: a report of three cases and review of the literature. Endocr Pathol. 24:229–33. PMID:24096806

827. Farndon JR, Leight GS, Dilley WG, et al. (1986). Familial medullary thyroid carcinoma without associated endocrinopathies: a distinct clinical entity. Br J Surg. 73:278–81. PMID:3697657

828. Farnebo F, Auer G, Farnebo LO, et al. (1999). Evaluation of retinoblastoma and Ki-67 immunostaining as diagnostic markers of benign and malignant parathyroid disease. World J Surg. 23:68–74. PMID:9841766

829. Farrag TY, Micchelli S, Tufano RP (2009). Solitary fibrous tumor of the thyroid gland. Laryngoscope. 119:2306–8. PMID:19806654

830. Farrell JM, Pang JC, Kim GE, et al. (2014). Pancreatic neuroendocrine tumors: accurate grading with Ki-67 index on fine-needle aspiration specimens using the WHO 2010/ENETS criteria. Cancer Cytopathol. 122:770–8. PMID:25044931

831. Farrell WE, Azevedo MF, Batista DL, et al. (2011). Unique gene expression profile associated with an early-onset multiple endocrine neoplasia (MEN1)-associated pituitary adenoma. J Clin Endocrinol Metab. 96:E1905–14. PMID:21917868

832. Fassett DR, Couldwell WT (2004). Metastases to the pituitary gland. Neurosurg Focus. 16:E8. PMID:15191337

833. Fassnacht M, Allolio B (2009). Clinical management of adrenocortical carcinoma. Best Pract Res Clin Endocrinol Metab. 23:273–89. PMID:19500769

834. Fassnacht M, Johanssen S, Quinkler M, et al. (2009). Limited prognostic value of the 2004 International Union Against Cancer staging classification for adrenocortical carcinoma: proposal for a revised TNM classification. Cancer. 115:243–50. PMID:19025987

835. Fassnacht M, Libé R, Kroiss M, et al. (2011). Adrenocortical carcinoma: a clinician's update. Nat Rev Endocrinol. 7:323–35. PMID:21386792

836. Fatemi N, Dusick JR, de Paiva Neto MA, et al. (2008). The endonasal microscopic approach for pituitary adenomas and other parasellar tumors: a 10-year experience. Neurosurgery. 63(4 Suppl 2):244–56, discussion 256. PMID:18981830

837. Favia G, Lumachi F, Polistina F, et al. (1998). Parathyroid carcinoma: sixteen new cases and suggestions for correct management. World J Surg. 22:1225–30. PMID:9841748

838. Favier J, Amar L, Gimenez-Roqueplo AP (2015). Paraganglioma and phaeochromocytoma: from genetics to personalized medicine. Nat Rev Endocrinol. 11:101–11. PMID:25385035

839. Feliberti E, Perry RR, Vinik A (2013). Multiple endocrine neoplasia type I and MEN II. In: De Groot LJ, Beck-Peccoz P, Chrousos G, et al., editors. Endotext. South Dartmouth: MDText.com, Inc. PMID:25905255

840. Fellegara G, Rosai J (2007). Signet ring cells in a poorly differentiated Hürthle cell carcinoma of the thyroid combined with two papillary microcarcinomas. Int J Surg Pathol. 15:388–90. PMID:17913947

841. Fellows IW, Leach IH, Smith PG, et al. (1990). Carcinoid tumour of the common bile duct–a novel complication of von Hippel-Lindau syndrome. Gut. 31:728–9. PMID:2379881

842. Fendrich V, Ramerth R, Waldmann J, et al. (2009). Sonic hedgehog and pancreatic-duodenal homeobox 1 expression distinguish between duodenal and pancreatic gastrinomas. Endocr Relat Cancer. 16:613–22. PMID:19240184

843. Feng J, Hong L, Wu Y, et al. (2014). Identification of a subtype-specific ENC1 gene related to invasiveness in human pituitary null cell adenoma and oncocytomas. J Neurooncol. 119:307–15. PMID:24916845

844. Feng X, Milas M, O'Malley M, et al. (2015). Characteristics of benign and malignant thyroid disease in familial adenomatous polyposis patients and recommendations for disease surveillance. Thyroid. 25:325–32. PMID:25585202

845. Fenton CL, Lukes Y, Nicholson D, et al. (2000). The ret/PTC mutations are common in sporadic papillary thyroid carcinoma of children and young adults. J Clin Endocrinol Metab. 85:1170–5. PMID:10720057

846. Fernandes-Rosa FL, Giscos-Douriez I, Amar L, et al. (2015). Different Somatic Mutations in Multinodular Adrenals With Aldosterone-Producing Adenoma. Hypertension. 66:1014–22. PMID:26351028

847. Fernandes-Rosa FL, Williams TA, Riester A, et al. (2014). Genetic spectrum and clinical correlates of somatic mutations in aldosterone-producing adenoma. Hypertension. 64:354–61. PMID:24866132

848. Fernández-Calvet L, García-Mayor RV (1994). Incidence of pheochromocytoma in South Galicia, Spain. J Intern Med. 236:675–7. PMID:7989903

849. Fernandez-Ranvier GG, Jensen K, Khanafshar E, et al. (2007). Nonfunctioning parathyroid carcinoma: case report and review of literature. Endocr Pract. 13:750–7. PMID:18194932

850. Fernandez-Ranvier GG, Khanafshar E, Jensen K, et al. (2007). Parathyroid carcinoma, atypical parathyroid adenoma, or parathyromatosis? Cancer. 110:255–64. PMID:17559137

851. Fernandez-Ranvier GG, Khanafshar E, Tacha D, et al. (2009). Defining a molecular phenotype for benign and malignant parathyroid tumors. Cancer. 115:334–44. PMID:19107770

852. Ferner RE, Huson SM, Thomas N, et al. (2007). Guidelines for the diagnosis and management of individuals with neurofibromatosis 1. J Med Genet. 44:81–8. PMID:17105749

853. Ferraz-Filho JR, Torres US, Teixeira AC, et al. (2012). Ectopic growth hormone-secreting pituitary adenoma involving the clivus treated with octreotide: role of magnetic resonance imaging in the diagnosis and clinical follow-up. Arq Neuropsiquiatr. 70:744–5. PMID:22990736

854. Ferrero S, Vaira V, Del Gobbo A, et al. (2015). Different expression of protein kinase A (PKA) regulatory subunits in normal and neoplastic thyroid tissues. Histol Histopathol. 30:473–8. PMID:25393625

855. Ferrone CR, Tang LH, Tomlinson J, et al. (2007). Determining prognosis in patients with pancreatic endocrine neoplasms: can the WHO classification system be simplified? J Clin Oncol. 25:5609–15. PMID:18065733

856. Fetsch PA, Powers CN, Zakowski MF, et al. (1999). Anti-alpha-inhibin: marker of choice for the consistent distinction between adrenocortical carcinoma and renal cell carcinoma in fine-needle aspiration. Cancer. 87:168–72. PMID:10385449

857. Filgueiras-Rama D, Oliver JM, Ruiz-Cantador J, et al. (2010). Pheochromocytoma in Eisenmenger's syndrome: a therapeutic challenge. Rev Port Cardiol. 29:1873–7. PMID:21428142

858. Fischer AH, Bond JA, Taysavang P, et al. (1998). Papillary thyroid carcinoma oncogene (RET/PTC) alters the nuclear envelope and chromatin structure. Am J Pathol. 153:1443–50. PMID:9811335

859. Fishbein L, Khare S, Wubbenhorst B, et al. (2015). Whole-exome sequencing identifies somatic ATRX mutations in pheochromocytomas and paragangliomas. Nat Commun. 6:6140. PMID:25608029

859A. Fishbein L et al. (2017) and The Cancer Genome Atlas Research Network. Comprehensive molecular characterization of pheochromocytoma and paraganglioma. Cancer Cell 31:181–193. PMID: 28162975

860. Fitko R, Roth SI, Hines JR, et al. (1990). Parathyromatosis in hyperparathyroidism. Hum Pathol. 21:234–7. PMID:2307452

861. Fletcher CD, Beham A, Bekir S, et al. (1991). Epithelioid angiosarcoma of deep soft tissue: a distinctive tumor readily mistaken for an epithelial neoplasm. Am J Surg Pathol. 15:915–24. PMID:1718176

862. Fletcher CDM, Bridge JA, Lee J-C (2013). Extrapleural solitary fibrous tumour. In: Fletcher CDM, Bridge JA, Hogendoorn PCW, et al., editors. WHO classification of tumours of soft tissue and bone. 4th ed. Lyon: IARC; pp 80–83.

863. Fliedner SM, Lehnert H, Pacak K (2010). Metastatic paraganglioma. Semin Oncol. 37:627–37. PMID:21167381

864. Flint A, Davenport RD, Lloyd RV, et al. (1988). Cytophotometric measurements of Hürthle cell tumors of the thyroid gland. Correlation with pathologic features and clinical behavior. Cancer. 61:110–3. PMID:3334936

865. Folpe AL, Lloyd RV, Bacchi CE, et al. (2009). Spindle epithelial tumor with thymus-like differentiation: a morphologic, immunohistochemical, and molecular genetic study of 11 cases. Am J Surg Pathol. 33:1179–86. PMID:19417583

866. Fonseca AL, Kugelberg J, Starker LF, et al. (2012). Comprehensive DNA methylation analysis of benign and malignant adrenocortical tumors. Genes Chromosomes Cancer. 51:949–60. PMID:22733721

867. Fontaine JF, Mirebeau-Prunier D, Franc B, et al. (2008). Microarray analysis refines classification of non-medullary thyroid tumours of uncertain malignancy. Oncogene. 27:2228–36. PMID:17968324

868. Fontanella S, Bongiovanni M, Nobile A, et al. (2016). Malignant Mucous Cells in a Thyroid Aspirate: Looking for a Source. Endocr Pathol. 27:79–82. PMID:26475625

869. Forman D, Bray F, Brewster DH, et al. (2013). Cancer incidence in five continents, Vol. X. Lyon: IARC. Available from: http://ci5.iarc.fr.

870. Fortson JK, Durden FL Jr, Patel V, et al. (2004). The coexistence of anaplastic and papillary carcinomas of the thyroid: a case presentation and literature review. Am Surg. 70:1116–9. PMID:15663057

871. Fougner SL, Casar-Borota O, Heck A, et al. (2012). Adenoma granulation pattern correlates with clinical variables and effect of somatostatin analogue treatment in a large series of patients with acromegaly. Clin Endocrinol (Oxf). 76:96–102. PMID:21722151

872. Foulkes WD (1995). A tale of four syndromes: familial adenomatous polyposis, Gardner syndrome, attenuated APC and Turcot syndrome. QJM. 88:853–63. PMID:8593545

873. Foulkes WD, Bahubeshi A, Hamel N, et al. (2011). Extending the phenotypes associated with DICER1 mutations. Hum Mutat. 32:1381–4. PMID:21882293

874. Foulkes WD, Priest JR, Duchaine TF (2014). DICER1: mutations, microRNAs and mechanisms. Nat Rev Cancer. 14:662–72. PMID:25176334

875. Fountas A, Giotaki Z, Ligkros N, et al. (2015). Cushing's Syndrome Due to CRH and ACTH Co-secreting Pancreatic Tumor—Presentation of a New Case Focusing on Diagnostic Pitfalls. Endocr Pathol. 26:239–42. PMID:26202047

876. Fraker DL, Travis WD, Merendino JJ Jr, et al. (1991). Locally recurrent parathyroid neoplasms as a cause for recurrent and persistent primary hyperparathyroidism. Ann Surg. 213:58–65. PMID:1985539

877. François P, Travers N, Lescanne E, et al. (2010). The interperiosteo-dural concept applied to the perisellar compartment: a microanatomical and electron microscopic study. J Neurosurg. 113:1045–52. PMID:20151780

878. Frank-Raue K, Döhring J, Scheumann G, et al. (2010). New mutations in the RET protooncogene-L881V – associated with medullary thyroid carcinoma and -R770Q – in a patient with mixed medullar/follicular thyroid tumour. Exp Clin Endocrinol Diabetes. 118:550–3. PMID:20013610

879. Frank-Raue K, Haag C, Schulze E, et al. (2011). CDC73-related hereditary hyperparathyroidism: five new mutations and the clinical spectrum. Eur J Endocrinol. 165:477–83. PMID:21652691

880. Frank-Raue K, Machens A, Leidig-Bruckner G, et al. (2013). Prevalence and clinical spectrum of nonsecretory medullary thyroid carcinoma in a series of 839 patients with sporadic medullary thyroid carcinoma. Thyroid. 23:294–300. PMID:22946486

881. Frank-Raue K, Raue F (2015). Hereditary Medullary Thyroid Cancer Genotype-Phenotype Correlation. Recent Results Cancer Res. 204:139–56. PMID:26494387

882. Frank-Raue K, Rybicki LA, Erlic Z, et al. (2011). Risk profiles and penetrance estimations in multiple endocrine neoplasia type 2A caused by germline RET mutations located in exon 10. Hum Mutat. 32:51–8. PMID:20979234

883. Franke WW, Grund C, Achtstätter T (1986). Co-expression of cytokeratins and neurofilament proteins in a permanent cell line: cultured rat PC12 cells combine neuronal and epithelial features. J Cell Biol. 103:1933–43. PMID:2430979

884. Franko J, Feng W, Yip L, et al. (2010). Non-functional neuroendocrine carcinoma of the pancreas: incidence, tumor biology, and outcomes in 2,158 patients. J Gastrointest Surg. 14:541–8. PMID:19997980

885. Franquemont DW, Mills SE, Lack EE (1994). Immunohistochemical detection of neuroblastomatous foci in composite adrenal pheochromocytoma-neuroblastoma. Am J Clin Pathol. 102:163–70. PMID:8042583

886. Franssila KO (1973). Is the differentiation between papillary and follicular thyroid carcinoma valid? Cancer. 32:853–64. PMID:4751916

887. Franssila KO, Harach HR, Wasenius VM (1984). Mucoepidermoid carcinoma of the thyroid. Histopathology. 8:847–60. PMID:6083973

888. Fraser WD (2009). Hyperparathyroidism. Lancet. 374:145–58. PMID:19595349

889. Frauenhoffer CM, Patchefsky AS, Cobanoglu A (1979). Thyroid carcinoma: a clinical and pathologic study of 125 cases. Cancer. 43:2414–21. PMID:455228

890. Frazier WD, Patel NP, Sullivan CA (2008). Pathology quiz case 1. Sclerosing mucoepidermoid carcinoma with eosinophilia (SMECE). Arch Otolaryngol Head Neck Surg. 134:333,335. PMID:18347265

891. Freda PU, Post KD (1999). Differential diagnosis of sellar masses. Endocrinol Metab Clin North Am. 28:81–117, vi. PMID:10207686

892. French AE, Grant R, Weitzman S, et al. (2003). Folic acid food fortification is associated with a decline in neuroblastoma. Clin Pharmacol Ther. 74:288–94. PMID:12966372

893. French CA, Alexander EK, Cibas ES, et al. (2003). Genetic and biological subgroups of low-stage follicular thyroid cancer. Am J Pathol. 162:1053–60. PMID:12651598

894. Frew IJ, Moch H (2015). A clearer view of the molecular complexity of clear cell renal cell carcinoma. Annu Rev Pathol. 10:263–89. PMID:25387056

895. Frew IJ, Smole Z, Thoma CR, et al. (2013). Genetic deletion of the long isoform of the von Hippel-Lindau tumour suppressor gene product alters microtubule dynamics. Eur J Cancer. 49:2433–40. PMID:23541568

896. Friedman E, Sakaguchi K, Bale AE, et al. (1989). Clonality of parathyroid tumors in familial multiple endocrine neoplasia type 1. N Engl J Med. 321:213–8. PMID:2568586

897. Friedman JM, Birch PH (1997). Type 1 neurofibromatosis: a descriptive analysis of the disorder in 1,728 patients. Am J Med Genet. 70:138–43. PMID:9128932

898. Frisk T, Foukakis T, Dwight T, et al. (2002). Silencing of the PTEN tumor-suppressor gene in anaplastic thyroid cancer. Genes Chromosomes Cancer. 35:74–80. PMID:12203792

898A. Fritz A, Percy C, Jack A, et al. (2000). International Classification of Diseases for Oncology. 3rd ed. Geneva: WHO Press.

899. Fujimori T, Okauchi M, Shindo A, et al. (2014). Intrapituitary adenoma metastasis from lung cancer with progressive cranial nerve palsies: a case report and literature review. No Shinkei Geka. [Japanese] 42:943–9. PMID:25266586

900. Fujimoto Y, Obara T, Ito Y, et al. (1990). Diffuse sclerosing variant of papillary carcinoma of the thyroid. Clinical importance, surgical treatment, and follow-up study. Cancer. 66:2306–12. PMID:2245385

901. Fujisawa H, Tohma Y, Muramatsu N, et al. (2012). Spindle cell oncocytoma of the adenohypophysis with marked hypervascularity. Case report. Neurol Med Chir (Tokyo). 52:594–8. PMID:22976144

902. Fujiwara S, Sposto R, Ezaki H, et al. (1992). Hyperparathyroidism among atomic bomb survivors in Hiroshima. Radiat Res. 130:372–8. PMID:1594765

903. Fujiwara T, Kawamura M, Sasou S, et al. (2000). Results of surgery for a compound adrenal tumor consisting of pheochromocytoma and ganglioneuroblastoma in an adult: 5-year follow-up. Intern Med. 39:58–62. PMID:10674851

904. Fujiya A, Kato M, Shibata T, et al. (2015). VIPoma with multiple endocrine neoplasia type 1 identified as an atypical gene mutation. BMJ Case Rep. 2015:2015. PMID:26564120

905. Fukushima M, Ito Y, Hirokawa M, et al. (2009). Clinicopathologic characteristics and prognosis of diffuse sclerosing variant of papillary thyroid carcinoma in Japan: an 18-year experience at a single institution. World J Surg. 33:958–62. PMID:19198928

906. Fulciniti F, Vuttariello E, Calise C, et al. (2015). Combined papillary and mucoepidermoid carcinoma of the thyroid gland: a possible collision tumor diagnosed on fine-needle cytology. Report of a case with immunocytochemical and molecular correlations. Endocr Pathol. 26:140–4. PMID:25771987

907. Funayama T, Sakane M, Yoshizawa T, et al. (2013). Tanycytic ependymoma of the filum terminale associated with multiple endocrine neoplasia type 1: first reported case. Spine J. 13:e49–54. PMID:23562332

908. Furlan D, Sahnane N, Bernasconi B, et al. (2014). APC alterations are frequently involved in the pathogenesis of acinar cell carcinoma of the pancreas, mainly through gene loss and promoter hypermethylation. Virchows Arch. 464:553–64. PMID:24590585

909. Furrer J, Hättenschwiler A, Komminoth P, et al. (2001). Carcinoid syndrome, acromegaly, and hypoglycemia due to an insulin-secreting neuroendocrine tumor of the liver. J Clin Endocrinol Metab. 86:2227–30. PMID:11344231

910. Furtado LV, Leventaki V, Layfield LJ, et al. (2011). Yolk sac tumor of the thyroid gland: a case report. Pediatr Dev Pathol. 14:475–9. PMID:21793665

911. Fusco A, Chiappetta G, Hui P, et al. (2002). Assessment of RET/PTC oncogene activation and clonality in thyroid nodules with incomplete morphological evidence of papillary carcinoma: a search for the early precursors of papillary cancer. Am J Pathol. 160:2157–67. PMID:12057919

912. Fuziwara CS, Kimura ET (2014). MicroRNA Deregulation in Anaplastic Thyroid Cancer Biology. Int J Endocrinol. 2014:743450. PMID:25202329

913. Gaal J, Burnichon N, Korpershoek E, et al. (2010). Isocitrate dehydrogenase mutations are rare in pheochromocytomas and paragangliomas. J Clin Endocrinol Metab. 95:1274–8. PMID:19915015

914. Gabrilove JL, Anderson PJ, Halmi NS (1986). Pituitary pro-opiomelanocortin-cell carcinoma occurring in conjunction with a glioblastoma in a patient with Cushing's disease and subsequent Nelson's syndrome. Clin Endocrinol (Oxf). 25:117–26. PMID:3024876

915. Gaffey MJ, Lack EE, Christ ML, et al. (1991). Anaplastic thyroid carcinoma with osteoclast-like giant cells. A clinicopathologic, immunohistochemical, and ultrastructural study. Am J Surg Pathol. 15:160–8. PMID:1989464

916. Gaffey TA, Scheithauer BW, Lloyd RV, et al. (2002). Corticotroph carcinoma of the pituitary: a clinicopathological study. Report of four cases. J Neurosurg. 96:352–60. PMID:11838811

917. Gaffney RL, Carney JA, Sebo TJ, et al. (2003). Galectin-3 expression in hyalinizing trabecular tumors of the thyroid gland. Am J Surg Pathol. 27:494–8. PMID:12657934

918. Galati LT, Barnes EL, Myers EN (1999). Dendritic cell sarcoma of the thyroid. Head Neck. 21:273–5. PMID:10208672

919. Galgano MT, Mills SE, Stelow EB (2006). Hyalinizing trabecular adenoma of the thyroid

revisited: a histologic and immunohistochemical study of thyroid lesions with prominent trabecular architecture and sclerosis. Am J Surg Pathol. 30:1269–73. PMID:17001158

920. Galland F, Lacroix L, Saulnier P, et al. (2010). Differential gene expression profiles of invasive and non-invasive non-functioning pituitary adenomas based on microarray analysis. Endocr Relat Cancer. 17:361–71. PMID:20228124

921. Gan HW, Bulwer C, Jeelani O, et al. (2015). Treatment-resistant pediatric giant prolactinoma and multiple endocrine neoplasia type 1. Int J Pediatr Endocrinol. 2015:15. PMID:26180530

922. Gandolfi G, Ragazzi M, Frasoldati A, et al. (2015). TERT promoter mutations are associated with distant metastases in papillary thyroid carcinoma. Eur J Endocrinol. 172:403–13. PMID:25583906

923. Ganly I, Ibrahimpasic T, Rivera M, et al. (2014). Prognostic implications of papillary thyroid carcinoma with tall-cell features. Thyroid. 24:662–70. PMID:24262069

924. Ganly I, Ricarte Filho J, Eng S, et al. (2013). Genomic dissection of Hürthle cell carcinoma reveals a unique class of thyroid malignancy. J Clin Endocrinol Metab. 98:E962–72. PMID:23543667

925. Ganly I, Wang L, Tuttle RM, et al. (2015). Invasion rather than nuclear features correlates with outcome in encapsulated follicular tumors: further evidence for the reclassification of the encapsulated papillary thyroid carcinoma follicular variant. Hum Pathol. 46:657–64. PMID:25721865

926. Gao B, Meng F, Bian W, et al. (2006). Development and validation of pheochromocytoma of the adrenal gland scaled score for predicting malignant pheochromocytomas. Urology. 68:282–6. PMID:16904437

927. Gara SK, Jia L, Merino MJ, et al. (2015). Germline HABP2 Mutation Causing Familial Nonmedullary Thyroid Cancer. N Engl J Med. 373:448–55. PMID:26222560

928. Gara SK, Kebebew E (2015). HABP2 Mutation and Nonmedullary Thyroid Cancer. N Engl J Med. 373:2086–7. PMID:26581001

929. Garbrecht N, Anlauf M, Schmitt A, et al. (2008). Somatostatin-producing neuroendocrine tumors of the duodenum and pancreas: incidence, types, biological behavior, association with inherited syndromes, and functional activity. Endocr Relat Cancer. 15:229–41. PMID:18310290

930. Garby L, Caron P, Claustrat F, et al. (2012). Clinical characteristics and outcome of acromegaly induced by ectopic secretion of growth hormone-releasing hormone (GHRH): a French nationwide series of 21 cases. J Clin Endocrinol Metab. 97:2093–104. PMID:22442262

931. Garcia-Rostan G, Camp RL, Herrero A, et al. (2001). Beta-catenin dysregulation in thyroid neoplasms: down-regulation, aberrant nuclear expression, and CTNNB1 exon 3 mutations are markers for aggressive tumor phenotypes and poor prognosis. Am J Pathol. 158:987–96. PMID:11238046

932. Garcia-Rostan G, Tallini G, Herrero A, et al. (1999). Frequent mutation and nuclear localization of beta-catenin in anaplastic thyroid carcinoma. Cancer Res. 59:1811–5. PMID:10213482

933. Garcia-Rostan G, Zhao H, Camp RL, et al. (2003). ras mutations are associated with aggressive tumor phenotypes and poor prognosis in thyroid cancer. J Clin Oncol. 21:3226–35. PMID:12947056

934. Garg K, Lee P, Ro JY, et al. (2005). Adenomatoid tumor of the adrenal gland: a clinicopathologic study of 3 cases. Ann Diagn Pathol. 9:11–5. PMID:15692945

935. Garnier S, Réguerre Y, Orbach D, et al. (2014). Pediatric pheochromocytoma and

paraganglioma: an update. Bull Cancer. 101:966–75. [French] PMID:25373696

936. Garrão AF, Sobrinho LG, Pedro-Oliveira, et al. (1997). ACTH-producing carcinoma of the pituitary with haematogenic metastases. Eur J Endocrinol. 137:176–80. PMID:9272107

937. Garty BZ, Laor A, Danon YL (1994). Neurofibromatosis type 1 in Israel: survey of young adults. J Med Genet. 31:853–7. PMID:7853369

938. Gasparre G, Bonora E, Tallini G, et al. (2010). Molecular features of thyroid oncocytic tumors. Mol Cell Endocrinol. 321:67–76. PMID:20184940

939. Gasparre G, Kurelac I, Capristo M, et al. (2011). A mutation threshold distinguishes the antitumorigenic effects of the mitochondrial gene MTND1, an oncojanus function. Cancer Res. 71:6220–9. PMID:21852384

940. Gasparre G, Porcelli AM, Bonora E, et al. (2007). Disruptive mitochondrial DNA mutations in complex I subunits are markers of oncocytic phenotype in thyroid tumors. Proc Natl Acad Sci U S A. 104:9001–6. PMID:17517629

941. Gatta-Cherifi B, Chabre O, Murat A, et al. (2012). Adrenal involvement in MEN1. Analysis of 715 cases from the Groupe d'etude des Tumeurs Endocrines database. Eur J Endocrinol. 166:269–79. PMID:22084155

942. Gaujoux S, Pinson S, Gimenez-Roqueplo AP, et al. (2010). Inactivation of the APC gene is constant in adrenocortical tumors from patients with familial adenomatous polyposis but not frequent in sporadic adrenocortical cancers. Clin Cancer Res. 16:5133–41. PMID:20978149

943. Gaujoux S, Salenave S, Ronot M, et al. (2014). Hepatobiliary and Pancreatic neoplasms in patients with McCune-Albright syndrome. J Clin Endocrinol Metab. 99:E97–101. PMID:24170100

944. Gaujoux S, Tissier F, Groussin L, et al. (2008). Wnt/beta-catenin and 3',5'-cyclic adenosine 5'-monophosphate/protein kinase A signaling pathways alterations and somatic beta-catenin gene mutations in the progression of adrenocortical tumors. J Clin Endocrinol Metab. 93:4135–40. PMID:18647815

945. Gaujoux S, Tissier F, Ragazzon B, et al. (2011). Pancreatic ductal and acinar cell neoplasms in Carney complex: a possible new association. J Clin Endocrinol Metab. 96:E1888–95. PMID:21900385

946. Geddes JF, Jansen GH, Robinson SF, et al. (2000). 'Gangliocytomas' of the pituitary: a heterogeneous group of lesions with differing histogenesis. Am J Surg Pathol. 24:607–13. PMID:10757410

947. Geisinger KR, Hartle EO, Warren T (2014). Eosinophilic replacement infiltrates in cystic Hashimoto's thyroiditis: a potential diagnostic pitfall. Endocr Pathol. 25:332–8. PMID:24639138

948. Geisinger KR, Steffee CH, McGee RS, et al. (1998). The cytomorphologic features of sclerosing mucoepidermoid carcinoma of the thyroid gland with eosinophilia. Am J Clin Pathol. 109:294–301. PMID:9495201

949. Geissmann F, Lepelletier Y, Fraitag S, et al. (2001). Differentiation of Langerhans cells in Langerhans cell histiocytosis. Blood. 97:1241–8. PMID:11222366

950. Gejman R, Batista DL, Zhong Y, et al. (2008). Selective loss of MEG3 expression and intergenic differentially methylated region hypermethylation in the MEG3/DLK1 locus in human clinically nonfunctioning pituitary adenomas. J Clin Endocrinol Metab. 93:4119–25. PMID:18628527

951. Geli J, Kiss N, Karimi M, et al. (2008). Global and regional CpG methylation in pheochromocytomas and abdominal paragangliomas: association to malignant behavior. Clin Cancer Res. 14:2551–9. PMID:18451216

952. Gennari M, Stratakis CA, Hovarth A, et al.

(2008). A novel PRKAR1A mutation associated with hepatocellular carcinoma in a young patient and a variable Carney complex phenotype in affected subjects in older generations. Clin Endocrinol (Oxf). 69:751–5. PMID:18445140

953. Gentilin E, Di Pasquale C, Gagliano T, et al. (2016). Protein Kinase C Delta restrains growth in ACTH-secreting pituitary adenoma cells. Mol Cell Endocrinol. 419:252–8. PMID:26522132

954. Gentilin E, Tagliati F, Filieri C, et al. (2013). miR-26a plays an important role in cell cycle regulation in ACTH-secreting pituitary adenomas by modulating protein kinase Cδ. Endocrinology. 154:1690–700. PMID:23525216

955. George RE, London WB, Cohn SL, et al. (2005). Hyperdiploidy plus nonamplified MYCN confers a favorable prognosis in children 12 to 18 months old with disseminated neuroblastoma: a Pediatric Oncology Group study. J Clin Oncol. 23:6466–73. PMID:16116152

956. George RE, Sanda T, Hanna M, et al. (2008). Activating mutations in ALK provide a therapeutic target in neuroblastoma. Nature. 455:975–8. PMID:18923525

957. George SR, Kovacs K, Asa SL, et al. (1987). Effect of SMS 201-995, a long-acting somatostatin analogue, on the secretion and morphology of a pituitary growth hormone cell adenoma. Clin Endocrinol (Oxf). 26:395–405. PMID:2888549

958. Ghaferi AA, Chojnacki KA, Long WD, et al. (2008). Pancreatic VIPomas: subject review and one institutional experience. J Gastrointest Surg. 12:382–93. PMID:17510774

959. Ghazi AA, Amirbaigloo A, Dezfooli AA, et al. (2013). Ectopic acromegaly due to growth hormone releasing hormone. Endocrine. 43:293–302. PMID:22983831

960. Ghazi AA, Dezfooli AA, Mohamadi F, et al. (2011). Cushing syndrome secondary to a thymic carcinoid tumor due to multiple endocrine neoplasia type 1. Endocr Pract. 17:e92–6. PMID:21550948

961. Ghazi AA, Rotondo F, Kovacs K, et al. (2015). Treatment of invasive silent somatotroph pituitary adenoma with temozolomide. Report of a case and review of the literature. Endocr Pathol. 26:135–9. PMID:25716461

962. Gherardi G (1987). Signet ring cell 'mucinous' thyroid adenoma: a follicle cell tumour with abnormal accumulation of thyroglobulin and a peculiar histochemical profile. Histopathology. 11:317–26. PMID:3428884

963. Ghorab Z, Jorda M, Ganjei P, et al. (2003). Melan A (A103) is expressed in adrenocortical neoplasms but not in renal cell and hepatocellular carcinomas. Appl Immunohistochem Mol Morphol. 11:330–3. PMID:14663359

964. Ghose A, Guha G, Kundu R, et al. (2014). CNS hemangiopericytoma: a systematic review of 523 patients. Am J Clin Oncol. EPUB 2014. PMID:25350465

965. Ghossein R, Ganly I, Biagini A, et al. (2014). Prognostic factors in papillary microcarcinoma with emphasis on histologic subtyping: a clinicopathologic study of 148 cases. Thyroid. 24:245–53. PMID:23745671

966. Ghossein R, Livolsi VA (2008). Papillary thyroid carcinoma tall cell variant. Thyroid. 18:1179–81. PMID:18925842

967. Ghossein RA, Hiltzik DH, Carlson DL, et al. (2006). Prognostic factors of recurrence in encapsulated Hürthle cell carcinoma of the thyroid gland: a clinicopathologic study of 50 cases. Cancer. 106:1669–76. PMID:16534796

968. Ghossein RA, Leboeuf R, Patel KN, et al. (2007). Tall cell variant of papillary thyroid carcinoma without extrathyroid extension: biologic behavior and clinical implications. Thyroid. 17:655–61. PMID:17696836

969. Giacomazzi J, Graudenz MS, Osorio CA, et al. (2014). Prevalence of the TP53 p.R337H

mutation in breast cancer patients in Brazil. PLoS One. 9:e99893. PMID:24936644

970. Gibril F, Jensen RT (2004). Zollinger-Ellison syndrome revisited: diagnosis, biologic markers, associated inherited disorders, and acid hypersecretion. Curr Gastroenterol Rep. 6:454–63. PMID:15527675

971. Gibril F, Schumann M, Pace A, et al. (2004). Multiple endocrine neoplasia type 1 and Zollinger-Ellison syndrome: a prospective study of 107 cases and comparison with 1009 cases from the literature. Medicine (Baltimore). 83:43–83. PMID:14747767

972. Gikas PW, Labow SS, DiGiulio W, et al. (1967). Occult metastasis from occult papillary carcinoma of the thyroid. Cancer. 20:2100–4. PMID:6073888

973. Gill AJ (2012). Succinate dehydrogenase (SDH) and mitochondrial driven neoplasia. Pathology. 44:285–92. PMID:22544211

974. Gill AJ (2014). Understanding the genetic basis of parathyroid carcinoma. Endocr Pathol. 25:30–4. PMID:24402736

975. Gill AJ, Benn DE, Chou A, et al. (2010). Immunohistochemistry for SDHB triages genetic testing of SDHB, SDHC, and SDHD in paraganglioma-pheochromocytoma syndromes. Hum Pathol. 41:805–14. PMID:20236688

976. Gill AJ, Chou A, Vilain R, et al. (2010). Immunohistochemistry for SDHB divides gastrointestinal stromal tumors (GISTs) into 2 distinct types. Am J Surg Pathol. 34:636–44. PMID:20305538

977. Gill AJ, Clarkson A, Gimm O, et al. (2006). Loss of nuclear expression of parafibromin distinguishes parathyroid carcinomas and hyperparathyroidism-jaw tumor (HPT-JT) syndrome-related adenomas from sporadic parathyroid adenomas and hyperplasias. Am J Surg Pathol. 30:1140–9. PMID:16931959

978. Gill AJ, Pachter NS, Chou A, et al. (2011). Renal tumors associated with germline SDHB mutation show distinctive morphology. Am J Surg Pathol. 35:1578–85. PMID:21934479

979. Gill AJ, Toon CW, Clarkson A, et al. (2014). Succinate dehydrogenase deficiency is rare in pituitary adenomas. Am J Surg Pathol. 38:560–6. PMID:24625421

980. Gimenez-Roqueplo AP, Dahia PL, Robledo M (2012). An update on the genetics of paraganglioma, pheochromocytoma, and associated hereditary syndromes. Horm Metab Res. 44:328–33. PMID:22328163

981. Gimm O, Marsh DJ, Andrew SD, et al. (1997). Germline dinucleotide mutation in codon 883 of the RET proto-oncogene in multiple endocrine neoplasia type 2B without codon 918 mutation. J Clin Endocrinol Metab. 82:3902–4. PMID:9360560

982. Ginn-Pease ME, Eng C (2003). Increased nuclear phosphatase and tensin homologue deleted on chromosome 10 is associated with G0-G1 in MCF-7 cells. Cancer Res. 63:282–6. PMID:12543774

983. Ginter PS, Scognamiglio T (2015). Papillary thyroid carcinoma with nodular fasciitis-like stroma: a usual entity with distinctive morphology. Int J Surg Pathol. 23:305–7. PMID:25663334

984. Giordano D, Frasoldati A, Kasperbauer JL, et al. (2015). Lateral neck recurrence from papillary thyroid carcinoma: Predictive factors and prognostic significance. Laryngoscope. 125:2226–31. PMID:25510637

985. Giordano TJ (2011). The argument for mitotic rate-based grading for the prognostication of adrenocortical carcinoma. Am J Surg Pathol. 35:471–3. PMID:21383612

986. Giordano TJ, Kuick R, Else T, et al. (2009). Molecular classification and prognostication of adrenocortical tumors by transcriptome profiling. Clin Cancer Res. 15:668–76. PMID:19147773

987. Giordano TJ, Kuick R, Thomas DG, et al. (2005). Molecular classification of papillary

thyroid carcinoma: distinct BRAF, RAS, and RET/PTC mutation-specific gene expression profiles discovered by DNA microarray analysis. Oncogene. 24:6646–56. PMID:16007166
988. Giordano TJ, Thomas DG, Kuick R, et al. (2003). Distinct transcriptional profiles of adrenocortical tumors uncovered by DNA microarray analysis. Am J Pathol. 162:521–31. PMID:12547710
989. Giubellino A, Lara K, Martucci V, et al. (2015). Urinary Bladder Paragangliomas: How Immunohistochemistry Can Assist to Identify Patients With SDHB Germline and Somatic Mutations. Am J Surg Pathol. 39:1488–92. PMID:26457353
990. Giusiano-Courcambeck S, Denizot A, Secq V, et al. (2008). Pure spindle cell follicular carcinoma of the thyroid. Thyroid. 18:1023–5. PMID:18788926
991. Giusti F, Marini F, Brandi ML (1993). Multiple endocrine neoplasia type 1. In: Pagon RA, Adam MP, Ardinger HH, et al., editors. GeneReviews®. Seattle: University of Washington, Seattle. PMID:20301710
992. Giustina A, Gola M, Doga M, et al. (2001). Clinical review 136: Primary lymphoma of the pituitary: an emerging clinical entity. J Clin Endocrinol Metab. 86:4567–75. PMID:11600505
993. Gläsker S, Lonser RR, Tran MG, et al. (2005). Effects of VHL deficiency on endolymphatic duct and sac. Cancer Res. 65:10847–53. PMID:16322231
994. Gläsker S, Tran MG, Shively SB, et al. (2006). Epididymal cystadenomas and epithelial tumourlets: effects of VHL deficiency on the human epididymis. J Pathol. 210:32–41. PMID:16841375
995. Glenn ST, Jones CA, Sexton S, et al. (2014). Conditional deletion of p53 and Rb in the renin-expressing compartment of the pancreas leads to a highly penetrant metastatic pancreatic neuroendocrine carcinoma. Oncogene. 33:5706–15. PMID:24292676
996. Glickman MH, Hart MJ, White TT (1980). Insulinoma in Seattle: 39 cases in 30 years. Am J Surg. 140:119–25. PMID:6249135
997. Gnemmi V, Renaud F, Do Cao C, et al. (2014). Poorly differentiated thyroid carcinomas: application of the Turin proposal provides prognostic results similar to those from the assessment of high-grade features. Histopathology. 64:263–73. PMID:24164362
998. Gnepp DR, Ogorzalek JM, Heffess CS (1989). Fat-containing lesions of the thyroid gland. Am J Surg Pathol. 13:605–12. PMID:2660611
999. Goasguen N, Chirica M, Roger N, et al. (2010). Primary hyperparathyroidism from parathyroid microadenoma: specific features and implications for a surgical strategy in the era of minimally invasive parathyroidectomy. J Am Coll Surg. 210:456–62. PMID:20347738
1000. Godbert Y, Henriques de Figueiredo B, Bonichon F, et al. (2015). Remarkable Response to Crizotinib in Woman With Anaplastic Lymphoma Kinase-Rearranged Anaplastic Thyroid Carcinoma. J Clin Oncol. 33:e84–7. PMID:24687827
1001. Goebel HH, Shimokawa K, Schaake T, et al. (1979). Schwannoma of the sellar region. Acta Neurochir (Wien). 48:191–7. PMID:484274
1002. Goffin A, Hoefsloot LH, Bosgoed E, et al. (2001). PTEN mutation in a family with Cowden syndrome and autism. Am J Med Genet. 105:521–4. PMID:11496368
1003. Goffredo P, Roman SA, Sosa JA (2013). Hürthle cell carcinoma: a population-level analysis of 3311 patients. Cancer. 119:504–11. PMID:22893587
1004. Goffredo P, Sosa JA, Roman SA (2013). Malignant pheochromocytoma and paraganglioma: a population level analysis of long-term survival over two decades. J Surg Oncol. 107:659–64. PMID:23233320
1005. Goh G, Scholl UI, Healy JM, et al. (2014). Recurrent activating mutation in PRKACA in cortisol-producing adrenal tumors. Nat Genet. 46:613–7. PMID:24747643
1006. Goh SG, Chuah KL, Goh HK, et al. (2003). Two cases of epithelioid angiosarcoma involving the thyroid and a brief review of non-Alpine epithelioid angiosarcoma of the thyroid. Arch Pathol Lab Med. 127:E70–3. PMID:12562256
1007. Gola M, Doga M, Bonadonna S, et al. (2006). Neuroendocrine tumors secreting growth hormone-releasing hormone: Pathophysiological and clinical aspects. Pituitary. 9:221–9. PMID:17036195
1008. Goldman RL (1964). Primary squamous cell carcinoma of the thyroid gland: report of a case and review of the literature. Am Surg. 30:247–52. PMID:14149689
1009. Goldstein J, Tovi F, Sidi J (1982). Primary Schwannoma of the thyroid gland. Int Surg. 67(4 Suppl):433–4. PMID:7183602
1010. Golouh R, Us-Krasovec M, Auersperg M, et al. (1985). Amphicrine–composite calcitonin and mucin-producing–carcinoma of the thyroid. Ultrastruct Pathol. 8:197–206. PMID:4060258
1011. Gomez-Hernandez K, Ezzat S, Asa SL, et al. (2015). Clinical implications of accurate subtyping of pituitary adenomas: perspectives from the treating physician. Turk Patoloji Derg. 31 Suppl 1:4–17. PMID:26177314
1012. Goodwin TL, Sainani K, Fisher PG (2009). Incidence patterns of central nervous system germ cell tumors: a SEER Study. J Pediatr Hematol Oncol. 31:541–4. PMID:19636276
1013. Gooskens SL, Furtwängler R, Spreafico F, et al. (2014). Treatment and outcome of patients with relapsed clear cell sarcoma of the kidney: a combined SIOP and AIEOP study. Br J Cancer. 111:227–33. PMID:24937667
1014. Gopal PP, Montone KT, Baloch Z, et al. (2011). The variable presentations of anaplastic spindle cell squamous carcinoma associated with tall cell variant of papillary thyroid carcinoma. Thyroid. 21:493–9. PMID:21309723
1015. Gorczyca W, Hardy J (1988). Microadenomas of the human pituitary and their vascularization. Neurosurgery. 22(1 Pt 1):1–6. PMID:2449627
1016. Gordon Cm, Majzoub JA, Marsh DJ, et al. (1998). Four cases of mucosal neuroma syndrome: multiple endocrine neoplasm 2B or not 2B? J Clin Endocrinol Metab. 83:17–20. PMID:9435410
1017. Gordon MV, Varma D, McLean CA, et al. (2007). Metastatic prolactinoma presenting as a cervical spinal cord tumour in multiple endocrine neoplasia type one (MEN-1). Clin Endocrinol (Oxf). 66:150–2. PMID:17201817
1018. Gorlin RJ, Sedano HO, Vickers RA, et al. (1968). Multiple mucosal neuromas, pheochromocytoma and medullary carcinoma of the thyroid–a syndrome. Cancer. 22:293–9, passim. PMID:5660196
1019. Görtz B, Roth J, Krähenmann A, et al. (1999). Mutations and allelic deletions of the MEN1 gene are associated with a subset of sporadic endocrine pancreatic and neuroendocrine tumors and not restricted to foregut neoplasms. Am J Pathol. 154:429–36. PMID:10027401
1020. Goto S, Umehara S, Gerbing RB, et al. (2001). Histopathology (International Neuroblastoma Pathology Classification) and MYCN status in patients with peripheral neuroblastic tumors: a report from the Children's Cancer Group. Cancer. 92:2699–708. PMID:11745206
1021. Gottschalk D, Fehn M, Patt S, et al. (2001). Matrix gene expression analysis and cellular phenotyping in chordoma reveals focal differentiation pattern of neoplastic cells mimicking nucleus pulposus development. Am J Pathol. 158:1571–8. PMID:11337353
1022. Goudet P, Bonithon-Kopp C, Murat A, et al. (2011). Gender-related differences in MEN1 lesion occurrence and diagnosis: a cohort study of 734 cases from the Groupe d'etude des Tumeurs Endocrines. Eur J Endocrinol. 165:97–105. PMID:21551167
1023. Goudet P, Dalac A, Le Bras M, et al. (2015). MEN1 disease occurring before 21 years old: a 160-patient cohort study from the Groupe d'étude des Tumeurs Endocrines. J Clin Endocrinol Metab. 100:1568–77. PMID:25594862
1024. Goudet P, Murat A, Binquet C, et al. (2010). Risk factors and causes of death in MEN1 disease. A GTE (Groupe d'Etude des Tumeurs Endocrines) cohort study among 758 patients. World J Surg. 34:249–55. PMID:19949948
1025. Gouveia P, Silva C, Magalhães F, et al. (2013). Non-Alpine thyroid angiosarcoma. Int J Surg Case Rep. 4:524–7. PMID:23570682
1026. Gowrishankar S, Pai SA, Carney JA (2008). Hyalinizing trabecular carcinoma of the thyroid gland. Histopathology. 52:529–31. PMID:18315612
1027. Gracanin A, Dreijerink KM, van der Luijt RB, et al. (2009). Tissue selectivity in multiple endocrine neoplasia type 1-associated tumorigenesis. Cancer Res. 69:6371–4. PMID:19654304
1028. Graff-Baker A, Roman SA, Thomas DC, et al. (2009). Prognosis of primary thyroid lymphoma: demographic, clinical, and pathologic predictors of survival in 1,408 cases. Surgery. 146:1105–15. PMID:19958938
1029. Graham RP, Shrestha B, Caron BL, et al. (2013). Islet-1 is a sensitive but not entirely specific marker for pancreatic neuroendocrine neoplasms and their metastases. Am J Surg Pathol. 37:399–405. PMID:23348208
1030. Grajower MM (2006). Malignant paraganglioma of thyroid. Endocr Pract. 12:696–7. PMID:17240539
1031. Grant CS (2005). Insulinoma. Best Pract Res Clin Gastroenterol. 19:783–98. PMID:16253900
1032. Granter SR, Cibas ES (1997). Cytologic findings in thyroid nodules after 131I treatment of hyperthyroidism. Am J Clin Pathol. 107:20–5. PMID:8980362
1033. Gray A, Doniach I (1969). Morphology of the nuclei of papillary carcinoma of the thyroid. Br J Cancer. 23:49–51. PMID:5768442
1034. Gray MH, Rosenberg AE, Dickersin GR, et al. (1990). Cytokeratin expression in epithelioid vascular neoplasms. Hum Pathol. 21:212–7. PMID:1689691
1035. Grebe SK, Hay ID (1996). Thyroid cancer nodal metastases: biologic significance and therapeutic considerations. Surg Oncol Clin N Am. 5:43–63. PMID:8789493
1036. Green BT, Rockey DC (2001). Duodenal somatostatinoma presenting with complete somatostatinoma syndrome. J Clin Gastroenterol. 33:415–7. PMID:11606861
1037. Greene AB, Butler RS, McIntyre S, et al. (2009). National trends in parathyroid surgery from 1998 to 2008: a decade of change. J Am Coll Surg. 209:332–43. PMID:19717037
1038. Greenman Y, Tordjman K, Osher E, et al. (2005). Postoperative treatment of clinically nonfunctioning pituitary adenomas with dopamine agonists decreases tumour remnant growth. Clin Endocrinol (Oxf). 63:39–44. PMID:15963059
1039. Grigg AP, Connors JM (2003). Primary adrenal lymphoma. Clin Lymphoma. 4:154–60. PMID:14715097
1040. Griniatsos JE, Dimitriou N, Zilos A, et al. (2011). Bilateral adrenocortical carcinoma in a patient with multiple endocrine neoplasia type 1 (MEN1) and a novel mutation in the MEN1 gene. World J Surg Oncol. 9:6. PMID:21266030
1041. Grogan RH, Kaplan SP, Cao H, et al. (2013). A study of recurrence and death from papillary thyroid cancer with 27 years of median follow-up. Surgery. 154:1436–46, discussion 1446–7. PMID:24075674
1042. Grubbs EG, Ng PK, Bui J, et al. (2015). RET fusion as a novel driver of medullary thyroid carcinoma. J Clin Endocrinol Metab. 100:788–93. PMID:25546157
1043. Gruppetta M, Mercieca C, Vassallo J (2013). Prevalence and incidence of pituitary adenomas: a population based study in Malta. Pituitary. 16:545–53. PMID:23239049
1044. Gryn A, Peyronnet B, Manunta A, et al. (2015). Patient selection for laparoscopic excision of adrenal metastases: A multicenter cohort study. Int J Surg. 24 Pt A:75–80. PMID:26542988
1045. Gucer H, Szentgyorgyi E, Ezzat S, et al. (2013). Inhibin-expressing clear cell neuroendocrine tumor of the ampulla: an unusual presentation of von Hippel-Lindau disease. Virchows Arch. 463:593–7. PMID:23913169
1046. Guigon CJ, Zhao L, Willingham MC, et al. (2009). PTEN deficiency accelerates tumour progression in a mouse model of thyroid cancer. Oncogene. 28:509–17. PMID:18997818
1047. Guiter GE, DeLellis RA (1996). Multinucleate giant cells in papillary thyroid carcinoma. A morphologic and immunohistochemical study. Am J Clin Pathol. 106:765–8. PMID:8980352
1048. Guiter GE, DeLellis RA (2002). Risk of recurrence or metastasis in atypical parathyroid adenomas. Mod Pathol. 15:115A.
1049. Gule MK, Chen Y, Sano D, et al. (2011). Targeted therapy of VEGFR2 and EGFR significantly inhibits growth of anaplastic thyroid cancer in an orthotopic murine model. Clin Cancer Res. 17:2281–91. PMID:21220477
1050. Gumbs AA, Moore PS, Falconi M, et al. (2002). Review of the clinical, histological, and molecular aspects of pancreatic endocrine neoplasms. J Surg Oncol. 81:45–53, discussion 54. PMID:12210027
1051. Gundry SR, Burney RE, Thompson NW, et al. (1983). Total thyroidectomy for Hürthle cell neoplasm of the thyroid. Arch Surg. 118:529–32. PMID:6838358
1052. Guo K, Wang Z (2014). Risk factors influencing the recurrence of papillary thyroid carcinoma: a systematic review and meta-analysis. Int J Clin Exp Pathol. 7:5393–403. PMID:25337182
1053. Guo M, Jia Y, Yu Z, et al. (2014). Epigenetic changes associated with neoplasms of the exocrine and endocrine pancreas. Discov Med. 17:67–73. PMID:24534469
1054. Gupta S, Ajise O, Dultz L, et al. (2012). Follicular variant of papillary thyroid cancer: encapsulated, nonencapsulated, and diffuse: distinct biologic and clinical entities. Arch Otolaryngol Head Neck Surg. 138:227–33. PMID:22431868
1055. Gurazada K, Ihuoma A, Galloway M, et al. (2014). Nasally located ectopic ACTH-secreting pituitary adenoma (EAPA) causing Nelson's syndrome: diagnostic challenges. Pituitary. 17:423–9. PMID:24065616
1056. Gurney JG, Ross JA, Wall DA, et al. (1997). Infant cancer in the U.S.: histology-specific incidence and trends, 1973 to 1992. J Pediatr Hematol Oncol. 19:428–32. PMID:9329464
1057. Gutmann DH, Rasmussen SA, Wolkenstein P, et al. (2002). Gliomas presenting after age 10 in individuals with neurofibromatosis type 1 (NF1). Neurology. 59:759–61. PMID:12221173
1058. Gutzeit A, Stuckmann G, Tosoni I, et al. (2011). A cavernous hemangioma of the thyroid gland: First documentation by ultrasound of a rare pathology. J Clin Ultrasound. 39:172–4. PMID:20806277
1059. Guyétant S, Dupre F, Bigorgne JC, et al. (1999). Medullary thyroid microcarcinoma: a clinicopathologic retrospective study of 38 patients with no prior familial disease. Hum Pathol. 30:957–63. PMID:10452509
1060. Guyétant S, Rousselet MC, Durigon M,

et al. (1997). Sex-related C cell hyperplasia in the normal human thyroid: a quantitative autopsy study. J Clin Endocrinol Metab. 82:42–7. PMID:8989230
1061. Ha EJ, Baek JH, Lee JH, et al. (2016). Core needle biopsy could reduce diagnostic surgery in patients with anaplastic thyroid cancer or thyroid lymphoma. Eur Radiol. 26:1031–6. PMID:26201291
1062. Haddad NM, Cavallerano JD, Silva PS (2013). Von hippel-lindau disease: a genetic and clinical review. Semin Ophthalmol. 28:377–86. PMID:24138046
1063. Hadoux J, Favier J, Scoazec JY, et al. (2014). SDHB mutations are associated with response to temozolomide in patients with metastatic pheochromocytoma or paraganglioma. Int J Cancer. 135:2711–20. PMID:24752622
1064. Hajdu M, Singer S, Maki RG, et al. (2010). IGF2 over-expression in solitary fibrous tumours is independent of anatomical location and is related to loss of imprinting. J Pathol. 221:300–7. PMID:20527023
1065. Halachmi N, Halachmi S, Evron E, et al. (1998). Somatic mutations of the PTEN tumor suppressor gene in sporadic follicular thyroid tumors. Genes Chromosomes Cancer. 23:239–43. PMID:9790504
1066. Hălălău F, Laky D (1983). Hemangiosarcoma of the thyroid gland. Histological diagnosis problems. Morphol Embryol (Bucur). 29:195–6. PMID:6199664
1067. Halfdanarson TR, Bamlet WR, McWilliams RR, et al. (2014). Risk factors for pancreatic neuroendocrine tumors: a clinic-based case-control study. Pancreas. 43:1219–22. PMID:25291526
1068. Halfdanarson TR, Rabe KG, Rubin J, et al. (2008). Pancreatic neuroendocrine tumors (PNETs): incidence, prognosis and recent trend toward improved survival. Ann Oncol. 19:1727–33. PMID:18515795
1069. Halfdanarson TR, Rubin J, Farnell MB, et al. (2008). Pancreatic endocrine neoplasms: epidemiology and prognosis of pancreatic endocrine tumors. Endocr Relat Cancer. 15:409–27. PMID:18508996
1070. Hall MJ, Innocent J, Rybak C, et al. (2015). Bilateral granulosa cell tumors: a novel malignant manifestation of multiple endocrine neoplasia 1 syndrome found in a patient with a rare menin in-frame deletion. Appl Clin Genet. 8:69–73. PMID:25733923
1071. Haller F, Moskalev EA, Faucz FR, et al. (2014). Aberrant DNA hypermethylation of SDHC: a novel mechanism of tumor development in Carney triad. Endocr Relat Cancer. 21:567–77. PMID:24859990
1072. Hamamatsu A, Arai T, Iwamoto M, et al. (2005). Adenomatoid tumor of the adrenal gland: case report with immunohistochemical study. Pathol Int. 55:665–9. PMID:16185299
1073. Hamatani K, Eguchi H, Ito R, et al. (2008). RET/PTC rearrangements preferentially occurred in papillary thyroid cancer among atomic bomb survivors exposed to high radiation dose. Cancer Res. 68:7176–82. PMID:18757433
1073A. Hameed A, Coleman RL (2000). Fine-needle aspiration cytology of primary granulosa cell tumor of the adrenal gland: a case report. Diagn Cytopathol. 22:107–9. PMID:10649522
1074. Hamilton NA, Liu TC, Cavatiao A, et al. (2012). Ki-67 predicts disease recurrence and poor prognosis in pancreatic neuroendocrine neoplasms. Surgery. 152:107–13. PMID:22503317
1075. Hammel PR, Vilgrain V, Terris B, et al. (2000). Pancreatic involvement in von Hippel-Lindau disease. The Groupe Francophone d'Etude de la Maladie de von Hippel-Lindau. Gastroenterology. 119:1087–95. PMID:11040195
1076. Hammond PJ, Murphy D, Carachi R, et al. (2010). Childhood phaeochromocytoma and paraganglioma: 100% incidence of genetic mutations and 100% survival. J Pediatr Surg. 45:383–6. PMID:20152357
1077. Hänggi D, Adams H, Hans VH, et al. (2005). Recurrent glomus tumor of the sellar region with malignant progression. Acta Neuropathol. 110:93–6. PMID:15952045
1078. Hann HW, Evans AE, Siegel SE, et al. (1985). Prognostic importance of serum ferritin in patients with Stages III and IV neuroblastoma: the Childrens Cancer Study Group experience. Cancer Res. 45:2843–8. PMID:3986811
1079. Hanna AN, Michael CW, Jing X (2011). Mixed medullary-follicular carcinoma of the thyroid: diagnostic dilemmas in fine-needle aspiration cytology. Diagn Cytopathol. 39:862–5. PMID:21994201
1080. Hansen TM, Batra S, Lim M, et al. (2014). Invasive adenoma and pituitary carcinoma: a SEER database analysis. Neurosurg Rev. 37:279–85, discussion 285–6. PMID:24526366
1081. Hao HX, Khalimonchuk O, Schraders M, et al. (2009). SDH5, a gene required for flavination of succinate dehydrogenase, is mutated in paraganglioma. Science. 325:1139–42. PMID:19628817
1082. Happle R (1986). The McCune-Albright syndrome: a lethal gene surviving by mosaicism. Clin Genet. 29:321–4. PMID:3720010
1083. Haq M, Harmer C (2005). Differentiated thyroid carcinoma with distant metastases at presentation: prognostic factors and outcome. Clin Endocrinol (Oxf). 63:87–93. PMID:15963067
1084. Harach HR (1991). Thyroglobulin in human thyroid follicles with acid mucin. J Pathol. 164:261–3. PMID:1679843
1085. Harach HR, Bergholm U (1988). Medullary (C cell) carcinoma of the thyroid with features of follicular oxyphilic cell tumours. Histopathology. 13:645–56. PMID:2466753
1086. Harach HR, Day ES, de Strizic NA (1986). Mucoepidermoid carcinoma of the thyroid. Report of a case with immunohistochemical studies. Medicina (B Aires). 46:213–6. PMID:3574073
1087. Harach HR, Soubeyran I, Brown A, et al. (1999). Thyroid pathologic findings in patients with Cowden disease. Ann Diagn Pathol. 3:331–40. PMID:10594284
1088. Harach HR, Williams ED (1983). Glandular (tubular and follicular) variants of medullary carcinoma of the thyroid. Histopathology. 7:83–97. PMID:6840715
1089. Harach HR, Williams GT, Williams ED (1994). Familial adenomatous polyposis associated thyroid carcinoma: a distinct type of follicular cell neoplasm. Histopathology. 25:549–61. PMID:7698732
1090. Harada K, Arita K, Kurisu K, et al. (2000). Telomerase activity and the expression of telomerase components in pituitary adenoma with malignant transformation. Surg Neurol. 53:267–74. PMID:10773260
1091. Harari A, Inabnet WB 3rd (2011). Malignant pheochromocytoma: a review. Am J Surg. 201:700–8. PMID:20870212
1092. Harari A, Waring A, Fernandez-Ranvier G, et al. (2011). Parathyroid carcinoma: a 43-year outcome and survival analysis. J Clin Endocrinol Metab. 96:3679–86. PMID:21937626
1093. Haresh KP, Prabhakar R, Anand Rajan KD, et al. (2009). A rare case of paraganglioma of the sella with bone metastases. Pituitary. 12:276–9. PMID:18320326
1094. Harrington KJ, Michalaki VJ, Vini L, et al. (2005). Management of non-Hodgkin's lymphoma of the thyroid: the Royal Marsden Hospital experience. Br J Radiol. 78:405–10. PMID:15845932
1095. Hart ES, Kelly MH, Brillante B, et al. (2007). Onset, progression, and plateau of skeletal lesions in fibrous dysplasia and the relationship to functional outcome. J Bone Miner Res. 22:1468–74. PMID:17501668
1096. Hasan M, Siddiqui F, Al-Ajmi M (2008). FNA diagnosis of adrenal myelolipoma: a rare entity. Diagn Cytopathol. 36:925–6. PMID:18855887
1097. Hassan I, Barth P, Celik I, et al. (2005). An authentic malignant epithelioid hemangioendothelioma of the thyroid: a case report and review of the literature. Thyroid. 15:1377–81. PMID:16405412
1098. Hasselblatt M, Jeibmann A, Gerss J, et al. (2005). Cellular and reticular variants of haemangioblastoma revisited: a clinicopathologic study of 88 cases. Neuropathol Appl Neurobiol. 31:618–22. PMID:16281910
1099. Hassoun AA, Hay ID, Goellner JR, et al. (1997). Insular thyroid carcinoma in adolescents: a potentially lethal endocrine malignancy. Cancer. 79:1044–8. PMID:9041169
1100. Hata JL, Correa H, Krishnan C, et al. (2015). Diagnostic utility of PHOX2B in primary and treated neuroblastoma and in neuroblastoma metastatic to the bone marrow. Arch Pathol Lab Med. 139:543–6. PMID:25822764
1101. Hattori Y, Tahara S, Ishii Y, et al. (2013). A case of prolactinoma with chordoma. Clin Neurol Neurosurg. 115:2537–9. PMID:24129004
1102. Haven CJ, van Puijenbroek M, Tan MH, et al. (2007). Identification of MEN1 and HRPT2 somatic mutations in paraffin-embedded (sporadic) parathyroid carcinomas. Clin Endocrinol (Oxf). 67:370–6. PMID:17555500
1103. Haven CJ, Wong FK, van Dam EW, et al. (2000). A genotypic and histopathological study of a large Dutch kindred with hyperparathyroidism-jaw tumor syndrome. J Clin Endocrinol Metab. 85:1449–54. PMID:10770180
1104. Hay ID (1990). Papillary thyroid carcinoma. Endocrinol Metab Clin North Am. 19:545–76. PMID:2261906
1105. Hay ID (2007). Management of patients with low-risk papillary thyroid carcinoma. Endocr Pract. 13:521–33. PMID:17872355
1106. Hay ID, Bergstralh EJ, Goellner JR, et al. (1993). Predicting outcome in papillary thyroid carcinoma: development of a reliable prognostic scoring system in a cohort of 1779 patients surgically treated at one institution during 1940 through 1989. Surgery. 114:1050–7, discussion 1057–8. PMID:8256208
1107. Hay ID, Grant CS, Bergstralh EJ, et al. (1998). Unilateral total lobectomy: is it sufficient surgical treatment for patients with AMES low-risk papillary thyroid carcinoma? Surgery. 124:958–64, discussion 964–6. PMID:9854569
1108. Hay ID, Grant CS, Taylor WF, et al. (1987). Ipsilateral lobectomy versus bilateral lobar resection in papillary thyroid carcinoma: a retrospective analysis of surgical outcome using a novel prognostic scoring system. Surgery. 102:1088–95. PMID:3686348
1109. Hay ID, Thompson GB, Grant CS, et al. (2002). Papillary thyroid carcinoma managed at the Mayo Clinic during six decades (1940–1999): temporal trends in initial therapy and long-term outcome in 2444 consecutively treated patients. World J Surg. 26:879–85. PMID:12016468
1110. Hayashi E, Takata K, Sato Y, et al. (2013). Distinct morphologic, phenotypic, and clinical-course characteristics of indolent peripheral T-cell lymphoma. Hum Pathol. 44:1927–36. PMID:23706909
1111. Hayashi K, Inoshita N, Kawaguchi K, et al. (2016). The USP8 mutational status may predict drug susceptibility in corticotroph adenomas of Cushing's disease. Eur J Endocrinol. 174:213–26. PMID:26578638
1112. Hayashi T, Gucer H, Mete O (2014). A mimic of sarcomatoid adrenal cortical carcinoma: epithelioid angiosarcoma occurring in adrenal cortical adenoma. Endocr Pathol. 25:404–9. PMID:25246132
1113. Hazard JB (1960). Small papillary carcinoma of the thyroid. A study with special reference to so-called nonencapsulated sclerosing tumor. Lab Invest. 9:86–97. PMID:14400378
1114. Hazard JB, Hawk WA, Crile G Jr (1959). Medullary (solid) carcinoma of the thyroid; a clinicopathologic entity. J Clin Endocrinol Metab. 19:152–61. PMID:13620740
1115. He H, Jazdzewski K, Li W, et al. (2005). The role of microRNA genes in papillary thyroid carcinoma. Proc Natl Acad Sci U S A. 102:19075–80. PMID:16365291
1116. He X, Wang L, Yan J, et al. (2016). Menin localization in cell membrane compartment. Cancer Biol Ther. 17:114–22. PMID:26560942
1117. Heaney A (2014). Management of aggressive pituitary adenomas and pituitary carcinomas. J Neurooncol. 117:459–68. PMID:24584748
1118. Heaney AP (2011). Clinical review: Pituitary carcinoma: difficult diagnosis and treatment. J Clin Endocrinol Metab. 96:3649–60. PMID:21956419
1119. Heaphy CM, de Wilde RF, Jiao Y, et al. (2011). Altered telomeres in tumors with ATRX and DAXX mutations. Science. 333:425. PMID:21719641
1120. Heck A, Ringstad G, Fougner SL, et al. (2012). Intensity of pituitary adenoma on T2-weighted magnetic resonance imaging predicts the response to octreotide treatment in newly diagnosed acromegaly. Clin Endocrinol (Oxf). 77:72–8. PMID:22066905
1121. Hedayati V, Thway K, Thomas JM, et al. (2014). MEN1 Syndrome and Hibernoma: An Uncommonly Recognised Association? Case Rep Med. 2014:804580. PMID:25309600
1122. Hedinger C (1981). Geographic pathology of thyroid diseases. Pathol Res Pract. 171:285–92. PMID:6895108
1123. Heetfeld M, Chougnet CN, Olsen IH, et al. (2015). Characteristics and treatment of patients with G3 gastroenteropancreatic neuroendocrine neoplasms. Endocr Relat Cancer. 22:657–64. PMID:26113608
1124. Heffess CS, Wenig BM, Thompson LD (2002). Metastatic renal cell carcinoma to the thyroid gland: a clinicopathologic study of 36 cases. Cancer. 95:1869–78. PMID:12404280
1125. Heide S, Masliah-Planchon J, Isidor B, et al. (2016). Oncologic Phenotype of Peripheral Neuroblastic Tumors Associated With PHOX2B Non-Polyalanine Repeat Expansion Mutations. Pediatr Blood Cancer. 63:71–7. PMID:26375764
1126. Heitz PU, Kasper M, Polak JM, et al. (1982). Pancreatic endocrine tumors. Hum Pathol. 13:263–71. PMID:7076209
1127. Hemmer S, Wasenius VM, Knuutila S, et al. (1998). Comparison of benign and malignant follicular thyroid tumours by comparative genomic hybridization. Br J Cancer. 78:1012–7. PMID:9792143
1128. Henderson SJ, Kearns PJ, Tong CM, et al. (2015). Patients with urinary bladder paragangliomas: a compiled case series from a literature review for clinical management. Urology. 85:e25–9. PMID:25618559
1129. Hendy GN, Cole DE (2013). Genetic defects associated with familial and sporadic hyperparathyroidism. Front Horm Res. 41:149–65. PMID:23652676
1130. Henopp T, Anlauf M, Schmitt A, et al. (2009). Glucagon cell adenomatosis: a newly recognized disease of the endocrine pancreas. J Clin Endocrinol Metab. 94:213–7. PMID:18957496
1131. Henry I, Jeanpierre M, Couillin P, et al. (1989). Molecular definition of the 11p15.5 region involved in Beckwith-Wiedemann syndrome and probably in predisposition to adrenocortical carcinoma. Hum Genet. 81:273–7. PMID:2921038
1132. Henzen-Logmans SC, Mullink H, Ramaekers FC, et al. (1987). Expression of cytokeratins and vimentin in epithelial cells of normal and pathologic thyroid tissue. Virchows

Arch A Pathol Anat Histopathol. 410:347–54. PMID:2433835
1133. Her YF, Maher LJ 3rd (2015). Succinate Dehydrogenase Loss in Familial Paraganglioma: Biochemistry, Genetics, and Epigenetics. Int J Endocrinol. 2015:296167. PMID:26294907
1134. Héritier S, Saffroy R, Radosevic-Robin N, et al. (2015). Common cancer-associated PIK3CA activating mutations rarely occur in Langerhans cell histiocytosis. Blood. 125:2448–9. PMID:25858893
1135. Hermann G, Konukiewitz B, Schmitt A, et al. (2011). Hormonally defined pancreatic and duodenal neuroendocrine tumors differ in their transcription factor signatures: expression of ISL1, PDX1, NGN3, and CDX2. Virchows Arch. 459:147–54. PMID:21739268
1136. Hernandez KG, Ezzat S, Morel CF, et al. (2015). Familial pheochromocytoma and renal cell carcinoma syndrome: TMEM127 as a novel candidate gene for the association. Virchows Arch. 466:727–32. PMID:25800244
1137. Hernández-Ramírez LC, Gabrovska P, Dénes J, et al. (2015). Landscape of Familial Isolated and Young-Onset Pituitary Adenomas: Prospective Diagnosis in AIP Mutation Carriers. J Clin Endocrinol Metab. 100:E1242–54. PMID:26186299
1138. Herrera MF, Stone E, Deitel M, et al. (1992). Pheochromocytoma producing multiple vasoactive peptides. Arch Surg. 127:105–8. PMID:1734841
1139. Herrmann MA, Hay ID, Bartelt DH Jr, et al. (1991). Cytogenetic and molecular genetic studies of follicular and papillary thyroid cancers. J Clin Invest. 88:1596–604. PMID:1939648
1140. Hicks DG, LiVolsi VA, Neidich JA, et al. (1990). Clonal analysis of solitary follicular nodules in the thyroid. Am J Pathol. 137:553–62. PMID:1975986
1141. Higgins DF, Kimura K, Bernhardt WM, et al. (2007). Hypoxia promotes fibrogenesis in vivo via HIF-1 stimulation of epithelial-to-mesenchymal transition. J Clin Invest. 117:3810–20. PMID:18037992
1142. Hijioka S, Hara K, Mizuno N, et al. (2016). Diagnostic performance and factors influencing the accuracy of EUS-FNA of pancreatic neuroendocrine neoplasms. J Gastroenterol. 51:923–30. PMID:26768605
1143. Hiltzik D, Carlson DL, Tuttle RM, et al. (2006). Poorly differentiated thyroid carcinomas defined on the basis of mitosis and necrosis: a clinicopathologic study of 58 patients. Cancer. 106:1286–95. PMID:16470605
1144. Hinton DR, Hahn JA, Weiss MH, et al. (1998). Loss of Rb expression in an ACTH-secreting pituitary carcinoma. Cancer Lett. 126:209–14. PMID:9585068
1145. Hirohata T, Asano K, Ogawa Y, et al. (2013). DNA mismatch repair protein (MSH6) correlated with the responses of atypical pituitary adenomas and pituitary carcinomas to temozolomide: the national cooperative study by the Japan Society for Hypothalamic and Pituitary Tumors. J Clin Endocrinol Metab. 98:1130–6. PMID:23365123
1146. Hirokawa M, Carney JA (2000). Cell membrane and cytoplasmic staining for MIB-1 in hyalinizing trabecular adenoma of the thyroid gland. Am J Surg Pathol. 24:575–8. PMID:10757406
1147. Hirokawa M, Miyauchi A, Minato H, et al. (2013). Intrathyroidal epithelial thymoma/carcinoma showing thymus-like differentiation; comparison with thymic lymphoepithelioma-like carcinoma and a possibility of development from a multipotential stem cell. APMIS. 121:523–30. PMID:23176314
1148. Ho KC, Meyer G, Garancis J, et al. (1982). Chemodectoma involving the cavernous sinus and semilunar ganglion. Hum Pathol. 13:942–3. PMID:6290369
1149. Hoang MP, Hruban RH, Albores-Saavedra J (2001). Clear cell endocrine pancreatic tumor mimicking renal cell carcinoma: a distinctive neoplasm of von Hippel-Lindau disease. Am J Surg Pathol. 25:602–9. PMID:11342771
1150. Hochwald SN, Zee S, Conlon KC, et al. (2002). Prognostic factors in pancreatic endocrine neoplasms: an analysis of 136 cases with a proposal for low-grade and intermediate-grade groups. J Clin Oncol. 20:2633–42. PMID:12039924
1151. Hoekstra AS, Devilee P, Bayley JP (2015). Models of parent-of-origin tumorigenesis in hereditary paraganglioma. Semin Cell Dev Biol. 43:117–24. PMID:26067997
1152. Hoellig A, Niehusmann P, Flacke S, et al. (2009). Metastasis to pituitary adenoma: case report and review of the literature. Cent Eur Neurosurg. 70:149–53. PMID:19701874
1153. Hofman V, Lassalle S, Bonnetaud C, et al. (2009). Thyroid tumours of uncertain malignant potential: frequency and diagnostic reproducibility. Virchows Arch. 455:21–33. PMID:19543912
1154. Hofmann BM, Kreutzer J, Saeger W, et al. (2006). Nuclear beta-catenin accumulation as reliable marker for the differentiation between cystic craniopharyngiomas and rathke cleft cysts: a clinico-pathologic approach. Am J Surg Pathol. 30:1595–603. PMID:17122517
1155. Hofstra RM, Landsvater RM, Ceccherini I, et al. (1994). A mutation in the RET proto-oncogene associated with multiple endocrine neoplasia type 2B and sporadic medullary thyroid carcinoma. Nature. 367:375–6. PMID:7906866
1156. Holland J, Chandurkar V (2014). A retrospective study of surgically excised phaeochromocytomas in Newfoundland, Canada. Indian J Endocrinol Metab. 18:542–5. PMID:25143914
1157. Hollander MC, Blumenthal GM, Dennis PA (2011). PTEN loss in the continuum of common cancers, rare syndromes and mouse models. Nat Rev Cancer. 11:289–301. PMID:21430697
1158. Holm LE, Blomgren H, Löwhagen T (1985). Cancer risks in patients with chronic lymphocytic thyroiditis. N Engl J Med. 312:601–4. PMID:3838363
1159. Hori A (1985). Suprasellar peri-infundibular ectopic adenohypophysis in fetal and adult brains. J Neurosurg. 63:113–5. PMID:4009259
1160. Horton ES, Dobin SM, Donner LR (2007). A clonal t(8;12)(p11.2;q24.3) as the sole abnormality in a solitary fibrous tumor of the pleura. Cancer Genet Cytogenet. 172:77–9. PMID:17175385
1161. Horvath E, Chalvardjian A, Kovacs K, et al. (1980). Leydig-like cells in the adrenals of a woman with ectopic ACTH syndrome. Hum Pathol. 11:284–7. PMID:7190543
1162. Horvath E, Kovacs K, Killinger DW, et al. (1980). Silent corticotropic adenomas of the human pituitary gland: a histologic, immunocytologic, and ultrastructural study. Am J Pathol. 98:617–38. PMID:6244736
1163. Horvath E, Kovacs K, Scheithauer BW (1999). Pituitary hyperplasia. Pituitary. 1:169–79. PMID:11081195
1164. Horvath E, Kovacs K, Scheithauer BW, et al. (1994). Pituitary adenoma with neuronal choristoma (PANCH): composite lesion or lineage infidelity? Ultrastruct Pathol. 18:565–74. PMID:7855931
1165. Horvath E, Kovacs K, Singer W, et al. (1981). Acidophil stem cell adenoma of the human pituitary: clinicopathologic analysis of 15 cases. Cancer. 47:761–71. PMID:6261917
1166. Horvath E, Kovacs K, Smyth HS, et al. (2005). Silent adenoma subtype 3 of the pituitary–immunohistochemical and ultrastructural classification: a review of 29 cases. Ultrastruct Pathol. 29:511–24. PMID:16316952
1167. Horvath E, Kovacs K, Smyth HS, et al. (1988). A novel type of pituitary adenoma: morphological features and clinical correlations. J Clin Endocrinol Metab. 66:1111–8. PMID:3372677
1168. Horwitz CA, Myers WP, Foote FW Jr (1972). Secondary malignant tumors of the parathyroid glands. Report of two cases with associated hypoparathyroidism. Am J Med. 52:797–808. PMID:4337783
1169. Hosaka N, Kitajiri S, Hiraumi H, et al. (2002). Ectopic pituitary adenoma with malignant transformation. Am J Surg Pathol. 26:1078–82. PMID:12170097
1170. Hosokawa Y, Pollak MR, Brown EM, et al. (1995). Mutational analysis of the extracellular Ca(2+)-sensing receptor gene in human parathyroid tumors. J Clin Endocrinol Metab. 80:3107–10. PMID:7593409
1171. Hou P, Liu D, Shan Y, et al. (2007). Genetic alterations and their relationship in the phosphatidylinositol 3-kinase/Akt pathway in thyroid cancer. Clin Cancer Res. 13:1161–70. PMID:17317825
1172. Hou P, Liu D, Xing M (2007). Functional characterization of the T1799-1801del and A1799-1816ins BRAF mutations in papillary thyroid cancer. Cell Cycle. 6:377–9. PMID:17297294
1173. Houck WA, Olson KB, Horton J (1970). Clinical features of tumor metastasis to the pituitary. Cancer. 26:656–9. PMID:5272295
1174. Houcke ML, Patey M (1998). Oxyphilic cell and clear cell carcinoma of the thyroid. Arch Anat Cytol Pathol. 46:79–85. [French] PMID:9754362
1175. Hough AJ, Hollifield JW, Page DL, et al. (1979). Prognostic factors in adrenal cortical tumors. A mathematical analysis of clinical and morphologic data. Am J Clin Pathol. 72:390–9. PMID:474519
1176. Howell VM, Gill A, Clarkson A, et al. (2009). Accuracy of combined protein gene product 9.5 and parafibromin markers for immunohistochemical diagnosis of parathyroid carcinoma. J Clin Endocrinol Metab. 94:434–41. PMID:19017757
1177. Howell VM, Haven CJ, Kahnoski K, et al. (2003). HRPT2 mutations are associated with malignancy in sporadic parathyroid tumours. J Med Genet. 40:657–63. PMID:12960210
1178. Howitt BE, Jia Y, Sholl LM, et al. (2013). Molecular alterations in partially-encapsulated or well-circumscribed follicular variant of papillary thyroid carcinoma. Thyroid. 23:1256–62. PMID:23477374
1179. Howlader N, Noone AM, Krapcho M, et al., editors (2015). SEER Cancer Statistics Review, 1975–2012. Bethesda: National Cancer Institute. Available: http://seer.cancer.gov/csr/1975_2012/.
1180. Howlett TA, Willis D, Walker G, et al. (UKAR-3) (2013). Control of growth hormone and IGF1 in patients with acromegaly in the UK: responses to medical treatment with somatostatin analogues and dopamine agonists. Clin Endocrinol (Oxf). 79:689–99. PMID:23574573
1181. Howson P, Kruijff S, Aniss A, et al. (2015). Oxyphil Cell Parathyroid Adenomas Causing Primary Hyperparathyroidism: a Clinico-Pathological Correlation. Endocr Pathol. 26:250–4. PMID:26091632
1182. Hruban RH, Pitman MB, Klimstra DS, et al. (2007). Tumors of the pancreas. In: AFIP atlas of tumor pathology. Series 4, Fascicle 6. Washington DC: American Registry of Pathology Press.
1183. Hsieh MS, Chen JH, Lin LW (2011). Myxoid adrenal cortical carcinoma presenting as primary hyperaldosteronism: case report and review of the literature. Int J Surg Pathol. 19:803–7. PMID:20444728
1184. Hsu SW, Shu K, Lee WC, et al. (2012). Adrenal myelolipoma: a 10-year single-center experience and literature review. Kaohsiung J Med Sci. 28:377–82. PMID:22726900
1185. Hu J, Wu J, Cai L, et al. (2013). Retroperitoneal composite pheochromocytoma-ganglioneuroma: a case report and review of literature. Diagn Pathol. 8:63. PMID:23587063
1186. Hu MI, Cote GJ (2012). Medullary thyroid carcinoma: who's on first? Thyroid. 22:451–3. PMID:22545752
1187. Huang AP, Yang SH, Yang CC, et al. (2008). Malignant prolactinoma with craniospinal metastasis in a 12-year-old boy. J Neurooncol. 90:41–6. PMID:18622581
1188. Huang C, Wang L, Wang Y, et al. (2013). Carcinoma showing thymus-like differentiation of the thyroid (CASTLE). Pathol Res Pract. 209:662–5. PMID:23920320
1189. Huang X, Zhang R, Mao Y, et al. (2010). Modified grading system for clinical outcome of intracranial non-germinomatous malignant germ cell tumors. Oncol Lett. 1:627–31. PMID:22966355
1190. Hubert JP Jr, Kiernan PD, Beahrs OH, et al. (1980). Occult papillary carcinoma of the thyroid. Arch Surg. 115:394–8. PMID:7362444
1191. Hug EB, Slater JD (2000). Proton radiation therapy for chordomas and chondrosarcomas of the skull base. Neurosurg Clin N Am. 11:627–38. PMID:11082173
1192. Hull MT, Warfel KA, Muller J, et al. (1979). Familial islet cell tumors in Von Hippel-Lindau's disease. Cancer. 44:1523–6. PMID:227568
1193. Hundahl SA, Cady B, Cunningham MP, et al. (2000). Initial results from a prospective cohort study of 5583 cases of thyroid carcinoma treated in the united states during 1996. U.S. and German Thyroid Cancer Study Group. An American College of Surgeons Commission on Cancer Patient Care Evaluation study. Cancer. 89:202–17. PMID:10897019
1194. Hundahl SA, Fleming ID, Fremgen AM, et al. (1998). A National Cancer Data Base report on 53,856 cases of thyroid carcinoma treated in the U.S., 1985–1995. Cancer. 83:2638–48. PMID:9874472
1195. Hunt JL, LiVolsi VA, Barnes EL (2004). p63 expression in sclerosing mucoepidermoid carcinomas with eosinophilia arising in the thyroid. Mod Pathol. 17:526–9.
1196. Hunter JA, Skelly RH, Aylwin SJ, et al. (2003). The relationship between pituitary tumour transforming gene (PTTG) expression and in vitro hormone and vascular endothelial growth factor (VEGF) secretion from human pituitary adenomas. Eur J Endocrinol. 148:203–11. PMID:12590639
1197. Hurel SJ, Harris PE, McNicol AM, et al. (1997). Metastatic prolactinoma: effect of octreotide, cabergoline, carboplatin and etoposide; immunocytochemical analysis of proto-oncogene expression. J Clin Endocrinol Metab. 82:2962–5. PMID:9284727
1198. Huson SM, Compston DA, Harper PS (1989). A genetic study of von Recklinghausen neurofibromatosis in south east Wales. II. Guidelines for genetic counselling. J Med Genet. 26:712–21. PMID:2511319
1199. Huss LJ, Mendelsohn G (1990). Medullary carcinoma of the thyroid gland: an encapsulated variant resembling the hyalinizing trabecular (paraganglioma-like) adenoma of thyroid. Mod Pathol. 3:581–5. PMID:2235983
1200. Huston TL, Simmons RM (2004). Ductal carcinoma in situ in a 27-year-old woman with McCune-Albright syndrome. Breast J. 10:440–2. PMID:15327499
1201. Hutcheon DF, Bayless TM, Cameron JL, et al. (1979). Hormone-mediated watery diarrhea in a family with multiple endocrine neoplasms. Ann Intern Med. 90:932–4. PMID:220898
1202. Hyjek E, Isaacson PG (1988). Primary B cell lymphoma of the thyroid and its relationship to Hashimoto's thyroiditis. Hum Pathol. 19:1315–26. PMID:3141260

1203. Iacobone M, Masi G, Barzon L, et al. (2009). Hyperparathyroidism-jaw tumor syndrome: a report of three large kindred. Langenbecks Arch Surg. 394:817–25. PMID:19529956
1204. Iacovazzo D, Carlsen E, Lugli F, et al. (2016). Factors predicting pasireotide responsiveness in somatotroph pituitary adenomas resistant to first-generation somatostatin analogues: an immunohistochemical study. Eur J Endocrinol. 174:241–50. PMID:26586796
1205. Ibrahimpasic T, Ghossein R, Carlson DL, et al. (2014). Outcomes in patients with poorly differentiated thyroid carcinoma. J Clin Endocrinol Metab. 99:1245–52. PMID:24512493
1206. Iczkowski KA, Butler SL, Shanks JH, et al. (2008). Trials of new germ cell immunohistochemical stains in 93 extragonadal and metastatic germ cell tumors. Hum Pathol. 39:275–81. PMID:18045648
1207. Idowu BD, Al-Adnani M, O'Donnell P, et al. (2007). A sensitive mutation-specific screening technique for GNAS1 mutations in cases of fibrous dysplasia: the first report of a codon 227 mutation in bone. Histopathology. 50:691–704. PMID:17493233
1208. Iglesias P, Díez JJ (2013). Macroprolactinoma: a diagnostic and therapeutic update. QJM. 106:495–504. PMID:23329574
1209. Igreja S, Chahal HS, King P, et al. (2010). Characterization of aryl hydrocarbon receptor interacting protein (AIP) mutations in familial isolated pituitary adenoma families. Hum Mutat. 31:950–60. PMID:20506337
1210. Ikegaki N, Shimada H, Fox AM, et al. (2013). Transient treatment with epigenetic modifiers yields stable neuroblastoma stem cells resembling aggressive large-cell neuroblastomas. Proc Natl Acad Sci U S A. 110:6097–102. PMID:23479628
1211. Ikota H, Tanimoto A, Komatsu H, et al. (2004). Ureteral leiomyoma causing hydronephrosis in Type 1 multiple endocrine neoplasia. Pathol Int. 54:457–9. PMID:15144407
1212. Ilett EE, Langer SW, Olsen IH, et al. (2015). Neuroendocrine Carcinomas of the Gastroenteropancreatic System: A Comprehensive Review. Diagnostics (Basel). 5:119–76. PMID:26854147
1213. Imam H, Eriksson B, Oberg K (2000). Expression of CD44 variant isoforms and association to the benign form of endocrine pancreatic tumours. Ann Oncol. 11:295–300. PMID:10811495
1214. Imamura H, Muroya K, Tanaka E, et al. (2016). Sporadic paraganglioma caused by de novo SDHB mutations in a 6-year-old girl. Eur J Pediatr. 175:137–41. PMID:26283294
1215. Imanishi Y, Hosokawa Y, Yoshimoto K, et al. (2001). Primary hyperparathyroidism caused by parathyroid-targeted overexpression of cyclin D1 in transgenic mice. J Clin Invest. 107:1093–102. PMID:11342573
1216. Imboden PN, Borruat FX, De Tribolet N, et al. (2004). Non-functioning pituitary carcinoma. Pituitary. 7:149–56. PMID:16010455
1216A. Imel EA, Econs MJ (2007). Fibrous dysplasia, phosphate wasting and fibroblast growth factor 23. Pediatr Endocrinol Rev. 4 Suppl 4:434–9. PMID:17982392
1217. Ingordo V, D'Andria G, Mendicini S, et al. (1995). Segmental neurofibromatosis: is it uncommon or underdiagnosed? Arch Dermatol. 131:959–60. PMID:7632074
1218. Ip JC, Pang TC, Glover AR, et al. (2015). Immunohistochemical validation of overexpressed genes identified by global expression microarrays in adrenocortical carcinoma reveals potential predictive and prognostic biomarkers. Oncologist. 20:247–56. PMID:25657202
1219. Ip YT, Dias Filho MA, Chan JK (2010). Nuclear inclusions and pseudoinclusions: friends or foes of the surgical pathologist? Int J Surg Pathol. 18:465–81. PMID:21081532
1220. Ippolito G, Palazzo FF, Sebag F, et al. (2007). Intraoperative diagnosis and treatment of parathyroid cancer and atypical parathyroid adenoma. Br J Surg. 94:566–70. PMID:17380564
1221. Ippolito S, Bellevicine C, Arpaia D, et al. (2016). Spindle epithelial tumor with thymus-like differentiation (SETTLE): clinical-pathological features, differential pathological diagnosis and therapy. Endocrine. 51:402–12. PMID:26289127
1222. Isa NM, James DT, Saw TH, et al. (2009). Primary angiosarcoma of the thyroid gland with recurrence diagnosed by fine needle aspiration: a case report. Diagn Cytopathol. 37:427–32. PMID:19306411
1223. Ishikawa Y, Sugano H, Matsumoto T, et al. (1999). Unusual features of thyroid carcinomas in Japanese patients with Werner syndrome and possible genotype-phenotype relations to cell type and race. Cancer. 85:1345–52. PMID:10189141
1224. Isidro ML, Iglesias Díaz P, Matías-Guiu X, et al. (2005). Acromegaly due to a growth hormone-releasing hormone-secreting intracranial gangliocytoma. J Endocrinol Invest. 28:162–5. PMID:15887863
1225. Isotalo PA, Keeney GL, Sebo TJ, et al. (2003). Adenomatoid tumor of the adrenal gland: a clinicopathologic study of five cases and review of the literature. Am J Surg Pathol. 27:969–77. PMID:12826889
1226. Ito E, Saito K, Okada T, et al. (2010). Long-term control of clival chordoma with initial aggressive surgical resection and gamma knife radiosurgery for recurrence. Acta Neurochir (Wien). 152:57–67, discussion 67. PMID:19826755
1227. Ito T, Igarashi H, Nakamura K, et al. (2015). Epidemiological trends of pancreatic and gastrointestinal neuroendocrine tumors in Japan: a nationwide survey analysis. J Gastroenterol. 50:58–64. PMID:24499825
1228. Ito T, Igarashi H, Uehara H, et al. (2013). Causes of death and prognostic factors in multiple endocrine neoplasia type 1: a prospective study: comparison of 106 MEN1/Zollinger-Ellison syndrome patients with 1613 literature MEN1 patients with or without pancreatic endocrine tumors. Medicine (Baltimore). 92:135–81. PMID:23645327
1229. Ito Y, Hirokawa M, Fukushima M, et al. (2008). Prevalence and prognostic significance of poor differentiation and tall cell variant in papillary carcinoma in Japan. World J Surg. 32:1535–43, discussion 1544–5. PMID:18224467
1230. Ito Y, Hirokawa M, Masuoka H, et al. (2013). Prognostic factors of minimally invasive follicular thyroid carcinoma: extensive vascular invasion significantly affects patient prognosis. Endocr J. 60:637–42. PMID:23327839
1231. Ito Y, Kakudo K, Hirokawa M, et al. (2009). Clinical significance of extrathyroid extension to the parathyroid gland of papillary thyroid carcinoma. Endocr J. 56:251–5. PMID:19122348
1232. Ito Y, Miyauchi A, Nakamura Y, et al. (2007). Clinicopathologic significance of intrathyroidal epithelial thymoma/carcinoma showing thymus-like differentiation: a collaborative study with Member Institutes of The Japanese Society of Thyroid Surgery. Am J Clin Pathol. 127:230–6. PMID:17210519
1233. Ito Y, Tomoda C, Uruno T, et al. (2006). Prognostic significance of extrathyroid extension of papillary thyroid carcinoma: massive but not minimal extension affects the relapse-free survival. World J Surg. 30:780–6. PMID:16411013
1234. Ivan M, Kondo K, Yang H, et al. (2001). HIFalpha targeted for VHL-mediated destruction by proline hydroxylation: implications for O2 sensing. Science. 292:464–8. PMID:11292862
1235. Ivanova R, Soares P, Castro P, et al. (2002). Diffuse (or multinodular) follicular variant of papillary thyroid carcinoma: a clinicopathologic and immunohistochemical analysis of ten cases of an aggressive form of differentiated thyroid carcinoma. Virchows Arch. 440:418–24. PMID:11956824
1236. Jaakkola P, Mole DR, Tian YM, et al. (2001). Targeting of HIF-alpha to the von Hippel-Lindau ubiquitylation complex by O2-regulated prolyl hydroxylation. Science. 292:468–72. PMID:11292861
1237. Jackson CE, Norum RA, Boyd SB, et al. (1990). Hereditary hyperparathyroidism and multiple ossifying jaw fibromas: a clinically and genetically distinct syndrome. Surgery. 108:1006–12, discussion 1012–3. PMID:2123361
1238. Jackson MA, Rich TA, Hu MI, et al. (2015). CDC73-related disorders. In: Pagon RA, Adam MP, Ardinger HH, et al., editors. GeneReviews®. Seattle: University of Washington, Seattle. PMID:20301744
1239. Jacoby LB, MacCollin M, Barone R, et al. (1996). Frequency and distribution of NF2 mutations in schwannomas. Genes Chromosomes Cancer. 17:45–55. PMID:8889506
1240. Jafri M, Whitworth J, Rattenberry E, et al. (2013). Evaluation of SDHB, SDHD and VHL gene susceptibility testing in the assessment of individuals with non-syndromic phaeochromocytoma, paraganglioma and head and neck paraganglioma. Clin Endocrinol (Oxf). 78:898–906. PMID:23072324
1241. Jahangiri A, Chin AT, Wagner JR, et al. (2015). Factors predicting recurrence after resection of clival chordoma using variable surgical approaches and radiation modalities. Neurosurgery. 76:179–85, discussion 185–6. PMID:25594191
1242. Jahangiri A, Wagner JR, Pekmezci M, et al. (2013). A comprehensive long-term retrospective analysis of silent corticotrophic adenomas vs hormone-negative adenomas. Neurosurgery. 73:8–17, discussion 17–8. PMID:23685641
1243. Jakowski JD, Wakely PE Jr, Jimenez RE (2008). An uncommon type of adrenal incidentaloma: a case report of a schwannoma of the adrenal medulla with cytological, histological, and ultrastructural correlation. Ann Diagn Pathol. 12:356–61. PMID:18774499
1244. Jamilloux Y, Favier J, Pertuit M, et al. (2014). A MEN1 syndrome with a paraganglioma. Eur J Hum Genet. 22:283–5. PMID:23778871
1245. Janoueix-Lerosey I, Lequin D, Brugières L, et al. (2008). Somatic and germline activating mutations of the ALK kinase receptor in neuroblastoma. Nature. 455:967–70. PMID:18923523
1246. Jansen JC, van den Berg R, Kuiper A, et al. (2000). Estimation of growth rate in patients with head and neck paragangliomas influences the treatment proposal. Cancer. 88:2811–6. PMID:10870065
1247. Janssen I, Blanchet EM, Adams K, et al. (2015). Superiority of [^{68}Ga]-DOTATATE PET/CT to other functional imaging modalities in the localization of SDHB-associated metastatic pheochromocytoma and paraganglioma. Clin Cancer Res. 21:3888–95. PMID:25873086
1248. Jarrar AM, Milas M, Mitchell J, et al. (2011). Screening for thyroid cancer in patients with familial adenomatous polyposis. Ann Surg. 253:515–21. PMID:21173694
1249. Jasperson KW, Burt RW (2014). APC-associated polyposis conditions. In: Pagon RA, Adam MP, Ardinger HH, et al., editors. GeneReviews®. Seattle: University of Washington, Seattle. PMID:20301519
1250. Jastania RA, Alsaad KO, Al-Shraim M, et al. (2005). Double adenomas of the pituitary: transcription factors Pit-1, T-pit, and SF-1 identify cytogenesis and differentiation. Endocr Pathol. 16:187–94. PMID:16299401
1251. Jayaram G, Cheah PL, Yip CH (2000). Malignant teratoma of the thyroid with predominantly neuroepithelial differentiation. Fine needle aspiration cytologic, histologic and immunocytochemical features of a case. Acta Cytol. 44:375–9. PMID:10833994
1252. Jayaram G, Wong KT, Jalaludin MA (1998). Mucoepidermoid carcinoma of the thyroid: a case report. Malays J Pathol. 20:45–8. PMID:10879264
1253. Jemal A, Siegel R, Ward E, et al. (2008). Cancer statistics, 2008. CA Cancer J Clin. 58:71–96. PMID:18287387
1254. Jenkins PJ, Satta MA, Simmgen M, et al. (1997). Metastatic parathyroid carcinoma in the MEN2A syndrome. Clin Endocrinol (Oxf). 47:747–51. PMID:9497883
1255. Jensen RT, Cadiot G, Brandi ML, et al. (2012). ENETS Consensus Guidelines for the management of patients with digestive neuroendocrine neoplasms: functional pancreatic endocrine tumor syndromes. Neuroendocrinology. 95:98–119. PMID:22261919
1256. Jensen RT, Niederle B, Mitry E, et al. (2006). Gastrinoma (duodenal and pancreatic). Neuroendocrinology. 84:173–82. PMID:17312377
1257. Jeong SH, Hong HS, Kwak JJ, et al. (2015). Analysis of RAS mutation and PAX8/PPARγ rearrangements in follicular-derived thyroid neoplasms in a Korean population: frequency and ultrasound findings. J Endocrinol Invest. 38:849–57. PMID:25999051
1258. Jeong YJ, Oh HK, Bong JG (2014). Multiple endocrine neoplasia type 1 associated with breast cancer: A case report and review of the literature. Oncol Lett. 8:230–4. PMID:24959251
1259. Ji JH, Oh YL, Hong M, et al. (2015). Identification of Driving ALK Fusion Genes and Genomic Landscape of Medullary Thyroid Cancer. PLoS Genet. 11:e1005467. PMID:26295973
1260. Jiang J, Zhang L, Wu Z, et al. (2014). A rare case of watery diarrhea, hypokalemia and achlorhydria syndrome caused by pheochromocytoma. BMC Cancer. 14:553. PMID:25081061
1261. Jiao Y, Shi C, Edil BH, et al. (2011). DAXX/ATRX, MEN1, and mTOR pathway genes are frequently altered in pancreatic neuroendocrine tumors. Science. 331:1199–203. PMID:21252315
1262. Jin LX, Moley JF (2016). Surgery for lymph node metastases of medullary thyroid carcinoma: A review. Cancer. 122:358–66. PMID:26539937
1263. Jin M, Roth R, Gayetsky V, et al. (2016). Grading pancreatic neuroendocrine neoplasms by Ki-67 staining on cytology cell blocks: manual count and digital image analysis of 58 cases. J Am Soc Cytopathol. 5:286–95.
1264. Jo JH, Chung TM, Youn H, et al. (2014). Cytoplasmic parafibromin/hCdc73 targets and destabilizes p53 mRNA to control p53-mediated apoptosis. Nat Commun. 5:5433. PMID:25388829
1265. Jochmanová I, Yang C, Zhuang Z, et al. (2013). Hypoxia-inducible factor signaling in pheochromocytoma: turning the rudder in the right direction. J Natl Cancer Inst. 105:1270–83. PMID:23940289
1266. Jochum W, Padberg BC, Schröder S (1994). Lymphoepithelial carcinoma of the thyroid gland. A thyroid gland carcinoma with thymus-like differentiation. Pathologe. 15:361–5. [German] PMID:7855107
1267. Johannessen JV, Sobrinho-Simões M (1980). The origin and significance of thyroid psammoma bodies. Lab Invest. 43:287–96. PMID:7401638
1268. Johnson KJ, Hussain I, Williams K, et al. (2013). Development of an international internet-based neurofibromatosis Type 1 patient registry. Contemp Clin Trials. 34:305–11. PMID:23246715
1269. Johnson PT, Horton KM, Fishman EK

(2009). Adrenal imaging with multidetector CT: evidence-based protocol optimization and interpretative practice. Radiographics. 29:1319–31. PMID:19755598

1270. Johnson PT, Horton KM, Fishman EK (2009). Adrenal mass imaging with multidetector CT: pathologic conditions, pearls, and pitfalls. Radiographics. 29:1333–51. PMID:19755599

1271. Johnston PC, Kennedy L, Weil RJ, et al. (2014). Ectopic ACTH-secreting pituitary adenomas within the sphenoid sinus. Endocrine. 47:717–24. PMID:24927792

1272. Jonkers YM, Claessen SM, Perren A, et al. (2007). DNA copy number status is a powerful predictor of poor survival in endocrine pancreatic tumor patients. Endocr Relat Cancer. 14:769–79. PMID:17914106

1273. Joung JY, Kim TH, Jeong DJ, et al. (2016). Diffuse sclerosing variant of papillary thyroid carcinoma: major genetic alterations and prognostic implications. Histopathology. 69:45–53. PMID:26568156

1274. Juco J, Horvath E, Smyth H, et al. (2007). Hemangiopericytoma of the sella mimicking pituitary adenoma: case report and review of the literature. Clin Neuropathol. 26:288–93. PMID:18232595

1275. Judkins AR, Roberts SA, Livolsi VA (1999). Utility of immunohistochemistry in the evaluation of necrotic thyroid tumors. Hum Pathol. 30:1373–6. PMID:10571520

1276. Juhlin CC, Goh G, Healy JM, et al. (2015). Whole-exome sequencing characterizes the landscape of somatic mutations and copy number alterations in adrenocortical carcinoma. J Clin Endocrinol Metab. 100:E493–502. PMID:25490274

1277. Juhlin CC, Haglund F, Villablanca A, et al. (2009). Loss of expression for the Wnt pathway components adenomatous polyposis coli and glycogen synthase kinase 3-beta in parathyroid carcinomas. Int J Oncol. 34:481–92. PMID:19148484

1278. Juhlin CC, Nilsson IL, Johansson K, et al. (2010). Parafibromin and APC as screening markers for malignant potential in atypical parathyroid adenomas. Endocr Pathol. 21:166–77. PMID:20473645

1279. Jun HH, Kim SM, Hong SW, et al. (2016). Warthin-like variant of papillary thyroid carcinoma: single institution experience. ANZ J Surg. 86:492–4. PMID:24981584

1280. Jun P, Chow LC, Jeffrey RB (2005). The sonographic features of papillary thyroid carcinomas: pictorial essay. Ultrasound Q. 21:39–45. PMID:15716757

1281. Jung CK, Little MP, Lubin JH, et al. (2014). The increase in thyroid cancer incidence during the last four decades is accompanied by a high frequency of BRAF mutations and a sharp increase in RAS mutations. J Clin Endocrinol Metab. 99:E276–85. PMID:24248188

1282. Jung YH, Kang MS (2010). Composite follicular variant of papillary carcinoma and mucoepidermoid carcinoma of thyroid gland: a case report. J Korean Med Sci. 25:1683–7. PMID:21060764

1283. Just PA, Guillevin R, Capron F, et al. (2008). An unusual clinical presentation of a rare tumor of the thyroid gland: report on one case of leiomyosarcoma and review of literature. Ann Diagn Pathol. 12:50–6. PMID:18164417

1284. Juweid M, O'Dorisio T, Milhem M (2008). Diagnosis of poorly differentiated thyroid cancer with radioiodine scanning after thyrotropin alfa stimulation. N Engl J Med. 359:1295–7. PMID:18799567

1285. Kaelin WG Jr (2002). Molecular basis of the VHL hereditary cancer syndrome. Nat Rev Cancer. 2:673–82. PMID:12209156

1286. Kaelin WG Jr (2008). The von Hippel-Lindau tumour suppressor protein: O2 sensing and cancer. Nat Rev Cancer. 8:865–73. PMID:18923434

1287. Kaelin WG Jr (2009). Treatment of kidney cancer: insights provided by the VHL tumor-suppressor protein. Cancer. 115(10 Suppl):2262–72. PMID:19402056

1288. Kaemmerer D, Wirtz RM, Fischer EK, et al. (2015). Analysis of somatostatin receptor 2A immunohistochemistry, RT-qPCR, and in vivo PET/CT data in patients with pancreatic neuroendocrine neoplasm. Pancreas. 44:648–54. PMID:25872131

1289. Kagawa T, Takamura M, Moritake K, et al. (1993). A case of sellar chordoma mimicking a non-functioning pituitary adenoma with survival of more than 10 years. Noshuyo Byori. 10:103–6. PMID:8220788

1290. Kageyama K, Ikeda H, Nigawara T, et al. (2007). Expression of adrenocorticotropic hormone, prolactin and transcriptional factors in clinically nonfunctioning pituitary adenoma. Endocr J. 54:961–8. PMID:18079591

1291. Kakkar A, Kaur K, Kumar T, et al. (2016). Pigmented Pheochromocytoma: an Unusual Variant of a Common Tumor. Endocr Pathol. 27:42–5. PMID:26578456

1292. Kakudo K, Bai Y, Liu Z, et al. (2012). Classification of thyroid follicular cell tumors: with special reference to borderline lesions. Endocr J. 59:1–12. PMID:21908930

1293. Kakudo K, Bai Y, Liu Z, et al. (2012). Encapsulated papillary thyroid carcinoma, follicular variant: a misnomer. Pathol Int. 62:155–60. PMID:22360502

1294. Kakudo K, Bai Y, Ozaki T, et al. (2013). Intrathyroid epithelial thymoma (ITET) and carcinoma showing thymus-like differentiation (CASTLE): CD5-positive neoplasms mimicking squamous cell carcinoma of the thyroid. Histol Histopathol. 28:543–56. PMID:23233417

1295. Kakudo K, Kameyama K, Hirokawa M, et al. (2015). Subclassification of follicular neoplasms recommended by the Japan thyroid association reporting system of thyroid cytology. Int J Endocrinol. 2015:938305. PMID:25722720

1296. Kakudo K, Miyauchi A, Ogihara T, et al. (1978). Medullary carcinoma of the thyroid. Giant cell type. Arch Pathol Lab Med. 102:445–7. PMID:210736

1297. Kakudo K, Miyauchi A, Takai S, et al. (1979). C cell carcinoma of the thyroid–papillary type. Acta Pathol Jpn. 29:653–9. PMID:463561

1298. Kakudo K, Mori I, Tamaoki N, et al. (1988). Carcinoma of possible thymic origin presenting as a thyroid mass: a new subgroup of squamous cell carcinoma of the thyroid. J Surg Oncol. 38:187–92. PMID:3260644

1299. Kakudo K, Wakasa T, Ohta Y, et al. (2015). Prognostic classification of thyroid follicular cell tumors using Ki-67 labeling index: risk stratification of thyroid follicular cell carcinomas. Endocr J. 62:1–12. PMID:25195708

1300. Kalitova P, Plzak J, Kodet R, et al. (2009). Angiosarcoma of the thyroid. Eur Arch Otorhinolaryngol. 266:903–5. PMID:18941766

1301. Kaltsas GA, Nomikos P, Kontogeorgos G, et al. (2005). Clinical review: Diagnosis and management of pituitary carcinomas. J Clin Endocrinol Metab. 90:3089–99. PMID:15741248

1302. Kamalanathan S, Mahesh DM, Muruganandham K, et al. (2012). Black adrenal adenoma: distinction from PPNAD. BMJ Case Rep. 2012:2012. PMID:22761223

1303. Kameyama K, Mukai M, Takami H, et al. (2004). Cribriform-morular variant of papillary thyroid carcinoma: ultrastructural study and somatic/germline mutation analysis of the APC gene. Ultrastruct Pathol. 28:97–102. PMID:15205109

1304. Kameyama K, Takami H (2005). Proposal for the histological classification of parathyroid carcinoma. Endocr Pathol. 16:49–52. PMID:16000846

1305. Kamisawa T, Tu Y, Egawa N, et al. (2002). Ductal and acinar differentiation in pancreatic endocrine tumors. Dig Dis Sci. 47:2254–61. PMID:12395898

1305A. Kamp K, Feelders RA, van Adrichem RC, et al. (2014). Parathyroid hormone-related peptide (PTHrP) secretion by gastroenteropancreatic neuroendocrine tumors (GEP-NETs): clinical features, diagnosis, management, and follow-up. J Clin Endocrinol Metab. 99:3060–9. PMID:24905065

1306. Kamphorst W, Wolbers JG, Ponssen H, et al. (1992). Ectopic parasellar pituitary adenoma with subarachnoid seeding. J Neurol Neurosurg Psychiatry. 55:73–4. PMID:1548504

1307. Kamura T, Koepp DM, Conrad MN, et al. (1999). Rbx1, a component of the VHL tumor suppressor complex and SCF ubiquitin ligase. Science. 284:657–61. PMID:10213691

1308. Kandil E, Abdel Khalek M, Abdullah O, et al. (2010). Primary peripheral nerve sheath tumors of the thyroid gland. Thyroid. 20:583–6. PMID:20553194

1309. Kane AJ, Sughrue ME, Rutkowski MJ, et al. (2012). Atypia predicting prognosis for intracranial extraventricular neurocytomas. J Neurosurg. 116:349–54. PMID:22054208

1310. Kannuki S, Matsumoto K, Sano T, et al. (1996). Double pituitary adenoma–two case reports. Neurol Med Chir (Tokyo). 36:818–21. PMID:9420436

1311. Kanter J, DeBlieux P (2014). Pressors and inotropes. Emerg Med Clin North Am. 32:823–34. PMID:25441037

1312. Kapran Y, Bauersfeld J, Anlauf M, et al. (2006). Multihormonality and entrapment of islets in pancreatic endocrine tumors. Virchows Arch. 448:394–8. PMID:16418841

1313. Karger S, Krause K, Engelhardt C, et al. (2012). Distinct pattern of oxidative DNA damage and DNA repair in follicular thyroid tumours. J Mol Endocrinol. 48:193–202. PMID:22331172

1314. Kars M, Dekkers OM, Pereira AM, et al. (2010). Update in prolactinomas. Neth J Med. 68:104–12. PMID:20308704

1315. Karvounaris DC, Symeonidis N, Triantafyllou A, et al. (2010). Ectopic parathyroid adenoma located inside the hypoglossal nerve. Head Neck. 32:1273–6. PMID:19691113

1316. Kasaian K, Wiseman SM, Thiessen N, et al. (2013). Complete genomic landscape of a recurring sporadic parathyroid carcinoma. J Pathol. 230:249–60. PMID:23616356

1317. Kasaliwal R, Goroshi M, Khadilkar K, et al. (2015). Primary adrenal lymphoma: a single-center experience. Endocr Pract. 21:719–24. PMID:25716633

1318. Kasem K, Lam AK (2014). Adrenal oncocytic phaeochromocytoma with putative adverse histologic features: a unique case report and review of the literature. Endocr Pathol. 25:416–21. PMID:25252620

1319. Kaserer K, Scheuba C, Neuhold N, et al. (2001). Sporadic versus familial medullary thyroid microcarcinoma: a histopathologic study of 50 consecutive patients. Am J Surg Pathol. 25:1245–51. PMID:11688458

1320. Kaserer K, Scheuba C, Neuhold N, et al. (1998). C-cell hyperplasia and medullary thyroid carcinoma in patients routinely screened for serum calcitonin. Am J Surg Pathol. 22:722–8. PMID:9630179

1321. Kaserer K, Scheuba C, Neuhold N, et al. (2002). Recommendations for reporting C cell pathology of the thyroid. Wien Klin Wochenschr. 114:274–8. PMID:12089863

1322. Kastelan D, Kraljevic I, Dusek T, et al. (2015). The clinical course of patients with adrenal incidentaloma: is it time to reconsider the current recommendations? Eur J Endocrinol. 173:275–82. PMID:26024670

1323. Kato I, Tajima K, Suchi T, et al. (1985). Chronic thyroiditis as a risk factor of B-cell lymphoma in the thyroid gland. Jpn J Cancer Res. 76:1085–90. PMID:3936828

1324. Katoh R, Sasaki J, Kurihara H, et al. (1992). Multiple thyroid involvement (intraglandular metastasis) in papillary thyroid carcinoma. A clinicopathologic study of 105 consecutive patients. Cancer. 70:1585–90. PMID:1516009

1325. Katoh R, Sugai T, Ono S, et al. (1990). Mucoepidermoid carcinoma of the thyroid gland. Cancer. 65:2020–7. PMID:1695544

1326. Katsuta T, Inoue T, Nakagaki H, et al. (2003). Distinctions between pituicytoma and ordinary pilocytic astrocytoma. Case report. J Neurosurg. 98:404–6. PMID:12593630

1327. Katznelson L, Laws ER Jr, Melmed S, et al. (2014). Acromegaly: an endocrine society clinical practice guideline. J Clin Endocrinol Metab. 99:3933–51. PMID:25356808

1328. Kaufmann O, Dietel M (2000). Expression of thyroid transcription factor-1 in pulmonary and extrapulmonary small cell carcinomas and other neuroendocrine carcinomas of various primary sites. Histopathology. 36:415–20. PMID:10792482

1329. Kaufmann TJ, Lopes MB, Laws ER Jr, et al. (2002). Primary sellar lymphoma: radiologic and pathologic findings in two patients. AJNR Am J Neuroradiol. 23:364–7. PMID:11901000

1330. Kaur A, Didolkar MS, Thomas A (2013). Angiosarcoma of the thyroid: a case report with review of the literature. Endocr Pathol. 24:156–61. PMID:23794134

1331. Kawahara E, Nakanishi I, Terahata S, et al. (1988). Leiomyosarcoma of the thyroid gland. A case report with a comparative study of five cases of anaplastic carcinoma. Cancer. 62:2558–63. PMID:3056606

1332. Kawaji H, Saito O, Amano S, et al. (2014). Extraventricular neurocytoma of the sellar region with spinal dissemination. Brain Tumor Pathol. 31:51–6. PMID:23250388

1333. Kawamoto S, Shi C, Hruban RH, et al. (2011). Small serotonin-producing neuroendocrine tumor of the pancreas associated with pancreatic duct obstruction. AJR Am J Roentgenol. 197:W482–8. PMID:21862776

1334. Kawanishi N, Norimatsu Y, Ohsaki H, et al. (2014). Diagnosis of pseudopapillary variant of medullary thyroid carcinoma by fine-needle aspiration cytology. Diagn Cytopathol. 42:823–6. PMID:23894022

1335. Kazaure HS, Roman SA, Sosa JA (2012). Insular thyroid cancer: a population-level analysis of patient characteristics and predictors of survival. Cancer. 118:3260–7. PMID:22252610

1336. Kebebew E, Greenspan FS, Clark OH, et al. (2005). Anaplastic thyroid carcinoma. Treatment outcome and prognostic factors. Cancer. 103:1330–5. PMID:15739211

1337. Kebebew E, Ituarte PH, Siperstein AE, et al. (2000). Medullary thyroid carcinoma: clinical characteristics, treatment, prognostic factors, and a comparison of staging systems. Cancer. 88:1139–48. PMID:10699905

1338. Kebebew E, Reiff E, Duh QY, et al. (2006). Extent of disease at presentation and outcome for adrenocortical carcinoma: have we made progress? World J Surg. 30:872–8. PMID:16680602

1339. Kebebew E, Weng J, Bauer J, et al. (2007). The prevalence and prognostic value of BRAF mutation in thyroid cancer. Ann Surg. 246:466–70, discussion 470–1. PMID:17717450

1340. Kelley MJ, Shi J, Ballew B, et al. (2014). Characterization of T gene sequence variants and germline duplications in familial and sporadic chordoma. Hum Genet. 133:1289–97. PMID:24990759

1341. Kellie SJ, Hayes FA, Bowman L, et al. (1991). Primary extracranial neuroblastoma with central nervous system metastases characterization by clinicopathologic findings and neuroimaging. Cancer. 68:1999–2006. PMID:1913549

1342. Kelly LM, Barila G, Liu P, et al. (2014). Identification of the transforming STRN-ALK

fusion as a potential therapeutic target in the aggressive forms of thyroid cancer. Proc Natl Acad Sci U S A. 111:4233–8. PMID:24613930
1343. Kemink SA, Wesseling P, Pieters GF, et al. (1999). Progression of a Nelson's adenoma to pituitary carcinoma; a case report and review of the literature. J Endocrinol Invest. 22:70–5. PMID:10090141
1344. Kemp DR (1967). Teratoma of the neck in the adult. Report of a case and review of the literature. Aust N Z J Surg. 36:323–7. PMID:5229783
1345. Kenney B, Singh G, Salem RR, et al. (2011). Pseudointraductal papillary mucinous neoplasia caused by microscopic periductal endocrine tumors of the pancreas: a report of 3 cases. Hum Pathol. 42:1034–41. PMID:21292301
1346. Kenny BD, Sloan JM, Hamilton PW, et al. (1989). The role of morphometry in predicting prognosis in pancreatic islet cell tumors. Cancer. 64:460–5. PMID:2544252
1347. Kent RB 3rd, van Heerden JA, Weiland LH (1981). Nonfunctioning islet cell tumors. Ann Surg. 193:185–90. PMID:6258500
1348. Khan AN, Solomon SS, Childress RD (2010). Composite pheochromocytoma-ganglioneuroma: a rare experiment of nature. Endocr Pract. 16:291–9. PMID:19833581
1349. Khan M, Caoili EM, Davenport MS, et al. (2014). CT imaging characteristics of oncocytic adrenal neoplasms (OANs): comparison with adrenocortical carcinomas. Abdom Imaging. 39:86–91. PMID:24271078
1350. Khan MS, Luong TV, Watkins J, et al. (2013). A comparison of Ki-67 and mitotic count as prognostic markers for metastatic pancreatic and midgut neuroendocrine neoplasms. Br J Cancer. 108:1838–45. PMID:23579216
1351. Khan N, Doros L, Schultz K-A, et al. (2015). PgmNr 2762: Thyroid nodules and multinodular goiter associated with germline mutations in DICER1 [abstract]. Paper presented at the 65th Annual Meeting of the American Society of Human Genetics, 6–10 October 2015, Baltimore, USA.
1352. Khunamornpong S, Settakorn J, Sukpan K, et al. (2015). Poorly Differentiated Thyroid Carcinoma Arising in Struma Ovarii. Case Rep Pathol. 2015:826978. PMID:26185700
1353. Khurana R, Agarwal A, Bajpai VK, et al. (2004). Unraveling the amyloid associated with human medullary thyroid carcinoma. Endocrinology. 145:5465–70. PMID:15459123
1354. Kie JH, Kim JY, Park YN, et al. (1997). Solitary fibrous tumour of the thyroid. Histopathology. 30:365–8. PMID:9147086
1355. Kier R, Silverman PM, Korobkin M, et al. (1985). Malignant teratoma of the thyroid in an adult: CT appearance. J Comput Assist Tomogr. 9:174–6. PMID:3968263
1356. Kikuchi K, Kowada M, Sasaki J, et al. (1994). Large pituitary adenoma of the sphenoid sinus and the nasopharynx: report of a case with ultrastructural evaluations. Surg Neurol. 42:330–4. PMID:7974131
1357. Kikuchi Y, Wada R, Sakihara S, et al. (2012). Pheochromocytoma with histologic transformation to composite type, complicated by watery diarrhea, hypokalemia, and achlorhydria syndrome. Endocr Pract. 18:e91–6. PMID:22440998
1358. Kilday JP, Laughlin S, Urbach S, et al. (2015). Diabetes insipidus in pediatric germinomas of the suprasellar region: characteristic features and significance of the pituitary bright spot. J Neurooncol. 121:167–75. PMID:25266413
1359. Kim AC, Reuter AL, Zubair M, et al. (2008). Targeted disruption of beta-catenin in Sf1-expressing cells impairs development and maintenance of the adrenal cortex. Development. 135:2593–602. PMID:18599507
1360. Kim GR, Kim MH, Moon HJ, et al. (2013). Sonographic characteristics suggesting papillary thyroid carcinoma according to nodule size. Ann Surg Oncol. 20:906–13. PMID:23266584
1361. Kim HJ, Hagan M, Butman JA, et al. (2013). Surgical resection of endolymphatic sac tumors in von Hippel-Lindau disease: findings, results, and indications. Laryngoscope. 123:477–83. PMID:23070752
1362. Kim HS, Yun KJ (2008). Adenolipoma of the thyroid gland: report of a case with diagnosis by fine-needle aspiration cytology. Diagn Cytopathol. 36:253–6. PMID:18335547
1363. Kim JY, Kim MS, Kim KS, et al. (2015). Clinicopathologic and prognostic significance of multiple hormone expression in pancreatic neuroendocrine tumors. Am J Surg Pathol. 39:592–601. PMID:25602797
1364. Kim K, Yamada S, Usui M, et al. (2004). Preoperative identification of clearly separated double pituitary adenomas. Clin Endocrinol (Oxf). 61:26–30. PMID:15212641
1365. Kim NR, Ko YH, Sung CO (2003). A case of coexistent angiosarcoma and follicular carcinoma of the thyroid. J Korean Med Sci. 18:908–13. PMID:14676455
1366. Kim T, Oh YL, Kim KM, et al. (2011). Diagnostic dilemmas of hyalinizing trabecular tumours on fine needle aspiration cytology: a study of seven cases with BRAF mutation analysis. Cytopathology. 22:407–13. PMID:21733000
1367. Kim TS, Asato R, Akamizu T, et al. (2007). A rare case of hyperfunctioning papillary carcinoma of the thyroid gland. Acta Otolaryngol Suppl. (557):55–7. PMID:17453446
1368. Kim YG, Park YS (2015). Second-stage transsphenoidal approach (TSA) for highly vascular pituicytomas in children. Childs Nerv Syst. 31:985–9. PMID:25771921
1369. Kimler SC, Muth WF (1978). Primary malignant teratoma of the thyroid: case report and literature review of cervical teratomas in adults. Cancer. 42:311–7. PMID:352506
1370. Kimmel DW, O'Neill BP (1983). Systemic cancer presenting as diabetes insipidus. Clinical and radiographic features of 11 patients with a review of metastatic-induced diabetes insipidus. Cancer. 52:2355–8. PMID:6640507
1371. Kimura ET, Nikiforova MN, Zhu Z, et al. (2003). High prevalence of BRAF mutations in thyroid cancer: genetic evidence for constitutive activation of the RET/PTC-RAS-BRAF signaling pathway in papillary thyroid carcinoma. Cancer Res. 63:1454–7. PMID:12670889
1372. Kimura N, Ishidate T, Kogawa T, et al. (2008). A retroperitoneal sympathetic paraganglioma invading the duodenum and mimicking a submucosal tumor. Endocr Pathol. 19:128–32. PMID:18438726
1373. Kimura N, Miura Y, Miura K, et al. (1991). Adrenal and retroperitoneal mixed neuroendocrine-neural tumors. Endocr Pathol. 2:139–47.
1374. Kimura N, Miura Y, Nagatsu I, et al. (1992). Catecholamine synthesizing enzymes in 70 cases of functioning and non-functioning phaeochromocytoma and extra-adrenal paraganglioma. Virchows Arch A Pathol Anat Histopathol. 421:25–32. PMID:1353277
1375. Kimura N, Nakazato Y, Nagura H, et al. (1990). Expression of intermediate filaments in neuroendocrine tumors. Arch Pathol Lab Med. 114:506–10. PMID:2159272
1376. Kimura N, Takayanagi R, Takizawa N, et al. (2014). Pathological grading for predicting metastasis in phaeochromocytoma and paraganglioma. Endocr Relat Cancer. 21:405–14. PMID:24521857
1377. Kimura N, Takekoshi K, Horii A, et al. (2014). Clinicopathological study of SDHB mutation-related pheochromocytoma and sympathetic paraganglioma. Endocr Relat Cancer. 21:L13–6. PMID:24659481
1378. Kimura N, Tateno H, Saijo S, et al. (2010). Familial cervical paragangliomas with lymph node metastasis expressing somatostatin receptor type 2A. Endocr Pathol. 21:139–43. PMID:19936639
1379. Kimura N, Watanabe T, Fukase M, et al. (2002). Neurofibromin and NF1 gene analysis in composite pheochromocytoma and tumors associated with von Recklinghausen's disease. Mod Pathol. 15:183–8. PMID:11904334
1380. Kimura N, Watanabe T, Noshiro T, et al. (2005). Histological grading of adrenal and extra-adrenal pheochromocytomas and relationship to prognosis: a clinicopathological analysis of 116 adrenal pheochromocytomas and 30 extra-adrenal sympathetic paragangliomas including 38 malignant tumors. Endocr Pathol. 16:23–32. PMID:16000843
1381. Kimura W, Kuroda A, Morioka Y (1991). Clinical pathology of endocrine tumors of the pancreas. Analysis of autopsy cases. Dig Dis Sci. 36:933–42. PMID:2070707
1382. Kindmark H, Sundin A, Granberg D, et al. (2007). Endocrine pancreatic tumors with glucagon hypersecretion: a retrospective study of 23 cases during 20 years. Med Oncol. 24:330–7. PMID:17873310
1383. King KS, Pacak K (2014). Familial pheochromocytomas and paragangliomas. Mol Cell Endocrinol. 386:92–100. PMID:23933153
1384. King KS, Prodanov T, Kantorovich V, et al. (2011). Metastatic pheochromocytoma/paraganglioma related to primary tumor development in childhood or adolescence: significant link to SDHB mutations. J Clin Oncol. 29:4137–42. PMID:21969497
1385. King R, Busam K, Rosai J (1999). Metastatic malignant melanoma resembling malignant peripheral nerve sheath tumor: report of 16 cases. Am J Surg Pathol. 23:1499–505. PMID:10584703
1386. Kini SR (1996). Post-fine-needle biopsy infarction of thyroid neoplasms: a review of 28 cases. Diagn Cytopathol. 15:211–20. PMID:8955603
1387. Kini SR, editor (2011). Color atlas of differential diagnosis in exfoliative and aspiration cytopathology. 2nd ed. Philadelphia: Wolters Kluwer/Lippincott Williams & Wilkins.
1388. Kinjo T, al-Mefty O, Ciric I (1995). Diaphragma sellae meningiomas. Neurosurgery. 36:1082–92. PMID:7643985
1389. Kirby PA, Ellison WA, Thomas PA (1999). Spindle epithelial tumor with thymus-like differentiation (SETTLE) of the thyroid with prominent mitotic activity and focal necrosis. Am J Surg Pathol. 23:712–6. PMID:10366154
1390. Kirk JM, Brain CE, Carson DJ, et al. (1999). Cushing's syndrome caused by nodular adrenal hyperplasia in children with McCune-Albright syndrome. J Pediatr. 134:789–92. PMID:10356155
1391. Kirkman MA, Jaunmuktane Z, Brandner S, et al. (2014). Active and silent thyroid-stimulating hormone-expressing pituitary adenomas: presenting symptoms, treatment, outcomes, and recurrence. World Neurosurg. 82:1224–31. PMID:24657816
1392. Kirkwood KS, Debas HT (1995). Neuroendocrine tumors: common presentations of uncommon diseases. Compr Ther. 21:719–25. PMID:8789136
1393. Kirschner LS, Carney JA, Pack SD, et al. (2000). Mutations of the gene encoding the protein kinase A type I-alpha regulatory subunit in patients with the Carney complex. Nat Genet. 26:89–92. PMID:10973256
1394. Kirschner LS, Sandrini F, Monbo J, et al. (2000). Genetic heterogeneity and spectrum of mutations of the PRKAR1A gene in patients with the carney complex. Hum Mol Genet. 9:3037–46. PMID:11115848
1395. Kissiedu JO, Prayson RA (2016). Sellar gangliocytoma with adrenocorticotropic and prolactin adenoma. J Clin Neurosci. 24:141–2. PMID:26314658
1396. Kjellman P, Lagercrantz S, Höög A, et al. (2001). Gain of 1q and loss of 9q21.3-q32 are associated with a less favorable prognosis in papillary thyroid carcinoma. Genes Chromosomes Cancer. 32:43–9. PMID:11477660
1397. Klein J, Zhuang Z, Lubensky I, et al. (2007). Multifocal microcysts and papillary cystadenoma of the lung in von Hippel-Lindau disease. Am J Surg Pathol. 31:1292–6. PMID:17667557
1398. Klein S, Lee H, Ghahremani S, et al. (2014). Expanding the phenotype of mutations in DICER1: mosaic missense mutations in the RNase IIIb domain of DICER1 cause GLOW syndrome. J Med Genet. 51:294–302. PMID:24676357
1399. Kleinschmidt-DeMasters BK, Lopes MB (2013). Update on hypophysitis and TTF-1 expressing sellar region masses. Brain Pathol. 23:495–514. PMID:23701182
1400. Kleinschmidt-DeMasters BK, Lopes MB, Prayson RA (2015). An algorithmic approach to sellar region masses. Arch Pathol Lab Med. 139:356–72. PMID:25724033
1401. Kleinschmidt-DeMasters BK, Winston KR, Rubinstein D, et al. (1990). Ectopic pituitary adenoma of the third ventricle. Case report. J Neurosurg. 72:139–42. PMID:2294174
1402. Klibanski A (2010). Clinical practice. Prolactinomas. N Engl J Med. 362:1219–26. PMID:20357284
1403. Kliewer KE, Cochran AJ (1989). A review of the histology, ultrastructure, immunohistology, and molecular biology of extra-adrenal paragangliomas. Arch Pathol Lab Med. 113:1209–18. PMID:2684087
1404. Klimstra DS (2007). Nonductal neoplasms of the pancreas. Mod Pathol. 20 Suppl 1:S94–112. PMID:17486055
1405. Klimstra DS (2016). Pathologic Classification of Neuroendocrine Neoplasms. Hematol Oncol Clin North Am. 30:1–19. PMID:26614366
1406. Klimstra DS, Rosai J, Heffess CS (1994). Mixed acinar-endocrine carcinomas of the pancreas. Am J Surg Pathol. 18:765–78. PMID:8037290
1407. Klimstra DS, Wenig BM, Heffess CS (2000). Solid-pseudopapillary tumor of the pancreas: a typically cystic carcinoma of low malignant potential. Semin Diagn Pathol. 17:66–80. PMID:10721808
1408. Klinck GH, Winship T (1955). Occult sclerosing carcinoma of the thyroid. Cancer. 8:701–6. PMID:13240651
1409. Klonoff DC, Greenspan FS (1982). The thyroid nodule. Adv Intern Med. 27:101–26. PMID:7041541
1410. Kloos RT, Eng C, Evans DB, et al. (2009). Medullary thyroid cancer: management guidelines of the American Thyroid Association. Thyroid. 19:565–612. PMID:19469690
1411. Klöppel G (2000). Mixed exocrine-endocrine tumors of the pancreas. Semin Diagn Pathol. 17:104–8. PMID:10839610
1412. Klöppel G (2003). Tumors of the adrenal medulla and the paraganglia. Pathologe. 24:280–6. [German] PMID:14513275
1413. Klöppel G, Anlauf M (2007). Gastrinoma–morphological aspects. Wien Klin Wochenschr. 119:579–84. PMID:17985091
1414. Klöppel G, Anlauf M, Perren A, et al. (2014). Hyperplasia to neoplasia sequence of duodenal and pancreatic neuroendocrine diseases and pseudohyperplasia of the PP-cells in the pancreas. Endocr Pathol. 25:181–5. PMID:24718881
1415. Klöppel G, Couvelard A, Perren A, et al. (2009). ENETS Consensus Guidelines for the Standards of Care in Neuroendocrine Tumors: towards a standardized approach to the diagnosis of gastroenteropancreatic neuroendocrine tumors and their prognostic stratification. Neuroendocrinology. 90:162–6. PMID:19060454
1416. Klöppel G, Heitz PU (1988). Pancreatic endocrine tumors. Pathol Res Pract. 183:155–68. PMID:2898775

1417. Klöppel G, Heitz PU (1990). Morphology and functional activity of gastroenteropancreatic neuroendocrine tumours. Recent Results Cancer Res. 118:27–36. PMID:1978380
1418. Klöppel G, Willemer S, Stamm B, et al. (1986). Pancreatic lesions and hormonal profile of pancreatic tumors in multiple endocrine neoplasia type I. An immunocytochemical study of nine patients. Cancer. 57:1824–32. PMID:2420439
1419. Kloub O, Perry A, Tu PH, et al. (2005). Spindle cell oncocytoma of the adenohypophysis: report of two recurrent cases. Am J Surg Pathol. 29:247–53. PMID:15644783
1420. Knauf JA, Ma X, Smith EP, et al. (2005). Targeted expression of BRAFV600E in thyroid cells of transgenic mice results in papillary thyroid cancers that undergo dedifferentiation. Cancer Res. 65:4238–45. PMID:15899815
1421. Kobayashi C, Monforte-Munoz HL, Gerbing RB, et al. (2005). Enlarged and prominent nucleoli may be indicative of MYCN amplification: a study of neuroblastoma (Schwannian stroma-poor), undifferentiated/poorly differentiated subtype with high mitosis-karyorrhexis index. Cancer. 103:174–80. PMID:15549714
1422. Kobayashi K, Imanishi Y, Koshiyama H, et al. (2006). Expression of FGF23 is correlated with serum phosphate level in isolated fibrous dysplasia. Life Sci. 78:2295–301. PMID:16337659
1423. Koch CA, Huang SC, Moley JF, et al. (2001). Allelic imbalance of the mutant and wild-type RET allele in MEN 2A-associated medullary thyroid carcinoma. Oncogene. 20:7809–11. PMID:11753660
1424. Koch CA, Mauro D, Walther MM, et al. (2002). Pheochromocytoma in von hippel-lindau disease: distinct histopathologic phenotype compared to pheochromocytoma in multiple endocrine neoplasia type 2. Endocr Pathol. 13:17–27. PMID:12114747
1425. Koch L (2011). Pediatric SDHB pheochromocytoma: a link to metastasis. Nat Rev Endocrinol. 7:692. PMID:22045106
1426. Kodama T, Okamoto T, Fujimoto Y, et al. (1988). C cell adenoma of the thyroid: a rare but distinct clinical entity. Surgery. 104:997–1003. PMID:3194851
1427. Koea JB, Shaw JH (1999). Parathyroid cancer: biology and management. Surg Oncol. 8:155–65. PMID:11113666
1428. Koga A, Tabata M, Kido H, et al. (1979). Successful treatment of ectopic insulinoma. Report of a case (author's transl). Nihon Shokakibyo Gakkai Zasshi. 76:279–84. [Japanese] PMID:220443
1429. Koike A, Naruse T, Kanemitsu T, et al. (1989). Clear cell carcinoma of the thyroid. A case report. Jpn J Surg. 19:237–40. PMID:2724724
1430. Komatsubara K, Tahara S, Umeoka K, et al. (2001). Immunohistochemical analysis of p27 (Kip1) in human pituitary glands and in various types of pituitary adenomas. Endocr Pathol. 12:181–8. PMID:11579684
1431. Komminoth P (2015). Somatostatin-producing tumor. In: La Rosa S, Sessa F, editors. Pancreatic neuroendocrine neoplasms: practical approach to diagnosis, classification, and therapy. Cham: Springer International Publishing AG; pp. 89–95.
1432. Komminoth P, Roth J, Schröder S, et al. (1995). Overlapping expression of immunohistochemical markers and synaptophysin mRNA in pheochromocytomas and adrenocortical carcinomas. Implications for the differential diagnosis of adrenal gland tumors. Lab Invest. 72:424–31. PMID:7723281
1433. Komninos J, Vlassopoulou V, Protopapa D, et al. (2004). Tumors metastatic to the pituitary gland: case report and literature review. J Clin Endocrinol Metab. 89:574–80. PMID:14764764
1434. Kondo T, Kato K, Nakazawa T, et al. (2005). Mucinous carcinoma (poorly differentiated carcinoma with extensive extracellular mucin deposition) of the thyroid: a case report with immunohistochemical studies. Hum Pathol. 36:698–701. PMID:16021578
1435. Kondo T, Matsuyama R, Ashihara H, et al. (2010). A case of ectopic adrenocorticotropic hormone-producing pancreatic neuroendocrine tumor with multiple liver metastases. Endocr J. 57:229–36. PMID:20032567
1436. Kong J, Wang O, Nie M, et al. (2014). Familial isolated primary hyperparathyroidism/hyperparathyroidism-jaw tumour syndrome caused by germline gross deletion or point mutations of CDC73 gene in Chinese. Clin Endocrinol (Oxf). 81:222–30. PMID:24716902
1437. Kontogeorgos G, Asa SL, Kovacs K, et al. (1993). Production of alpha-subunit of glycoprotein hormones by pituitary somatotroph adenomas in vitro. Acta Endocrinol (Copenh). 129:565–72. PMID:7509101
1438. Kontogeorgos G, Kapranos N, Orphanidis G, et al. (1999). Molecular cytogenetics of chromosome 11 in pituitary adenomas: a comparison of fluorescence in situ hybridization and DNA ploidy study. Hum Pathol. 30:1377–82. PMID:10571521
1439. Kontogeorgos G, Kovacs K, Horvat E, et al. (1993). Null cell adenomas, oncocytomas, and gonadotroph adenomas of the human pituitary: an immunocytochemical and ultrastructural analysis of 300 cases. Endocrinol Pathol. 4:20–7.
1440. Kontogeorgos G, Kovacs K, Horvath E, et al. (1991). Multiple adenomas of the human pituitary. A retrospective autopsy study with clinical implications. J Neurosurg. 74:243–7. PMID:1988594
1441. Kontogeorgos G, Mourouti G, Kyrodimou E, et al. (2006). Ganglion cell containing pituitary adenomas: signs of neuronal differentiation in adenoma cells. Acta Neuropathol. 112:21–8. PMID:16699777
1442. Kontogeorgos G, Sambaziotis D, Piaditis G, et al. (1997). Apoptosis in human pituitary adenomas: a morphologic and in situ end-labeling study. Mod Pathol. 10:921–6. PMID:9310956
1443. Kontogeorgos G, Scheithauer BW, Horvath E, et al. (1992). Double adenomas of the pituitary: a clinicopathological study of 11 tumors. Neurosurgery. 31:840–9, discussion 849. PMID:1331847
1444. Kontogeorgos G, Thodou E (2016). The gonadotroph origin of null cell adenomas. Hormones (Athens). 15:243–7. PMID:27376427
1445. Konukiewitz B, Enosawa T, Klöppel G (2011). Glucagon expression in cystic pancreatic neuroendocrine neoplasms: an immunohistochemical analysis. Virchows Arch. 458:47–53. PMID:20922407
1445A. Konukiewitz B, Schlitter AM, Jesinghaus M, et al. (2017). Somatostatin receptor expression related to TP53 and RB1 alterations in pancreatic and extrapancreatic neuroendocrine neoplasms with a Ki67-index above 20%. Mod Pathol. 30:587–98. PMID:28059098
1446. Koo JS, Hong S, Park CS (2009). Diffuse sclerosing variant is a major subtype of papillary thyroid carcinoma in the young. Thyroid. 19:1225–31. PMID:19888860
1447. Koo JS, Shin E, Hong SW (2010). Immunohistochemical characteristics of diffuse sclerosing variant of papillary carcinoma: comparison with conventional papillary carcinoma. APMIS. 118:744–52. PMID:20854468
1448. Kooijman CD (1988). Immature teratomas in children. Histopathology. 12:491–502. PMID:3397045
1449. Koperek O, Asari R, Niederle B, et al. (2011). Desmoplastic stromal reaction in papillary thyroid microcarcinoma. Histopathology. 58:919–24. PMID:21477259
1450. Koperek O, Scheuba C, Cherenko M, et al. (2008). Desmoplasia in medullary thyroid carcinoma: a reliable indicator of metastatic potential. Histopathology. 52:623–30. PMID:18370959
1451. Korbonits M (2015). Genetics of acromegaly. Endocr Rev. S01–1.
1452. Korbonits M, Chahal HS, Kaltsas G, et al. (2002). Expression of phosphorylated p27(Kip1) protein and Jun activation domain-binding protein 1 in human pituitary tumors. J Clin Endocrinol Metab. 87:2635–43. PMID:12050228
1453. Koren R, Bernheim J, Schachter P, et al. (2000). Black thyroid adenoma. Clinical, histochemical, and ultrastructural features. Appl Immunohistochem Mol Morphol. 8:80–4. PMID:10937053
1454. Korevaar TI, Grossman AB (2011). Pheochromocytomas and paragangliomas: assessment of malignant potential. Endocrine. 40:354–65. PMID:22038451
1455. Körner M, Waser B, Schonbrunn A, et al. (2012). Somatostatin receptor subtype 2A immunohistochemistry using a new monoclonal antibody selects tumors suitable for in vivo somatostatin receptor targeting. Am J Surg Pathol. 36:242–52. PMID:22251942
1456. Korpershoek E, Favier J, Gaal J, et al. (2011). SDHA immunohistochemistry detects germline SDHA gene mutations in apparently sporadic paragangliomas and pheochromocytomas. J Clin Endocrinol Metab. 96:E1472–6. PMID:21752896
1457. Korpershoek E, Petri BJ, Post E, et al. (2014). Adrenal medullary hyperplasia is a precursor lesion for pheochromocytoma in MEN2 syndrome. Neoplasia. 16:868–73. PMID:25379023
1458. Korpi-Hyövälti E, Cranston T, Ryhänen E, et al. (2014). CDC73 intragenic deletion in familial primary hyperparathyroidism associated with parathyroid carcinoma. J Clin Endocrinol Metab. 99:3044–8. PMID:24823466
1459. Kosary CL (2007). Cancer of the thyroid. In: Ries LAG, Young JL, Keel GE, et al., editors. SEER survival monograph: cancer survival among adults: U.S. SEER Program, 1998–2001, patient and tumor characteristics. NIH Pub. No. 07–6215. Bethesda: National Cancer Institute, SEER Program; pp 217–226.
1460. Kostoglou-Athanassiou I, Athanassiou P, Vecchini G, et al. (2004). Mixed medullary-follicular thyroid carcinoma. Report of a case and review of the literature. Horm Res. 61:300–4. PMID:15153799
1461. Koutourousiou M, Kontogeorgos G, Wesseling P, et al. (2010). Collision sellar lesions: experience with eight cases and review of the literature. Pituitary. 13:8–17. PMID:19551516
1462. Koutourousiou M, Seretis A, Kontogeorgos G (2009). Intra-sellar schwannoma co-existing with GH-secreting pituitary adenoma. Acta Neurochir (Wien). 151:1693–7. PMID:19350200
1463. Kovács GL, Góth M, Rotondo F, et al. (2013). ACTH-secreting Crooke cell carcinoma of the pituitary. Eur J Clin Invest. 43:20–6. PMID:23134557
1464. Kovacs K (1973). Metastatic cancer of the pituitary gland. Oncology. 27:533–42. PMID:4355105
1465. Kovacs K, Horvath E, Rewcastle NB, et al. (1980). Gonadotroph cell adenoma of the pituitary in a women with long-standing hypogonadism. Arch Gynecol. 229:57–65. PMID:7362277
1466. Kovacs K, Horvath E, Ryan N, et al. (1980). Null cell adenoma of the human pituitary. Virchows Arch A Pathol Anat Histol. 387:165–74. PMID:7456308
1467. Kovacs K, Horvath E, Thorner MO, et al. (1984). Mammosomatotroph hyperplasia associated with acromegaly and hyperprolactinemia in a patient with the McCune-Albright syndrome. A histologic, immunocytologic and ultrastructural study of the surgically-removed adenohypophysis. Virchows Arch A Pathol Anat Histopathol. 403:77–86. PMID:6426154
1468. Kovacs K, Ryan N, Horvath E, et al. (1980). Pituitary adenomas in old age. J Gerontol. 35:16–22. PMID:6243145
1469. Kovacs K, Scheithauer BW, Lombardero M, et al. (2008). MGMT immunoexpression predicts responsiveness of pituitary tumors to temozolomide therapy. Acta Neuropathol. 115:261–2. PMID:17926052
1470. Kovacs KA, Gay JD (1998). Remission of primary hyperparathyroidism due to spontaneous infarction of a parathyroid adenoma. Case report and review of the literature. Medicine (Baltimore). 77:398–402. PMID:9854603
1471. Kragel PJ, Johnston CA (1985). Pheochromocytoma-ganglioneuroma of the adrenal. Arch Pathol Lab Med. 109:470–2. PMID:3838664
1472. Krampitz GW, Norton JA (2013). Current management of the Zollinger-Ellison syndrome. Adv Surg. 47:59–79. PMID:24298844
1473. Krampitz GW, Norton JA (2014). RET gene mutations (genotype and phenotype) of multiple endocrine neoplasia type 2 and familial medullary thyroid carcinoma. Cancer. 120:1920–31. PMID:24699901
1474. Krausz Y, Freedman N, Rubinstein R, et al. (2011). ^{68}Ga-DOTA-NOC PET/CT imaging of neuroendocrine tumors: comparison with ^{111}In-DTPA-octreotide (OctreoScan®). Mol Imaging Biol. 13:583–93. PMID:20652423
1475. Krayenbühl N, Heppner F, Yonekawa Y, et al. (2007). Intrasellar malignant peripheral nerve sheath tumor (MPNST). Acta Neurochir (Wien). 149:201–5, discussion 205–6. PMID:17195046
1476. Krebs LJ, Shattuck TM, Arnold A (2005). HRPT2 mutational analysis of typical sporadic parathyroid adenomas. J Clin Endocrinol Metab. 90:5015–7. PMID:15956079
1477. Krgović K, Paunović I, Diklić A, et al. (2003). Follicular carcinoma of the thyroid gland. Acta Chir Iugosl. 50:107–11. [Serbian] PMID:15179765
1478. Krohn K, Führer D, Holzapfel HP, et al. (1998). Clonal origin of toxic thyroid nodules with constitutively activating thyrotropin receptor mutations. J Clin Endocrinol Metab. 83:130–4. PMID:9435429
1479. Krohn K, Maier J, Paschke R (2007). Mechanisms of disease: hydrogen peroxide, DNA damage and mutagenesis in the development of thyroid tumors. Nat Clin Pract Endocrinol Metab. 3:713–20. PMID:17893690
1480. Krohn K, Reske A, Ackermann F, et al. (2001). Ras mutations are rare in solitary cold and toxic thyroid nodules. Clin Endocrinol (Oxf). 55:241–8. PMID:11531932
1481. Kroll TG, Sarraf P, Pecciarini L, et al. (2000). PAX8-PPARgamma1 fusion oncogene in human thyroid carcinoma. Science. 289:1357–60. PMID:10958784 [Erratum in: Science. 2000;289:1474.]
1482. Krueger JE, Maitra A, Albores-Saavedra J (2000). Inherited medullary microcarcinoma of the thyroid: a study of 11 cases. Am J Surg Pathol. 24:853–8. PMID:10843288
1483. Kruijff S, Sidhu SB, Sywak MS, et al. (2014). Negative parafibromin staining predicts malignant behavior in atypical parathyroid adenomas. Ann Surg Oncol. 21:426–33. PMID:24081804
1484. Kuhel WI, Gonzales D, Hoda SA, et al. (2001). Synchronous water-clear cell double parathyroid adenomas a hitherto uncharacterized entity? Arch Pathol Lab Med. 125:256–9. PMID:11175646
1485. Kuhlen M, Hönscheid A, Schemme J, et al. (2016). Hodgkin lymphoma as a novel presentation of familial DICER1 syndrome. Eur J Pediatr. 175:593–7. PMID:26526666

1486. Kuhn E, Teller L, Piana S, et al. (2012). Different clonal origin of bilateral papillary thyroid carcinoma, with a review of the literature. Endocr Pathol. 23:101–7. PMID:22434481
1487. Kulaksiz H, Eissele R, Rössler D, et al. (2002). Identification of somatostatin receptor subtypes 1, 2A, 3, and 5 in neuroendocrine tumours with subtype specific antibodies. Gut. 50:52–60. PMID:11772967
1488. Kulig E, Jin L, Qian X, et al. (1999). Apoptosis in nontumorous and neoplastic human pituitaries: expression of the Bcl-2 family of proteins. Am J Pathol. 154:767–74. PMID:10079254
1489. Kulke MH, Anthony LB, Bushnell DL, et al. (NANETS) (2010). NANETS treatment guidelines: well-differentiated neuroendocrine tumors of the stomach and pancreas. Pancreas. 39:735–52. PMID:20664472
1490. Kulke MH, Hornick JL, Frauenhoffer C, et al. (2009). O6-methylguanine DNA methyltransferase deficiency and response to temozolomide-based therapy in patients with neuroendocrine tumors. Clin Cancer Res. 15:338–45. PMID:19118063
1491. Kuma S, Hirokawa M, Xu B, et al. (2004). Cribriform-morular variant of papillary thyroid carcinoma. Report of a case showing morules with peculiar nuclear clearing. Acta Cytol. 48:431–6. PMID:15192965
1492. Kumar K, Macaulay RJ, Kelly M, et al. (2001). Absent p53 immunohistochemical staining in a pituitary carcinoma. Can J Neurol Sci. 28:174–8. PMID:11383946
1493. Kumar PV, Torabinejad S, Omrani GH (1997). Osteoclastomalike anaplastic carcinoma of the thyroid gland diagnosed by fine needle aspiration cytology. Report of two cases. Acta Cytol. 41(4 Suppl):1345–8. PMID:9990272
1494. Kumar R, Gupta R, Khullar S, et al. (2000). Thyroid hemangioma: a case report with a review of the literature. Clin Nucl Med. 25:769–71. PMID:11043713
1495. Kumar S, Jayant K, Prasad S, et al. (2015). Rare adrenal gland emergencies: a case series of giant myelolipoma presenting with massive hemorrhage and abscess. Nephrourol Mon. 7:e22671. PMID:25738127
1496. Kumar S, Nanjappa B (2012). Giant benign adrenal adenoma. Urology. 80:e25–6. PMID:22840871
1497. Kunst HP, Rutten MH, de Mönnink JP, et al. (2011). SDHAF2 (PGL2-SDH5) and hereditary head and neck paraganglioma. Clin Cancer Res. 17:247–54. PMID:21224366
1498. Kunstman JW, Juhlin CC, Goh G, et al. (2015). Characterization of the mutational landscape of anaplastic thyroid cancer via whole-exome sequencing. Hum Mol Genet. 24:2318–29. PMID:25576899
1499. Kunwar S, Wilson CB (1999). Pediatric pituitary adenomas. J Clin Endocrinol Metab. 84:4385–9. PMID:10599692
1500. Kuper H, Boffetta P, Adami HO (2002). Tobacco use and cancer causation: association by tumour type. J Intern Med. 252:206–24. PMID:12270001
1501. Kurosaki M, Kambe A, Ishibashi M, et al. (2014). Case report of sarcoma of the sella caused by postoperative radiotherapy for a prolactin-producing pituitary adenoma. Brain Tumor Pathol. 31:187–91. PMID:24446079
1502. Kurosaki M, Saeger W, Lüdecke DK (2002). Intrasellar gangliocytomas associated with acromegaly. Brain Tumor Pathol. 19:63–7. PMID:12622135
1503. Kurtkaya-Yapicier O, Scheithauer BW, Carney JA, et al. (2002). Pituitary adenoma in Carney complex: an immunohistochemical, ultrastructural, and immunoelectron microscopic study. Ultrastruct Pathol. 26:345–53. PMID:12537759
1504. Kurzrock R, Sherman SI, Ball DW, et al. (2011). Activity of XL184 (Cabozantinib), an oral tyrosine kinase inhibitor, in patients with medullary thyroid cancer. J Clin Oncol. 29:2660–6. PMID:21606412
1505. Kusada N, Hara Y, Kobayashi S, et al. (2005). A case of aggressive carcinoma showing thymus-like differentiation with distant metastases. Thyroid. 15:1383–8. PMID:16405413
1506. Kwancharoen R, Blitz AM, Tavares F, et al. (2014). Clinical features of sellar and suprasellar meningiomas. Pituitary. 17:342–8. PMID:23975080
1507. Kwon MJ, Rho YS, Jeong JC, et al. (2015). Cribriform-morular variant of papillary thyroid carcinoma: a study of 3 cases featuring the PIK3CA mutation. Hum Pathol. 46:1180–8. PMID:26054797
1508. Kwon T, Jeong IG, Pak S, et al. (2014). Renal tumor size is an independent prognostic factor for overall survival in von Hippel-Lindau disease. J Cancer Res Clin Oncol. 140:1171–7. PMID:24671227
1509. Kwon Y, Hong EK, Koo HL, et al. (2006). Clinicopathological and immunohistochemical studies of thymic-related tumours in thyroid gland: report of five cases. Histopathology. 48:312–5. PMID:16430482
1510. Kytölä S, Farnebo F, Obara T, et al. (2000). Patterns of chromosomal imbalances in parathyroid carcinomas. Am J Pathol. 157:579–86. PMID:10934160
1511. La Rosa S, Adsay V, Albarello L, et al. (2012). Clinicopathologic study of 62 acinar cell carcinomas of the pancreas: insights into the morphology and immunophenotype and search for prognostic markers. Am J Surg Pathol. 36:1782–95. PMID:23026929
1512. La Rosa S, Franzi F, Albarello L, et al. (2011). Serotonin-producing enterochromaffin cell tumors of the pancreas: clinicopathologic study of 15 cases and comparison with intestinal enterochromaffin cell tumors. Pancreas. 40:883–95. PMID:21705949
1513. La Rosa S, Franzi F, Marchet S, et al. (2009). The monoclonal anti-BCL10 antibody (clone 331.1) is a sensitive and specific marker of pancreatic acinar cell carcinoma and pancreatic metaplasia. Virchows Arch. 454:133–42. PMID:19066953
1514. La Rosa S, Furlan D, Sessa F, et al. (2010). The endocrine pancreas. In: Lloyd RV, editor. Endocrine pathology: differential diagnosis and molecular advances. 2nd ed. New York: Springer-Verlag; pp. 367–413.
1515. La Rosa S, Pariani D, Calandra C, et al. (2013). Ectopic duodenal insulinoma: a very rare and challenging tumor type. Description of a case and review of the literature. Endocr Pathol. 24:213–9. PMID:24006218
1516. La Vecchia C, Malvezzi M, Bosetti C, et al. (2015). Thyroid cancer mortality and incidence: a global overview. Int J Cancer. 136:2187–95. PMID:25284703
1517. Lach B, Rippstein P, Benott BG, et al. (1996). Differentiating neuroblastoma of pituitary gland: neuroblastic transformation of epithelial adenoma cells. Case report. J Neurosurg. 85:953–60. PMID:8893739
1518. Lack EE (2008). Tumors of the adrenal glands and extraadrenal paraganglia. In: AFIP atlas of tumor pathology. Series 4, Fascicle 8. Washington DC: American Registry of Pathology Press.
1519. Lack EE, Delay S, Linnoila RI (1988). Ectopic parathyroid tissue within the vagus nerve. Incidence and possible clinical significance. Arch Pathol Lab Med. 112:304–6. PMID:3345129
1520. Ladroue C, Carcenac R, Leporrier M, et al. (2008). PHD2 mutation and congenital erythrocytosis with paraganglioma. N Engl J Med. 359:2685–92. PMID:19092153
1521. Ladurner D, Tötsch M, Luze T, et al. (1990). Malignant hemangioendothelioma of the thyroid gland. Pathology, clinical aspects and prognosis. Wien Klin Wochenschr. [German] 102:256–9. PMID:2375113
1522. Laforga JB, Aranda FI (2007). Pseudoangiosarcomatous features in medullary thyroid carcinoma spindle-cell variant. Report of a case studied by FNA and immunohistochemistry. Diagn Cytopathol. 35:424–8. PMID:17580345
1523. LaGuette J, Matias-Guiu X, Rosai J (1997). Thyroid paraganglioma: a clinicopathologic and immunohistochemical study of three cases. Am J Surg Pathol. 21:748–53. PMID:9236830
1524. Lai CY, Chao TC, Lin JD, et al. (2015). Sclerosing mucoepidermoid carcinoma with eosinophilia of thyroid gland in a male patient: a case report and literature review. Int J Clin Exp Pathol. 8:5947–51. PMID:26191325
1525. Lai JP, Mertens RB, Mirocha J, et al. (2015). Comparison of PAX6 and PAX8 as immunohistochemical markers for pancreatic neuroendocrine tumors. Endocr Pathol. 26:54–62. PMID:25433656
1526. Lai ML, Faa G, Serra S, et al. (2005). Rhabdoid tumor of the thyroid gland: a variant of anaplastic carcinoma. Arch Pathol Lab Med. 129:e55–7. PMID:15737050
1527. Lall RR, Shafizadeh SF, Lee KH, et al. (2013). Orbital metastasis of pituitary growth hormone secreting carcinoma causing lateral gaze palsy. Surg Neurol Int. 4:59. PMID:23646269
1528. Lam AK, Lo CY (2006). Diffuse sclerosing variant of papillary carcinoma of the thyroid: a 35-year comparative study at a single institution. Ann Surg Oncol. 13:176–81. PMID:16411146
1529. Lam AK, Lo CY, Lam KS (2005). Papillary carcinoma of thyroid: A 30-yr clinicopathological review of the histological variants. Endocr Pathol. 16:323–30. PMID:16627919
1530. Lam KY (1992). Adrenal tumours in Chinese. Virchows Arch A Pathol Anat Histopathol. 421:13–6. PMID:1636245
1531. Lam KY, Chan AC, Ng IO (1997). Giant adrenal lipoma: a report of two cases and review of literature. Scand J Urol Nephrol. 31:89–90. PMID:9060090
1532. Lam KY, Lo CY (1999). Composite Pheochromocytoma-Ganglioneuroma of the Adrenal Gland: An Uncommon Entity with Distinctive Clinicopathologic Features. Endocr Pathol. 10:343–52. PMID:12114771
1533. Lam KY, Lo CY (2001). Adrenal lipomatous tumours: a 30 year clinicopathological experience at a single institution. J Clin Pathol. 54:707–12. PMID:11533079
1534. Lam KY, Lo CY (2002). Metastatic tumours of the adrenal glands: a 30-year experience in a teaching hospital. Clin Endocrinol (Oxf). 56:95–101. PMID:11849252
1535. Lam KY, Lo CY, Chan KW, et al. (2000). Insular and anaplastic carcinoma of the thyroid: a 45-year comparative study at a single institution and a review of the significance of p53 and p21. Ann Surg. 231:329–38. PMID:10714625
1536. Lam KY, Lo CY, Liu MC (2001). Primary squamous cell carcinoma of the thyroid gland: an entity with aggressive clinical behaviour and distinctive cytokeratin expression profiles. Histopathology. 39:279–86. PMID:11532039
1537. Lam KY, Loong F, Shek TW, et al. (1998). Composite Paraganglioma-Ganglioneuroma of the Urinary Bladder: A Clinicopathologic, Immunohistochemical, and Ultrastructural Study of a Case and Review of the Literature. Endocr Pathol. 9:353–61. PMID:12114785
1538. Lam KY, Lui MC, Lo CY (2001). Cytokeratin expression profiles in thyroid carcinomas. Eur J Surg Oncol. 27:631–5. PMID:11669590
1539. Lamovec J, Zidar A, Zidanik B (1994). Epithelioid angiosarcoma of the thyroid gland. Report of two cases. Arch Pathol Lab Med. 118:642–6. PMID:8204012
1540. Lampertico P (1993). Anaplastic (sarcomatoid) carcinoma of the thyroid gland. Semin Diagn Pathol. 10:159–68. PMID:8367624
1541. Landa I, Ganly I, Chan TA, et al. (2013). Frequent somatic TERT promoter mutations in thyroid cancer: higher prevalence in advanced forms of the disease. J Clin Endocrinol Metab. 98:E1562–6. PMID:23833040
1542. Landa I, Ibrahimpasic T, Boucai L, et al. (2016). Genomic and transcriptomic hallmarks of poorly differentiated and anaplastic thyroid cancers. J Clin Invest. 126:1052–66. PMID:26878173
1543. Landis CA, Masters SB, Spada A, et al. (1989). GTPase inhibiting mutations activate the alpha chain of Gs and stimulate adenylyl cyclase in human pituitary tumours. Nature. 340:692–6. PMID:2549426
1544. Landman RE, Horwith M, Peterson RE, et al. (2002). Long-term survival with ACTH-secreting carcinoma of the pituitary: a case report and review of the literature. J Clin Endocrinol Metab. 87:3084–9. PMID:12107205
1545. Landon G, Ordóñez NG (1985). Clear cell variant of medullary carcinoma of the thyroid. Hum Pathol. 16:844–7. PMID:4018781
1545A. Landry CS, Wang TS, Asare EA et al. (2017). Parathyroid. In: AJCC Cancer Staging Manual, 8th Edition, Chapter 75, p. 903–910, edited by MB Amin. AJCC/Springer.
1546. Lang W, Borrusch H, Bauer L (1988). Occult carcinomas of the thyroid. Evaluation of 1,020 sequential autopsies. Am J Clin Pathol. 90:72–6. PMID:3389346
1547. Lang W, Georgii A, Stauch G, et al. (1980). The differentiation of atypical adenomas and encapsulated follicular carcinomas in the thyroid gland. Virchows Arch A Pathol Anat Histol. 385:125–41. PMID:7355566
1548. Langer P, Cupisti K, Bartsch DK, et al. (2002). Adrenal involvement in multiple endocrine neoplasia type 1. World J Surg. 26:891–6. PMID:12016472
1549. Langerman A, Athavale SM, Rangarajan SV, et al. (2012). Natural history of cervical paragangliomas: outcomes of observation of 43 patients. Arch Otolaryngol Head Neck Surg. 138:341–5. PMID:22431860
1550. Lapinski JE, Chen L, Zhou M (2010). Distinguishing clear cell renal cell carcinoma, retroperitoneal paraganglioma, and adrenal cortical lesions on limited biopsy material: utility of immunohistochemical markers. Appl Immunohistochem Mol Morphol. 18:414–21. PMID:20861762
1551. Larkin S, Reddy R, Karavitaki N, et al. (2013). Granulation pattern, but not GSP or GHR mutation, is associated with clinical characteristics in somatostatin-naive patients with somatotroph adenomas. Eur J Endocrinol. 168:491–9. PMID:23288882
1552. Larkin SJ, Preda V, Karavitaki N, et al. (2014). BRAF V600E mutations are characteristic for papillary craniopharyngioma and may coexist with CTNNB1-mutated adamantinomatous craniopharyngioma. Acta Neuropathol. 127:927–9. PMID:24715106
1553. Larsen SR, Godballe C, Krogdahl A (2010). Solitary fibrous tumor arising in an intrathoracic goiter. Thyroid. 20:435–7. PMID:20373988
1554. Larson RS, Wick MR (1993). Primary mucoepidermoid carcinoma of the thyroid: diagnosis by fine-needle aspiration biopsy. Diagn Cytopathol. 9:438–43. PMID:8261851
1555. Larsson C, Skogseid B, Oberg K, et al. (1988). Multiple endocrine neoplasia type 1 gene maps to chromosome 11 and is lost in insulinoma. Nature. 332:85–7. PMID:2894610
1556. Lassalle S, Hofman V, Ilie M, et al. (2011). Can the microRNA signature distinguish between thyroid tumors of uncertain malignant potential and other well-differentiated tumors of the thyroid gland? Endocr Relat Cancer. 18:579–94. PMID:21778212

1557. Lastoria S, Marciello F, Faggiano A, et al. (2016). Role of (68)Ga-DOTATATE PET/CT in patients with multiple endocrine neoplasia type 1 (MEN1). Endocrine. 52:488–94. PMID:26242621
1558. Lattin GE Jr, Sturgill ED, Tujo CA, et al. (2014). From the radiologic pathology archives: Adrenal tumors and tumor-like conditions in the adult: radiologic-pathologic correlation. Radiographics. 34:805–29. PMID:24819798
1559. Lau Q, Scheithauer B, Kovacs K, et al. (2010). MGMT immunoexpression in aggressive pituitary adenoma and carcinoma. Pituitary. 13:367–79. PMID:20740317
1560. Lau SK, Spagnolo DV, Weiss LM (2006). Schwannoma of the adrenal gland: report of two cases. Am J Surg Pathol. 30:630–4. PMID:16699318
1560A. Lau SK, Weiss LM (2009). The Weiss system for evaluating adrenocortical neoplasms: 25 years later. Hum Pathol. 40(6):757–68. PMID:19442788
1561. Laug WE, Siegel SE, Shaw KN, et al. (1978). Initial urinary catecholamine metabolite concentrations and prognosis in neuroblastoma. Pediatrics. 62:77–83. PMID:683787
1562. Laurell C, Velázquez-Fernández D, Lindsten K, et al. (2009). Transcriptional profiling enables molecular classification of adrenocortical tumours. Eur J Endocrinol. 161:141–52. PMID:19411298
1563. Laury AR, Bongiovanni M, Tille JC, et al. (2011). Thyroid pathology in PTEN-hamartoma tumor syndrome: characteristic findings of a distinct entity. Thyroid. 21:135–44. PMID:21190448
1564. Lawrence B, Gustafsson BI, Chan A, et al. (2011). The epidemiology of gastroenteropancreatic neuroendocrine tumors. Endocrinol Metab Clin North Am. 40:1–18, vii. PMID:21349409
1565. Le Bodic MF, Heymann MF, Lecomte M, et al. (1996). Immunohistochemical study of 100 pancreatic tumors in 28 patients with multiple endocrine neoplasia, type I. Am J Surg Pathol. 20:1378–84. PMID:8898842
1566. Leath CA 3rd, Huh WK, Straughn JM Jr, et al. (2002). Uterine leiomyosarcoma metastatic to the thyroid. Obstet Gynecol. 100(5 Pt 2):1122–4. PMID:12423830
1567. Lecomte-Houcke M, Parent M, Carnaille B, et al. (1992). Primary malignant teratoma of the thyroid. Two cases involving immunohistochemical and ultrastructural studies. Ann Pathol. 12:12–9. [French] PMID:1580935
1568. Lee DH, Kang WJ, Seo HS, et al. (2009). Detection of metastatic cervical lymph nodes in recurrent papillary thyroid carcinoma: computed tomography versus positron emission tomography-computed tomography. J Comput Assist Tomogr. 33:805–10. PMID:19820516
1569. Lee DH, Lee GK, Kong SY, et al. (2007). Epidermal growth factor receptor status in anaplastic thyroid carcinoma. J Clin Pathol. 60:881–4. PMID:17079354
1570. Lee EB, Tihan T, Scheithauer BW, et al. (2009). Thyroid transcription factor 1 expression in sellar tumors: a histogenetic marker? J Neuropathol Exp Neurol. 68:482–8. PMID:19525896
1571. Lee FY, Jan YJ, Chou G, et al. (2007). Thyroid involvement in Rosai-Dorfman disease. Thyroid. 17:471–6. PMID:17542678
1572. Lee J, Yun JS, Nam KH, et al. (2007). Huge cavernous hemangioma of the thyroid gland. Thyroid. 17:375–6. PMID:17465872
1573. Lee JH, Barich F, Karnell LH, et al. (2002). National Cancer Data Base report on malignant paragangliomas of the head and neck. Cancer. 94:730–7. PMID:11857306
1574. Lee JI, Chung YJ, Park SJ, et al. (2012). Euthyroid status after total thyroidectomy due to functioning lung metastases from a clear cell variant of papillary thyroid carcinoma. Thyroid. 22:1084–7. PMID:22873179
1575. Lee M, Pellegata NS (2013). Multiple endocrine neoplasia syndromes associated with mutation of p27. J Endocrinol Invest. 36:781–7. PMID:23800691
1576. Lee M, Pellegata NS (2013). Multiple endocrine neoplasia type 4. Front Horm Res. 41:63–78. PMID:23652671
1577. Lee PK, Jarosek SL, Virnig BA, et al. (2007). Trends in the incidence and treatment of parathyroid cancer in the United States. Cancer. 109:1736–41. PMID:17372919
1578. Lee S, Han BK, Ko EY, et al. (2011). The ultrasonography features of hyalinizing trabecular tumor of the thyroid are more consistent with its benign behavior than cytology or frozen section readings. Thyroid. 21:253–9. PMID:21190434
1579. Lee S, Hong SW, Shin SJ, et al. (2004). Papillary thyroid carcinoma associated with familial adenomatous polyposis: molecular analysis of pathogenesis in a family and review of the literature. Endocr J. 51:317–23. PMID:15256777
1580. Lee SW, Shin EA, Kwon KW, et al. (2009). Primary lymphangioma of the thyroid gland. Thyroid. 19:915–6. PMID:19500020
1581. Lee WS, Koh YS, Kim JC, et al. (2005). Zollinger-Ellison syndrome associated with neurofibromatosis type 1: a case report. BMC Cancer. 5:85. PMID:16042772
1582. Lee YY, Wang WC, Li CF (2015). Aspiration cytology of an ectopic cervical thymoma misinterpreted as a lymphoproliferative lesion of the thyroid: A case report. Oncol Lett. 10:1255–8. PMID:26622659
1583. Leet AI, Chebli C, Kushner H, et al. (2004). Fracture incidence in polyostotic fibrous dysplasia and the McCune-Albright syndrome. J Bone Miner Res. 19:571–7. PMID:15005844
1584. Lefebvre M, Foulkes WD (2014). Pheochromocytoma and paraganglioma syndromes: genetics and management update. Curr Oncol. 21:e8–17. PMID:24523625
1585. Lehman NL, Horoupian DS, Harsh GR 4th (2003). Synchronous subarachnoid drop metastases from a pituitary adenoma with multiple recurrences. Case report. J Neurosurg. 98:1120–3. PMID:12744376
1586. Lemoine NR, Mayall ES, Wyllie FS, et al. (1989). High frequency of ras oncogene activation in all stages of human thyroid tumorigenesis. Oncogene. 4:159–64. PMID:2648253
1587. Lenders JW, Duh QY, Eisenhofer G, et al. (2014). Pheochromocytoma and paraganglioma: an endocrine society clinical practice guideline. J Clin Endocrinol Metab. 99:1915–42. PMID:24893135
1588. Lenders JW, Eisenhofer G, Mannelli M, et al. (2005). Phaeochromocytoma. Lancet. 366:665–75. PMID:16112304
1589. Lenggenhager D, Maggio EM, Moch H, et al. (2013). HBME-1 expression in hyalinizing trabecular tumours of the thyroid gland. Histopathology. 62:1092–7. PMID:23617709
1590. Leonardo E, Volante M, Barbareschi M, et al. (2007). Cell membrane reactivity of MIB-1 antibody to Ki67 in human tumors: fact or artifact? Appl Immunohistochem Mol Morphol. 15:220–3. PMID:17525638
1591. Leoncini E, Carioli G, La Vecchia C, et al. (2016). Risk factors for neuroendocrine neoplasms: a systematic review and meta-analysis. Ann Oncol. 27:68–81. PMID:26487581
1592. Leong AS, Chawla JC, Teh EC (1976). Pituitary thyrotropic tumour secondary to long-standing primary hypothyroidism. Pathol Eur. 11:49–55. PMID:934699
1593. Leontiou CA, Gueorguiev M, van der Spuy J, et al. (2008). The role of the aryl hydrocarbon receptor-interacting protein gene in familial and sporadic pituitary adenomas. J Clin Endocrinol Metab. 93:2390–401. PMID:18381572
1594. Lepage C, Rachet B, Coleman MP (2007). Survival from malignant digestive endocrine tumors in England and Wales: a population-based study. Gastroenterology. 132:899–904. PMID:17383419
1595. Letouzé E, Martinelli C, Loriot C, et al. (2013). SDH mutations establish a hypermethylator phenotype in paraganglioma. Cancer Cell. 23:739–52. PMID:23707781
1596. Levin KE, Galante M, Clark OH (1987). Parathyroid carcinoma versus parathyroid adenoma in patients with profound hypercalcemia. Surgery. 101:649–60. PMID:3589961
1597. Levy A, Hall L, Yeudall WA, et al. (1994). p53 gene mutations in pituitary adenomas: rare events. Clin Endocrinol (Oxf). 41:809–14. PMID:7889618
1598. Levy MT, Braun JT, Pennant M, et al. (2010). Primary paraganglioma of the parathyroid: a case report and clinicopathologic review. Head Neck Pathol. 4:37–43. PMID:20237987
1599. Levy RA, Hui VW, Sood R, et al. (2014). Cribriform-morular variant of papillary thyroid carcinoma: an indication to screen for occult FAP. Fam Cancer. 13:547–51. PMID:24934245
1600. Li C, Lee KC, Schneider EB, et al. (2012). BRAF V600E mutation and its association with clinicopathological features of papillary thyroid cancer: a meta-analysis. J Clin Endocrinol Metab. 97:4559–70. PMID:23055546
1601. Li H, Hes O, MacLennan GT, et al. (2015). Immunohistochemical distinction of metastases of renal cell carcinoma to the adrenal from primary adrenal nodules, including oncocytic tumor. Virchows Arch. 466:581–8. PMID:25690138
1602. Li JY, Racadot O, Kujas M, et al. (1989). Immunocytochemistry of four mixed pituitary adenomas and intrasellar gangliocytomas associated with different clinical syndromes: acromegaly, amenorrhea-galactorrhea, Cushing's disease and isolated tumoral syndrome. Acta Neuropathol. 77:320–8. PMID:2922994
1603. Li M, Carcangiu ML, Rosai J (1997). Abnormal intracellular and extracellular distribution of basement membrane material in papillary carcinoma and hyalinizing trabecular tumors of the thyroid: implication for deregulation of secretory pathways. Hum Pathol. 28:1366–72. PMID:9416692
1604. Li M, Song J, Pytel P (2014). Expression of HIF-1 regulated proteins vascular endothelial growth factor, carbonic anhydrase IX and hypoxia inducible gene 2 in hemangioblastomas. Folia Neuropathol. 52:234–42. PMID:25310734
1605. Li SQ, Zhang YS, Shi J, et al. (2015). Clinical features and retroperitoneal laparoscopic resection of adrenal schwannoma in 19 patients. Endocr Pract. 21:323–9. PMID:25932565
1606. Li X, Su J, Zhao L, et al. (2014). Familial Cushing syndrome due to thymic carcinoids in a multiple endocrine neoplasia type 1 kindred. Endocrine. 47:183–90. PMID:24452869
1607. Li ZJ, Sun P, Guo Y, et al. (2010). Primary pituitary fibrosarcoma presenting with multiple metastases: a case report and literature review. Neurol India. 58:316–8. PMID:20508360
1608. Liang J, Shao SH, Xu ZX, et al. (2007). The energy sensing LKB1-AMPK pathway regulates p27(kip1) phosphorylation mediating the decision to enter autophagy or apoptosis. Nat Cell Biol. 9:218–24. PMID:17237771
1609. Liao S, Song W, Liu Y, et al. (2013). Familial multinodular goiter syndrome with papillary thyroid carcinomas: mutational analysis of the associated genes in 5 cases from 1 Chinese family. BMC Endocr Disord. 13:48. PMID:24144365
1610. Libé R, Borget I, Ronchi CL, et al. (2015). Prognostic factors in stage III-IV adrenocortical carcinomas (ACC): an European Network for the Study of Adrenal Tumor (ENSAT) study. Ann Oncol. 26:2119–25. PMID:26392430
1611. Libè R, Dall'Asta C, Barbetta L, et al. (2002). Long-term follow-up study of patients with adrenal incidentalomas. Eur J Endocrinol. 147:489–94. PMID:12370111
1612. Libutti SK, Crabtree JS, Lorang D, et al. (2003). Parathyroid gland-specific deletion of the mouse Men1 gene results in parathyroid neoplasia and hypercalcemic hyperparathyroidism. Cancer Res. 63:8022–8. PMID:14633735
1613. Lichtenauer UD, Di Dalmazi G, Slater EP, et al. (2015). Frequency and clinical correlates of somatic Ying Yang 1 mutations in sporadic insulinomas. J Clin Endocrinol Metab. 100:E776–82. PMID:25763608
1614. Lidhar K, Korbonits M, Jordan S, et al. (1999). Low expression of the cell cycle inhibitor p27Kip1 in normal corticotroph cells, corticotroph tumors, and malignant pituitary tumors. J Clin Endocrinol Metab. 84:3823–30. PMID:10523037
1615. Lièvre A, Leboulleux S, Boige V, et al. (2006). Thyroid metastases from colorectal cancer: the Institut Gustave Roussy experience. Eur J Cancer. 42:1756–9. PMID:16762542
1616. Lifante JC, Blanchard C, Mirallié E, et al. (2014). Role of preoperative basal calcitonin levels in the timing of prophylactic thyroidectomy in patients with germline RET mutations. World J Surg. 38:576–81. PMID:24357249
1617. Ligneau B, Lombard-Bohas C, Partensky C, et al. (2001). Cystic endocrine tumors of the pancreas: clinical, radiologic, and histopathologic features in 13 cases. Am J Surg Pathol. 25:752–60. PMID:11395552
1618. Lim JS, Ku CR, Lee MK, et al. (2010). A case of fugitive acromegaly, initially presented as invasive prolactinoma. Endocrine. 38:1–5. PMID:20960094
1619. Lim S, Shahinian H, Maya MM, et al. (2006). Temozolomide: a novel treatment for pituitary carcinoma. Lancet Oncol. 7:518–20. PMID:16750503
1620. Lima J, Feijão T, Ferreira da Silva A, et al. (2007). High frequency of germline succinate dehydrogenase mutations in sporadic cervical paragangliomas in northern Spain: mitochondrial succinate dehydrogenase structure-function relationships and clinical-pathological correlations. J Clin Endocrinol Metab. 92:4853–64. PMID:17848412
1621. Lin BT, Bonsib SM, Mierau GW, et al. (1998). Oncocytic adrenocortical neoplasms: a report of seven cases and review of the literature. Am J Surg Pathol. 22:603–14. PMID:9591731
1622. Lin HW, Shih SR, Yao M, et al. (2012). Relapse of acute myeloid leukemia at the pituitary gland: a case report and review of literature. Endocr Pathol. 23:172–6. PMID:22527946
1623. Lin JH, Tsai DH, Chiang YH (2009). A primary sellar esthesioneuroblastomas with unusual presentations: a case report and reviews of literatures. Pituitary. 12:70–5. PMID:18176843
1624. Lin MW, Wu CT, Lee YH, et al. (2014). Intrathoracic thyroid solitary fibrous tumor presenting with respiratory failure. Ann Thorac Cardiovasc Surg. 20 Suppl:427–9. PMID:23445791
1625. Lin O, Gerhard R, Coelho Siqueira SA, et al. (2002). Cytologic findings of epithelioid angiosarcoma of the thyroid. A case report. Acta Cytol. 46:767–71. PMID:12146050
1626. Lin X, Zhu B, Liu Y, et al. (2010). Follicular thyroid carcinoma invades venous rather than lymphatic vessels. Diagn Pathol. 5:8. PMID:20205756
1627. Lindboe CF, Unsgård G, Myhr G, et al. (1993). ACTH and TSH producing ectopic suprasellar pituitary adenoma of the hypothalamic region: case report. Clin Neuropathol. 12:138–41. PMID:8391955
1628. Linnoila RI, Keiser HR, Steinberg SM, et al. (1990). Histopathology of benign versus malignant sympathoadrenal paragangliomas: clinicopathologic study of 120

cases including unusual histologic features. Hum Pathol. 21:1168–80. PMID:2172151
1629. Lino-Silva LS, Domínguez-Malagón HR, Caro-Sánchez CH, et al. (2012). Thyroid gland papillary carcinomas with "micropapillary pattern," a recently recognized poor prognostic finding: clinicopathologic and survival analysis of 7 cases. Hum Pathol. 43:1596–600. PMID:22425190
1630. Listernick R, Charrow J, Greenwald M, et al. (1994). Natural history of optic pathway tumors in children with neurofibromatosis type 1: a longitudinal study. J Pediatr. 125:63–6. PMID:8021787
1631. Liu H, Shi J, Wilkerson M, et al. (2013). Immunohistochemical evaluation of ERG expression in various benign and malignant tissues. Ann Clin Lab Sci. 43:3–9. PMID:23462600
1632. Liu J, Singh B, Tallini G, et al. (2006). Follicular variant of papillary thyroid carcinoma: a clinicopathologic study of a problematic entity. Cancer. 107:1255–64. PMID:16900519
1633. Liu JK, Couldwell WT (2004). Contemporary management of prolactinomas. Neurosurg Focus. 16:E2. PMID:15191331
1634. Liu R, Xing M (2016). TERT promoter mutations in thyroid cancer. Endocr Relat Cancer. 23:R143–55. PMID:26733501
1635. Liu S, Tian Y, Chlenski A, et al. (2005). Cross-talk between Schwann cells and neuroblasts influences the biology of neuroblastoma xenografts. Am J Pathol. 166:891–900. PMID:15743800
1636. Liu TC, Hamilton N, Hawkins W, et al. (2013). Comparison of WHO Classifications (2004, 2010), the Hochwald grading system, and AJCC and ENETS staging systems in predicting prognosis in locoregional well-differentiated pancreatic neuroendocrine tumors. Am J Surg Pathol. 37:853–9. PMID:23598967
1637. Liu W, Asa SL, Ezzat S (2002). Vitamin D and its analog EB1089 induce p27 accumulation and diminish association of p27 with Skp2 independent of PTEN in pituitary corticotroph cells. Brain Pathol. 12:412–9. PMID:12408227
1638. Liu X, Bishop J, Shan Y, et al. (2013). Highly prevalent TERT promoter mutations in aggressive thyroid cancers. Endocr Relat Cancer. 20:603–10. PMID:23766237
1639. Liu Y, Chotai S, Ming C, et al. (2014). Characteristics of midline suprasellar meningiomas based on their origin and growth pattern. Clin Neurol Neurosurg. 125:173–81. PMID:25171391
1640. Liu Y, Yao Y, Xing B, et al. (2015). Prolactinomas in children under 14. Clinical presentation and long-term follow-up. Childs Nerv Syst. 31:909–16. PMID:25771923
1641. Liu YQ, Zhang HX, Wang GL, et al. (2010). A giant cystic adenomatoid tumor of the adrenal gland: a case report. Chin Med J (Engl). 123:372–4. PMID:20193264
1642. Liu Z, Hou P, Ji M, et al. (2008). Highly prevalent genetic alterations in receptor tyrosine kinases and phosphatidylinositol 3-kinase/akt and mitogen-activated protein kinase pathways in anaplastic and follicular thyroid cancers. J Clin Endocrinol Metab. 93:3106–16. PMID:18492751
1643. Liu Z, Teng XY, Sun DX, et al. (2013). Clinical analysis of thyroid carcinoma showing thymus-like differentiation: report of 8 cases. Int Surg. 98:95–100. PMID:23701142
1644. Liu Z, Zhou G, Nakamura M, et al. (2011). Encapsulated follicular thyroid tumor with equivocal nuclear changes, so-called well-differentiated tumor of uncertain malignant potential: a morphological, immunohistochemical, and molecular appraisal. Cancer Sci. 102:288–94. PMID:21070478
1645. LiVolsi VA (1992). Papillary neoplasms of the thyroid. Pathologic and prognostic features. Am J Clin Pathol. 97:426–34. PMID:1543168
1646. LiVolsi VA (1997). C cell hyperplasia/neoplasia. J Clin Endocrinol Metab. 82:39–41. PMID:8989229
1647. LiVolsi VA, Abrosimov AA, Bogdanova T, et al. (2011). The Chernobyl thyroid cancer experience: pathology. Clin Oncol (R Coll Radiol). 23:261–7. PMID:21333507
1648. LiVolsi VA, Asa SL (1994). The demise of follicular carcinoma of the thyroid gland. Thyroid. 4:233–6. PMID:7920009
1649. Livolsi VA, Feind CR (1979). Incidental medullary thyroid carcinoma in sporadic hyperparathyroidism. An expansion of the concept of C-cell hyperplasia. Am J Clin Pathol. 71:595–9. PMID:377940
1650. LiVolsi VA, LoGerfo P, Feind CR (1978). Coexistent parathyroid adenomas and thyroid carcinoma. Can radiation be blamed? Arch Surg. 113:285–6. PMID:637693
1651. LiVolsi VA, Merino MJ (1994). Worrisome histologic alterations following fine-needle aspiration of the thyroid (WHAFFT). Pathol Annu. 29(Pt 2):99–120. PMID:7936753
1652. Lloyd RV (1987). Use of molecular probes in the study of endocrine diseases. Hum Pathol. 18:1199–211. PMID:2445649
1653. Lloyd RV, Blaivas M, Wilson BS (1985). Distribution of chromogranin and S100 protein in normal and abnormal adrenal medullary tissues. Arch Pathol Lab Med. 109:633–5. PMID:3839362
1654. Lloyd RV, Chandler WF, Kovacs K, et al. (1986). Ectopic pituitary adenomas with normal anterior pituitary glands. Am J Surg Pathol. 10:546–52. PMID:3017137
1655. Lloyd RV, Erickson LA, Casey MB, et al. (2004). Observer variation in the diagnosis of follicular variant of papillary thyroid carcinoma. Am J Surg Pathol. 28:1336–40. PMID:15371949
1656. Lloyd RV, Mervak T, Schmidt K, et al. (1984). Immunohistochemical detection of chromogranin and neuron-specific enolase in pancreatic endocrine neoplasms. Am J Surg Pathol. 8:607–14. PMID:6205601
1657. Lloyd RV, Osamura RY (1997). Transcription factors in normal and neoplastic pituitary tissues. Microsc Res Tech. 39:168–81. PMID:9361268
1658. Lloyd RV, Scheithauer BW, Kuroki T, et al. (1999). Vascular Endothelial Growth Factor (VEGF) Expression in Human Pituitary Adenomas and Carcinomas. Endocr Pathol. 10:229–35. PMID:12114703
1659. Lo CP, Chen CY, Lin CK, et al. (2004). Parasellar solitary fibrous tumor of meninges: magnetic resonance imaging features with pathologic correlation. J Neuroimaging. 14:281–4. PMID:15228772
1660. Lodewijk L, Bongers PJ, Kist JW, et al. (2015). Thyroid incidentalomas in patients with multiple endocrine neoplasia type 1. Eur J Endocrinol. 172:337–42. PMID:25572387
1661. Lodish MB, Trivellin G, Stratakis CA (2016). Pituitary gigantism: update on molecular biology and management. Curr Opin Endocrinol Diabetes Obes. 23:72–80. PMID:26574647
1662. Loehry CA, Kingham JG, Whorwell PJ (1975). Watery diarrhoea and hypokalaemia associated with a phaeochromocytoma. Postgrad Med J. 51:416–9. PMID:175362
1663. Loh KC, Greenspan FS, Gee L, et al. (1997). Pathological tumor-node-metastasis (pTNM) staging for papillary and follicular thyroid carcinomas: a retrospective analysis of 700 patients. J Clin Endocrinol Metab. 82:3553–62. PMID:9360506
1664. Lollar K, Farrag TY, Cao D, et al. (2008). Langerhans cell histiocytosis of the thyroid gland. Am J Otolaryngol. 29:201–4. PMID:18439957
1665. Lombardi CP, Raffaelli M, Pani G, et al. (2006). Gene expression profiling of adrenal cortical tumors by cDNA macroarray analysis. Results of a preliminary study. Biomed Pharmacother. 60:186–90. PMID:16677799
1666. London WB, Castleberry RP, Matthay KK, et al. (2005). Evidence for an age cutoff greater than 365 days for neuroblastoma risk group stratification in the Children's Oncology Group. J Clin Oncol. 23:6459–65. PMID:16116153
1667. Lonser RR, Kindzelski BA, Mehta GU, et al. (2010). Acromegaly without imaging evidence of pituitary adenoma. J Clin Endocrinol Metab. 95:4192–6. PMID:20610592
1668. Look AT, Hayes FA, Nitschke R, et al. (1984). Cellular DNA content as a predictor of response to chemotherapy in infants with unresectable neuroblastoma. N Engl J Med. 311:231–5. PMID:6738617
1669. Lopes MB, Lanzino G, Cloft HJ, et al. (1998). Primary fibrosarcoma of the sella unrelated to previous radiation therapy. Mod Pathol. 11:579–84. PMID:9647597
1670. López CL, Langer P, Waldmann J, et al. (2013). Shortness: an unknown phenotype of multiple endocrine neoplasia type 1. Eur J Endocrinol. 169:133–7. PMID:23828958
1671. Lopez JA, Kleinschmidt-Demasters Bk Bk, Sze CI, et al. (2004). Silent corticotroph adenomas: further clinical and pathological observations. Hum Pathol. 35:1137–47. PMID:15343517
1672. López JI, Gaafar A, Garmendia M, et al. (2008). Sclerosing mucoepidermoid carcinoma of the thyroid gland: cytohistological findings of a case. Hematol Oncol Stem Cell Ther. 1:62–5. PMID:20063531
1673. Lorenzo FR, Yang C, Ng Tang Fui M, et al. (2013). A novel EPAS1/HIF2A germline mutation in a congenital polycythemia with paraganglioma. J Mol Med (Berl). 91:507–12. PMID:23090011
1674. Louis DN, Ohgaki H, Wiestler OD, et al. (2016). WHO Classification of Tumours of the Central Nervous System. Revised 4th edition. IARC: Lyon 2016. ISBN: 978-92-832-4492-9
1674A. Louis DN, Ohgaki H, Wiestler OD, et al. (2016). The 2016 World Health Organization classification of tumors of the central nervous system: a summary. Acta Neuropathol. 131:803–20. PMID: 27157931
1675. Lowery MA, Klimstra DS, Shia J, et al. (2011). Acinar cell carcinoma of the pancreas: new genetic and treatment insights into a rare malignancy. Oncologist. 16:1714–20. PMID:22042785
1676. Lubensky IA, Debelenko LV, Zhuang Z, et al. (1996). Allelic deletions on chromosome 11q13 in multiple tumors from individual MEN1 patients. Cancer Res. 56:5272–8. PMID:8912868
1677. Lubensky IA, Gnarra JR, Bertheau P, et al. (1996). Allelic deletions of the VHL gene detected in multiple microscopic clear cell renal lesions in von Hippel-Lindau disease patients. Am J Pathol. 149:2089–94. PMID:8952541
1678. Lubensky IA, Pack S, Ault D, et al. (1998). Multiple neuroendocrine tumors of the pancreas in von Hippel-Lindau disease patients: histopathological and molecular genetic analysis. Am J Pathol. 153:223–31. PMID:9665483
1679. Lubitz CC, Economopoulos KP, Pawlak AC, et al. (2014). Hobnail variant of papillary thyroid carcinoma: an institutional case series and molecular profile. Thyroid. 24:958–65. PMID:24417340
1680. Luboshitzky R, Dharan M (2004). Mixed follicular-medullary thyroid carcinoma: a case report. Diagn Cytopathol. 30:122–4. PMID:14755766
1681. Lucas DG Jr, Lockett MA, Cole DJ (2002). Spontaneous infarction of a parathyroid adenoma: two case reports and review of the literature. Am Surg. 68:173–6. PMID:11842966
1682. Luchetti A, Walsh D, Rodger F, et al. (2015). Profiling of somatic mutations in phaeochromocytoma and paraganglioma by targeted next generation sequencing analysis. Int J Endocrinol. 2015:138573. PMID:25883647
1683. Lüdecke D, Kautzky R, Saeger W, et al. (1976). Selective removal of hypersecreting pituitary adenomas? An analysis of endocrine function, operative and microscopical findings in 101 cases. Acta Neurochir (Wien). 35:27–42. PMID:183463
1684. Ludvíková M, Ryska A, Korabecná M, et al. (2001). Oncocytic papillary carcinoma with lymphoid stroma (Warthin-like tumour) of the thyroid: a distinct entity with favourable prognosis. Histopathology. 39:17–24. PMID:11454040
1685. Lughezzani G, Sun M, Perrotte P, et al. (2010). The European Network for the Study of Adrenal Tumors staging system is prognostically superior to the international union against cancer-staging system: a North American validation. Eur J Cancer. 46:713–9. PMID:20044246
1686. Lugli A, Forster Y, Haas P, et al. (2003). Calretinin expression in human normal and neoplastic tissues: a tissue microarray analysis on 5233 tissue samples. Hum Pathol. 34:994–1000. PMID:14608532
1687. Lugli A, Terracciano LM, Oberholzer M, et al. (2004). Macrofollicular variant of papillary carcinoma of the thyroid: a histologic, cytologic, and immunohistochemical study of 3 cases and review of the literature. Arch Pathol Lab Med. 128:54–8. PMID:14692811
1688. Lui WO, Zeng L, Rehrmann V, et al. (2008). CREB3L2-PPARgamma fusion mutation identifies a thyroid signaling pathway regulated by intramembrane proteolysis. Cancer Res. 68:7156–64. PMID:18757431
1689. Lumbroso S, Paris F, Sultan C, et al. (2004). Activating Gsalpha mutations: analysis of 113 patients with signs of McCune-Albright syndrome–a European Collaborative Study. J Clin Endocrinol Metab. 89:2107–13. PMID:15126527
1690. Luna IE, Monrad N, Binderup T, et al. (2016). Somatostatin-immunoreactive pancreaticoduodenal neuroendocrine neoplasms: twenty-three cases evaluated according to the WHO 2010 classification. Neuroendocrinology. 103:567–77. PMID:26505735
1691. Lupi C, Giannini R, Ugolini C, et al. (2007). Association of BRAF V600E mutation with poor clinicopathological outcomes in 500 consecutive cases of papillary thyroid carcinoma. J Clin Endocrinol Metab. 92:4085–90. PMID:17785355
1692. Lupoli G, Vitale G, Caraglia M, et al. (1999). Familial papillary thyroid microcarcinoma: a new clinical entity. Lancet. 353:637–9. PMID:10030330
1693. Luton JP, Cerdas S, Billaud L, et al. (1990). Clinical features of adrenocortical carcinoma, prognostic factors, and the effect of mitotane therapy. N Engl J Med. 322:1195–201. PMID:2325710
1694. Luze T, Tötsch M, Bangerl I, et al. (1990). Fine needle aspiration cytodiagnosis of anaplastic carcinoma and malignant haemangioendothelioma of the thyroid in an endemic goitre area. Cytopathology. 1:305–10. PMID:2101676
1695. Luzi P, Miracco C, Lio R, et al. (1987). Endocrine inactive pituitary carcinoma metastasizing to cervical lymph nodes: a case report. Hum Pathol. 18:90–2. PMID:3817801
1696. Ma W, Ikeda H, Yoshimoto T (2002). Clinicopathologic study of 123 cases of prolactin-secreting pituitary adenomas with special reference to multihormone production and clonality of the adenomas. Cancer. 95:258–66. PMID:12124824
1697. Ma X, Xia C, Liu H, et al. (2015). Primary thyroid spindle cell tumors: spindle cell variant of papillary thyroid carcinoma? Int J Clin Exp Pathol. 8:13528–31. PMID:26722568
1698. Ma ZY, Song ZJ, Chen JH, et al. (2015). Recurrent gain-of-function USP8 mutations in Cushing's disease. Cell Res. 25:306–17. PMID:25675982

1699. Maartens NF, Ellegala DB, Vance ML, et al. (2003). Intrasellar schwannomas: report of two cases. Neurosurgery. 52:1200–5, discussion 1205–6. PMID:12699566
1700. Machens A, Dralle H (2010). Biomarker-based risk stratification for previously untreated medullary thyroid cancer. J Clin Endocrinol Metab. 95:2655–63. PMID:20339026
1701. Machens A, Lorenz K, Dralle H (2013). Peak incidence of pheochromocytoma and primary hyperparathyroidism in multiple endocrine neoplasia 2: need for age-adjusted biochemical screening. J Clin Endocrinol Metab. 98:E336–45. PMID:23284010
1702. Machens A, Niccoli-Sire P, Hoegel J, et al. (EUROMEN) Study Group (2003). Early malignant progression of hereditary medullary thyroid cancer. N Engl J Med. 349:1517–25. PMID:14561794
1703. Maciel LM, Gomes PM, Magalhães PK, et al. (2011). A giant primary hemangioma of the thyroid gland. J Clin Endocrinol Metab. 96:1623–4. PMID:21602455
1704. Mackay B, Ordóñez NG, Huang WL (1989). Ultrastructural and immunocytochemical observations on angiosarcomas. Ultrastruct Pathol. 13:97–110. PMID:2499967
1705. Maddock IR, Moran A, Maher ER, et al. (1996). A genetic register for von Hippel-Lindau disease. J Med Genet. 33:120–7. PMID:8929948
1706. Magalhães JF, Bacchin RP, Costa PS, et al. (2014). Breast cancer metastasis to the pituitary gland. Arq Bras Endocrinol Metabol. 58:869–72. PMID:25465612
1707. Magalhães PK, Antonini SR, de Paula FJ, et al. (2011). Primary hyperparathyroidism as the first clinical manifestation of multiple endocrine neoplasia type 2A in a 5-year-old child. Thyroid. 21:547–50. PMID:21449769
1708. Magiakou MA, Mastorakos G, Oldfield EH, et al. (1994). Cushing's syndrome in children and adolescents. Presentation, diagnosis, and therapy. N Engl J Med. 331:629–36. PMID:8052272
1709. Maguire JA, Bilbao JM, Kovacs K, et al. (1992). Hypothalamic neurocytoma with vasopressin immunoreactivity: immunohistochemical and ultrastructural observations. Endocr Pathol. 3:99–104.
1710. Mahajan A, Lin X, Nayar R (2013). Thyroid Bethesda reporting category, 'suspicious for papillary thyroid carcinoma', pitfalls and clues to optimize the use of this category. Cytopathology. 24:85–91. PMID:22356185
1711. Mahdi H, Mester JL, Nizialek EA, et al. (2015). Germline PTEN, SDHB-D, and KLLN alterations in endometrial cancer patients with Cowden and Cowden-like syndromes: an international, multicenter, prospective study. Cancer. 121:688–96. PMID:25376524
1712. Maher ER, Neumann HP, Richard S (2011). von Hippel-Lindau disease: a clinical and scientific review. Eur J Hum Genet. 19:617–23. PMID:21386872
1713. Maher ER, Webster AR, Richards FM, et al. (1996). Phenotypic expression in von Hippel-Lindau disease: correlations with germline VHL gene mutations. J Med Genet. 33:328–32. PMID:8730290
1714. Maher ER, Yates JR, Harries R, et al. (1990). Clinical features and natural history of von Hippel-Lindau disease. Q J Med. 77:1151–63. PMID:2274658
1715. Mahoney NR, Liu GT, Menacker SJ, et al. (2006). Pediatric horner syndrome: etiologies and roles of imaging and urine studies to detect neuroblastoma and other responsible mass lesions. Am J Ophthalmol. 142:651–9. PMID:17011859
1716. Mai KT, Landry DC, Thomas J, et al. (2001). Follicular adenoma with papillary architecture: a lesion mimicking papillary thyroid carcinoma. Histopathology. 39:25–32. PMID:11454041
1717. Mai KT, Thomas J, Yazdi HM, et al. (2004). Pathologic study and clinical significance of Hürthle cell papillary thyroid carcinoma. Appl Immunohistochem Mol Morphol. 12:329–37. PMID:15536332
1718. Maiorana A, Collina G, Cesinaro AM, et al. (1996). Epithelioid angiosarcoma of the thyroid. Clinicopathological analysis of seven cases from non-Alpine areas. Virchows Arch. 429:131–7. PMID:8917714
1719. Maiter D, Delgrange E (2014). Therapy of endocrine disease: the challenges in managing giant prolactinomas. Eur J Endocrinol. 170:R213–27. PMID:24536090
1720. Majewski JT, Wilson SD (1979). The MEA-I syndrome: an all or none phenomenon? Surgery. 86:475–84. PMID:38521
1721. Maki M, Kaneko Y, Ohta Y, et al. (1995). Somatostatinoma of the pancreas associated with von Hippel-Lindau disease. Intern Med. 34:661–5. PMID:7496080
1722. Malaguarnera R, Vella V, Vigneri R, et al. (2007). p53 family proteins in thyroid cancer. Endocr Relat Cancer. 14:43–60. PMID:17395974
1723. Maleszewski JJ, Larsen BT, Kip NS, et al. (2014). PRKAR1A in the development of cardiac myxoma: a study of 110 cases including isolated and syndromic tumors. Am J Surg Pathol. 38:1079–87. PMID:24618615
1724. Maletta F, Massa F, Torregrossa L, et al. (2016). Cytological features of "noninvasive follicular thyroid neoplasm with papillary-like nuclear features" and their correlation with tumor histology. Hum Pathol. 54:134–42. PMID:27085556
1725. Mallya SM, Gallagher JJ, Wild YK, et al. (2005). Abnormal parathyroid cell proliferation precedes biochemical abnormalities in a mouse model of primary hyperparathyroidism. Mol Endocrinol. 19:2603–9. PMID:15928311
1726. Maloberti A, Meani P, Pirola R, et al. (2015). Acute coronary syndrome: a rare case of multiple endocrine neoplasia syndromes with pheochromocytoma and medullary thyroid carcinoma. Cancer Biol Med. 12:255–8. PMID:26487970
1727. Mandriota SJ, Turner KJ, Davies DR, et al. (2002). HIF activation identifies early lesions in VHL kidneys: evidence for site-specific tumor suppressor function in the nephron. Cancer Cell. 1:459–68. PMID:12124175
1728. Mannelli M, Castellano M, Schiavi F, et al. (2009). Clinically guided genetic screening in a large cohort of italian patients with pheochromocytomas and/or functional or nonfunctional paragangliomas. J Clin Endocrinol Metab. 94:1541–7. PMID:19223516
1729. Mannina EM, Xiong Z, Self R, et al. (2014). Resection of a catecholamine-elaborating retroperitoneal paraganglioma invading the inferior vena cava. Case Rep Surg. 2014:837054. PMID:25610696
1730. Manolidis S, Shohet JA, Jackson CG, et al. (1999). Malignant glomus tumors. Laryngoscope. 109:30–4. PMID:9917036
1731. Manski TJ, Heffner DK, Glenn GM, et al. (1997). Endolymphatic sac tumors. A source of morbid hearing loss in von Hippel-Lindau disease. JAMA. 277:1461–6. PMID:9145719
1732. Mansmann G, Lau J, Balk E, et al. (2004). The clinically inapparent adrenal mass: update in diagnosis and management. Endocr Rev. 25:309–40. PMID:15082524
1733. Maragliano R, Vanoli A, Albarello L, et al. (2015). ACTH-secreting pancreatic neoplasms associated with Cushing syndrome: clinicopathologic study of 11 cases and review of the literature. Am J Surg Pathol. 39:374–82. PMID:25353285
1734. Marchesa P, Fazio VW, Church JM, et al. (1997). Adrenal masses in patients with familial adenomatous polyposis. Dis Colon Rectum. 40:1023–8. PMID:9293929
1735. Marcocci C, Cetani F (2011). Clinical practice. Primary hyperparathyroidism. N Engl J Med. 365:2389–97. PMID:22187986
1736. Marinoni I, Kurrer AS, Vassella E, et al. (2014). Loss of DAXX and ATRX are associated with chromosome instability and reduced survival of patients with pancreatic neuroendocrine tumors. Gastroenterology. 146:453–60.e5. PMID:24148618
1737. Maris JM (2010). Recent advances in neuroblastoma. N Engl J Med. 362:2202–11. PMID:20558371
1738. Maris JM, Mosse YP, Bradfield JP, et al. (2008). Chromosome 6p22 locus associated with clinically aggressive neuroblastoma. N Engl J Med. 358:2585–93. PMID:18463370
1739. Maris JM, Weiss MJ, Mosse Y, et al. (2002). Evidence for a hereditary neuroblastoma predisposition locus at chromosome 16p12-13. Cancer Res. 62:6651–8. PMID:12438263
1740. Mark D, Boyd C, Eatock F (2014). Adrenal sarcomatoid carcinoma: a case report and review of the literature. Ulster Med J. 83:89–92. PMID:25075137
1741. Marks IN, Bank S, Louw JH (1967). Islet cell tumor of the pancreas with reversible watery diarrhea and achylorhydraia. Gastroenterology. 52:695–708. PMID:4290095
1742. Marques P, Mafra M, Calado C, et al. (2014). Aggressive pituitary lesion with a remarkably high Ki-67. Arq Bras Endocrinol Metabol. 58:656–60. PMID:25211450
1743. Marsh DJ, Hahn MA, Howell VM, et al. (2007). Molecular diagnosis of primary hyperparathyroidism in familial cancer syndromes. Expert Opin Med Diagn. 1:377–92. PMID:23489357
1744. Martucci VL, Emaminia A, del Rivero J, et al. (2015). Succinate dehydrogenase gene mutations in cardiac paragangliomas. Am J Cardiol. 115:1753–9. PMID:25896150
1745. Marupudi KC, Karanth SS, Thomas J (2014). Langerhans cell histiocytosis presenting as hypothyroid goitre: a unique presentation. BMJ Case Rep. 2014:2014. PMID:25465459
1746. Maruta J, Hashimoto H, Suehisa Y, et al. (2011). Improving the diagnostic accuracy of thyroid follicular neoplasms: cytological features in fine-needle aspiration cytology. Diagn Cytopathol. 39:28–34. PMID:20091899
1747. Marx SJ, Nieman LK (2002). Aggressive pituitary tumors in MEN1: do they refute the two-hit model of tumorigenesis? J Clin Endocrinol Metab. 87:453–6. PMID:11836267
1748. Masala MV, Scapaticci S, Olivieri C, et al. (2007). Epidemiology and clinical aspects of Werner's syndrome in North Sardinia: description of a cluster. Eur J Dermatol. 17:213–6. PMID:17478382
1749. Masi G, Barzon L, Iacobone M, et al. (2008). Clinical, genetic, and histopathologic investigation of CDC73-related familial hyperparathyroidism. Endocr Relat Cancer. 15:1115–26. PMID:18755853
1750. Massironi S, Rossi RE, Ferrero S, et al. (2014). An esophageal gastrointestinal stromal tumor in a patient with MEN1-related pancreatic gastrinoma: an unusual association and review of the literature. J Cancer Res Ther. 10:443–5. PMID:25022420
1751. Massironi S, Zilli A, Rossi RE, et al. (2014). Gastrinoma and neurofibromatosis type 2: the first case report and review of the literature. BMC Gastroenterol. 14:110. PMID:24961548
1751A. Masson P (1970). Human tumors. 2nd ed. Detroit: Wayne State University Press.
1752. Mastorakos G, Mitsiades NS, Doufas AG, et al. (1997). Hyperthyroidism in McCune-Albright syndrome with a review of thyroid abnormalities sixty years after the first report. Thyroid. 7:433–9. PMID:9226216
1753. Matarazzo P, Lala R, Andreo M, et al. (2006). McCune-Albright syndrome: persistence of autonomous ovarian hyperfunction during adolescence and early adult age. J Pediatr Endocrinol Metab. 19 Suppl 2:607–17. PMID:16789624
1754. Mateus C, Palangié A, Franck N, et al. (2008). Heterogeneity of skin manifestations in patients with Carney complex. J Am Acad Dermatol. 59:801–10. PMID:18804312
1755. Matias-Guiu X, De Lellis R (2014). Medullary thyroid carcinoma: a 25-year perspective. Endocr Pathol. 25:21–9. PMID:24343523
1756. Matias-Guiu X, Garrastazu MT (1998). Composite phaeochromocytoma-ganglioneuroblastoma in a patient with multiple endocrine neoplasia type IIA. Histopathology. 32:281–2. PMID:9568520
1757. Matias-Guiu X, LaGuette J, Puras-Gil AM, et al. (1997). Metastatic neuroendocrine tumors to the thyroid gland mimicking medullary carcinoma: a pathologic and immunohistochemical study of six cases. Am J Surg Pathol. 21:754–62. PMID:9236831
1758. Matias-Guiu X, Villanueva A, Cuatrecasas M, et al. (1996). p53 in a thyroid follicular carcinoma with foci of poorly differentiated and anaplastic carcinoma. Pathol Res Pract. 192:1242–9, discussion 1250–1. PMID:9182295
1759. Matsui I, Tanimura M, Kobayashi N, et al. (1993). Neurofibromatosis type 1 and childhood cancer. Cancer. 72:2746–54. PMID:8402499
1760. Matsuki M, Kaji Y, Matsuo M, et al. (2000). MR findings of subarachnoid dissemination of a pituitary adenoma. Br J Radiol. 73:783–5. PMID:11089473
1761. Matsumura A, Meguro K, Doi M, et al. (1990). Suprasellar ectopic pituitary adenoma: case report and review of the literature. Neurosurgery. 26:681–5. PMID:2184378
1762. Matsuno A, Murakami M, Hoya K, et al. (2014). Molecular status of pituitary carcinoma and atypical adenoma that contributes the effectiveness of temozolomide. Med Mol Morphol. 47:1–7. PMID:23955641
1763. Matyakhina L, Pack S, Kirschner LS, et al. (2003). Chromosome 2 (2p16) abnormalities in Carney complex tumours. J Med Genet. 40:268–77. PMID:12676898
1764. Matyja E, Maksymowicz M, Grajkowska W, et al. (2015). Ganglion cell tumours in the sella turcica in close morphological connection with pituitary adenomas. Folia Neuropathol. 53:203–18. PMID:26443311
1765. Max MB, Deck MD, Rottenberg DA (1981). Pituitary metastasis: incidence in cancer patients and clinical differentiation from pituitary adenoma. Neurology. 31:998–1002. PMID:7196526
1766. Máximo V, Botelho T, Capela J, et al. (2005). Somatic and germline mutation in GRIM-19, a dual function gene involved in mitochondrial metabolism and cell death, is linked to mitochondrion-rich (Hürthle cell) tumours of the thyroid. Br J Cancer. 92:1892–8. PMID:15841082
1767. Máximo V, Lima J, Prazeres H, et al. (2012). The biology and the genetics of Hürthle cell tumors of the thyroid. Endocr Relat Cancer. 19:R131–47. PMID:22514109
1768. Máximo V, Soares P, Lima J, et al. (2002). Mitochondrial DNA somatic mutations (point mutations and large deletions) and mitochondrial DNA variants in human thyroid pathology: a study with emphasis on Hürthle cell tumors. Am J Pathol. 160:1857–65. PMID:12000737
1769. Máximo V, Sobrinho-Simões M (2000). Hürthle cell tumours of the thyroid. A review with emphasis on mitochondrial abnormalities with clinical relevance. Virchows Arch. 437:107–15. PMID:10993269
1770. Máximo V, Sobrinho-Simões M (2000). Mitochondrial DNA 'common' deletion in Hürthle cell lesions of the thyroid. J Pathol. 192:561–2. PMID:11113879
1771. Máximo V, Sores P, Rocha AS, et al.

(1998). The common deletion of mitochondrial DNA is found in goiters and thyroid tumors with and without oxyphil cell change. Ultrastruct Pathol. 22:271–3. PMID:9793208

1772. Maxwell PH, Wiesener MS, Chang GW, et al. (1999). The tumour suppressor protein VHL targets hypoxia-inducible factors for oxygen-dependent proteolysis. Nature. 399:271–5. PMID:10353251

1773. Mayo-Smith WW, Boland GW, Noto RB, et al. (2001). State-of-the-art adrenal imaging. Radiographics. 21:995–1012. PMID:11452074

1774. Mayr B, Buslei R, Theodoropoulou M, et al. (2013). Molecular and functional properties of densely and sparsely granulated GH-producing pituitary adenomas. Eur J Endocrinol. 169:391–400. PMID:23847328

1775. Mayr JA, Meierhofer D, Zimmermann F, et al. (2008). Loss of complex I due to mitochondrial DNA mutations in renal oncocytoma. Clin Cancer Res. 14:2270–5. PMID:18413815

1776. Mazarakis N, Kontogeorgos G, Kovacs K, et al. (2001). Composite somatotroph–ACTH-immunoreactive pituitary adenoma with transformation of hyperplasia to adenoma. Pituitary. 4:215–21. PMID:12501971

1777. Mazzaferri EL, Jhiang SM (1994). Long-term impact of initial surgical and medical therapy on papillary and follicular thyroid cancer. Am J Med. 97:418–28. PMID:7977430

1778. Mazzaferri EL, Kloos RT (2001). Clinical review 128: Current approaches to primary therapy for papillary and follicular thyroid cancer. J Clin Endocrinol Metab. 86:1447–63. PMID:11297567

1779. Mazzuco TL, Durand J, Chapman A, et al. (2012). Genetic aspects of adrenocortical tumours and hyperplasias. Clin Endocrinol (Oxf). 77:1–10. PMID:22471738

1780. McCall CM, Shi C, Klein AP, et al. (2012). Serotonin expression in pancreatic neuroendocrine tumors correlates with a trabecular histologic pattern and large duct involvement. Hum Pathol. 43:1169–76. PMID:22221702

1781. McCluggage WG, Burton J, Maxwell P, et al. (1998). Immunohistochemical staining of normal, hyperplastic, and neoplastic adrenal cortex with a monoclonal antibody against alpha inhibin. J Clin Pathol. 51:114–6. PMID:9602683

1782. McCluggage WG, Sloan JM (1996). Hyalinizing trabecular carcinoma of thyroid gland. Histopathology. 28:357–62. PMID:8732345

1783. McConahey WM, Hay ID, Woolner LB, et al. (1986). Papillary thyroid cancer treated at the Mayo Clinic, 1946 through 1970: initial manifestations, pathologic findings, therapy, and outcome. Mayo Clin Proc. 61:978–96. PMID:3773569

1784. McCormick PC, Post KD, Kandji AD, et al. (1989). Metastatic carcinoma to the pituitary gland. Br J Neurosurg. 3:71–9. PMID:2789715

1785. McCoy KL, Seethala RR, Armstrong MJ, et al. (2015). The clinical importance of parathyroid atypia: is long-term surveillance necessary? Surgery. 158:929–35, discussion 935–6. PMID:26210223

1786. McCutcheon IE, Pieper DR, Fuller GN, et al. (2000). Pituitary carcinoma containing gonadotropins: treatment by radical excision and cytotoxic chemotherapy: case report. Neurosurgery. 46:1233–9, discussion 1239–40. PMID:10807257

1787. McDermott MB, Swanson PE, Wick MR (1995). Immunostains for collagen type IV discriminate between C-cell hyperplasia and microscopic medullary carcinoma in multiple endocrine neoplasia, type 2a. Hum Pathol. 26:1308–12. PMID:8522302

1788. McFadden DG, Vernon A, Santiago PM, et al. (2014). p53 constrains progression to anaplastic thyroid carcinoma in a Braf-mutant mouse model of papillary thyroid cancer. Proc Natl Acad Sci U S A. 111:E1600–9. PMID:24711431

1789. McGaughran JM, Harris DI, Donnai D, et al. (1999). A clinical study of type 1 neurofibromatosis in north west England. J Med Genet. 36:197–203. PMID:10204844

1790. McKeeby JL, Li X, Zhuang Z, et al. (2001). Multiple leiomyomas of the esophagus, lung, and uterus in multiple endocrine neoplasia type 1. Am J Pathol. 159:1121–7. PMID:11549605

1791. McLaughlin DM, Gray WJ, Jones FG, et al. (2004). Plasmacytoma: an unusual cause of a pituitary mass lesion. A case report and a review of the literature. Pituitary. 7:179–81. PMID:16328566

1792. McMaster ML, Goldstein AM, Bromley CM, et al. (2001). Chordoma: incidence and survival patterns in the United States, 1973-1995. Cancer Causes Control. 12:1–11. PMID:11227920

1793. Medeiros LJ, Wolf BC, Balogh K, et al. (1985). Adrenal pheochromocytoma: a clinicopathologic review of 60 cases. Hum Pathol. 16:580–9. PMID:3997135

1794. Medina-Arana V, Delgado L, González L, et al. (2011). Adrenocortical carcinoma, an unusual extracolonic tumor associated with Lynch II syndrome. Fam Cancer. 10:265–71. PMID:21225464

1795. Mediouni A, Ammari S, Wassef M, et al. (2014). Malignant head/neck paragangliomas. Comparative study. Eur Ann Otorhinolaryngol Head Neck Dis. 131:159–66. PMID:24239180

1796. Mehrabi A, Fischer L, Hafezi M, et al. (2014). A systematic review of localization, surgical treatment options, and outcome of insulinoma. Pancreas. 43:675–86. PMID:24921202

1797. Mehta A, Patel D, Rosenberg A, et al. (2014). Hyperparathyroidism-jaw tumor syndrome: Results of operative management. Surgery. 156:1315–24, discussion 1324–5. PMID:25444225

1798. Mei K, Liu A, Allan RW, et al. (2009). Diagnostic utility of SALL4 in primary germ cell tumors of the central nervous system: a study of 77 cases. Mod Pathol. 22:1628–36. PMID:19820689

1799. Meij BP, Lopes MB, Ellegala DB, et al. (2002). The long-term significance of microscopic dural invasion in 354 patients with pituitary adenomas treated with transsphenoidal surgery. J Neurosurg. 96:195–208. PMID:11838791

1800. Meij BP, Lopes MB, Vance ML, et al. (2000). Double pituitary lesions in three patients with Cushing's disease. Pituitary. 3:159–68. PMID:11383480

1801. Meijer JA, le Cessie S, van den Hout WB, et al. (2010). Calcitonin and carcinoembryonic antigen doubling times as prognostic factors in medullary thyroid carcinoma: a structured meta-analysis. Clin Endocrinol (Oxf). 72:534–42. PMID:19563448

1802. Melmed S (2006). Medical progress: Acromegaly. N Engl J Med. 355:2558–73. PMID:17167139

1803. Melmed S (2011). Pathogenesis of pituitary tumors. Nat Rev Endocrinol. 7:257–66. PMID:21423242

1804. Melmed S, Casanueva FF, Klibanski A, et al. (2013). A consensus on the diagnosis and treatment of acromegaly complications. Pituitary. 16:294–302. PMID:22903574

1805. Melmed S, Popovic V, Bidlingmaier M, et al. (2015). Safety and efficacy of oral octreotide in acromegaly: results of a multicenter phase III trial. J Clin Endocrinol Metab. 100:1699–708. PMID:25664604

1806. Melo M, da Rocha AG, Vinagre J, et al. (2014). TERT promoter mutations are a major indicator of poor outcome in differentiated thyroid carcinomas. J Clin Endocrinol Metab. 99:E754–65. PMID:24476079

1807. Mendelsohn G (1984). Signet-cell-simulating microfollicular adenoma of the thyroid. Am J Surg Pathol. 8:705–8. PMID:6383090

1808. Mendelsohn G, Baylin SB, Bigner SH, et al. (1980). Anaplastic variants of medullary thyroid carcinoma: a light-microscopic and immunohistochemical study. Am J Surg Pathol. 4:333–41. PMID:6999920

1809. Mendelsohn G, Wells SA Jr, Baylin SB (1984). Relationship of tissue carcinoembryonic antigen and calcitonin to tumor virulence in medullary thyroid carcinoma. An immunohistochemical study in early, localized, and virulent disseminated stages of disease. Cancer. 54:657–62. PMID:6378353

1810. Mendola M, Dolci A, Piscopello L, et al. (2014). Rare case of Cushing's disease due to double ACTH-producing adenomas, one located in the pituitary gland and one into the stalk. Hormones (Athens). 13:574–8. PMID:25402386

1811. Menegaux F, Olshan AF, Neglia JP, et al. (2004). Day care, childhood infections, and risk of neuroblastoma. Am J Epidemiol. 159:843–51. PMID:15105177

1812. Menke JR, Raleigh DR, Gown AM, et al. (2015). Somatostatin receptor 2a is a more sensitive diagnostic marker of meningioma than epithelial membrane antigen. Acta Neuropathol. 130:441–3. PMID:26195322

1813. Menon RK, Ferrau F, Kurzawinski TR, et al. (2014). Adrenal cancer in neurofibromatosis type 1: case report and DNA analysis. Endocrinol Diabetes Metab Case Rep. 2014:140074. PMID:25520849

1814. Mercante G, Frasoldati A, Pedroni C, et al. (2009). Prognostic factors affecting neck lymph node recurrence and distant metastasis in papillary microcarcinoma of the thyroid: results of a study in 445 patients. Thyroid. 19:707–16. PMID:19348581

1815. Merino MJ, Chuaqui R, Fernandez P (1996). Parathyroid Hemangioma: A Report of Two Cases. Endocr Pathol. 7:319–22. PMID:12114803

1816. Messiaen LM, Callens T, Mortier G, et al. (2000). Exhaustive mutation analysis of the NF1 gene allows identification of 95% of mutations and reveals a high frequency of unusual splicing defects. Hum Mutat. 15:541–55. PMID:10862084

1817. Messinger YH, Stewart DR, Priest JR, et al. (2015). Pleuropulmonary blastoma: a report on 350 central pathology-confirmed pleuropulmonary blastoma cases by the International Pleuropulmonary Blastoma Registry. Cancer. 121:276–85. PMID:25209242

1818. Mester J, Eng C (2012). Estimate of de novo mutation frequency in probands with PTEN hamartoma tumor syndrome. Genet Med. 14:819–22. PMID:22595938

1819. Mete O, Asa SL (2011). Pathological definition and clinical significance of vascular invasion in thyroid carcinomas of follicular epithelial derivation. Mod Pathol. 24:1545–52. PMID:21804527

1820. Mete O, Asa SL (2012). Clinicopathological correlations in pituitary adenomas. Brain Pathol. 22:443–53. PMID:22697380

1821. Mete O, Asa SL (2012). Pitfalls in the diagnosis of follicular epithelial proliferations of the thyroid. Adv Anat Pathol. 19:363–73. PMID:23060062

1822. Mete O, Asa SL (2013). Precursor lesions of endocrine system neoplasms. Pathology. 45:316–30. PMID:23478233

1823. Mete O, Asa SL (2013). Therapeutic implications of accurate classification of pituitary adenomas. Semin Diagn Pathol. 30:158–64. PMID:24144285

1824. Mete O, Ezzat S, Asa SL (2012). Biomarkers of aggressive pituitary adenomas. J Mol Endocrinol. 49:R69–78. PMID:22822048

1825. Mete O, Gomez-Hernandez K, Kucharczyk W, et al. (2016). Silent subtype 3 pituitary adenomas are not always silent and represent poorly differentiated monomorphous plurihormonal Pit-1 lineage adenomas. Mod Pathol. 29:131–42. PMID:26743473

1826. Mete O, Hayhurst C, Alahmadi H, et al. (2013). The role of mediators of cell invasiveness, motility, and migration in the pathogenesis of silent corticotroph adenomas. Endocr Pathol. 24:191–8. PMID:24091601

1827. Mete O, Lopes MB, Asa SL (2013). Spindle cell oncocytomas and granular cell tumors of the pituitary are variants of pituicytoma. Am J Surg Pathol. 37:1694–9. PMID:23887161

1828. Mete O, Ng T, Christie-David D, et al. (2013). Silent corticotroph adenoma with adrenal cortical choristoma: a rare but distinct morphological entity. Endocr Pathol. 24:162–6. PMID:23872913

1829. Mete O, Tischler AS, de Krijger R, et al. (2014). Protocol for the examination of specimens from patients with pheochromocytomas and extra-adrenal paragangliomas. Arch Pathol Lab Med. 138:182–8. PMID:24476517

1830. Mhawech-Fauceglia P, Herrmann FR, Bshara W, et al. (2007). Friend leukaemia integration-1 expression in malignant and benign tumours: a multiple tumour tissue microarray analysis using polyclonal antibody. J Clin Pathol. 60:694–700. PMID:16917000

1831. Mian C, Barollo S, Zambonin L, et al. (2009). Characterization of the largest kindred with MEN2A due to a Cys609Ser RET mutation. Fam Cancer. 8:379–82. PMID:19475497

1832. Mian C, Pennelli G, Barollo S, et al. (2011). Combined RET and Ki-67 assessment in sporadic medullary thyroid carcinoma: a useful tool for patient risk stratification. Eur J Endocrinol. 164:971–6. PMID:21422198

1833. Mian M, Gaidano G, Conconi A, et al. (2011). High response rate and improvement of long-term survival with combined treatment modalities in patients with poor-risk primary thyroid diffuse large B-cell lymphoma: an International Extranodal Lymphoma Study Group and Intergruppo Italiano Linfomi study. Leuk Lymphoma. 52:823–32. PMID:21338283

1834. Michalkiewicz E, Sandrini R, Figueiredo B, et al. (2004). Clinical and outcome characteristics of children with adrenocortical tumors: a report from the International Pediatric Adrenocortical Tumor Registry. J Clin Oncol. 22:838–45. PMID:14990639

1835. Miermeister CP, Petersenn S, Buchfelder M, et al. (2015). Histological criteria for atypical pituitary adenomas - data from the German pituitary adenoma registry suggests modifications. Acta Neuropathol Commun. 3:50. PMID:26285571

1836. Miettinen M, Chatten J, Paetau A, et al. (1998). Monoclonal antibody NB84 in the differential diagnosis of neuroblastoma and other small round cell tumors. Am J Surg Pathol. 22:327–32. PMID:9500774

1837. Miettinen M, Franssila K, Lehto VP, et al. (1984). Expression of intermediate filament proteins in thyroid gland and thyroid tumors. Lab Invest. 50:262–70. PMID:6199582

1838. Miettinen M, Lehto VP, Virtanen I (1985). Immunofluorescence microscopic evaluation of the intermediate filament expression of the adrenal cortex and medulla and their tumors. Am J Pathol. 118:360–6. PMID:3883796

1839. Miettinen M, McCue PA, Sarlomo-Rikala M, et al. (2015). Sox10–a marker for not only schwannian and melanocytic neoplasms but also myoepithelial cell tumors of soft tissue: a systematic analysis of 5134 tumors. Am J Surg Pathol. 39:826–35. PMID:25724000

1840. Miettinen M, Wang ZF, Sarlomo-Rikala M, et al. (2011). Succinate dehydrogenase-deficient GISTs: a clinicopathologic, immunohistochemical, and molecular genetic study of 66 gastric GISTs with predilection to young age. Am J Surg Pathol. 35:1712–21. PMID:21997692

1841. Migliorini D, Haller S, Merkler D, et al. (2015). Recurrent multiple CNS hemangioblastomas with VHL disease treated with pazopanib: a case report and literature review. CNS Oncol. 4:387–92. PMID:26497655

1842. Mikami S, Kameyama K, Takahashi S, et al. (2008). Combined gangliocytoma and prolactinoma of the pituitary gland. Endocr Pathol. 19:117–21. PMID:18651251
1843. Miki H, Sumitomo M, Inoue H, et al. (1996). Parathyroid carcinoma in patients with chronic renal failure on maintenance hemodialysis. Surgery. 120:897–901. PMID:8909528
1844. Milas M, Wagner K, Easley KA, et al. (2003). Double adenomas revisited: nonuniform distribution favors enlarged superior parathyroids (fourth pouch disease). Surgery. 134:995–1003, discussion 1003–4. PMID:14668733
1845. Millar AC, Mete O, Cusimano RJ, et al. (2014). Functional cardiac paraganglioma associated with a rare SDHC mutation. Endocr Pathol. 25:315–20. PMID:24402737
1846. Miller HC, Kidd M, Modlin IM, et al. (2015). Glucagon receptor gene mutations with hyperglucagonemia but without the glucagonoma syndrome. World J Gastrointest Surg. 7:60–6. PMID:25914784
1847. Mills SE, Gaffey MJ, Watts JC, et al. (1994). Angiomatoid carcinoma and 'angiosarcoma' of the thyroid gland. A spectrum of endothelial differentiation. Am J Clin Pathol. 102:322–30. PMID:8085556
1848. Mills SE, Stallings RG, Austin MB (1986). Angiomatoid carcinoma of the thyroid gland. Anaplastic carcinoma with follicular and medullary features mimicking angiosarcoma. Am J Clin Pathol. 86:674–8. PMID:3776922
1849. Minagawa A, Iitaka M, Suzuki M, et al. (2002). A case of primary mucoepidermoid carcinoma of the thyroid: molecular evidence of its origin. Clin Endocrinol (Oxf). 57:551–6. PMID:12354139
1850. Minematsu T, Miyai S, Kajiya H, et al. (2005). Recent progress in studies of pituitary tumor pathogenesis. Endocrine. 28:37–41. PMID:16311408
1851. Minniti G, Traish D, Ashley S, et al. (2005). Risk of second brain tumor after conservative surgery and radiotherapy for pituitary adenoma: update after an additional 10 years. J Clin Endocrinol Metab. 90:800–4. PMID:15562021
1852. Minniti G, Traish D, Ashley S, et al. (2006). Fractionated stereotactic conformal radiotherapy for secreting and nonsecreting pituitary adenomas. Clin Endocrinol (Oxf). 64:542–8. PMID:16649974
1853. Mir SA, Masoodi SR, Bashir MI, et al. (2013). Dissociated hypopituitarism after spontaneous pituitary apoplexy in acromegaly. Indian J Endocrinol Metab. 17 Suppl 1:S102–4. PMID:24251123
1854. Miranda RN, Myint MA, Gnepp DR (1995). Composite follicular variant of papillary carcinoma and mucoepidermoid carcinoma of the thyroid. Report of a case and review of the literature. Am J Surg Pathol. 19:1209–15. PMID:7573680
1855. Miranda RN, Wu CD, Nayak RN, et al. (1995). Amyloid in adrenal gland pheochromocytomas. Arch Pathol Lab Med. 119:827–30. PMID:7545387
1856. Missiaglia E, Dalai I, Barbi S, et al. (2010). Pancreatic endocrine tumors: expression profiling evidences a role for AKT-mTOR pathway. J Clin Oncol. 28:245–55. PMID:19917848
1857. Mitsuya K, Nakasu Y, Nioka H, et al. (2004). Ectopic growth hormone-releasing adenoma in the cavernous sinus–case report. Neurol Med Chir (Tokyo). 44:380–5. PMID:15347217
1858. Mixson AJ, Friedman TC, Katz DA, et al. (1993). Thyrotropin-secreting pituitary carcinoma. J Clin Endocrinol Metab. 76:529–33. PMID:8432799
1859. Miyauchi A, Futami H, Hai N, et al. (1999). Two germline missense mutations at codons 804 and 806 of the RET proto-oncogene in the same allele in a patient with multiple endocrine neoplasia type 2B without codon 918 mutation. Jpn J Cancer Res. 90:1–5. PMID:10076558
1860. Miyauchi A, Kudo T, Hirokawa M, et al. (2013). Ki-67 labeling index is a predictor of postoperative persistent disease and cancer growth and a prognostic indicator in papillary thyroid carcinoma. Eur Thyroid J. 2:57–64. PMID:24783039
1861. Miyauchi A, Kudo T, Miya A, et al. (2011). Prognostic impact of serum thyroglobulin doubling-time under thyrotropin suppression in patients with papillary thyroid carcinoma who underwent total thyroidectomy. Thyroid. 21:707–16. PMID:21649472
1862. Miyauchi A, Kuma K, Matsuzuka F, et al. (1985). Intrathyroidal epithelial thymoma: an entity distinct from squamous cell carcinoma of the thyroid. World J Surg. 9:128–35. PMID:3984364
1863. Mizukami Y, Kurumaya H, Kitagawa T, et al. (1995). Papillary carcinoma of the thyroid gland with fibromatosis-like stroma: a case report and review of the literature. Mod Pathol. 8:366–70. PMID:7567932
1864. Mizukami Y, Kurumaya H, Nonomura A, et al. (1992). Sporadic medullary microcarcinoma of the thyroid. Histopathology. 21:375–7. PMID:1398540
1865. Mizukami Y, Michigishi T, Nonomura A, et al. (1993). Mixed medullary-follicular carcinoma of the thyroid occurring in familial form. Histopathology. 22:284–7. PMID:8495962
1866. Mizukami Y, Michigishi T, Nonomura A, et al. (1995). Adenolipoma of the thyroid gland. Pathol Int. 45:247–9. PMID:7787996
1867. Mizukami Y, Michigishi T, Nonomura A, et al. (1994). Autonomously functioning (hot) nodule of the thyroid gland. A clinical and histopathologic study of 17 cases. Am J Clin Pathol. 101:29–35. PMID:8279452
1868. Mizukami Y, Noguchi M, Michigishi T, et al. (1992). Papillary thyroid carcinoma in Kanazawa, Japan: prognostic significance of histological subtypes. Histopathology. 20:243–50. PMID:1563711
1869. Mizukami Y, Nonomura A, Michigishi T, et al. (1996). Encapsulated follicular thyroid carcinoma exhibiting glandular and spindle cell components. A case report. Pathol Res Pract. 192:67–71, discussion 72–4. PMID:8685044
1870. Mizukami Y, Nonomura A, Michigishi T, et al. (1995). Diffuse follicular variant of papillary carcinoma of the thyroid. Histopathology. 27:575–7. PMID:8838340
1871. Mizutani K, Onda M, Asaka S, et al. (2005). Overexpressed in anaplastic thyroid carcinoma-1 (OEATC-1) as a novel gene responsible for anaplastic thyroid carcinoma. Cancer. 103:1785–90. PMID:15789362
1872. Mizuuchi Y, Yamamoto H, Nakamura K, et al. (2014). Solitary fibrous tumor of the thyroid gland. Med Mol Morphol. 47:117–22. PMID:24013381
1873. Mnif H, Chakroun A, Charfi S, et al. (2013). Primary mucinous carcinoma of the thyroid gland: case report with review of the literature. Pathologica. 105:128–31. PMID:24466763
1874. Modigliani E, Cohen R, Campos JM, et al. (1998). Prognostic factors for survival and for biochemical cure in medullary thyroid carcinoma: results in 899 patients. The GETC Study Group. Groupe d'étude des tumeurs à calcitonine. Clin Endocrinol (Oxf). 48:265–73. PMID:9578814
1875. Modigliani E, Vasen HM, Raue K, et al. (1995). Pheochromocytoma in multiple endocrine neoplasia type 2: European study. J Intern Med. 238:363–7. PMID:7595173
1876. Mohajeri A, Tayebwa J, Collin A, et al. (2013). Comprehensive genetic analysis identifies a pathognomonic NAB2/STAT6 fusion gene, nonrandom secondary genomic imbalances, and a characteristic gene expression profile in solitary fibrous tumor. Genes Chromosomes Cancer. 52:873–86. PMID:23761323
1877. Mohammed S, Cusimano MD, Scheithauer BW, et al. (2010). O-methylguanine-DNA methyltransferase immunoexpression in a double pituitary adenoma: case report. Neurosurgery. 66:E421–2, discussion E422. PMID:20087113
1878. Mohiuddin Y, Gilliland MG (2013). Adrenal schwannoma: a rare type of adrenal incidentaloma. Arch Pathol Lab Med. 137:1009–14. PMID:23808475
1879. Mohr VH, Vortmeyer AO, Zhuang Z, et al. (2000). Histopathology and molecular genetics of multiple cysts and microcystic (serous) adenomas of the pancreas in von Hippel-Lindau patients. Am J Pathol. 157:1615–21. PMID:11073821
1880. Mohyuddin N, Ferrer K, Patel U (2013). Malignant paraganglioma of the thyroid gland with synchronous bilateral carotid body tumors. Ear Nose Throat J. 92:E20–3. PMID:23460222
1881. Mokry M, Kleinert R, Clarici G, et al. (1998). Primary paraganglioma simulating pituitary macroadenoma: a case report and review of the literature. Neuroradiology. 40:233–7. PMID:9592793
1882. Molatore S, Kiermaier E, Jung CB, et al. (2010). Characterization of a naturally-occurring p27 mutation predisposing to multiple endocrine tumors. Mol Cancer. 9:116. PMID:20492666
1883. Molatore S, Marinoni I, Lee M, et al. (2010). A novel germline CDKN1B mutation causing multiple endocrine tumors: clinical, genetic and functional characterization. Hum Mutat. 31:E1825–35. PMID:20824794
1884. Molatore S, Pellegata NS (2010). The MENX syndrome and p27: relationships with multiple endocrine neoplasia. Prog Brain Res. 182:295–320. PMID:20541671
1885. Moline J, Eng C (2011). Multiple endocrine neoplasia type 2: an overview. Genet Med. 13:755–64. PMID:21552134
1886. Molitch ME (2012). Management of incidentally found nonfunctional pituitary tumors. Neurosurg Clin N Am. 23:543–53. PMID:23040742
1887. Molloy PT, Bilaniuk LT, Vaughan SN, et al. (1995). Brainstem tumors in patients with neurofibromatosis type 1: a distinct clinical entity. Neurology. 45:1897–902. PMID:7477989
1888. Monclair T, Brodeur GM, Ambros PF, et al. (2009). The International Neuroblastoma Risk Group (INRG) staging system: an INRG Task Force report. J Clin Oncol. 27:298–303. PMID:19047290
1889. Monclair T, Ruud E, Holmstrøm H, et al. (2015). Extra-adrenal composite phaeochromocytoma/neuroblastoma in a 15-month-old child. J Pediatr Surg Case Rep. 3:348–50.
1890. Mondal SK, Dasgupta S, Jain P, et al. (2013). Histopathological study of adrenocortical carcinoma with special reference to the Weiss system and TNM staging and the role of immunohistochemistry to differentiate it from renal cell carcinoma. J Cancer Res Ther. 9:436–41. PMID:24125979
1891. Mondal SK, Dasgupta S, Mandal PK, et al. (2014). Cytodiagnosis of myxoid adrenocortical carcinoma and role of immunocytochemistry to differentiate it from renal cell carcinoma. J Cytol. 31:111–3. PMID:25210244
1892. Monroe MM, Sauer DA, Samuels MH, et al. (2009). Pathology quiz case 1. Coexistent conventional mucoepidermoid carcinoma of the thyroid (MECT) and papillary thyroid carcinoma. Arch Otolaryngol Head Neck Surg. 135:720,722. PMID:19620598
1893. Montani M, Heinimann K, von Teichman A, et al. (2010). VHL-gene deletion in single renal tubular epithelial cells and renal tubular cysts: further evidence for a cyst-dependent progression pathway of clear cell renal carcinoma in von Hippel-Lindau disease. Am J Surg Pathol. 34:806–15. PMID:20431476
1894. Montero-Conde C, Martín-Campos JM, Lerma E, et al. (2008). Molecular profiling related to poor prognosis in thyroid carcinoma. Combining gene expression data and biological information. Oncogene. 27:1554–61. PMID:17873908
1895. Monticone S, Else T, Mulatero P, et al. (2015). Understanding primary aldosteronism: impact of next generation sequencing and expression profiling. Mol Cell Endocrinol. 399:311–20. PMID:25240470
1896. Montone KT (2015). The differential diagnosis of sinonasal/nasopharyngeal neuroendocrine/neuroectodermally derived tumors. Arch Pathol Lab Med. 139:1498–507. PMID:26619022
1897. Montone KT, Baloch ZW, LiVolsi VA (2008). The thyroid Hürthle (oncocytic) cell and its associated pathologic conditions: a surgical pathology and cytopathology review. Arch Pathol Lab Med. 132:1241–50. PMID:18684023
1898. Montone KT, Rosen M, Siegelman ES, et al. (2009). Adrenocortical neoplasms with myelolipomatous and lipomatous metaplasia: report of 3 cases. Endocr Pract. 15:128–33. PMID:19289323
1899. Moo-Young TA, Traugott AL, Moley JF (2009). Sporadic and familial medullary thyroid carcinoma: state of the art. Surg Clin North Am. 89:1193–204. PMID:19836492
1900. Moraitis AG, Martucci VL, Pacak K (2014). Genetics, diagnosis, and management of medullary thyroid carcinoma and pheochromocytoma/paraganglioma. Endocr Pract. 20:176–87. PMID:24449662
1901. Moran A, Asa SL, Kovacs K, et al. (1990). Gigantism due to pituitary mammosomatotroph hyperplasia. N Engl J Med. 323:322–7. PMID:2164153
1902. Moreno S, Guillermo M, Decoulx M, et al. (2006). Feminizing adreno-cortical carcinomas in male adults. A dire prognosis. Three cases in a series of 801 adrenalectomies and review of the literature. Ann Endocrinol (Paris). 67:32–8. PMID:16596055
1903. Morgan KA, Adams DB (2010). Solid tumors of the body and tail of the pancreas. Surg Clin North Am. 90:287–307. PMID:20362787
1904. Morimoto R, Satoh F, Murakami O, et al. (2008). Immunohistochemistry of a proliferation marker Ki67/MIB1 in adrenocortical carcinomas: Ki67/MIB1 labeling index is a predictor for recurrence of adrenocortical carcinomas. Endocr J. 55:49–55. PMID:18187873
1905. Morin E, Mete O, Wasserman JD, et al. (2012). Carney complex with adrenal cortical carcinoma. J Clin Endocrinol Metab. 97:E202–6. PMID:22112809
1906. Morita A, Meyer FB, Laws ER Jr (1998). Symptomatic pituitary metastases. J Neurosurg. 89:69–73. PMID:9647174
1907. Morris LG, Shaha AR, Tuttle RM, et al. (2010). Tall-cell variant of papillary thyroid carcinoma: a matched-pair analysis of survival. Thyroid. 20:153–8. PMID:20151822
1908. Moschovi M, Adamaki M, Vlahopoulos S, et al. (2015). Synchronous and metachronous thyroid cancer in relation to Langerhans cell histiocytosis; involvement of V600E BRAF-mutation? Pediatr Blood Cancer. 62:173–4. PMID:25156525
1909. Moshkin O, Syro LV, Scheithauer BW, et al. (2011). Aggressive silent corticotroph adenoma progressing to pituitary carcinoma: the role of temozolomide therapy. Hormones (Athens). 10:162–7. PMID:21724542
1910. Moshynska OV, Saxena A (2008). Clonal relationship between Hashimoto thyroiditis and thyroid lymphoma. J Clin Pathol. 61:438–44. PMID:18006670
1911. Moskovic DJ, Smolarz JR, Stanley D, et al. (2010). Malignant head and neck

paragangliomas: is there an optimal treatment strategy? Head Neck Oncol. 2:23. PMID:20863367
1912. Mossé YP (2016). Anaplastic Lymphoma Kinase as a Cancer Target in Pediatric Malignancies. Clin Cancer Res. 22:546–52. PMID:26503946
1913. Mossé YP, Laudenslager M, Longo L, et al. (2008). Identification of ALK as a major familial neuroblastoma predisposition gene. Nature. 455:930–5. PMID:18724359
1914. Motokura T, Bloom T, Kim HG, et al. (1991). A novel cyclin encoded by a bcl1-linked candidate oncogene. Nature. 350:512–5. PMID:1826542
1915. Motosugi U, Murata S, Nagata K, et al. (2009). Thyroid papillary carcinoma with micropapillary and hobnail growth pattern: a histological variant with intermediate malignancy? Thyroid. 19:535–7. PMID:19348583
1916. Moura MM, Cavaco BM, Leite V (2015). RAS proto-oncogene in medullary thyroid carcinoma. Endocr Relat Cancer. 22:R235–52. PMID:26285815
1917. Moura MM, Cavaco BM, Pinto AE, et al. (2009). Correlation of RET somatic mutations with clinicopathological features in sporadic medullary thyroid carcinomas. Br J Cancer. 100:1777–83. PMID:19401695
1918. Moura MM, Cavaco BM, Pinto AE, et al. (2011). High prevalence of RAS mutations in RET-negative sporadic medullary thyroid carcinomas. J Clin Endocrinol Metab. 96:E863–8. PMID:21325462
1919. Movahedi-Lankarani S, Hruban RH, Westra WH, et al. (2002). Primitive neuroectodermal tumors of the pancreas: a report of seven cases of a rare neoplasm. Am J Surg Pathol. 26:1040–7. PMID:12170091
1920. Mozos A, Ye H, Chuang WY, et al. (2009). Most primary adrenal lymphomas are diffuse large B-cell lymphomas with non-germinal center B-cell phenotype, BCL6 gene rearrangement and poor prognosis. Mod Pathol. 22:1210–7. PMID:19525926
1921. Mrad K, Charfi L, Dhouib R, et al. (2004). Extra-nodal Rosai-Dorfman disease: a case report with thyroid involvement. Ann Pathol. 24:446–9. [French] PMID:15738872
1922. Mu Q, Yu J, Qu L, et al. (2015). Spindle cell oncocytoma of the adenohypophysis: two case reports and a review of the literature. Mol Med Rep. 12:871–6. PMID:25777996
1923. Mukai K, Grotting JC, Greider MH, et al. (1982). Retrospective study of 77 pancreatic endocrine tumors using the immunoperoxidase method. Am J Surg Pathol. 6:387–99. PMID:6127037
1924. Mukhida K, Asa S, Gentili F, et al. (2006). Ependymoma of the pituitary fossa. Case report and review of the literature. J Neurosurg. 105:616–20. PMID:17044567
1925. Müller S, Kupka S, Königsrainer I, et al. (2012). MSH2 and CXCR4 involvement in malignant VIPoma. World J Surg Oncol. 10:264. PMID:23231927
1926. Müller U, Troidl C, Niemann S (2005). SDHC mutations in hereditary paraganglioma/pheochromocytoma. Fam Cancer. 4:9–12. PMID:15883704
1927. Mulligan LM, Eng C, Healey CS, et al. (1994). Specific mutations of the RET proto-oncogene are related to disease phenotype in MEN 2A and FMTC. Nat Genet. 6:70–4. PMID:7907913
1928. Mulligan LM, Kwok JB, Healey CS, et al. (1993). Germ-line mutations of the RET proto-oncogene in multiple endocrine neoplasia type 2A. Nature. 363:458–60. PMID:8099202
1929. Murakami I, Matsushita M, Iwasaki T, et al. (2014). Merkel cell polyomavirus DNA sequences in peripheral blood and tissues from patients with Langerhans cell histiocytosis. Hum Pathol. 45:119–26. PMID:24321520
1930. Murakami I, Matsushita M, Iwasaki T, et al. (2015). Interleukin-1 loop model for pathogenesis of Langerhans cell histiocytosis. Cell Commun Signal. 13:13. PMID:25889448
1931. Murakami M, Kamiya Y, Yanagita Y, et al. (1999). Gs alpha mutations in hyperfunctioning thyroid adenomas. Arch Med Res. 30:514–21. PMID:10714366
1932. Murakami M, Mizutani A, Asano S, et al. (2011). A mechanism of acquiring temozolomide resistance during transformation of atypical prolactinoma into prolactin-producing pituitary carcinoma: case report. Neurosurgery. 68:E1761–7, discussion E1767. PMID:21389894
1933. Murat A, Heymann MF, Bernat S, et al. (1997). Thymic and bronchial neuroendocrine tumors in multiple endocrine neoplasia type 1. GENEM1. Presse Med. 26:1616–21. [French] PMID:9452725
1934. Muro M, Yoshioka T, Idani H, et al. (2009). Pulmonary hilar lymph node metastasis from cancer of unknown origin; report of a case. Kyobu Geka. 62:427–9. [Japanese] PMID:19425388
1935. Murugan AK, Xing M (2011). Anaplastic thyroid cancers harbor novel oncogenic mutations of the ALK gene. Cancer Res. 71:4403–11. PMID:21596819
1936. Muth A, Hammarstedt L, Hellström M, et al. (2011). Cohort study of patients with adrenal lesions discovered incidentally. Br J Surg. 98:1383–91. PMID:21618498
1937. Mylonis I, Sembongi H, Befani C, et al. (2012). Hypoxia causes triglyceride accumulation by HIF-1-mediated stimulation of lipin 1 expression. J Cell Sci. 125(Pt 14):3485–93. PMID:22467849
1938. Myssiorek D, Rinaldo A, Barnes L, et al. (2004). Laryngeal paraganglioma: an updated critical review. Acta Otolaryngol. 124:995–9. PMID:15513540
1939. Na KY, Kim HS, Sung JY, et al. (2013). Papillary Carcinoma of the Thyroid Gland with Nodular Fasciitis-like Stroma. Korean J Pathol. 47:167–71. PMID:23667377
1940. Nakagawara A, Azar CG, Scavarda NJ, et al. (1994). Expression and function of TRK-B and BDNF in human neuroblastomas. Mol Cell Biol. 14:759–67. PMID:8264643
1941. Nakagawara A, Ikeda K, Tsuneyoshi M, et al. (1985). Malignant pheochromocytoma with ganglioneuroblastoma elements in a patient with von Recklinghausen's disease. Cancer. 55:2794–8. PMID:3922614
1942. Nakamura N, Erickson LA, Jin L, et al. (2006). Immunohistochemical separation of follicular variant of papillary thyroid carcinoma from follicular adenoma. Endocr Pathol. 17:213–23. PMID:17308358
1943. Nakamura T, Moriyama S, Nariya S, et al. (1998). Macrofollicular variant of papillary thyroid carcinoma. Pathol Int. 48:467–70. PMID:9702860
1944. Nakamura Y, Maekawa T, Felizola SJ, et al. (2014). Adrenal CYP11B1/2 expression in primary aldosteronism: immunohistochemical analysis using novel monoclonal antibodies. Mol Cell Endocrinol. 392:73–9. PMID:24837548
1945. Nakatani Y, Masudo K, Nozawa A, et al. (2004). Biotin-rich, optically clear nuclei express estrogen receptor-beta: tumors with morules may develop under the influence of estrogen and aberrant beta-catenin expression. Hum Pathol. 35:869–74. PMID:15257551
1946. Nakazawa T, Cameselle-Teijeiro J, Vinagre J, et al. (2014). C-cell-derived calcitonin-free neuroendocrine carcinoma of the thyroid: the diagnostic importance of CGRP immunoreactivity. Int J Surg Pathol. 22:530–5. PMID:24599901
1947. Nakazawa T, Celestino R, Machado JC, et al. (2013). Cribriform-morular variant of papillary thyroid carcinoma displaying poorly differentiated features. Int J Surg Pathol. 21:379–89. PMID:23349472
1948. Nakhjavani MK, Gharib H, Goellner JR, et al. (1997). Metastasis to the thyroid gland. A report of 43 cases. Cancer. 79:574–8. PMID:9028370
1949. Namba H, Matsuo K, Fagin JA (1990). Clonal composition of benign and malignant human thyroid tumors. J Clin Invest. 86:120–5. PMID:1973172
1950. Namba H, Rubin SA, Fagin JA (1990). Point mutations of ras oncogenes are an early event in thyroid tumorigenesis. Mol Endocrinol. 4:1474–9. PMID:2283998
1951. Nanba K, Tsuiki M, Sawai K, et al. (2013). Histopathological diagnosis of primary aldosteronism using CYP11B2 immunohistochemistry. J Clin Endocrinol Metab. 98:1567–74. PMID:23443813
1952. Nandagopal R, Vortmeyer A, Oldfield EH, et al. (2007). Cushing's syndrome due to a pituitary corticotropinoma in a child with tuberous sclerosis: an association or a coincidence? Clin Endocrinol (Oxf). 67:639–41. PMID:17596199
1953. Nangue C, Bron L, Portmann L, et al. (2009). Mixed medullary-papillary carcinoma of the thyroid: report of a case and review of the literature. Head Neck. 31:968–74. PMID:19260112
1954. Naruse T, Koike A, Suzumura K, et al. (1991). Malignant "triton" tumor in the thyroid–a case report. Jpn J Surg. 21:466–70. PMID:1960908
1955. Nasr C, Mason A, Mayberg M, et al. (2006). Acromegaly and somatotroph hyperplasia with adenomatous transformation due to pituitary metastasis of a growth hormone-releasing hormone-secreting pulmonary endocrine carcinoma. J Clin Endocrinol Metab. 91:4776–80. PMID:16968791
1956. Nasuti JF, Benedict C, Hurford M, et al. (1999). Differential diagnosis of oncocytic lesions of the breast and thyroid utilizing a semiquantitative approach. Acta Cytol. 43:544–51. PMID:10432873
1957. Nath V, Parks GE, Baliga M, et al. (2014). Mucoepidermoid carcinoma of the thyroid with concomitant papillary carcinoma: comparison of findings on fine-needle aspiration biopsy and histology. Endocr Pathol. 25:427–32. PMID:25307114
1958. Näthke I (2006). Cytoskeleton out of the cupboard: colon cancer and cytoskeletal changes induced by loss of APC. Nat Rev Cancer. 6:967–74. PMID:17093505
1959. National Institutes of Health Consensus Development Conference (1988). Neurofibromatosis. Conference statement. National Institutes of Health Consensus Development Conference. Arch Neurol 45: 575–8. PMID:3128965
1960. Navas M, Martinez P, Shakur SF, et al. (2015). Intrasellar chordoma associated with a primitive persistent trigeminal artery. Turk Neurosurg. 25:146–53. PMID:25640561
1961. Nawata H, Higuchi K, Ikuyama S, et al. (1990). Corticotropin-releasing hormone- and adrenocorticotropin-producing pituitary carcinoma with metastases to the liver and lung in a patient with Cushing's disease. J Clin Endocrinol Metab. 71:1068–73. PMID:1698198
1962. Naziat A, Karavitaki N, Thakker R, et al. (2013). Confusing genes: a patient with MEN2A and Cushing's disease. Clin Endocrinol (Oxf). 78:966–8. PMID:23072303
1963. Nelen MR, van Staveren WC, Peeters EA, et al. (1997). Germline mutations in the PTEN/MMAC1 gene in patients with Cowden disease. Hum Mol Genet. 6:1383–7. PMID:9259288
1964. Nelson AC, Pillay N, Henderson S, et al. (2012). An integrated functional genomics approach identifies the regulatory network directed by brachyury (T) in chordoma. J Pathol. 228:274–85. PMID:22847733
1965. Nelson DS, Quispel W, Badalian-Very G, et al. (2014). Somatic activating ARAF mutations in Langerhans cell histiocytosis. Blood. 123:3152–5. PMID:24652991
1966. Nelson DS, van Halteren A, Quispel WT, et al. (2015). MAP2K1 and MAP3K1 mutations in Langerhans cell histiocytosis. Genes Chromosomes Cancer. 54:361–8. PMID:25899310
1967. Nelson S, Näthke IS (2013). Interactions and functions of the adenomatous polyposis coli (APC) protein at a glance. J Cell Sci. 126(Pt 4):873–7. PMID:23589686
1968. Neumann HP, Bausch B, McWhinney SR, et al. (2002). Germ-line mutations in nonsyndromic pheochromocytoma. N Engl J Med. 346:1459–66. PMID:12000816
1969. Neumann HP, Eng C, Mulligan LM, et al. (1995). Consequences of direct genetic testing for germline mutations in the clinical management of families with multiple endocrine neoplasia, type II. JAMA. 274:1149–51. PMID:7563486
1970. Neumann HP, Erlic Z, Boedeker CC, et al. (2009). Clinical predictors for germline mutations in head and neck paraganglioma patients: cost reduction strategy in genetic diagnostic process as fall-out. Cancer Res. 69:3650–6. PMID:19351833
1971. Nevoux J, Nowak C, Vellin JF, et al. (2014). Management of endolymphatic sac tumors: sporadic cases and von Hippel-Lindau disease. Otol Neurotol. 35:899–904. PMID:24662627
1972. Newey PJ, Bowl MR, Cranston T, et al. (2010). Cell division cycle protein 73 homolog (CDC73) mutations in the hyperparathyroidism-jaw tumor syndrome (HPT-JT) and parathyroid tumors. Hum Mutat. 31:295–307. PMID:20052758
1973. Newey PJ, Nesbit MA, Rimmer AJ, et al. (2013). Whole-exome sequencing studies of nonfunctioning pituitary adenomas. J Clin Endocrinol Metab. 98:E796–800. PMID:23450047
1974. Ng WK, Collins RJ, Shek WH, et al. (1996). Cytologic Diagnosis of "CASTLE" of thyroid gland: report of a case with histologic correlation. Diagn Cytopathol. 15:224–7. PMID:8955605
1975. Ngeow J, He X, Mester JL, et al. (2012). Utility of PTEN protein dosage in predicting for underlying germline PTEN mutations among patients presenting with thyroid cancer and Cowden-like phenotypes. J Clin Endocrinol Metab. 97:E2320–7. PMID:23066114
1976. Nguyen LB, Diskin SJ, Capasso M, et al. (2011). Phenotype restricted genome-wide association study using a gene-centric approach identifies three low-risk neuroblastoma susceptibility loci. PLoS Genet. 7:e1002026. PMID:21436895
1977. Nguyen PL, Poetker DM, Zambrano E (2011). Parathyroid hemangioma: a case report in proof of its existence. Endocr Pathol. 22:53–6. PMID:21286857
1978. Ni Y, He X, Chen J, et al. (2012). Germline SDHx variants modify breast and thyroid cancer risks in Cowden and Cowden-like syndrome via FAD/NAD-dependant destabilization of p53. Hum Mol Genet. 21:300–10. PMID:21979946
1979. Nibu Y, José-Edwards DS, Di Gregorio A (2013). From notochord formation to hereditary chordoma: the many roles of Brachyury. Biomed Res Int. 2013:826435. PMID:23662285
1980. Nicolis G, Shimshi M, Allen C, et al. (1988). Gonadotropin-producing pituitary adenoma in a man with long-standing primary hypogonadism. J Clin Endocrinol Metab. 66:237–41. PMID:2447114
1981. Niederle MB, Hackl M, Kaserer K, et al. (2010). Gastroenteropancreatic neuroendocrine tumours: the current incidence and staging based on the WHO and European Neuroendocrine Tumour Society classification: an analysis based on prospectively collected

parameters. Endocr Relat Cancer. 17:909–18. PMID:20702725

1982. Nielsen EH, Feldt-Rasmussen U, Poulsgaard L, et al. (2011). Incidence of craniopharyngioma in Denmark (n = 189) and estimated world incidence of craniopharyngioma in children and adults. J Neurooncol. 104:755–63. PMID:21336771

1983. Nieman LK (2015). Cushing's syndrome: update on signs, symptoms and biochemical screening. Eur J Endocrinol. 173:M33–8. PMID:26156970

1984. Niemeijer ND, Papathomas TG, Korpershoek E, et al. (2015). Succinate Dehydrogenase (SDH)-Deficient Pancreatic Neuroendocrine Tumor Expands the SDH-Related Tumor Spectrum. J Clin Endocrinol Metab. 100:E1386–93. PMID:26259135

1984A. Nieuwenhuis MH, Kets CM, Murphy-Ryan M, et al. (2014). Cancer risk and genotype-phenotype correlations in PTEN hamartoma tumor syndrome. Fam Cancer 13:57-63. PMID:23934601

1985. Nigawara K, Suzuki T, Tazawa H, et al. (1987). A case of recurrent malignant pheochromocytoma complicated by watery diarrhea, hypokalemia, achlorhydria syndrome. J Clin Endocrinol Metab. 65:1053–6. PMID:3667875

1986. Niitsu N, Okamoto M, Nakamura N, et al. (2007). Clinicopathologic correlations of stage IE/IIE primary thyroid diffuse large B-cell lymphoma. Ann Oncol. 18:1203–8. PMID:17429099

1987. Nijhoff MF, Dekkers OM, Vleming LJ, et al. (2009). ACTH-producing pheochromocytoma: clinical considerations and concise review of the literature. Eur J Intern Med. 20:682–5. PMID:19818286

1988. Nikfarjam M, Warshaw AL, Axelrod L, et al. (2008). Improved contemporary surgical management of insulinomas: a 25-year experience at the Massachusetts General Hospital. Ann Surg. 247:165–72. PMID:18156937

1989. Nikiforov Y, Gnepp DR (1994). Pediatric thyroid cancer after the Chernobyl disaster. Pathomorphologic study of 84 cases (1991-1992) from the Republic of Belarus. Cancer. 74:748–66. PMID:8033057

1990. Nikiforov YE, Carty SE, Chiosea SI, et al. (2015). Impact of the Multi-Gene ThyroSeq Next-Generation Sequencing Assay on Cancer Diagnosis in Thyroid Nodules with Atypia of Undetermined Significance/Follicular Lesion of Undetermined Significance Cytology. Thyroid. 25:1217–23. PMID:26356635

1991. Nikiforov YE, Erickson LA, Nikiforova MN, et al. (2001). Solid variant of papillary thyroid carcinoma: incidence, clinical-pathologic characteristics, molecular analysis, and biologic behavior. Am J Surg Pathol. 25:1478–84. PMID:11717536

1992. Nikiforov YE, Nikiforova MN (2011). Molecular genetics and diagnosis of thyroid cancer. Nat Rev Endocrinol. 7:569–80. PMID:21878896

1993. Nikiforov YE, Rowland JM, Bove KE, et al. (1997). Distinct pattern of ret oncogene rearrangements in morphological variants of radiation-induced and sporadic thyroid papillary carcinomas in children. Cancer Res. 57:1690–4. PMID:9135009

1994. Nikiforov YE, Seethala RR, Tallini G, et al. (2016). Nomenclature Revision for Encapsulated Follicular Variant of Papillary Thyroid Carcinoma: A Paradigm Shift to Reduce Overtreatment of Indolent Tumors. JAMA Oncol. 2:1023–9. PMID:27078145

1995. Nikiforova MN, Biddinger PW, Caudill CM, et al. (2002). PAX8-PPARgamma rearrangement in thyroid tumors: RT-PCR and immunohistochemical analyses. Am J Surg Pathol. 26:1016–23. PMID:12170088

1996. Nikiforova MN, Kimura ET, Gandhi M, et al. (2003). BRAF mutations in thyroid tumors are restricted to papillary carcinomas and

anaplastic or poorly differentiated carcinomas arising from papillary carcinomas. J Clin Endocrinol Metab. 88:5399–404. PMID:14602780

1997. Nikiforova MN, Lynch RA, Biddinger PW, et al. (2003). RAS point mutations and PAX8-PPAR gamma rearrangement in thyroid tumors: evidence for distinct molecular pathways in thyroid follicular carcinoma. J Clin Endocrinol Metab. 88:2318–26. PMID:12727991

1998. Nikiforova MN, Wald AI, Roy S, et al. (2013). Targeted next-generation sequencing panel (ThyroSeq) for detection of mutations in thyroid cancer. J Clin Endocrinol Metab. 98:E1852–60. PMID:23979959

1999. Ning S, Song X, Xiang L, et al. (2011). Malignant solitary fibrous tumor of the thyroid gland: report of a case and review of the literature. Diagn Cytopathol. 39:694–9. PMID:21837658

2000. Nishida T, Katayama S, Tsujimoto M, et al. (1999). Clinicopathological significance of poorly differentiated thyroid carcinoma. Am J Surg Pathol. 23:205–11. PMID:9989848

2001. Nishigami K, Liu Z, Taniguchi E, et al. (2012). Cytological features of well-differentiated tumors of uncertain malignant potential: Indeterminate cytology and WDT-UMP. Endocr J. 59:483–7. PMID:22484994

2002. Nishimoto K, Nakagawa K, Li D, et al. (2010). Adrenocortical zonation in humans under normal and pathological conditions. J Clin Endocrinol Metab. 95:2296–305. PMID:20200334

2003. Nishimoto K, Seki T, Kurihara I, et al. (2016). Case Report: Nodule Development From Subcapsular Aldosterone-Producing Cell Clusters Causes Hyperaldosteronism. J Clin Endocrinol Metab. 101:6–9. PMID:26580238

2004. Nishimoto K, Tomlins SA, Kuick R, et al. (2015). Aldosterone-stimulating somatic gene mutations are common in normal adrenal glands. Proc Natl Acad Sci U S A. 112:E4591–9. PMID:26240369

2005. Nishioka H, Fukuhara N, Horiguchi K, et al. (2014). Aggressive transsphenoidal resection of tumors invading the cavernous sinus in patients with acromegaly: predictive factors, strategies, and outcomes. J Neurosurg. 121:505–10. PMID:25014437

2006. Nishioka H, Haraoka J, Akada K, et al. (2002). Gender-related differences in prolactin secretion in pituitary prolactinomas. Neuroradiology. 44:407–10. PMID:12012125

2007. Nishioka H, Inoshita N, Mete O, et al. (2015). The Complementary Role of Transcription Factors in the Accurate Diagnosis of Clinically Nonfunctioning Pituitary Adenomas. Endocr Pathol. 26:349–55. PMID:26481628

2008. Nishioka H, Inoshita N, Sano T, et al. (2012). Correlation between histological subtypes and MRI findings in clinically nonfunctioning pituitary adenomas. Endocr Pathol. 23:151–6. PMID:22569896

2009. Nishioka H, Ito H, Hirano A, et al. (1997). Immunocytochemical study of pituitary oncocytic adenomas. Acta Neuropathol. 94:42–7. PMID:9224529

2010. Nishioka H, Shibuya M, Izawa H, et al. (2009). Primary suprasellar malignant tumor with odontogenic features: case report. Neurosurgery. 65:E380–2, discussion E382. PMID:19625894

2011. Nishizawa H, Fukuoka H, Iguchi G, et al. (2013). AIP mutation identified in a patient with acromegaly caused by pituitary somatotroph adenoma with neuronal choristoma. Exp Clin Endocrinol Diabetes. 121:295–9. PMID:23674160

2012. Nixon IJ, Whitcher MM, Palmer FL, et al. (2012). The impact of distant metastases at presentation on prognosis in patients with differentiated carcinoma of the thyroid gland. Thyroid. 22:884–9. PMID:22827579

2013. Njim L, Moussa A, Hadhri R, et al. (2008). Angiomatoid tumor of the thyroid gland:

primitive angiosarcoma or variant of anaplastic carcinoma? Ann Pathol. 28:221–4. [French] PMID:18706366

2014. Nobuoka Y, Hirokawa M, Kuma S, et al. (2014). Cytologic findings and differential diagnoses of primary thyroid MALT lymphoma with striking plasma cell differentiation and amyloid deposition. Diagn Cytopathol. 42:73–7. PMID:23636898

2015. Noctor E, Gupta S, Brown T, et al. (2015). Paediatric cyclical Cushing's disease due to corticotroph cell hyperplasia. BMC Endocr Disord. 15:27. PMID:26063496

2016. Nogales FF, Goyenaga P, Preda O, et al. (2012). An analysis of five clear cell papillary cystadenomas of mesosalpinx and broad ligament: four associated with von Hippel-Lindau disease and one aggressive sporadic type. Histopathology. 60:748–57. PMID:22296276

2017. Noh JM, Ha SY, Ahn YC, et al. (2015). Potential Role of Adjuvant Radiation Therapy in Cervical Thymic Neoplasm Involving Thyroid Gland or Neck. Cancer Res Treat. 47:436–40. PMID:25648096

2018. Nomori H, Morinaga S, Kobayashi R, et al. (1994). Cervical thymic cancer infiltrating the trachea and thyroid. Eur J Cardiothorac Surg. 8:222–4. PMID:8031568

2019. Nonaka D (2011). Study of parathyroid transcription factor Gcm2 expression in parathyroid lesions. Am J Surg Pathol. 35:145–51. PMID:21164298

2020. Nonaka D, Chiriboga L, Rubin BP (2008). Sox10: a pan-schwannian and melanocytic marker. Am J Surg Pathol. 32:1291–8. PMID:18636017

2021. Nonaka D, Rodriguez J, Rosai J (2007). Extraneural hemangioblastoma: a report of 5 cases. Am J Surg Pathol. 31:1545–51. PMID:17895756

2022. Nonaka D, Tang Y, Chiriboga L, et al. (2008). Diagnostic utility of thyroid transcription factors Pax8 and TTF-2 (FoxE1) in thyroid epithelial neoplasms. Mod Pathol. 21:192–200. PMID:18084247

2023. Nord B, Platz A, Smoczynski K, et al. (2000). Malignant melanoma in patients with multiple endocrine neoplasia type 1 and involvement of the MEN1 gene in sporadic melanoma. Int J Cancer. 87:463–7. PMID:10918183

2024. Norton JA, Froome LC, Farrell RE, et al. (1979). Multiple endocrine neoplasia type IIb: the most aggressive form of medullary thyroid carcinoma. Surg Clin North Am. 59:109–18. PMID:441904

2025. Norton JA, Melcher ML, Gibril F, et al. (2004). Gastric carcinoid tumors in multiple endocrine neoplasia-1 patients with Zollinger-Ellison syndrome can be symptomatic, demonstrate aggressive growth, and require surgical treatment. Surgery. 136:1267–74. PMID:15657586

2026. Nosé V (2011). Familial thyroid cancer: a review. Mod Pathol. 24 Suppl 2:S19–33. PMID:21455198

2027. Nosé V, Paner GP, Geenson JK, et al., editors (2013). Diagnostic pathology: familial cancer syndromes. Salt Lake City: Amirsys Publishing, Inc.

2028. Nosé V, Erickson LA, Tischler AS, et al., editors (2012). Diagnostic pathology: endocrine. Salt Lake City: Amirsys Publishing, Inc.

2029. Nosé V, Ezzat S, Horvath E, et al. (2011). Protocol for the examination of specimens from patients with primary pituitary tumors. Arch Pathol Lab Med. 135:640–6. PMID:21526962

2030. Novello M, Coli A, Della Pepa GM, et al. (2014). Myeloid sarcoma with megakaryoblastic differentiation mimicking a sellar tumor. Neuropathology. 34:179–84. PMID:24118374

2031. Ntali G, Capatina C, Grossman A,

et al. (2014). Clinical review: Functioning gonadotroph adenomas. J Clin Endocrinol Metab. 99:4423–33. PMID:25166722

2032. Nucera C, Porrello A, Antonello ZA, et al. (2010). B-Raf(V600E) and thrombospondin-1 promote thyroid cancer progression. Proc Natl Acad Sci U S A. 107:10649–54. PMID:20498063

2033. Nwokoro NA, Korytkowski MT, Rose S, et al. (1997). Spectrum of malignancy and premalignancy in Carney syndrome. Am J Med Genet. 73:369–77. PMID:9415461

2034. O'Brien T, Young WF Jr, Davila DG, et al. (1992). Cushing's syndrome associated with ectopic production of corticotrophin-releasing hormone, corticotrophin and vasopressin by a phaeochromocytoma. Clin Endocrinol (Oxf). 37:460–7. PMID:1283118

2035. O'Brien WM, Lynch JH (1987). Adrenal metastases by renal cell carcinoma. Incidence at nephrectomy. Urology. 29:605–7. PMID:3576885

2036. O'Gorman CS, Hamilton J, Rachmiel M, et al. (2010). Thyroid cancer in childhood: a retrospective review of childhood course. Thyroid. 20:375–80. PMID:20373982

2037. O'Neill CJ, Vaughan L, Learoyd DL, et al. (2011). Management of follicular thyroid carcinoma should be individualised based on degree of capsular and vascular invasion. Eur J Surg Oncol. 37:181–5. PMID:21144693

2038. O'Neill S, O'Donnell M, Harkin D, et al. (2011). A 22-year Northern Irish experience of carotid body tumours. Ulster Med J. 80:133–40. PMID:23526121

2039. O'Riordain DS, Young WF Jr, Grant CS, et al. (1996). Clinical spectrum and outcome of functional extraadrenal paraganglioma. World J Surg. 20:916–21, discussion 922. PMID:8678971

2040. O'Toole SM, Dénes J, Robledo M, et al. (2015). 15 YEARS OF PARAGANGLIOMA: The association of pituitary adenomas and phaeochromocytomas or paragangliomas. Endocr Relat Cancer. 22:T105–22. PMID:26113600

2041. Obara T (1992). Diagnosis and treatment of primary hyperparathyroidism. Nihon Naibunpi Gakkai Zasshi. 68:1167–76. [Japanese] PMID:1468593

2042. Obari A, Sano T, Ohyama K, et al. (2008). Clinicopathological features of growth hormone-producing pituitary adenomas: difference among various types defined by cytokeratin distribution pattern including a transitional form. Endocr Pathol. 19:82–91. PMID:18629656

2043. Öberg K, Knigge U, Kwekkeboom D, et al. (2012). Neuroendocrine gastro-entero-pancreatic tumors: ESMO Clinical Practice Guidelines for diagnosis, treatment and follow-up. Ann Oncol. 23 Suppl 7:vii124–30. PMID:22997445

2044. Ogrin C (2013). A rare case of double parathyroid lipoadenoma with hyperparathyroidism. Am J Med Sci. 346:432–4. PMID:24157966

2045. Oh YL, Ko YH, Ree HJ (1998). Aspiration cytology of ectopic cervical thymoma mimicking a thyroid mass. A case report. Acta Cytol. 42:1167–71. PMID:9755676

2046. Ohike N, Jürgensen A, Pipeleers-Marichal M, et al. (2003). Mixed ductal-endocrine carcinomas of the pancreas and ductal adenocarcinomas with scattered endocrine cells: characterization of the endocrine cells. Virchows Arch. 442:258–65. PMID:12647216

2047. Ohike N, Kosmahl M, Klöppel G (2004). Mixed acinar-endocrine carcinoma of the pancreas. A clinicopathological study and comparison with acinar-cell carcinoma. Virchows Arch. 445:231–5. PMID:15517367

2048. Ohtsuki Y, Kimura M, Murao S, et al. (2009). Immunohistochemical and electron

microscopy studies of a case of hyalinizing trabecular tumor of the thyroid gland, with special consideration of the hyalinizing mass associated with it. Med Mol Morphol. 42:189–94. PMID:19784748
2049. Okada Y, Nishikawa R, Matsutani M, et al. (2002). Hypomethylated X chromosome gain and rare isochromosome 12p in diverse intracranial germ cell tumors. J Neuropathol Exp Neurol. 61:531–8. PMID:12071636
2050. Onozawa M, Fukuhara T, Minoguchi M, et al. (2005). Hypokalemic rhabdomyolysis due to WDHA syndrome caused by VIP-producing composite pheochromocytoma: a case in neurofibromatosis type 1. Jpn J Clin Oncol. 35:559–63. PMID:16027147
2051. Ooi A, Kameya T, Tsumuraya M, et al. (1985). Pancreatic endocrine tumours associated with WDHA syndrome. An immunohistochemical and electron microscopic study. Virchows Arch A Pathol Anat Histopathol. 405:311–23. PMID:2579503
2052. Opotowsky AR, Moko LE, Ginns J, et al. (2015). Pheochromocytoma and paraganglioma in cyanotic congenital heart disease. J Clin Endocrinol Metab. 100:1325–34. PMID:25581599
2053. Orbach D, Sarnacki S, Brisse HJ, et al. (2013). Neonatal cancer. Lancet Oncol. 14:e609–20. PMID:24275134
2054. Orbeal R, Jimeno J, Monroy G, et al. (2015). Sclerosing mucoepidermoid carcinoma of the thyroid gland with eosinophilia. Cir Esp. 93:e137–8. [Spanish] PMID:25064518
2055. Ordóñez NG (2003). Application of mesothelin immunostaining in tumor diagnosis. Am J Surg Pathol. 27:1418–28. PMID:14576474
2056. Ordóñez NG (2014). Value of GATA3 immunostaining in the diagnosis of parathyroid tumors. Appl Immunohistochem Mol Morphol. 22:756–61. PMID:25046229
2057. Orrico A, Galli L, Buoni S, et al. (2009). Novel PTEN mutations in neurodevelopmental disorders and macrocephaly. Clin Genet. 75:195–8. PMID:18759867
2058. Orselli RC, Bassler TJ (1973). Theca granuloma cell tumor arising in adrenal. Cancer. 31:474–7. PMID:4687888
2059. Ortiz J, Villabona C, Bengoechea O, et al. (2008). Primary epithelioid angiosarcoma of the thyroid: an infrequent malignant thyroid tumor. Endocrinol Nutr. 55:181–3. PMID:22975456
2059A. Osamura RY, Tahara S, Komatsubara K et al. (1999). Pit-1 positive alpha-subunit positive nonfunctioning human pituitary adenomas: a dedifferentiated GH cell lineage? Pituitary 1:269-71. PMID:11081207
2060. Osamura RY, Watanabe K, Komatsu N, et al. (1982). Amorphous and stellate amyloid in functioning human pituitary adenomas: histochemical, immunohistochemical and electron microscopic studies. Acta Pathol Jpn. 32:605–11. PMID:7113700
2061. Oshima J, Martin GM, Hisama FM (2014). Werner syndrome In: Pagon RA, Adam MP, Ardinger HH, et al., editors. GeneReviews®. Seattle: University of Washington, Seattle. PMID:20301687
2062. Oshmyansky AR, Mahammedi A, Dackiw A, et al. (2013). Serendipity in the diagnosis of pheochromocytoma. J Comput Assist Tomogr. 37:820–3. PMID:24045263
2063. Osinga TE, Korpershoek E, de Krijger RR, et al. (2015). Catecholamine-Synthesizing Enzymes Are Expressed in Parasympathetic Head and Neck Paraganglioma Tissue. Neuroendocrinology. 101:289–95. PMID:25677368
2064. Ostrom QT, Gittleman H, Fulop J, et al. (2015). CBTRUS Statistical Report: Primary Brain and Central Nervous System Tumors Diagnosed in the United States in 2008-2012. Neuro Oncol. 17 Suppl 4:iv1–62. PMID:26511214
2065. Ostrom QT, Gittleman H, Liao P, et al. (2014). CBTRUS statistical report: primary brain and central nervous system tumors diagnosed in the United States in 2007–2011. Neuro Oncol. 16 Suppl 4:iv1–63. PMID:25304271
2066. Otto AI, Marschalko M, Zalatnai A, et al. (2011). Glucagon cell adenomatosis: a new entity associated with necrolytic migratory erythema and glucagonoma syndrome. J Am Acad Dermatol. 65:458–9. PMID:21763589
2067. Oudijk L, de Krijger RR, Rapa I, et al. (2014). H-RAS mutations are restricted to sporadic pheochromocytomas lacking specific clinical or pathological features: data from a multi-institutional series. J Clin Endocrinol Metab. 99:E1376–80. PMID:24684458
2068. Oudijk L, van Nederveen F, Badoual C, et al. (2015). Vascular pattern analysis for the prediction of clinical behaviour in pheochromocytomas and paragangliomas. PLoS One. 10:e0121361. PMID:25794004
2069. Oyama K, Sanno N, Teramoto A, et al. (2001). Expression of neuro D1 in human normal pituitaries and pituitary adenomas. Mod Pathol. 14:892–9. PMID:11557786
2070. Oyama K, Yamada S, Usui M, et al. (2005). Sellar neuroblastoma mimicking pituitary adenoma. Pituitary. 8:109–14. PMID:16501893
2071. Özata DM, Caramuta S, Velázquez-Fernández D, et al. (2011). The role of microRNA deregulation in the pathogenesis of adrenocortical carcinoma. Endocr Relat Cancer. 18:643–55. PMID:21859927
2072. Ozsari L, Kutahyalioglu M, Elsayes KM, et al. (2016). Preexisting adrenal masses in patients with adrenocortical carcinoma: clinical and radiological factors contributing to delayed diagnosis. Endocrine. 51:351–9. PMID:26206754
2073. Ozüm U, Eğilmez R, Yildirim A (2008). Paraganglioma in pituitary fossa. Neuropathology. 28:547–50. PMID:18410271
2074. Pacak K, Chew EY, Pappo AS, et al. (2014). Ocular manifestations of hypoxia-inducible factor-2α paraganglioma-somatostatinoma-polycythemia syndrome. Ophthalmology. 121:2291–3. PMID:25109928
2075. Pacak K, Eisenhofer G, Ahlman H, et al. (2007). Pheochromocytoma: recommendations for clinical practice from the First International Symposium. October 2005. Nat Clin Pract Endocrinol Metab. 3:92–102. PMID:17237836
2076. Pacak K, Jochmanova I, Prodanov T, et al. (2013). New syndrome of paraganglioma and somatostatinoma associated with polycythemia. J Clin Oncol. 31:1690–8. PMID:23509317
2077. Pacak K, Wimalawansa SJ (2015). Pheochromocytoma and paraganglioma. Endocr Pract. 21:406–12. PMID:25716634
2078. Pack SD, Kirschner LS, Pak E, et al. (2000). Genetic and histologic studies of somatomammotropic pituitary tumors in patients with the "complex of spotty skin pigmentation, myxomas, endocrine overactivity and schwannomas" (Carney complex). J Clin Endocrinol Metab. 85:3860–5. PMID:11061550
2079. Pagano M, Tam SW, Theodoras AM, et al. (1995). Role of the ubiquitin-proteasome pathway in regulating abundance of the cyclin-dependent kinase inhibitor p27. Science. 269:682–5. PMID:7624798
2080. Pagotto U, Arzberger T, Theodoropoulou M, et al. (2000). The expression of the antiproliferative gene ZAC is lost or highly reduced in nonfunctioning pituitary adenomas. Cancer Res. 60:6794–9. PMID:11156367
2081. Palculict TB, Ruteshouser EC, Fan Y, et al. (2016). Identification of germline DICER1 mutations and loss of heterozygosity in familial Wilms tumour. J Med Genet. 53:385–8. PMID:26566882
2082. Pallares J, Perez-Ruiz L, Ros S, et al. (2004). Malignant peripheral nerve sheath tumor of the thyroid: a clinicopathological and ultrastructural study of one case. Endocr Pathol. 15:167–74. PMID:15299203
2083. Palmedo H, Bucerius J, Joe A, et al. (2006). Integrated PET/CT in differentiated thyroid cancer: diagnostic accuracy and impact on patient management. J Nucl Med. 47:616–24. PMID:16595495
2084. Palos-Paz F, Perez-Guerra O, Cameselle-Teijeiro J, et al. (2008). Prevalence of mutations in TSHR, GNAS, PRKAR1A and RAS genes in a large series of toxic thyroid adenomas from Galicia, an iodine-deficient area in NW Spain. Eur J Endocrinol. 159:623–31. PMID:18694911
2085. Pandya C, Uzilov AV, Bellizzi J, et al. (2015). PgmNr 365: The driver landscape of parathyroid carcinoma [abstract]. Paper presented at the 65th Annual Meeting of the American Society of Human Genetics, 6–10 October 2015, Baltimore, USA.
2086. Pantelia E, Kontogeorgos G, Piaditis G, et al. (1998). Triple pituitary adenoma in Cushing's disease: case report. Acta Neurochir (Wien). 140:190–3. PMID:10399001
2087. Papanastasiou L, Pappa T, Dasou A, et al. (2012). Case report: Primary pituitary non-Hodgkin's lymphoma developed following surgery and radiation of a pituitary macroadenoma. Hormones (Athens). 11:488–94. PMID:23422773
2088. Papanikolaou A, Michala L (2015). Autonomous Ovarian Cysts in Prepubertal Girls. How Aggressive Should We Be? A Review of the Literature. J Pediatr Adolesc Gynecol. 28:292–6. PMID:26228588
2089. Papaparaskeva K, Nagel H, Droese M (2000). Cytologic diagnosis of medullary carcinoma of the thyroid gland. Diagn Cytopathol. 22:351–8. PMID:10820528
2090. Papathomas TG, de Krijger RR, Tischler AS (2013). Paragangliomas: update on differential diagnostic considerations, composite tumors, and recent genetic developments. Semin Diagn Pathol. 30:207–23. PMID:24144290
2091. Papathomas TG, Gaal J, Corssmit EP, et al. (2013). Non-pheochromocytoma (PCC)/paraganglioma (PGL) tumors in patients with succinate dehydrogenase-related PCC-PGL syndromes: a clinicopathological and molecular analysis. Eur J Endocrinol. 170:1–12. PMID:24096523
2092. Papathomas TG, Oudijk L, Persu A, et al. (2015). SDHB/SDHA immunohistochemistry in pheochromocytomas and paragangliomas: a multicenter interobserver variation analysis using virtual microscopy: a Multinational Study of the European Network for the Study of Adrenal Tumors (ENS@T). Mod Pathol. 28:807–21. PMID:25720320
2093. Papathomas TG, Pucci E, Giordano TJ, et al. (2016). An International Ki67 Reproducibility Study in Adrenal Cortical Carcinoma. Am J Surg Pathol. 40:569–76. PMID:26685085
2094. Papi G, Corrado S, LiVolsi VA (2006). Primary spindle cell lesions of the thyroid gland; an overview. Am J Clin Pathol. 125 Suppl:S95–123. PMID:16830961
2095. Papi G, Corrado S, Ruggiero C, et al. (2006). Solitary fibrous tumor of the thyroid gland associated with papillary thyroid carcinoma. Thyroid. 16:319–20. PMID:16571098
2096. Papi G, Fadda G, Corsello SM, et al. (2007). Metastases to the thyroid gland: prevalence, clinicopathological aspects and prognosis: a 10-year experience. Clin Endocrinol (Oxf). 66:565–71. PMID:17371476
2097. Papotti M, Arrondini M, Tavaglione V, et al. (2008). Diagnostic controversies in vascular proliferations of the thyroid gland. Endocr Pathol. 19:175–83. PMID:18766472
2098. Papotti M, Bongiovanni M, Volante M, et al. (2002). Expression of somatostatin receptor types 1-5 in 81 cases of gastrointestinal and pancreatic endocrine tumors. A correlative immunohistochemical and reverse-transcriptase polymerase chain reaction analysis. Virchows Arch. 440:461–75. PMID:12021920
2099. Papotti M, Botto Micca F, Favero A, et al. (1993). Poorly differentiated thyroid carcinomas with primordial cell component. A group of aggressive lesions sharing insular, trabecular, and solid patterns. Am J Surg Pathol. 17:291–301. PMID:8434709
2100. Papotti M, Duregon E, Volante M, et al. (2014). Pathology of the adrenal cortex: a reappraisal of the past 25 years focusing on adrenal cortical tumors. Endocr Pathol. 25:35–48. PMID:24382573
2101. Papotti M, Negro F, Carney JA, et al. (1997). Mixed medullary-follicular carcinoma of the thyroid. A morphological, immunohistochemical and in situ hybridization analysis of 11 cases. Virchows Arch. 430:397–405. PMID:9174630
2102. Papotti M, Riella P, Montemurro F, et al. (1997). Immunophenotypic heterogeneity of hyalinizing trabecular tumours of the thyroid. Histopathology. 31:525–33. PMID:9447383
2103. Papotti M, Rodriguez J, De Pompa R, et al. (2005). Galectin-3 and HBME-1 expression in well-differentiated thyroid tumors with follicular architecture of uncertain malignant potential. Mod Pathol. 18:541–6. PMID:15529186
2104. Papotti M, Sapino A, Abbona G, et al. (1995). Pseudoangiosarcomatous features in medullary carcinomas of the thyroid: report of two cases. Int J Surg Pathol. 3:29–34.
2105. Papotti M, Torchio B, Grassi L, et al. (1996). Poorly differentiated oxyphilic (Hürthle cell) carcinomas of the thyroid. Am J Surg Pathol. 20:686–94. PMID:8651347
2106. Papotti M, Volante M, Duregon E, et al. (2010). Adrenocortical tumors with myxoid features: a distinct morphologic and phenotypical variant exhibiting malignant behavior. Am J Surg Pathol. 34:973–83. PMID:20534995
2107. Papotti M, Volante M, Giuliano A, et al. (2000). RET/PTC activation in hyalinizing trabecular tumors of the thyroid. Am J Surg Pathol. 24:1615–21. PMID:11117781
2108. Papotti M, Volante M, Komminoth P, et al. (2000). Thyroid carcinomas with mixed follicular and C-cell differentiation patterns. Semin Diagn Pathol. 17:109–19. PMID:10839611
2109. Papotti M, Volante M, Negro F, et al. (2000). Thyroglobulin mRNA expression helps to distinguish anaplastic carcinoma from angiosarcoma of the thyroid. Virchows Arch. 437:635–42. PMID:11193475
2110. Pardi E, Mariotti S, Pellegata NS, et al. (2015). Functional characterization of a CDKN1B mutation in a Sardinian kindred with multiple endocrine neoplasia type 4 (MEN4). Endocr Connect. 4:1–8. PMID:25416039
2111. Parfitt AM, Wang Q, Palnitkar S (1998). Rates of cell proliferation in adenomatous, suppressed, and normal parathyroid tissue: implications for pathogenesis. J Clin Endocrinol Metab. 83:863–9. PMID:9506741
2112. Parish JM, Bonnin JM, Goodman JM, et al. (2015). Intrasellar ependymoma: clinical, imaging, pathological, and surgical findings. J Clin Neurosci. 22:638–41. PMID:25744072
2113. Park HW, Jung S, Jung TY, et al. (2009). Intra-suprasellar schwannoma originating from the diaphragma sellae. J Korean Neurosurg Soc. 45:375–7. PMID:19609422
2114. Park JR, Bagatell R, London WB, et al. (2013). Children's Oncology Group's 2013 blueprint for research: neuroblastoma. Pediatr Blood Cancer. 60:985–93. PMID:23255319
2115. Park SH, Kim SJ, Jung HK (2014). Thyroid hemangiomas diagnosed on sonography. J Ultrasound Med. 33:729–33. PMID:24658955
2116. Park SY, Park YJ, Lee YJ, et al. (2006). Analysis of differential BRAF(V600E) mutational status in multifocal papillary thyroid carcinoma: evidence of independent clonal origin in distinct tumor foci. Cancer. 107:1831–8. PMID:16983703

2117. Park Y, Kim H, Kim EH, et al. (2016). Effective Treatment of Solitary Pituitary Metastasis with Panhypopituitarism in HER2-Positive Breast Cancer by Lapatinib. Cancer Res Treat. 48:403–8. PMID:25715765
2118. Parker LN, Kollin J, Wu SY, et al. (1985). Carcinoma of the thyroid with a mixed medullary, papillary, follicular, and undifferentiated pattern. Arch Intern Med. 145:1507–9. PMID:3896182
2119. Parma J, Duprez L, Van Sande J, et al. (1997). Diversity and prevalence of somatic mutations in the thyrotropin receptor and Gs alpha genes as a cause of toxic thyroid adenomas. J Clin Endocrinol Metab. 82:2695–701. PMID:9253356
2120. Parodi S, Merlo DF, Ranucci A, et al. (2014). Risk of neuroblastoma, maternal characteristics and perinatal exposures: the SETIL study. Cancer Epidemiol. 38:686–94. PMID:25280392
2121. Partington MD, Davis DH, Laws ER Jr, et al. (1994). Pituitary adenomas in childhood and adolescence. Results of transsphenoidal surgery. J Neurosurg. 80:209–16. PMID:8283258
2122. Parvanescu A, Cros J, Ronot M, et al. (2014). Lessons from McCune-Albright syndrome-associated intraductal papillary mucinous neoplasms: GNAS-activating mutations in pancreatic carcinogenesis. JAMA Surg. 149:858–62. PMID:24898823
2123. Parwani AV, Galindo R, Steinberg DM, et al. (2003). Solitary fibrous tumor of the thyroid: cytopathologic findings and differential diagnosis. Diagn Cytopathol. 28:213–6. PMID:12672098
2124. Pasini B, Stratakis CA (2009). SDH mutations in tumorigenesis and inherited endocrine tumours: lesson from the phaeochromocytoma-paraganglioma syndromes. J Intern Med. 266:19–42. PMID:19522823
2125. Patel D, Boufraqech M, Jain M, et al. (2013). MiR-34a and miR-483-5p are candidate serum biomarkers for adrenocortical tumors. Surgery. 154:1224–8, discussion 1229. PMID:24238045
2126. Patel J, Eloy JA, Liu JK (2015). Nelson's syndrome: a review of the clinical manifestations, pathophysiology, and treatment strategies. Neurosurg Focus. 38:E14. PMID:25639316
2127. Patten DK, Wani Z, Tolley N (2012). Solitary langerhans histiocytosis of the thyroid gland: a case report and literature review. Head Neck Pathol. 6:279–89. PMID:22198822
2128. Patterson EE, Holloway AK, Weng J, et al. (2011). MicroRNA profiling of adrenocortical tumors reveals miR-483 as a marker of malignancy. Cancer. 117:1630–9. PMID:21472710
2129. Pausova Z, Soliman E, Amizuka N, et al. (1996). Role of the RET proto-oncogene in sporadic hyperparathyroidism and in hyperparathyroidism of multiple endocrine neoplasia type 2. J Clin Endocrinol Metab. 81:2711–8. PMID:8675600
2130. Pavlovich CP, Schmidt LS, Phillips JL (2003). The genetic basis of renal cell carcinoma. Urol Clin North Am. 30:437–54, vii. PMID:12953747
2131. Pazienza V, la Torre A, Baorda F, et al. (2013). Identification and functional characterization of three NoLS (nucleolar localisation signals) mutations of the CDC73 gene. PLoS One. 8:e82292. PMID:24340015
2132. Pea A, Hruban RH, Wood LD (2015). Genetics of pancreatic neuroendocrine tumors: implications for the clinic. Expert Rev Gastroenterol Hepatol. 9:1407–19. PMID:26413978
2133. Pease M, Ling C, Mack WJ, et al. (2013). The role of epigenetic modification in tumorigenesis and progression of pituitary adenomas: a systematic review of the literature. PLoS One. 8:e82619. PMID:24367530
2134. Pęczkowska M, Kowalska A, Sygut J, et al. (2013). Testing new susceptibility genes in the cohort of apparently sporadic phaeochromocytoma/paraganglioma patients with clinical characteristics of hereditary syndromes. Clin Endocrinol (Oxf). 79:817–23. PMID:23551045
2135. Pedersen RK, Pedersen NT (1996). Primary non-Hodgkin's lymphoma of the thyroid gland: a population based study. Histopathology. 28:25–32. PMID:8838117
2136. Pei L, Melmed S, Scheithauer B, et al. (1994). H-ras mutations in human pituitary carcinoma metastases. J Clin Endocrinol Metab. 78:842–6. PMID:8157709
2137. Peifer M, Fernández-Cuesta L, Sos ML, et al. (2012). Integrative genome analyses identify key somatic driver mutations of small-cell lung cancer. Nat Genet. 44:1104–10. PMID:22941188
2138. Peifer M, Hertwig F, Roels F, et al. (2015). Telomerase activation by genomic rearrangements in high-risk neuroblastoma. Nature. 526:700–4. PMID:26466568
2139. Pekmezci M, Louie J, Gupta N, et al. (2010). Clinicopathological characteristics of adamantinomatous and papillary craniopharyngiomas: University of California, San Francisco experience 1985-2005. Neurosurgery. 67:1341–9, discussion 1349. PMID:20871436
2140. Pelizzo MR, Torresan F, Boschin IM, et al. (2015). Early, Prophylactic Thyroidectomy in Hereditary Medullary Thyroid Carcinoma: A 26-year Monoinstitutional Experience. Am J Clin Oncol. 38:508–13. PMID:24064755
2141. Pellegata NS, Quintanilla-Martinez L, Siggelkow H, et al. (2006). Germ-line mutations in p27Kip1 cause a multiple endocrine neoplasia syndrome in rats and humans. Proc Natl Acad Sci U S A. 103:15558–63. PMID:17030811
2142. Pelletier G, Cortot A, Launay JM, et al. (1984). Serotonin-secreting and insulin-secreting ileal carcinoid tumor and the use of in vitro culture of tumoral cells. Cancer. 54:319–22. PMID:6372987
2143. Pelletier J, Bellot G, Gounon P, et al. (2012). Glycogen Synthesis is Induced in Hypoxia by the Hypoxia-Inducible Factor and Promotes Cancer Cell Survival. Front Oncol. 2:18. PMID:22649778
2144. Pelosi G, Bresaola E, Bogina G, et al. (1996). Endocrine tumors of the pancreas: Ki-67 immunoreactivity on paraffin sections is an independent predictor for malignancy: a comparative study with proliferating-cell nuclear antigen and progesterone receptor protein immunostaining, mitotic index, and other clinicopathologic variables. Hum Pathol. 27:1124–34. PMID:8912819
2145. Pemov A, Sung H, Hyland PL, et al. (2014). Genetic modifiers of neurofibromatosis type 1-associated café-au-lait macule count identified using multi-platform analysis. PLoS Genet. 10:e1004575. PMID:25329635
2146. Peng P, Chen F, Zhou D, et al. (2015). Neurocytoma of the pituitary gland: A case report and literature review. Biomed Rep. 3:301–3. PMID:26137226
2147. Peng SY, Li JT, Liu YB, et al. (2004). Diagnosis and treatment of VIPoma in China: (case report and 31 cases review) diagnosis and treatment of VIPoma. Pancreas. 28:93–7. PMID:14707737
2147A. Pennanen M, Heiskanen I, Sane T, et al. (2015). Helsinki score-a novel model for prediction of metastases in adrenocortical carcinomas. Hum Pathol. 46(3):404–10. PMID:25582500
2148. Pereira BD, Raimundo L, Mete O, et al. (2016). Monomorphous Plurihormonal Pituitary Adenoma of Pit-1 Lineage in a Giant Adolescent with Central Hyperthyroidism. Endocr Pathol. 27:25–33. PMID:26330191
2149. Perez-Montiel MD, Frankel WL, Suster S (2003). Neuroendocrine carcinomas of the pancreas with 'Rhabdoid' features. Am J Surg Pathol. 27:642–9. PMID:12717248
2150. Perez-Rivas LG, Theodoropoulou M, Ferraù F, et al. (2015). The Gene of the Ubiquitin-Specific Protease 8 Is Frequently Mutated in Adenomas Causing Cushing's Disease. J Clin Endocrinol Metab. 100:E997–1004. PMID:25942478
2151. Périgny M, Hammel P, Corcos O, et al. (2009). Pancreatic endocrine microadenomatosis in patients with von Hippel-Lindau disease: characterization by VHL/HIF pathway proteins expression. Am J Surg Pathol. 33:739–48. PMID:19238077
2152. Permanetter W, Nathrath WB, Löhrs U (1982). Immunohistochemical analysis of thyroglobulin and keratin in benign and malignant thyroid tumours. Virchows Arch A Pathol Anat Histopathol. 398:221–8. PMID:6187120
2153. Pernicone PJ, Scheithauer BW, Sebo TJ, et al. (1997). Pituitary carcinoma: a clinicopathologic study of 15 cases. Cancer. 79:804–12. PMID:9024719
2154. Perone TP, Robinson B, Holmes SM (1984). Intrasellar schwannoma: case report. Neurosurgery. 14:71–3. PMID:6694795
2155. Perren A, Anlauf M, Henopp T, et al. (2007). Multiple endocrine neoplasia type 1 (MEN1): loss of one MEN1 allele in tumors and monohormonal endocrine cell clusters but not in islet hyperplasia of the pancreas. J Clin Endocrinol Metab. 92:1118–28. PMID:17179192
2156. Perren A, Barghorn A, Schmid S, et al. (2002). Absence of somatic SDHD mutations in sporadic neuroendocrine tumors and detection of two germline variants in paraganglioma patients. Oncogene. 21:7605–8. PMID:12386824
2157. Perry A, Molberg K, Albores-Saavedra J (1996). Physiologic versus neoplastic C-cell hyperplasia of the thyroid: separation of distinct histologic and biologic entities. Cancer. 77:750–6. PMID:8616768
2158. Péter I, Besznyák I, Szántó J, et al. (1989). Clear cell thyroid cancer–undifferentiated type–an immunohistochemical and electron microscopical study. Arch Geschwulstforsch. 59:121–8. PMID:2719532
2159. Petterson T, MacFarlane IA, MacKenzie JM, et al. (1992). Prolactin secreting pituitary carcinoma. J Neurol Neurosurg Psychiatry. 55:1205–6. PMID:1479402
2160. Peuchmaur M, d'Amore ES, Joshi VV, et al. (2003). Revision of the International Neuroblastoma Pathology Classification: confirmation of favorable and unfavorable prognostic subsets in ganglioneuroblastoma, nodular. Cancer. 98:2274–81. PMID:14601099
2161. Pezzolo A, Rossi E, Gimelli S, et al. (2009). Presence of 1q gain and absence of 7p gain are new predictors of local or metastatic relapse in localized resectable neuroblastoma. Neuro Oncol. 11:192–200. PMID:18923191
2162. Pfaltz M, Hedinger C, Saremaslani P, et al. (1983). Malignant hemangioendothelioma of the thyroid and factor VIII-related antigen. Virchows Arch A Pathol Anat Histopathol. 401:177–84. PMID:6415902
2163. Pfister C (2014). Adrenal biopsy is recommended to differentiate benign versus malignant metastasis of primary adrenal lesions. AJR Am J Roentgenol. 203:W340-1. PMID:25148194
2164. Phillips JJ, Misra A, Feuerstein BG, et al. (2010). Pituicytoma: characterization of a unique neoplasm by histology, immunohistochemistry, ultrastructure, and array-based comparative genomic hybridization. Arch Pathol Lab Med. 134:1063–9. PMID:20586639
2165. Piana S, Frasoldati A, Di Felice E, et al. (2010). Encapsulated well-differentiated follicular-patterned thyroid carcinomas do not play a significant role in the fatality rates from thyroid carcinoma. Am J Surg Pathol. 34:868–72. PMID:20463572
2166. Piana S, Ragazzi M, Tallini G, et al. (2013). Papillary thyroid microcarcinoma with fatal outcome: evidence of tumor progression in lymph node metastases: report of 3 cases, with morphological and molecular analysis. Hum Pathol. 44:556–65. PMID:23079204
2167. Piccini V, Rapizzi E, Bacca A, et al. (2012). Head and neck paragangliomas: genetic spectrum and clinical variability in 79 consecutive patients. Endocr Relat Cancer. 19:149–55. PMID:22241717
2168. Piccirilli M, Maiola V, Salvati M, et al. (2014). Granular cell tumor of the neurohypophysis: a single-institution experience. Tumori. 100:160e–4e. PMID:25296610
2169. Pichard DC, Boyce AM, Collins MT, et al. (2014). Oral pigmentation in McCune-Albright syndrome. JAMA Dermatol. 150:760–3. PMID:24671640
2170. Pieterman CR, Conemans EB, Dreijerink KM, et al. (2014). Thoracic and duodenopancreatic neuroendocrine tumors in multiple endocrine neoplasia type 1: natural history and function of menin in tumorigenesis. Endocr Relat Cancer. 21:R121–42. PMID:24389729
2171. Pieterman CR, van Hulsteijn LT, den Heijer M, et al. (2012). Primary hyperparathyroidism in MEN1 patients: a cohort study with longterm follow-up on preferred surgical procedure and the relation with genotype. Ann Surg. 255:1171–8. PMID:22470073
2172. Pilato FP, D'Adda T, Banchini E, et al. (1988). Nonrandom expression of polypeptide hormones in pancreatic endocrine tumors. An immunohistochemical study in a case of multiple islet cell neoplasia. Cancer. 61:1815–20. PMID:2895680
2173. Pillarisetty VG, Katz SC, Ghossein RA, et al. (2009). Micromedullary thyroid cancer: how micro is truly micro? Ann Surg Oncol. 16:2875–81. PMID:19568813
2174. Pilotti S, Collini P, Del Bo R, et al. (1994). A novel panel of antibodies that segregates immunocytochemically poorly differentiated carcinoma from undifferentiated carcinoma of the thyroid gland. Am J Surg Pathol. 18:1054–64. PMID:7522412
2175. Pimenta FJ, Gontijo Silveira LF, Tavares GC, et al. (2006). HRPT2 gene alterations in ossifying fibroma of the jaws. Oral Oncol. 42:735–9. PMID:16458039
2176. Pinato DJ, Ramachandran R, Toussi ST, et al. (2013). Immunohistochemical markers of the hypoxic response can identify malignancy in phaeochromocytomas and paragangliomas and optimize the detection of tumours with VHL germline mutations. Br J Cancer. 108:429–37. PMID:23257898
2177. Pinto EM, Chen X, Easton J, et al. (2015). Genomic landscape of paediatric adrenocortical tumours. Nat Commun. 6:6302. PMID:25743702
2178. Pipeleers-Marichal M, Somers G, Willems G, et al. (1990). Gastrinomas in the duodenums of patients with multiple endocrine neoplasia type 1 and the Zollinger-Ellison syndrome. N Engl J Med. 322:723–7. PMID:1968616
2179. Pippa R, Espinosa L, Gundem G, et al. (2012). p27Kip1 represses transcription by direct interaction with p130/E2F4 at the promoters of target genes. Oncogene. 31:4207–20. PMID:22179826
2180. Pita JM, Figueiredo IF, Moura MM, et al. (2014). Cell cycle deregulation and TP53 and RAS mutations are major events in poorly differentiated and undifferentiated thyroid carcinomas. J Clin Endocrinol Metab. 99:E497–507. PMID:24423316
2181. Pithukpakorn M, Toro JR (2015). Hereditary leiomyomatosis and renal cell cancer. In: Pagon RA, Adam MP, Ardinger HH, et al., editors. GeneReviews®. Seattle: University of Washington, Seattle. PMID:20301430
2182. Pivonello R, De Leo M, Cozzolino A, et al. (2015). The Treatment of Cushing's Disease. Endocr Rev. 36:385–486. PMID:26067718
2183. Pizzi S, D'Adda T, Azzoni C, et al. (2002).

Malignancy-associated allelic losses on the X-chromosome in foregut but not in midgut endocrine tumours. J Pathol. 196:401–7. PMID:11920735
2184. Pluta RM, Wait SD, Butman JA, et al. (2003). Sacral hemangioblastoma in a patient with von Hippel-Lindau disease. Case report and review of the literature. Neurosurg Focus. 15:E11. PMID:15350042
2185. Polak M (1999). Hyperfunctioning thyroid adenoma and activating mutations in the TSH receptor gene. Arch Med Res. 30:510–3. PMID:10714365
2186. Poli F, Trezzi R, Rosai J (2009). Images in pathology. Single thyroid follicle involved by papillary carcinoma: partially classic and partially oncocytic. Int J Surg Pathol. 17:272–3. PMID:18805871
2187. Pollack IF, Shultz B, Mulvihill JJ (1996). The management of brainstem gliomas in patients with neurofibromatosis 1. Neurology. 46:1652–60. PMID:8649565
2188. Pollock WJ, McConnell CF, Hilton C, et al. (1986). Virilizing Leydig cell adenoma of adrenal gland. Am J Surg Pathol. 10:816–22. PMID:3022613
2189. Potorac I, Petrossians P, Daly AF, et al. (2015). Pituitary MRI characteristics in 297 acromegaly patients based on T2-weighted sequences. Endocr Relat Cancer. 22:169–77. PMID:25556181
2190. Poulsen ML, Gimsing S, Kosteljanetz M, et al. (2011). von Hippel-Lindau disease: surveillance strategy for endolymphatic sac tumors. Genet Med. 13:1032–41. PMID:21912262
2191. Powell JG, Goellner JR, Nowak LE, et al. (2003). Rosai-Dorfman disease of the thyroid masquerading as anaplastic carcinoma. Thyroid. 13:217–21. PMID:12699598
2192. Powell SZ (2005). Intraoperative consultation, cytologic preparations, and frozen section in the central nervous system. Arch Pathol Lab Med. 129:1635–52. PMID:16329736
2193. Powers JF, Brachold JM, Tischler AS (2003). Ret protein expression in adrenal medullary hyperplasia and pheochromocytoma. Endocr Pathol. 14:351–61. PMID:14739491
2194. Powers JF, Korgaonkar PG, Fliedner S, et al. (2014). Cytocidal activities of topoisomerase 1 inhibitors and 5-azacytidine against pheochromocytoma/paraganglioma cells in primary human tumor cultures and mouse cell lines. PLoS One. 9:e87807. PMID:24516563
2195. Poyhonen M, Kytölä S, Leisti J (2000). Epidemiology of neurofibromatosis type 1 (NF1) in northern Finland. J Med Genet. 37:632–6. PMID:10991696
2196. Pradhan D, Sharma A, Mohanty SK (2015). Cribriform-morular variant of papillary thyroid carcinoma. Pathol Res Pract. 211:712–6. PMID:26293799
2197. Prall JA, McGavran L, Greffe BS, et al. (1995). Intracranial malignant germ cell tumor and the Klinefelter syndrome. Case report and review of the literature. Pediatr Neurosurg. 23:219–24. PMID:8835213
2198. Prasad ML, Pellegata NS, Huang Y, et al. (2005). Galectin-3, fibronectin-1, CITED-1, HBME1 and cytokeratin-19 immunohistochemistry is useful for the differential diagnosis of thyroid tumors. Mod Pathol. 18:48–57. PMID:15272279
2199. Preda V, Korbonits M, Cudlip S, et al. (2014). Low rate of germline AIP mutations in patients with apparently sporadic pituitary adenomas before the age of 40: a single-centre adult cohort. Eur J Endocrinol. 171:659–66. PMID:25184284
2200. Preda V, Sywak M, Learoyd D (2015). A new association - multiple endocrine neoplasia type 1 and malignant peripheral nerve sheath tumor. Clin Case Rep. 3:29–31. PMID:25678969
2201. Presneau N, Shalaby A, Ye H, et al. (2011). Role of the transcription factor T (brachyury) in the pathogenesis of sporadic chordoma: a genetic and functional-based study. J Pathol. 223:327–35. PMID:21171078
2202. Preto A, Cameselle-Teijeiro J, Moldes-Boullosa J, et al. (2004). Telomerase expression and proliferative activity suggest a stem cell role for thyroid solid cell nests. Mod Pathol. 17:819–26. PMID:15044923
2203. Prichard RS, Lee JC, Gill AJ, et al. (2012). Mucoepidermoid carcinoma of the thyroid: a report of three cases and postulated histogenesis. Thyroid. 22:205–9. PMID:22224821
2204. Priest JR, Hill DA, Williams GM, et al. (2006). Type I pleuropulmonary blastoma: a report from the International Pleuropulmonary Blastoma Registry. J Clin Oncol. 24:4492–8. PMID:16983119
2205. Priest JR, Watterson J, Strong L, et al. (1996). Pleuropulmonary blastoma: a marker for familial disease. J Pediatr. 128:220–4. PMID:8636815
2206. Priest JR, Williams GM, Manera R, et al. (2011). Ciliary body medulloepithelioma: four cases associated with pleuropulmonary blastoma–a report from the International Pleuropulmonary Blastoma Registry. Br J Ophthalmol. 95:1001–5. PMID:21156700
2207. Pritchard CC, Smith C, Marushchak T, et al. (2013). A mosaic PTEN mutation causing Cowden syndrome identified by deep sequencing. Genet Med. 15:1004–7. PMID:23619277
2208. Proppe KH, Scully RE (1980). Large-cell calcifying Sertoli cell tumor of the testis. Am J Clin Pathol. 74:607–19. PMID:7446466
2209. Puchner MJ, Lüdecke DK, Saeger W, et al. (1995). Gangliocytomas of the sellar region–a review. Exp Clin Endocrinol Diabetes. 103:129–49. PMID:7584515
2210. Puchner MJ, Lüdecke DK, Valdueza JM, et al. (1993). Cushing's disease in a child caused by a corticotropin-releasing hormone-secreting intrasellar gangliocytoma associated with an adrenocorticotropic hormone-secreting pituitary adenoma. Neurosurgery. 33:920–4, discussion 924–5. PMID:8264895
2211. Pugh TJ, Morozova O, Attiyeh EF, et al. (2013). The genetic landscape of high-risk neuroblastoma. Nat Genet. 45:279–84. PMID:23334666
2212. Puri P, Motwani N, Pande M (2001). Squamous carcinoma of the thyroid metastatic to the choroid: a report. Eur J Cancer Care (Engl). 10:63–4. PMID:11827270
2213. Pusel J, Rodier JF, Auge B, et al. (1993). Malignant hemangioendothelioma of the thyroid. Pathologic study of a case. Ann Pathol. 13:253–5. [French] PMID:8280300
2214. Pusztaszeri M, Wang H, Cibas ES, et al. (2015). Fine-needle aspiration biopsy of secondary neoplasms of the thyroid gland: a multi-institutional study of 62 cases. Cancer Cytopathol. 123:19–29. PMID:25369542
2215. Pusztaszeri MP, Bongiovanni M, Faquin WC (2014). Update on the cytologic and molecular features of medullary thyroid carcinoma. Adv Anat Pathol. 21:26–35. PMID:24316908
2216. Pytel P, Krausz T, Wollmann R, et al. (2005). Ganglioneuromatous paraganglioma of the cauda equina–a pathological case study. Hum Pathol. 36:444–6. PMID:15892009
2217. Qasem E, Murugan AK, Al-Hindi H, et al. (2015). TERT promoter mutations in thyroid cancer: a report from a Middle Eastern population. Endocr Relat Cancer. 22:901–8. PMID:26354077
2218. Qiao N, Ye Z, Wang Y, et al. (2014). Gangliocytomas in the sellar region. Clin Neurol Neurosurg. 126:156–61. PMID:25259876
2219. Qin N, de Cubas AA, Garcia-Martin R, et al. (2014). Opposing effects of HIF1α and HIF2α on chromaffin cell phenotypic features and tumor cell proliferation: Insights from MYC-associated factor X. Int J Cancer. 135:2054–64. PMID:24676840
2220. Qin Y, Deng Y, Ricketts CJ, et al. (2014). The tumor susceptibility gene TMEM127 is mutated in renal cell carcinomas and modulates endolysosomal function. Hum Mol Genet. 23:2428–39. PMID:24334765
2221. Queipo G, Aguirre D, Nieto K, et al. (2008). Intracranial germ cell tumors: association with Klinefelter syndrome and sex chromosome aneuploidies. Cytogenet Genome Res. 121:211–4. PMID:18758161
2222. Quinn TR, Duncan LM, Zembowicz A, et al. (2005). Cutaneous metastases of follicular thyroid carcinoma: a report of four cases and a review of the literature. Am J Dermatopathol. 27:306–12. PMID:16121050
2223. Quiroga-Garza G, Lee JH, El-Naggar A, et al. (2015). Sclerosing mucoepidermoid carcinoma with eosinophilia of the thyroid: more aggressive than previously reported. Hum Pathol. 46:725–31. PMID:25754017
2224. Quiros RM, Ding HG, Gattuso P, et al. (2005). Evidence that one subset of anaplastic thyroid carcinomas are derived from papillary carcinomas due to BRAF and p53 mutations. Cancer. 103:2261–8. PMID:15880523
2225. Quist EE, Javadzadeh BM, Johannesen E, et al. (2015). Malignant paraganglioma of the bladder: a case report and review of the literature. Pathol Res Pract. 211:183–8. PMID:25512259
2226. Raaf HN, Grant LD, Santoscoy C, et al. (1996). Adenomatoid tumor of the adrenal gland: a report of four new cases and a review of the literature. Mod Pathol. 9:1046–51. PMID:8933514
2227. Rabban JT, Zaloudek CJ (2013). A practical approach to immunohistochemical diagnosis of ovarian germ cell tumours and sex cord-stromal tumours. Histopathology. 62:71–88. PMID:23240671
2228. Raco A, Bristot R, Domenicucci M, et al. (1999). Meningiomas of the tuberculum sellae. Our experience in 69 cases surgically treated between 1973 and 1993. J Neurosurg Sci. 43:253–60, discussion 260–2. PMID:10864387
2229. Radi MJ, Fenoglio-Preiser CM, Chiffelle T (1985). Functioning oncocytic islet-cell carcinoma. Report of a case with electron-microscopic and immunohistochemical confirmation. Am J Surg Pathol. 9:517–24. PMID:3004244
2230. Radotra B, Apostolopoulos V, Sandison A, et al. (2010). Primary sellar neuroblastoma presenting with syndrome of inappropriate secretion of anti-diuretic hormone. Endocr Pathol. 21:266–73. PMID:21053097
2231. Ragel BT, Couldwell WT (2004). Pituitary carcinoma: a review of the literature. Neurosurg Focus. 16:E7. PMID:15191336
2232. Rahman A, Maitra A, Ashfaq R, et al. (2003). Loss of p27 nuclear expression in a prognostically favorable subset of well-differentiated pancreatic endocrine neoplasms. Am J Clin Pathol. 120:685–90. PMID:14608893
2233. Rainsbury P, Mitchell-Innes A, Clifton Nj, et al. (2012). Primary lymphoma of the pituitary gland: an unusual cause of hemianopia in an immunocompetent patient. JRSM Short Rep. 3:55. PMID:23301143
2234. Rainwater LM, Farrow GM, Hay ID, et al. (1986). Oncocytic tumours of the salivary gland, kidney, and thyroid: nuclear DNA patterns studied by flow cytometry. Br J Cancer. 53:799–804. PMID:3718832
2235. Rajasoorya C, Holdaway IM, Wrightson P, et al. (1994). Determinants of clinical outcome and survival in acromegaly. Clin Endocrinol (Oxf). 41:95–102. PMID:8050136
2236. Rajendran R, Naik S, Sandeman DD, et al. (2013). Pasireotide therapy in a rare and unusual case of plurihormonal pituitary macroadenoma. Endocrinol Diabetes Metab Case Rep. 2013:130026. PMID:24616766
2237. Rakheja D, Chen KS, Liu Y, et al. (2014). Somatic mutations in DROSHA and DICER1 impair microRNA biogenesis through distinct mechanisms in Wilms tumours. Nat Commun. 2:4802. PMID:25190313
2238. Ramírez C, Cheng S, Vargas G, et al. (2012). Expression of Ki-67, PTTG1, FGFR4, and SSTR 2, 3, and 5 in nonfunctioning pituitary adenomas: a high throughput TMA, immunohistochemical study. J Clin Endocrinol Metab. 97:1745–51. PMID:22419713
2239. Ramírez C, Hernández-Ramirez LC, Espinosa-de-los-Monteros AL, et al. (2013). Ectopic acromegaly due to a GH-secreting pituitary adenoma in the sphenoid sinus: a case report and review of the literature. BMC Res Notes. 6:411. PMID:24119925
2240. Ranade R, Rachh S, Basu S (2015). Late Manifestation of Struma Peritonei and Widespread Functioning Lesions in the Setting of Struma Ovarii Simulating Highly Differentiated Follicular Carcinoma. J Nucl Med Technol. 43:231–3. PMID:25537757
2241. Rasbach DA, Monchik JM, Geelhoed GW, et al. (1984). Solitary parathyroid microadenoma. Surgery. 96:1092–8. PMID:6505961
2242. Rashidi A, Fisher SI (2013). Primary adrenal lymphoma: a systematic review. Ann Hematol. 92:1583–93. PMID:23771429
2243. Raskin A, Castro-Dominguez Y, Mirani N, et al. (2016). Incidental ectopic thyroid follicular adenoma on myocardial perfusion imaging. J Nucl Cardiol. 23:153–4. PMID:26122882
2244. Rasmuson T, Tavelin B (2006). Risk of parathyroid adenomas in patients with thyrotoxicosis exposed to radioactive iodine. Acta Oncol. 45:1059–61. PMID:17118839
2245. Rasmussen P, Lindholm J (1979). Ectopic pituitary adenomas. Clin Endocrinol (Oxf). 11:69–74. PMID:519872
2246. Rasul FT, Jaunmuktane Z, Khan AA, et al. (2014). Plurihormonal pituitary adenoma with concomitant adrenocorticotropic hormone (ACTH) and growth hormone (GH) secretion: a report of two cases and review of the literature. Acta Neurochir (Wien). 156:141–6. PMID:24081787
2247. Rath SR, Bartley A, Charles A, et al. (2014). Multinodular Goiter in children: an important pointer to a germline DICER1 mutation. J Clin Endocrinol Metab. 99:1947–8. PMID:24628552
2248. Ratliff JK, Oldfield EH (2000). Multiple pituitary adenomas in Cushing's disease. J Neurosurg. 93:753–61. PMID:11059654
2249. Ratner N, Miller SJ (2015). A RASopathy gene commonly mutated in cancer: the neurofibromatosis type 1 tumour suppressor. Nat Rev Cancer. 15:290–301. PMID:25877329
2250. Rattner DW, Marrone GC, Kasdon E, et al. (1985). Recurrent hyperparathyroidism due to implantation of parathyroid tissue. Am J Surg. 149:745–8. PMID:4014550
2251. Raue F, Frank-Raue K (2010). Update multiple endocrine neoplasia type 2. Fam Cancer. 9:449–57. PMID:20087666
2252. Raue F, Frank-Raue K (2015). Epidemiology and Clinical Presentation of Medullary Thyroid Carcinoma. Recent Results Cancer Res. 204:61–90. PMID:26494384
2253. Raue F, Kotzerke J, Reinwein D, et al. (1993). Prognostic factors in medullary thyroid carcinoma: evaluation of 741 patients from the German Medullary Thyroid Carcinoma Register. Clin Investig. 71:7–12. PMID:8095831
2254. Raverot G, Arnous W, Calender A, et al. (2007). Familial pituitary adenomas with a heterogeneous functional pattern: clinical and genetic features. J Endocrinol Invest. 30:787–90. PMID:17993773
2255. Raverot G, Castinetti F, Jouanneau E, et al. (2012). Pituitary carcinomas and aggressive pituitary tumours: merits and pitfalls of temozolomide treatment. Clin Endocrinol (Oxf). 76:769–75. PMID:22404748
2256. Raverot G, Jouanneau E, Trouillas J (2014). Management of endocrine disease:

clinicopathological classification and molecular markers of pituitary tumours for personalized therapeutic strategies. Eur J Endocrinol. 170:R121–32. PMID:24431196
2257. Raverot G, Sturm N, de Fraipont F, et al. (2010). Temozolomide treatment in aggressive pituitary tumors and pituitary carcinomas: a French multicenter experience. J Clin Endocrinol Metab. 95:4592–9. PMID:20660056
2258. Raymond VM, Everett JN, Furtado LV, et al. (2013). Adrenocortical carcinoma is a lynch syndrome-associated cancer. J Clin Oncol. 31:3012–8. PMID:23752102
2259. Raz DJ, Lanuti M, Gaissert HC, et al. (2011). Outcomes of patients with isolated adrenal metastasis from non-small cell lung carcinoma. Ann Thorac Surg. 92:1788–92, discussion 1793. PMID:21944257
2260. Recavarren RA, Yang J (2010). Cytomorphologic features of primary anaplastic large cell lymphoma of the psoas muscle: a case report and literature review. Diagn Cytopathol. 38:208–12. PMID:19760764
2261. Rechache NS, Wang Y, Stevenson HS, et al. (2012). DNA methylation profiling identifies global methylation differences and markers of adrenocortical tumors. J Clin Endocrinol Metab. 97:E1004–13. PMID:22472567
2262. Recondo G Jr, Busaidy N, Erasmus J, et al. (2015). Spindle epithelial tumor with thymus-like differentiation: A case report and comprehensive review of the literature and treatment options. Head Neck. 37:746–54. PMID:24677409
2263. Reddick RL, Costa JC, Marx SJ (1977). Parathyroid hyperplasia and parathyromatosis. Lancet. 1:549. PMID:65648
2264. Reddy R, Cudlip S, Byrne JV, et al. (2011). Can we ever stop imaging in surgically treated and radiotherapy-naive patients with non-functioning pituitary adenoma? Eur J Endocrinol. 165:739–44. PMID:21900406
2265. Redman BG, Pazdur R, Zingas AP, et al. (1987). Prospective evaluation of adrenal insufficiency in patients with adrenal metastasis. Cancer. 60:103–7. PMID:3581024
2266. Regalbuto C, Malandrino P, Tumminia A, et al. (2011). A diffuse sclerosing variant of papillary thyroid carcinoma: clinical and pathologic features and outcomes of 34 consecutive cases. Thyroid. 21:383–9. PMID:21309722
2266A. Rehfeld JF, Federspiel B, Bardram L. (2013). A neuroendocrine tumor syndrome from cholecystokinin secretion. N Engl J Med. 368:1165–6. PMID:23514309
2267. Reid MD, Bagci P, Ohike N, et al. (2015). Calculation of the Ki67 index in pancreatic neuroendocrine tumors: a comparative analysis of four counting methodologies. Mod Pathol. 28:686–94. PMID:25412850
2268. Reid MD, Balci S, Saka B, et al. (2014). Neuroendocrine tumors of the pancreas: current concepts and controversies. Endocr Pathol. 25:65–79. PMID:24430597
2269. Reimann JD, Dorfman DM, Nosé V (2006). Carcinoma showing thymus-like differentiation of the thyroid (CASTLE): a comparative study: evidence of thymic differentiation and solid cell nest origin. Am J Surg Pathol. 30:994–1001. PMID:16861971
2270. Reincke M (2000). Subclinical Cushing's syndrome. Endocrinol Metab Clin North Am. 29:43–56. PMID:10732263
2271. Reincke M, Sbiera S, Hayakawa A, et al. (2015). Mutations in the deubiquitinase gene USP8 cause Cushing's disease. Nat Genet. 47:31–8. PMID:25485838
2272. Rejnmark L, Vestergaard P, Mosekilde L (2011). Nephrolithiasis and renal calcifications in primary hyperparathyroidism. J Clin Endocrinol Metab. 96:2377–85. PMID:21646371
2273. Relles D, Baek J, Witkiewicz A, et al. (2010). Periampullary and duodenal neoplasms in neurofibromatosis type 1: two cases and an updated 20-year review of the literature yielding 76 cases. J Gastrointest Surg. 14:1052–61. PMID:20300877
2274. Renshaw AA (2001). Accuracy of thyroid fine-needle aspiration using receiver operator characteristic curves. Am J Clin Pathol. 116:477–82. PMID:11601131
2275. Renshaw AA, Gould EW (2002). Why there is the tendency to "overdiagnose" the follicular variant of papillary thyroid carcinoma. Am J Clin Pathol. 117:19–21. PMID:11789725
2276. Reubi JC, Heitz PU, Gyr K (1987). Vasoactive intestinal peptide producing tumour contains high density of somatostatin receptors. Lancet. 1:741–2. PMID:2882148
2277. Reyes CV, Wang T (1981). Undifferentiated small cell carcinoma of the pancreas: a report of five cases. Cancer. 47:2500–2. PMID:6268272
2278. Rhatigan RM, Roque JL, Bucher RL (1977). Mucoepidermoid carcinoma of the thyroid gland. Cancer. 39:210–4. PMID:832236
2279. Ribeiro-Oliveira A Jr, Barkan A (2012). The changing face of acromegaly–advances in diagnosis and treatment. Nat Rev Endocrinol. 8:605–11. PMID:22733271
2280. Ricarte-Filho JC, Li S, Garcia-Rendueles ME, et al. (2013). Identification of kinase fusion oncogenes in post-Chernobyl radiation-induced thyroid cancers. J Clin Invest. 123:4935–44. PMID:24135138
2281. Ricarte-Filho JC, Ryder M, Chitale DA, et al. (2009). Mutational profile of advanced primary and metastatic radioactive iodine-refractory thyroid cancers reveals distinct pathogenetic roles for BRAF, PIK3CA, and AKT1. Cancer Res. 69:4885–93. PMID:19487299
2282. Richard S, Gardie B, Couvé S, et al. (2013). Von Hippel-Lindau: how a rare disease illuminates cancer biology. Semin Cancer Biol. 23:26–37. PMID:22659535
2283. Richter KK, Premkumar R, Yoon HS, et al. (2011). Laparoscopic adrenalectomy for a rare 14-cm adrenal schwannoma. Surg Laparosc Endosc Percutan Tech. 21:e339–43. PMID:22146188
2284. Richter S, Peitzsch M, Rapizzi E, et al. (2014). Krebs cycle metabolite profiling for identification and stratification of pheochromocytomas/paragangliomas due to succinate dehydrogenase deficiency. J Clin Endocrinol Metab. 99:3903–11. PMID:25014000
2285. Rickert CH, Dockhorn-Dworniczak B, Busch G, et al. (2001). Increased chromosomal imbalances in recurrent pituitary adenomas. Acta Neuropathol. 102:615–20. PMID:11761722
2286. Rickert CH, Scheithauer BW, Paulus W (2001). Chromosomal aberrations in pituitary carcinoma metastases. Acta Neuropathol. 102:117–20. PMID:11563625
2287. Ricketts CJ, Forman JR, Rattenberry E, et al. (2010). Tumor risks and genotype-phenotype-proteotype analysis in 358 patients with germline mutations in SDHB and SDHD. Hum Mutat. 31:41–51. PMID:19802898
2288. Riddle PE, Dincsoy HP (1987). Primary squamous cell carcinoma of the thyroid associated with leukocytosis and hypercalcemia. Arch Pathol Lab Med. 111:373–4. PMID:3827545
2289. Riester A, Weismann D, Quinkler M, et al. (2015). Life-threatening events in patients with pheochromocytoma. Eur J Endocrinol. 173:757–64. PMID:26346138
2290. Rigaud G, Missiaglia E, Moore PS, et al. (2001). High resolution allelotype of nonfunctional pancreatic endocrine tumors: identification of two molecular subgroups with clinical implications. Cancer Res. 61:285–92. PMID:11196176
2291. Righi A, Morandi L, Leonardi E, et al. (2013). Galectin-3 expression in pituitary adenomas as a marker of aggressive behavior. Hum Pathol. 44:2400–9. PMID:24007691
2292. Riminucci M, Collins MT, Fedarko NS, et al. (2003). FGF-23 in fibrous dysplasia of bone and its relationship to renal phosphate wasting. J Clin Invest. 112:683–92. PMID:12952917
2293. Rindi G, Arnold R, Bosman FT, et al. (2010). Nomenclature and classification of neuroendocrine neoplasms of the digestive system. In: Bosman FT, Carneiro F, Hruban RH, et al., editors. WHO classification of tumours of the digestive system. 4th ed. Lyon: IARC; pp. 13–4.
2294. Rindi G, Falconi M, Klersy C, et al. (2012). TNM staging of neoplasms of the endocrine pancreas: results from a large international cohort study. J Natl Cancer Inst. 104:764–77. PMID:22525418
2295. Rindi G, Klöppel G, Alhman H, et al. (ENETS) (2006). TNM staging of foregut (neuro)endocrine tumors: a consensus proposal including a grading system. Virchows Arch. 449:395–401. PMID:16967267
2296. Ringel MD, Schwindinger WF, Levine MA (1996). Clinical implications of genetic defects in G proteins. The molecular basis of McCune-Albright syndrome and Albright hereditary osteodystrophy. Medicine (Baltimore). 75:171–84. PMID:8699958
2297. Rinke A, Müller HH, Schade-Brittinger C, et al. (2009). Placebo-controlled, double-blind, prospective, randomized study on the effect of octreotide LAR in the control of tumor growth in patients with metastatic neuroendocrine midgut tumors: a report from the PROMID Study Group. J Clin Oncol. 27:4656–63. PMID:19704057
2298. Rio Frio T, Bahubeshi A, Kanellopoulou C, et al. (2011). DICER1 mutations in familial multinodular goiter with and without ovarian Sertoli-Leydig cell tumors. JAMA. 305:68–77. PMID:21205968
2299. Ríos A, Rodríguez JM, Acosta JM, et al. (2010). Prognostic value of histological and immunohistochemical characteristics for predicting the recurrence of medullary thyroid carcinoma. Ann Surg Oncol. 17:2444–51. PMID:20224859
2300. Ríos A, Rodríguez JM, Martínez E, et al. (2001). Cavernous hemangioma of the thyroid. Thyroid. 11:279–80. PMID:11327620
2301. Rippe V, Belge G, Meiboom M, et al. (1999). A KRAB zinc finger protein gene is the potential target of 19q13 translocation in benign thyroid tumors. Genes Chromosomes Cancer. 26:229–36. PMID:10502321
2302. Rippe V, Dittberner L, Lorenz VN, et al. (2010). The two stem cell microRNA gene clusters C19MC and miR-371-3 are activated by specific chromosomal rearrangements in a subgroup of thyroid adenomas. PLoS One. 5:e9485. PMID:20209130
2303. Rippe V, Drieschner N, Meiboom M, et al. (2003). Identification of a gene rearranged by 2p21 aberrations in thyroid adenomas. Oncogene. 22:6111–4. PMID:12955091
2304. Riss D, Jin L, Qian X, et al. (2003). Differential expression of galectin-3 in pituitary tumors. Cancer Res. 63:2251–5. PMID:12727847
2305. Ritter JH, Mills SE, Nappi O, et al. (1995). Angiosarcoma-like neoplasms of epithelial organs: true endothelial tumors or variants of carcinoma? Semin Diagn Pathol. 12:270–82. PMID:8545593
2306. Rivera M, Ghossein RA, Schoder H, et al. (2008). Histopathologic characterization of radioactive iodine-refractory fluorodeoxyglucose-positron emission tomography-positive thyroid carcinoma. Cancer. 113:48–56. PMID:18484584
2307. Rivera M, Ricarte-Filho J, Knauf J, et al. (2010). Molecular genotyping of papillary thyroid carcinoma follicular variant according to its histological subtypes (encapsulated vs infiltrative) reveals distinct BRAF and RAS mutation patterns. Mod Pathol. 23:1191–200. PMID:20526288
2308. Rivera M, Ricarte-Filho J, Patel S, et al. (2010). Encapsulated thyroid tumors of follicular cell origin with high grade features (high mitotic rate/tumor necrosis): a clinicopathologic and molecular study. Hum Pathol. 41:172–80. PMID:19913280
2309. Rivera M, Ricarte-Filho J, Tuttle RM, et al. (2010). Molecular, morphologic, and outcome analysis of thyroid carcinomas according to degree of extrathyroid extension. Thyroid. 20:1085–93. PMID:20860430
2310. Robinson DR, Wu YM, Kalyana-Sundaram S, et al. (2013). Identification of recurrent NAB2-STAT6 gene fusions in solitary fibrous tumor by integrative sequencing. Nat Genet. 45:180–5. PMID:23313952
2311. Rocha AS, Soares P, Machado JC, et al. (2002). Mucoepidermoid carcinoma of the thyroid: a tumour histotype characterised by P-cadherin neoexpression and marked abnormalities of E-cadherin/catenins complex. Virchows Arch. 440:498–504. PMID:12021924
2312. Rodd C, Millette M, Iacovazzo D, et al. (2016). Somatic GPR101 Duplication Causing X-Linked Acrogigantism (XLAG)-Diagnosis and Management. J Clin Endocrinol Metab. 101:1927–30. PMID:26982009
2313. Roden AC, Hu X, Kip S, et al. (2014). BRAF V600E expression in Langerhans cell histiocytosis: clinical and immunohistochemical study on 25 pulmonary and 54 extrapulmonary cases. Am J Surg Pathol. 38:548–51. PMID:24625419
2314. Rodrigues MG, Matos Lima L, Fonseca G, et al. (2015). Mucoepidermoid carcinoma of the thyroid. A case report. Thyroid. 25(S1):A-262–3.
2315. Rodriguez FJ, Folpe AL, Giannini C, et al. (2012). Pathology of peripheral nerve sheath tumors: diagnostic overview and update on selected diagnostic problems. Acta Neuropathol. 123:295–319. PMID:22327363
2316. Rodriguez I, Ayala E, Caballero C, et al. (2001). Solitary fibrous tumor of the thyroid gland: report of seven cases. Am J Surg Pathol. 25:1424–8. PMID:11684960
2317. Rodríguez-Cuevas S, López-Garza J, Labastida-Almendaro S (1998). Carotid body tumors in inhabitants of altitudes higher than 2000 meters above sea level. Head Neck. 20:374–8. PMID:9663663
2318. Rojiani AM, Owen DA, Berry K, et al. (1991). Hepatic hemangioblastoma. An unusual presentation in a patient with von Hippel-Lindau disease. Am J Surg Pathol. 15:81–6. PMID:1898683
2319. Roka S, Kornek G, Schüller J, et al. (2004). Carcinoma showing thymic-like elements–a rare malignancy of the thyroid gland. Br J Surg. 91:142–5. PMID:14760659
2320. Roldo C, Missiaglia E, Hagan JP, et al. (2006). MicroRNA expression abnormalities in pancreatic endocrine and acinar tumors are associated with distinctive pathologic features and clinical behavior. J Clin Oncol. 24:4677–84. PMID:16966691
2321. Roman S, Lin R, Sosa JA (2006). Prognosis of medullary thyroid carcinoma: demographic, clinical, and pathologic predictors of survival in 1252 cases. Cancer. 107:2134–42. PMID:17019736
2322. Romei C, Fugazzola L, Puxeddu E, et al. (2012). Modifications in the papillary thyroid cancer gene profile over the last 15 years. J Clin Endocrinol Metab. 97:E1758–65. PMID:22745248
2323. Romei C, Ugolini C, Cosci B, et al. (2012). Low prevalence of the somatic M918T RET mutation in micro-medullary thyroid cancer. Thyroid. 22:476–81. PMID:22404432
2324. Romero Arenas MA, Ryu H, Lee S, et al. (2014). The role of thyroidectomy in metastatic disease to the thyroid gland. Ann Surg Oncol. 21:434–9. PMID:24081800

2325. Romero Arenas MA, Sui D, Grubbs EG, et al. (2014). Adrenal metastectomy is safe in selected patients. World J Surg. 38:1336–42. PMID:24452292
2326. Romero-Rojas AE, Diaz-Perez JA, Mastrodimos M, et al. (2013). Follicular thyroid carcinoma with signet ring cell morphology: fine-needle aspiration cytology, histopathology, and immunohistochemistry. Endocr Pathol. 24:239–45. PMID:24068558
2327. Romero-Rojas AE, Melo-Uribe MA, Barajas-Solano PA, et al. (2011). Spindle cell oncocytoma of the adenohypophysis. Brain Tumor Pathol. 28:359–64. PMID:21833579
2328. Roncaroli F, Nosé V, Scheithauer BW, et al. (2003). Gonadotropic pituitary carcinoma: HER-2/neu expression and gene amplification. Report of two cases. J Neurosurg. 99:402–8. PMID:12924717
2329. Roncaroli F, Scheithauer BW, Cenacchi G, et al. (2002). 'Spindle cell oncocytoma' of the adenohypophysis: a tumor of folliculostellate cells? Am J Surg Pathol. 26:1048–55. PMID:12170092
2330. Roncaroli F, Scheithauer BW, Horvath E, et al. (2010). Silent subtype 3 carcinoma of the pituitary: a case report. Neuropathol Appl Neurobiol. 36:90–4. PMID:19811617
2331. Roncaroli F, Scheithauer BW, Young WF, et al. (2003). Silent corticotroph carcinoma of the adenohypophysis: a report of five cases. Am J Surg Pathol. 27:477–86. PMID:12657932
2332. Ronchi CL, Peverelli E, Herterich S, et al. (2016). Landscape of somatic mutations in sporadic GH-secreting pituitary adenomas. Eur J Endocrinol. 174:363–72. PMID:26701869
2333. Ronchi CL, Sbiera S, Leich E, et al. (2013). Single nucleotide polymorphism array profiling of adrenocortical tumors–evidence for an adenoma carcinoma sequence? PLoS One. 8:e73959. PMID:24066089
2334. Ronchi CL, Sbiera S, Volante M, et al. (2014). CYP2W1 is highly expressed in adrenal glands and is positively associated with the response to mitotane in adrenocortical carcinoma. PLoS One. 9:e105855. PMID:25144458
2335. Roque L, Clode A, Belge G, et al. (1998). Follicular thyroid carcinoma: chromosome analysis of 19 cases. Genes Chromosomes Cancer. 21:250–5. PMID:9523201
2336. Roque L, Rodrigues R, Pinto A, et al. (2003). Chromosome imbalances in thyroid follicular neoplasms: a comparison between follicular adenomas and carcinomas. Genes Chromosomes Cancer. 36:292–302. PMID:12557229
2337. Rosai J (2005). Handling of thyroid follicular patterned lesions. Endocr Pathol. 16:279–83. PMID:16627915
2338. Rosai J (2010). The encapsulated follicular variant of papillary thyroid carcinoma: back to the drawing board. Endocr Pathol. 21:7–11. PMID:20066572
2339. Rosai J, DeLellis RA, Carcangiu ML, et al. (2015). Tumors of the thyroid and parathyroid glands. In: AFIP Atlas of Tumor Pathology. Series 4, Fascicle 21. Washington DC: American Registry of Pathology Press.
2340. Rosai J, DeLellis RA, Carcangiu ML, et al. (2015). Tumors of the thyroid and parathyroid glands. In: AFIP atlas of tumor pathology. Series 4, Fascicle 21. Washington DC: American Registry of Pathology Press; pp. 96-8.
2341. Rosai J, DeLellis RA, Carcangiu ML, et al. (2015). Tumors of the thyroid and parathyroid glands. In: AFIP atlas of tumor pathology. Series 4, Fascicle 21. Washington DC: American Registry of Pathology Press; pp. 543–60.
2342. Rosai J, DeLellis RA, Carcangiu ML, et al. (2015). Tumors of the thyroid and parathyroid glands. In: AFIP atlas of tumor pathology. Series 4, Fascicle 21. Washington DC: American Registry of Pathology Press; pp. 513–42.
2343. Rosai J, LiVolsi VA, Sobrinho-Simoes M, et al. (2003). Renaming papillary microcarcinoma of the thyroid gland: the Porto proposal. Int J Surg Pathol. 11:249–51. PMID:14615819
2344. Rosai J, Zampi G, Carcangiu ML (1983). Papillary carcinoma of the thyroid. A discussion of its several morphologic expressions, with particular emphasis on the follicular variant. Am J Surg Pathol. 7:809–17. PMID:6660353
2345. Rossi D (2009). Thyroid lymphoma: beyond antigen stimulation. Leuk Res. 33:607–9. PMID:19128828
2346. Rossi ED, Martini M, Straccia P, et al. (2015). Is thyroid gland only a "land" for primary malignancies? role of morphology and immunocytochemistry. Diagn Cytopathol. 43:374–80. PMID:25427948
2347. Rossi ED, Straccia P, Martini M, et al. (2014). The role of thyroid fine-needle aspiration cytology in the pediatric population: an institutional experience. Cancer Cytopathol. 122:359–67. PMID:24474727
2348. Rostomyan L, Daly AF, Petrossians P, et al. (2015). Clinical and genetic characterization of pituitary gigantism: an international collaborative study in 208 patients. Endocr Relat Cancer. 22:745–57. PMID:26187128
2349. Roth J, Komminoth P, Heitz PU (1995). Topographic abnormalities of proinsulin to insulin conversion in functioning human insulinomas. Comparison of immunoelectron microscopic and clinical data. Am J Pathol. 147:489–502. PMID:7639339
2350. Roth SI, Gallagher MJ (1976). The rapid identification of "normal" parathyroid glands by the presence of intracellular fat. Am J Pathol. 84:521–8. PMID:60884
2351. Rothenberg AB, Berdon WE, D'Angio GJ, et al. (2009). The association between neuroblastoma and opsoclonus-myoclonus syndrome: a historical review. Pediatr Radiol. 39:723–6. PMID:19430769
2352. Rothenberg HJ, Goellner JR, Carney JA (1999). Hyalinizing trabecular adenoma of the thyroid gland: recognition and characterization of its cytoplasmic yellow body. Am J Surg Pathol. 23:118–25. PMID:9888712
2353. Rotondo F, Khatun N, Scheithauer BW, et al. (2011). Unusual double pituitary adenoma: a case report. Pathol Int. 61:42–6. PMID:21166942
2354. Rowland KJ, Moley JF (2015). Hereditary thyroid cancer syndromes and genetic testing. J Surg Oncol. 111:51–60. PMID:25351655
2355. Roy A, Timothy J, Anthony R, et al. (2000). Correspondence: aesthesioneuroblastoma arising in pituitary gland. Neuropathol Appl Neurobiol. 26:177–9. PMID:10840281
2356. Roy J, Pompilio M, Samama G (1996). Pancreatic somatostatinoma and MEN 1. Apropos of a case. Review of the literature. Ann Endocrinol (Paris). 57:71–6. [French] PMID:8734292
2357. Ruebel KH, Jin L, Qian X, et al. (2005). Effects of DNA methylation on galectin-3 expression in pituitary tumors. Cancer Res. 65:1136–40. PMID:15734994
2358. Ruebel KH, Jin L, Zhang S, et al. (2001). Inactivation of the p16 gene in human pituitary nonfunctioning tumors by hypermethylation is more common in null cell adenomas. Endocr Pathol. 12:281–9. PMID:11740049
2359. Ruebel KH, Leontovich AA, Jin L, et al. (2006). Patterns of gene expression in pituitary carcinomas and adenomas analyzed by high-density oligonucleotide arrays, reverse transcriptase-quantitative PCR, and protein expression. Endocrine. 29:435–44. PMID:16943582
2360. Ruelle A, Palladino M, Andrioli GC (1992). Pituitary metastases as presenting lesions of malignancy. J Neurosurg Sci. 36:51–4. PMID:1323647
2361. Ruggieri P, Sim FH, Bond JR, et al. (1994). Malignancies in fibrous dysplasia. Cancer. 73:1411–24. PMID:8111708
2362. Russell WO, Ibanez ML, Clark RL, et al. (1963). Thyroid carcinoma. Classification, intraglandular dissemination, and clinicopathological study based upon whole organ sections of 80 glands. Cancer. 16:1425–60. PMID:14086580
2363. Rutkowski MJ, Sughrue ME, Kane AJ, et al. (2010). Predictors of mortality following treatment of intracranial hemangiopericytoma. J Neurosurg. 113:333–9. PMID:20367074
2364. Rutter MM, Jha P, Schultz KA, et al. (2016). DICER1 Mutations and Differentiated Thyroid Carcinoma: Evidence of a Direct Association. J Clin Endocrinol Metab. 101:1–5. PMID:26555935
2365. Ryder M, Ghossein RA, Ricarte-Filho JC, et al. (2008). Increased density of tumor-associated macrophages is associated with decreased survival in advanced thyroid cancer. Endocr Relat Cancer. 15:1069–74. PMID:18719091
2366. Ryska A, Ludvíková M, Szépe P, et al. (2004). Epithelioid haemangiosarcoma of the thyroid gland. Report of six cases from a non-Alpine region. Histopathology. 44:40–6. PMID:14717668
2367. Sadot E, Reidy-Lagunes DL, Tang LH, et al. (2016). Observation versus Resection for Small Asymptomatic Pancreatic Neuroendocrine Tumors: A Matched Case-Control Study. Ann Surg Oncol. 23:1361–70. PMID:26597365
2368. Sadow PM, Hunt JL (2010). Mixed Medullary-follicular-derived carcinomas of the thyroid gland. Adv Anat Pathol. 17:282–5. PMID:20574174
2369. Saeed Kamil Z, Sinson G, Gucer H, et al. (2014). TTF-1 expressing sellar neoplasm with ependymal rosettes and oncocytic change: mixed ependymal and oncocytic variant pituicytoma. Endocr Pathol. 25:436–8. PMID:24242699
2370. Saeger W, Lüdecke DK, Buchfelder M, et al. (2007). Pathohistological classification of pituitary tumors: 10 years of experience with the German Pituitary Tumor Registry. Eur J Endocrinol. 156:203–16. PMID:17287410
2371. Saeger W, Puchner MJ, Lüdecke DK (1994). Combined sellar gangliocytoma and pituitary adenoma in acromegaly or Cushing's disease. A report of 3 cases. Virchows Arch. 425:93–9. PMID:7921420
2372. Saggiorato E, De Pompa R, Volante M, et al. (2005). Characterization of thyroid 'follicular neoplasms' in fine-needle aspiration cytological specimens using a panel of immunohistochemical markers: a proposal for clinical application. Endocr Relat Cancer. 12:305–17. PMID:15947105
2373. Saggiorato E, Rapa I, Garino F, et al. (2007). Absence of RET gene point mutations in sporadic thyroid C-cell hyperplasia. J Mol Diagn. 9:214–9. PMID:17384213
2374. Sağlıcan Y, Kurtulmus N, Tunca F, et al. (2015). Mesothelial derived adenomatoid tumour in a location devoid of mesothelium: adrenal adenomatoid tumour. BMJ Case Rep. 2015:2015. PMID:26243749
2375. Sahagian-Edwards A, Holland JF (1956). Metastatic carcinoma to the adrenal glands with cortical hypofunction. Acta Unio Int Contra Cancrum. 12:57–61. PMID:13339527
2376. Sahakitrungruang T, Srichomthong C, Pornkunwilai S, et al. (2014). Germline and somatic DICER1 mutations in a pituitary blastoma causing infantile-onset Cushing's disease. J Clin Endocrinol Metab. 99:E1487–92. PMID:24823459
2377. Sahasrabudhe R, Stultz J, Williamson J, et al. (2015). The HABP2 G534E variant is an unlikely cause of familial non-medullary thyroid cancer. J Clin Endocrinol Metab. EPUB 2015. PMID:26691890
2378. Sahin A, Robinson RA (1988). Papillae formation in parathyroid adenoma. A source of possible diagnostic error. Arch Pathol Lab Med. 112:99–100. PMID:3337625
2379. Sahin M, Allard BL, Yates M, et al. (2005). PPARgamma staining as a surrogate for PAX8/PPARgamma fusion oncogene expression in follicular neoplasms: clinicopathological correlation and histopathological diagnostic value. J Clin Endocrinol Metab. 90:463–8. PMID:15483076
2380. Sahoo S, Hoda SA, Rosai J, et al. (2001). Cytokeratin 19 immunoreactivity in the diagnosis of papillary thyroid carcinoma: a note of caution. Am J Clin Pathol. 116:696–702. PMID:11710686
2381. Saito K, Kuratomi Y, Yamamoto K, et al. (1981). Primary squamous cell carcinoma of the thyroid associated with marked leukocytosis and hypercalcemia. Cancer. 48:2080–3. PMID:7296515
2382. Saito Y, Sugitani I, Toda K, et al. (2014). Metastatic thyroid tumors: ultrasonographic features, prognostic factors and outcomes in 29 cases. Surg Today. 44:55–61. PMID:23355002
2383. Sajid MS, Hamilton G, Baker DM; Joint Vascular Research Group (2007). A multicenter review of carotid body tumour management. Eur J Vasc Endovasc Surg. 34:127–30. PMID:17400487
2384. Sakaki S, Yokoyama S, Mamitsuka K, et al. (1999). A case of pituitary adenoma associated with McCune-Albright syndrome. Pituitary. 1:297–302. PMID:11081212
2385. Sakamoto A, Kasai N, Sugano H (1983). Poorly differentiated carcinoma of the thyroid. A clinicopathologic entity for a high-risk group of papillary and follicular carcinomas. Cancer. 52:1849–55. PMID:6313176
2386. Sakorafas GH, Giannopoulos GA, Parasi A, et al. (2008). Large somatostatin-producing endocrine carcinoma of the ampulla of vater in association with GIST in a patient with von Recklinghausen's disease. Case report and review of the literature. JOP. 9:633–9. PMID:18762695
2387. Sakurai A, Imai T, Kikumori T, et al. (2013). Thymic neuroendocrine tumour in multiple endocrine neoplasia type 1: female patients are not rare exceptions. Clin Endocrinol (Oxf). 78:248–54. PMID:22690831
2388. Sakurai A, Matsumoto K, Ikeo Y, et al. (2000). Frequency of facial angiofibromas in Japanese patients with multiple endocrine neoplasia type 1. Endocr J. 47:569–73. PMID:11200937
2389. Salame K, Ouaknine GE, Yossipov J, et al. (2001). Paraganglioma of the pituitary fossa: diagnosis and management. J Neurooncol. 54:49–52. PMID:11763422
2390. Salehi F, Agur A, Scheithauer BW, et al. (2009). Ki-67 in pituitary neoplasms: a review–part I. Neurosurgery. 65:429–37, discussion 437. PMID:19687686
2391. Salehi F, Agur A, Scheithauer BW, et al. (2010). Biomarkers of pituitary neoplasms: a review (Part II). Neurosurgery. 67:1790–8, discussion 1798. PMID:21107210
2392. Salehi F, Scheithauer BW, Kros JM, et al. (2011). MGMT promoter methylation and immunoexpression in aggressive pituitary adenomas and carcinomas. J Neurooncol. 104:647–57. PMID:21311951
2393. Salehi F, Scheithauer BW, Moyes VJ, et al. (2010). Low immunohistochemical expression of MGMT in ACTH secreting pituitary tumors of patients with Nelson syndrome. Endocr Pathol. 21:227–9. PMID:21061089
2394. Salenave S, Ancelle D, Bahougne T, et al. (2015). Macroprolactinomas in children and adolescents: factors associated with the response to treatment in 77 patients. J Clin Endocrinol Metab. 100:1177–86. PMID:25532043
2395. Salenave S, Boyce AM, Collins MT, et al. (2014). Acromegaly and McCune-Albright

syndrome. J Clin Endocrinol Metab. 99:1955–69. PMID:24517150
2396. Salpea P, Stratakis CA (2014). Carney complex and McCune Albright syndrome: an overview of clinical manifestations and human molecular genetics. Mol Cell Endocrinol. 386:85–91. PMID:24012779
2397. Salvatore G, Chiappetta G, Nikiforov YE, et al. (2005). Molecular profile of hyalinizing trabecular tumours of the thyroid: high prevalence of RET/PTC rearrangements and absence of B-raf and N-ras point mutations. Eur J Cancer. 41:816–21. PMID:15763659
2398. Salvatore G, Nappi TC, Salerno P, et al. (2007). A cell proliferation and chromosomal instability signature in anaplastic thyroid carcinoma. Cancer Res. 67:10148–58. PMID:17981789
2399. Samaan NA, Schultz PN, Ordonez NG, et al. (1987). A comparison of thyroid carcinoma in those who have and have not had head and neck irradiation in childhood. J Clin Endocrinol Metab. 64:219–23. PMID:3793847
2400. Samander EH, Arnold A (2006). Mutational analysis of the vitamin D receptor does not support its candidacy as a tumor suppressor gene in parathyroid adenomas. J Clin Endocrinol Metab. 91:5019–21. PMID:17003089
2401. Sambade C, Baldaque-Faria A, Cardoso-Oliveira M, et al. (1988). Follicular and papillary variants of medullary carcinoma of the thyroid. Pathol Res Pract. 184:98–107. PMID:3068650
2402. Sambade C, Franssila K, Basilio-de-Oliveira CA, et al. (1990). Mucoepidermoid carcinoma of the thyroid revisited. Surg Pathol. 3:317–24.
2403. Sambaziotis D, Kontogeorgos G, Kovacs K, et al. (1999). Intrasellar paraganglioma presenting as nonfunctioning pituitary adenoma. Arch Pathol Lab Med. 123:429–32. PMID:10235503
2404. Samson SL (2015). Pasireotide in Acromegaly: An Overview of Current Mechanistic and Clinical Data. Neuroendocrinology. 102:8–17. PMID:25792118
2405. Samulski TD, Bai S, LiVolsi VA, et al. (2013). Malignant potential of small oncocytic follicular carcinoma/Hürthle cell carcinoma: an institutional experience. Histopathology. 63:568–73. PMID:23952654
2406. Sandler M, Rubin PC, Reid JL, et al. (1992). Oat cell carcinoma in the pancreas: an unusual cause of Cushing's syndrome. Br J Hosp Med. 47:537–8. PMID:1316198
2407. Sandrini F, Matyakhina L, Sarlis NJ, et al. (2002). Regulatory subunit type I-alpha of protein kinase A (PRKAR1A): a tumor-suppressor gene for sporadic thyroid cancer. Genes Chromosomes Cancer. 35:182–92. PMID:12203783
2408. Sangoi AR, Fujiwara M, West RB, et al. (2011). Immunohistochemical distinction of primary adrenal cortical lesions from metastatic clear cell renal cell carcinoma: a study of 248 cases. Am J Surg Pathol. 35:678–86. PMID:21490444
2409. Sangoi AR, McKenney JK (2010). A tissue microarray-based comparative analysis of novel and traditional immunohistochemical markers in the distinction between adrenal cortical lesions and pheochromocytoma. Am J Surg Pathol. 34:423–32. PMID:20154585
2410. Sanno N, Teramoto A, Osamura RY, et al. (1997). A growth hormone-releasing hormone-producing pancreatic islet cell tumor metastasized to the pituitary is associated with pituitary somatotroph hyperplasia and acromegaly. J Clin Endocrinol Metab. 82:2731–7. PMID:9253362
2411. Sanno N, Teramoto A, Sugiyama M, et al. (1996). Application of catalyzed signal amplification in immunodetection of gonadotropin subunits in clinically nonfunctioning pituitary adenomas. Am J Clin Pathol. 106:16–21. PMID:8701926
2412. Sanno N, Teramoto A, Sugiyama M, et al. (1998). Expression of Pit-1 mRNA and activin/inhibin subunits in clinically nonfunctioning pituitary adenomas. In situ hybridization and immunohistochemical analysis. Horm Res. 50:11–7. PMID:9691207
2413. Sano K, Matsutani M, Seto T (1989). So-called intracranial germ cell tumours: personal experiences and a theory of their pathogenesis. Neurol Res. 11:118–26. PMID:2569683
2414. Sano T, Horiguchi H, Xu B, et al. (1999). Double pituitary adenomas: six surgical cases. Pituitary. 1:243–50. PMID:11081204
2415. Santarpia L, El-Naggar AK, Cote GJ, et al. (2008). Phosphatidylinositol 3-kinase/akt and ras/raf-mitogen-activated protein kinase pathway mutations in anaplastic thyroid cancer. J Clin Endocrinol Metab. 93:278–84. PMID:17989125
2416. Santeusanio G, Schiaroli S, Ortenzi A, et al. (2008). Solitary fibrous tumour of thyroid: report of two cases with immunohistochemical features and literature review. Head Neck Pathol. 2:231–5. PMID:20614321
2417. Santini F, Bottici V, Elisei R, et al. (2002). Cytotoxic effects of carboplatinum and epirubicin in the setting of an elevated serum thyrotropin for advanced poorly differentiated thyroid cancer. J Clin Endocrinol Metab. 87:4160–5. PMID:12213865
2418. Santoro M, Carlomagno F, Romano A, et al. (1995). Activation of RET as a dominant transforming gene by germline mutations of MEN2A and MEN2B. Science. 267:381–3. PMID:7824936
2419. Santoro M, Papotti M, Chiappetta G, et al. (2002). RET activation and clinicopathologic features in poorly differentiated thyroid tumors. J Clin Endocrinol Metab. 87:370–9. PMID:11788678
2420. Sapino A, Papotti M, Macrì L, et al. (1995). Intranodular reactive endothelial hyperplasia in adenomatous goitre. Histopathology. 26:457–62. PMID:7657314
2421. Sarquis MS, Silveira LG, Pimenta FJ, et al. (2008). Familial hyperparathyroidism: surgical outcome after 30 years of follow-up in three families with germline HRPT2 mutations. Surgery. 143:630–40. PMID:18436011
2422. Sasagawa Y, Tachibana O, Iizuka H (2013). Undifferentiated sarcoma of the cavernous sinus after γ knife radiosurgery for pituitary adenoma. J Clin Neurosci. 20:1152–4. PMID:23587603
2423. Sasaki A, Daa T, Kashima K, et al. (1996). Insular component as a risk factor of thyroid carcinoma. Pathol Int. 46:939–46. PMID:9110345
2424. Sasano H, Shizawa S, Nagura H (1995). Adrenocortical cytopathology. Am J Clin Pathol. 104:161–6. PMID:7639190
2425. Sasano H, Shizawa S, Suzuki T, et al. (1995). Ad4BP in the human adrenal cortex and its disorders. J Clin Endocrinol Metab. 80:2378–80. PMID:7629233
2426. Sasano H, Shizawa S, Suzuki T, et al. (1995). Transcription factor adrenal 4 binding protein as a marker of adrenocortical malignancy. Hum Pathol. 26:1154–6. PMID:7557951
2427. Sasano H, Suzuki T, Moriya T (2006). Recent advances in histopathology and immunohistochemistry of adrenocortical carcinoma. Endocr Pathol. 17:345–54. PMID:17525483
2428. Sasano H, Suzuki T, Sano T, et al. (1991). Adrenocortical oncocytoma. A true nonfunctioning adrenocortical tumor. Am J Surg Pathol. 15:949–56. PMID:1928551
2429. Sastry P, Tocock A, Coonar AS (2014). Adrenalectomy for isolated metastasis from operable non-small-cell lung cancer. Interact Cardiovasc Thorac Surg. 18:495–7. PMID:24357471
2430. Satake H, Inoue K, Kamada M, et al. (2001). Malignant composite pheochromocytoma of the adrenal gland in a patient with von Recklinghausen's disease. J Urol. 165:1199–200. PMID:11257670
2431. Sathananthan M, Sathananthan A, Scheithauer BW, et al. (2013). Sellar meningiomas: an endocrinologic perspective. Pituitary. 16:182–8. PMID:22644157
2432. Sato Y, Maekawa S, Ishii R, et al. (2014). Recurrent somatic mutations underlie corticotropin-independent Cushing's syndrome. Science. 344:917–20. PMID:24855271
2433. Sato Y, Nakamura N, Nakamura S, et al. (2006). Deviated VH4 immunoglobulin gene usage is found among thyroid mucosa-associated lymphoid tissue lymphomas, similar to the usage at other sites, but is not found in thyroid diffuse large B-cell lymphomas. Mod Pathol. 19:1578–84. PMID:16980947
2434. Satoh H, Saito R, Hisata S, et al. (2012). An ectopic ACTH-producing small cell lung carcinoma associated with enhanced corticosteroid biosynthesis in the peritumoral areas of adrenal metastasis. Lung Cancer. 76:486–90. PMID:22251774
2435. Satoh M, Imai M, Sugimoto M, et al. (1999). Prevalence of Werner's syndrome heterozygotes in Japan. Lancet. 353:1766. PMID:10347997
2436. Sausen M, Leary RJ, Jones S, et al. (2013). Integrated genomic analyses identify ARID1A and ARID1B alterations in the childhood cancer neuroblastoma. Nat Genet. 45:12–7. PMID:23202128
2437. Sawamura Y, Ikeda J, Shirato H, et al. (1998). Germ cell tumours of the central nervous system: treatment consideration based on 111 cases and their long-term clinical outcomes. Eur J Cancer. 34:104–10. PMID:9624246
2438. Sawant S, Snyman C, Bhoola K (2001). Comparison of tissue kallikrein and kinin receptor expression in gastric ulcers and neoplasms. Int Immunopharmacol. 1:2063–80. PMID:11710536
2439. Sayar I, Peker K, Gelincik I, et al. (2014). Clear cell variant of follicular thyroid carcinoma with normal thyroid-stimulating hormone value: a case report. J Med Case Rep. 8:160. PMID:24884725
2439A. Saygin C, Uzunaslan D, Ozguroglu M, et al. (2013). Dendritic cell sarcoma: a pooled analysis including 462 cases with presentation of our case series. Crit Rev Oncol Hematol 88: 253-71. PMID: 23755890
2440. Sbiera S, Schmull S, Assie G, et al. (2010). High diagnostic and prognostic value of steroidogenic factor-1 expression in adrenal tumors. J Clin Endocrinol Metab. 95:E161–71. PMID:20660055
2440A. Scarpa A, Chang DK, Nones K et al. (2017). Whole-genome landscape of pancreatic neuroendocrine tumours. Nature. 543:65-71. PMID:28199314
2441. Scarpa A, Mantovani W, Capelli P, et al. (2010). Pancreatic endocrine tumors: improved TNM staging and histopathological grading permit a clinically efficient prognostic stratification of patients. Mod Pathol. 23:824–33. PMID:20305616
2442. Schalin-Jäntti C, Asa SL, Arola J, et al. (2013). Recurrent acute-onset Cushing's syndrome 6 years after removal of a thymic neuroendocrine carcinoma: from ectopic ACTH to CRH. Endocr Pathol. 24:25–9. PMID:23233312
2443. Schaller B, Kirsch E, Tolnay M, et al. (1998). Symptomatic granular cell tumor of the pituitary gland: case report and review of the literature. Neurosurgery. 42:166–70, discussion 170–1. PMID:9442519
2444. Schantz A, Castleman B (1973). Parathyroid carcinoma. A study of 70 cases. Cancer. 31:600–5. PMID:4693587
2445. Scheithauer BW, Fereidooni F, Horvath E, et al. (2001). Pituitary carcinoma: an ultrastructural study of eleven cases. Ultrastruct Pathol. 25:227–42. PMID:11465479
2446. Scheithauer BW, Gaffey TA, Lloyd RV, et al. (2006). Pathobiology of pituitary adenomas and carcinomas. Neurosurgery. 59:341–53, discussion 341–53. PMID:16883174
2447. Scheithauer BW, Horvath E, Abel TW, et al. (2012). Pituitary blastoma: a unique embryonal tumor. Pituitary. 15:365–73. PMID:21805093
2448. Scheithauer BW, Horvath E, Kovacs K, et al. (1999). Prolactin-producing pituitary adenoma and carcinoma with neuronal components–a metaplastic lesion. Pituitary. 1:197–205. PMID:11081198
2449. Scheithauer BW, Jaap AJ, Horvath E, et al. (2000). Clinically silent corticotroph tumors of the pituitary gland. Neurosurgery. 47:723–9, discussion 729–30. PMID:10981760
2450. Scheithauer BW, Kovacs K, Horvath E, et al. (2008). Pituitary blastoma. Acta Neuropathol. 116:657–66. PMID:18551299
2451. Scheithauer BW, Kovacs K, Nose V, et al. (2009). Multiple endocrine neoplasia type 1-associated thyrotropin-producing pituitary carcinoma: report of a probable de novo example. Hum Pathol. 40:270–8. PMID:18755492
2452. Scheithauer BW, Kovacs K, Randall RV, et al. (1985). Pituitary gland in hypothyroidism. Histologic and immunocytologic study. Arch Pathol Lab Med. 109:499–504. PMID:2986571
2453. Scheithauer BW, Parameswaran A, Burdick B (1996). Intrasellar paraganglioma: report of a case in a sibship of von Hippel-Lindau disease. Neurosurgery. 38:395–9. PMID:8869071
2454. Scheithauer BW, Randall RV, Laws ER Jr, et al. (1985). Prolactin cell carcinoma of the pituitary. Clinicopathologic, immunohistochemical, and ultrastructural study of a case with cranial and extracranial metastases. Cancer. 55:598–604. PMID:3965110
2455. Scheithauer BW, Sano T, Kovacs KT, et al. (1990). The pituitary gland in pregnancy: a clinicopathologic and immunohistochemical study of 69 cases. Mayo Clin Proc. 65:461–74. PMID:2159093
2456. Scheithauer BW, Swearingen B, Whyte ET, et al. (2009). Ependymoma of the sella turcica: a variant of pituicytoma. Hum Pathol. 40:435–40. PMID:18992914
2457. Schernthaner-Reiter MH, Trivellin G, Stratakis CA (2016). MEN1, MEN4, and Carney Complex: Pathology and Molecular Genetics. Neuroendocrinology. 103:18–31. PMID:25592387
2458. Scherübl H, Jensen RT, Cadiot G, et al. (2011). Management of early gastrointestinal neuroendocrine neoplasms. World J Gastrointest Endosc. 3:133–9. PMID:21860682
2459. Schimke RN (1984). Genetic aspects of multiple endocrine neoplasia. Annu Rev Med. 35:25–31. PMID:6144286
2460. Schleiermacher G, Delattre O, Peter M, et al. (1996). Clinical relevance of loss heterozygosity of the short arm of chromosome 1 in neuroblastoma: a single-institution study. Int J Cancer. 69:73–8. PMID:8608986
2461. Schlisio S, Kenchappa RS, Vredeveld LC, et al. (2008). The kinesin KIF1Bbeta acts downstream from EglN3 to induce apoptosis and is a potential 1p36 tumor suppressor. Genes Dev. 22:884–93. PMID:18334619
2462. Schlumberger M, Gicquel C, Lumbroso J, et al. (1992). Malignant pheochromocytoma: clinical, biological, histologic and therapeutic data in a series of 20 patients with distant metastases. J Endocrinol Invest. 15:631–42. PMID:1479146
2463. Schmalisch K, Psaras T, Beschorner R, et al. (2009). Sellar neuroblastoma mimicking a pituitary tumour: case report and review of the literature. Clin Neurol Neurosurg. 111:774–8. PMID:19640636
2464. Schmid KW (2015). Histopathology of C Cells and Medullary Thyroid Carcinoma.

Recent Results Cancer Res. 204:41–60. PMID:26494383
2465. Schmitt AM, Anlauf M, Rousson V, et al. (2007). WHO 2004 criteria and CK19 are reliable prognostic markers in pancreatic endocrine tumors. Am J Surg Pathol. 31:1677–82. PMID:18059224
2466. Schmitt AM, Pavel M, Rudolph T, et al. (2014). Prognostic and predictive roles of MGMT protein expression and promoter methylation in sporadic pancreatic neuroendocrine neoplasms. Neuroendocrinology. 100:35–44. PMID:25012122
2467. Schmitt AM, Schmid S, Rudolph T, et al. (2009). VHL inactivation is an important pathway for the development of malignant sporadic pancreatic endocrine tumors. Endocr Relat Cancer. 16:1219–27. PMID:19690016
2468. Schmitz KJ, Helwig J, Bertram S, et al. (2011). Differential expression of microRNA-675, microRNA-139-3p and microRNA-335 in benign and malignant adrenocortical tumours. J Clin Pathol. 64:529–35. PMID:21471143
2469. Schneikert J, Grohmann A, Behrens J (2007). Truncated APC regulates the transcriptional activity of beta-catenin in a cell cycle dependent manner. Hum Mol Genet. 16:199–209. PMID:17189293
2470. Scholl UI, Goh G, Stölting G, et al. (2013). Somatic and germline CACNA1D calcium channel mutations in aldosterone-producing adenomas and primary aldosteronism. Nat Genet. 45:1050–4. PMID:23913001
2471. Schovanek J, Martucci V, Wesley R, et al. (2014). The size of the primary tumor and age at initial diagnosis are independent predictors of the metastatic behavior and survival of patients with SDHB-related pheochromocytoma and paraganglioma: a retrospective cohort study. BMC Cancer. 14:523. PMID:25048685
2472. Schreiber CS, Sakon JR, Simião FP, et al. (2008). Primary adrenal lymphoma: a case series study. Ann Hematol. 87:859–61. PMID:18458904
2473. Schreinemakers JM, Pieterman CR, Scholten A, et al. (2011). The optimal surgical treatment for primary hyperparathyroidism in MEN1 patients: a systematic review. World J Surg. 35:1993–2005. PMID:21713580
2474. Schröder S, Böcker W (1985). Signet-ring-cell thyroid tumors. Follicle cell tumors with arrest of folliculogenesis. Am J Surg Pathol. 9:619–29. PMID:2996373
2475. Schröder S, Böcker W (1986). Clear-cell carcinomas of thyroid gland: a clinicopathological study of 13 cases. Histopathology. 10:75–89. PMID:3957248
2476. Schröder S, Böcker W, Dralle H, et al. (1984). The encapsulated papillary carcinoma of the thyroid. A morphologic subtype of the papillary thyroid carcinoma. Cancer. 54:90–3. PMID:6722747
2477. Schröder S, Böcker W, Hüsselmann H, et al. (1984). Adenolipoma (thyrolipoma) of the thyroid gland report of two cases and review of literature. Virchows Arch A Pathol Anat Histopathol. 404:99–103. PMID:6433552
2478. Schröder S, Hüsselmann H, Böcker W (1984). Lipid-rich cell adenoma of the thyroid gland. Report of a peculiar thyroid tumour. Virchows Arch A Pathol Anat Histopathol. 404:105–8. PMID:6433543
2479. Schuffenecker I, Virally-Monod M, Brohet R, et al. (1998). Risk and penetrance of primary hyperparathyroidism in multiple endocrine neoplasia type 2A families with mutations at codon 634 of the RET proto-oncogene. Groupe D'etude des Tumeurs à Calcitonine. J Clin Endocrinol Metab. 83:487–91. PMID:9467562
2480. Schuijers J, Clevers H (2012). Adult mammalian stem cells: the role of Wnt, Lgr5 and R-spondins. EMBO J. 31:2685–96. PMID:22617424
2481. Schultz AB, Brat DJ, Oyesiku NM, et al. (2001). Intrasellar pituicytoma in a patient with other endocrine neoplasms. Arch Pathol Lab Med. 125:527–30. PMID:11260629
2482. Schultz KA, Pacheco MC, Yang J, et al. (2011). Ovarian sex cord-stromal tumors, pleuropulmonary blastoma and DICER1 mutations: a report from the International Pleuropulmonary Blastoma Registry. Gynecol Oncol. 122:246–50. PMID:21501861
2483. Schultz KA, Yang J, Doros L, et al. (2014). DICER1-pleuropulmonary blastoma familial tumor predisposition syndrome: a unique constellation of neoplastic conditions. Pathol Case Rev. 19:90–100. PMID:25356068
2484. Schussheim DH, Skarulis MC, Agarwal SK, et al. (2001). Multiple endocrine neoplasia type 1: new clinical and basic findings. Trends Endocrinol Metab. 12:173–8. PMID:11295574
2485. Schwarzkopf G, Pfisterer J (1994). Metastasizing gastrinoma and tuberous sclerosis complex. Association or coincidence? Zentralbl Pathol. 139:477–81. [German] PMID:8161496
2486. Schweizer L, Koelsche C, Sahm F, et al. (2013). Meningeal hemangiopericytoma and solitary fibrous tumors carry the NAB2-STAT6 fusion and can be diagnosed by nuclear expression of STAT6 protein. Acta Neuropathol. 125:651–8. PMID:23575898
2487. Sclafani LM, Woodruff JM, Brennan MF (1990). Extraadrenal retroperitoneal paragangliomas: natural history and response to treatment. Surgery. 108:1124–9, discussion 1129–30. PMID:2174194
2488. Scognamiglio T, Hyjek E, Kao J, et al. (2006). Diagnostic usefulness of HBME1, galectin-3, CK19, and CITED1 and evaluation of their expression in encapsulated lesions with questionable features of papillary thyroid carcinoma. Am J Clin Pathol. 126:700–8. PMID:17050067
2489. Scollo C, Baudin E, Travagli JP, et al. (2003). Rationale for central and bilateral lymph node dissection in sporadic and hereditary medullary thyroid cancer. J Clin Endocrinol Metab. 88:2070–5. PMID:12727956
2490. Scopa CD, Melachrinou M, Saradopoulou C, et al. (1993). The significance of the grooved nucleus in thyroid lesions. Mod Pathol. 6:691–4. PMID:8302810
2491. Scopsi L, Castellani MR, Gullo M, et al. (1996). Malignant pheochromocytoma in multiple endocrine neoplasia type 2B syndrome. Case report and review of the literature. Tumori. 82:480–4. PMID:9063528
2492. Scopsi L, Sampietro G, Boracchi P, et al. (1996). Multivariate analysis of prognostic factors in sporadic medullary carcinoma of the thyroid. A retrospective study of 109 consecutive patients. Cancer. 78:2173–83. PMID:8918412
2493. Sedney CL, Morris JM, Giannini C, et al. (2012). Radiation-associated sarcoma of the skull base after irradiation for pituitary adenoma. Rare Tumors. 4:e7. PMID:22532923
2494. Seefelder C, Sparks JW, Chirnomas D, et al. (2005). Perioperative management of a child with severe hypertension from a catecholamine secreting neuroblastoma. Paediatr Anaesth. 15:606–10. PMID:15960647
2495. Seeger RC, Brodeur GM, Sather H, et al. (1985). Association of multiple copies of the N-myc oncogene with rapid progression of neuroblastomas. N Engl J Med. 313:1111–6. PMID:4047115
2496. Seethala RR, Asa SL, Carty SE, et al. (2014). Protocol for the examination of specimens from patients with carcinomas of the thyroid gland, Version 3.1.0.0. Washington, DC: College of American Pathologists. Available from: http://www.cap.org/ShowProperty?nodePath=/UCMCon/Contribution%20Folders/WebContent/pdf/thyroid_2014protocol.pdf.
2497. Seidenwurm DJ, Elmer EB, Kaplan LM, et al. (1984). Metastases to the adrenal glands and the development of Addison's disease. Cancer. 54:552–7. PMID:6733685
2498. Seigne C, Auret M, Treilleux I, et al. (2013). High incidence of mammary intraepithelial neoplasia development in Men1-disrupted murine mammary glands. J Pathol. 229:546–58. PMID:23180448
2499. Sekine S, Takata T, Shibata T, et al. (2004). Expression of enamel proteins and LEF1 in adamantinomatous craniopharyngioma: evidence for its odontogenic epithelial differentiation. Histopathology. 45:573–9. PMID:15569047
2500. Seltzer J, Ashton CE, Scotton TC, et al. (2015). Gene and protein expression in pituitary corticotroph adenomas: a systematic review of the literature. Neurosurg Focus. 38:E17. PMID:25639319
2501. Seltzer J, Lucas J, Commins D, et al. (2015). Ectopic ACTH-secreting pituitary adenoma of the sphenoid sinus: case report of endoscopic endonasal resection and systematic review of the literature. Neurosurg Focus. 38:E10. PMID:25639312
2502. Serres MP, Kossatz U, Chi Y, et al. (2012). p27(Kip1) controls cytokinesis via the regulation of citron kinase activation. J Clin Invest. 122:844–58. PMID:22293177
2503. Serres MP, Zlotek-Zlotkiewicz E, Concha C, et al. (2011). Cytoplasmic p27 is oncogenic and cooperates with Ras both in vivo and in vitro. Oncogene. 30:2846–58. PMID:21317921
2504. Service FJ (1999). Diagnostic approach to adults with hypoglycemic disorders. Endocrinol Metab Clin North Am. 28:519–32, vi. PMID:10500929
2505. Service FJ, Dale AJ, Elveback LR, et al. (1976). Insulinoma: clinical and diagnostic features of 60 consecutive cases. Mayo Clin Proc. 51:417–29. PMID:180358
2506. Service FJ, McMahon MM, O'Brien PC, et al. (1991). Functioning insulinoma–incidence, recurrence, and long-term survival of patients: a 60-year study. Mayo Clin Proc. 66:711–9. PMID:1677058
2507. Sethi RV, Sethi RK, Herr MW, et al. (2013). Malignant head and neck paragangliomas: treatment efficacy and prognostic indicators. Am J Otolaryngol. 34:431–8. PMID:23642313
2508. Settakorn J, Sirivanichai C, Rangdaeng S, et al. (1999). Fine-needle aspiration cytology of adrenal myelolipoma: case report and review of the literature. Diagn Cytopathol. 21:409–12. PMID:10572274
2509. Shah R, Schniederjan M, DelGaudio JM, et al. (2011). Visual vignette. Ectopic ACTH-secreting pituitary adenoma. Endocr Pract. 17:966. PMID:21803709
2510. Shaha AR, Shah JP (1999). Parathyroid carcinoma: a diagnostic and therapeutic challenge. Cancer. 86:378–80. PMID:10430243
2511. Shaha AR, Shah JP, Loree TR (1996). Risk group stratification and prognostic factors in papillary carcinoma of thyroid. Ann Surg Oncol. 3:534–8. PMID:8915484
2512. Shahani S, Nudelman RJ, Nalini R, et al. (2010). Ectopic corticotropin-releasing hormone (CRH) syndrome from metastatic small cell carcinoma: a case report and review of the literature. Diagn Pathol. 5:56. PMID:20807418
2513. Shames JM, Dhurandhar NR, Blackard WG (1968). Insulin-secreting bronchial carcinoid tumor with widespread metastases. Am J Med. 44:632–7. PMID:4296076
2514. Shan L, Nakamura Y, Nakamura M, et al. (1998). Somatic mutations of multiple endocrine neoplasia type 1 gene in the sporadic endocrine tumors. Lab Invest. 78:471–5. PMID:9564891
2515. Shane E (2001). Clinical review 122: Parathyroid carcinoma. J Clin Endocrinol Metab. 86:485–93. PMID:11157996
2516. Shankar GM, Chen L, Kim AH, et al. (2010). Composite ganglioneuroma-paraganglioma of the filum terminale. J Neurosurg Spine. 12:709–13. PMID:20515359
2517. Shankavaram U, Fliedner SM, Elkahloun AG, et al. (2013). Genotype and tumor locus determine expression profile of pseudohypoxic pheochromocytomas and paragangliomas. Neoplasia. 15:435–47. PMID:23555188
2518. Sharma D, Sharma S, Jhobta A, et al. (2012). Virilizing adrenal oncocytoma. J Clin Imaging Sci. 2:76. PMID:23393632
2519. Sharma K, Nigam S, Khurana N, et al. (2003). Sclerosing mucoepidermoid carcinoma with eosinophilia of the thyroid–a case report. Indian J Pathol Microbiol. 46:660–1. PMID:15025372
2520. Sharma S, Salehi F, Scheithauer BW, et al. (2009). Role of MGMT in tumor development, progression, diagnosis, treatment and prognosis. Anticancer Res. 29:3759–68. PMID:19846906
2521. Sharretts JM, Kebebew E, Simonds WF (2010). Parathyroid cancer. Semin Oncol. 37:580–90. PMID:21167377
2522. Shattuck TM, Kim TS, Costa J, et al. (2003). Mutational analyses of RB and BRCA2 as candidate tumour suppressor genes in parathyroid carcinoma. Clin Endocrinol (Oxf). 59:180–9. PMID:12864795
2523. Shattuck TM, Välimäki S, Obara T, et al. (2003). Somatic and germ-line mutations of the HRPT2 gene in sporadic parathyroid carcinoma. N Engl J Med. 349:1722–9. PMID:14585940
2524. Shehadeh NJ, Vernick J, Lonardo F, et al. (2004). Sclerosing mucoepidermoid carcinoma with eosinophilia of the thyroid: a case report and review of the literature. Am J Otolaryngol. 25:48–53. PMID:15011206
2525. Shen GM, Zhao YZ, Chen MT, et al. (2012). Hypoxia-inducible factor-1 (HIF-1) promotes LDL and VLDL uptake through inducing VLDLR under hypoxia. Biochem J. 441:675–83. PMID:21970364
2526. Shen T, Zhuang Z, Gersell DJ, et al. (2000). Allelic Deletion of VHL Gene Detected in Papillary Tumors of the Broad Ligament, Epididymis, and Retroperitoneum in von Hippel-Lindau Disease Patients. Int J Surg Pathol. 8:207–12. PMID:11493991
2527. Shen WH, Balajee AS, Wang J, et al. (2007). Essential role for nuclear PTEN in maintaining chromosomal integrity. Cell. 128:157–70. PMID:17218262
2528. Shenker A, Weinstein LS, Moran A, et al. (1993). Severe endocrine and nonendocrine manifestations of the McCune-Albright syndrome associated with activating mutations of stimulatory G protein GS. J Pediatr. 123:509–18. PMID:8410501
2529. Shenker Y, LLoyd RV, Weatherbee L, et al. (1986). Ectopic prolactinoma in a patient with hyperparathyroidism and abnormal sellar radiography. J Clin Endocrinol Metab. 62:1065–9. PMID:3958123
2530. Shenoy BV, Carpenter PC, Carney JA (1984). Bilateral primary pigmented nodular adrenocortical disease. Rare cause of the Cushing syndrome. Am J Surg Pathol. 8:335–44. PMID:6329005
2531. Shenoy VG, Thota A, Shankar R, et al. (2015). Adrenal myelolipoma: Controversies in its management. Indian J Urol. 31:94–101. PMID:25878407
2532. Sherman SI (2013). Lessons learned and questions unanswered from use of multitargeted kinase inhibitors in medullary thyroid cancer. Oral Oncol. 49:707–10. PMID:23582411
2533. Sherr CJ, Roberts JM (1995). Inhibitors of mammalian G1 cyclin-dependent kinases. Genes Dev. 9:1149–63. PMID:7758941
2534. Shetty S, Varghese RT, Shanthly N, et al. (2014). Toxic Thyroid Adenoma in McCune-Albright Syndrome. J Clin Diagn Res. 8:281–2. PMID:24701557
2535. Shetty T, Chase TN (1976). Central monoamines and hyperkinase of childhood. Neurology. 26:1000–2. PMID:986582

2536. Sheu SY, Schwertheim S, Worm K, et al. (2007). Diffuse sclerosing variant of papillary thyroid carcinoma: lack of BRAF mutation but occurrence of RET/PTC rearrangements. Mod Pathol. 20:779–87. PMID:17464312
2537. Sheu SY, Vogel E, Worm K, et al. (2010). Hyalinizing trabecular tumour of the thyroid-differential expression of distinct miRNAs compared with papillary thyroid carcinoma. Histopathology. 56:632–40. PMID:20459574
2538. Shi C, Klimstra DS (2014). Pancreatic neuroendocrine tumors: pathologic and molecular characteristics. Semin Diagn Pathol. 31:498–511. PMID:25441311
2539. Shibata Y, Yamazaki M, Takei M, et al. (2015). Early-onset, severe, and recurrent primary hyperparathyroidism associated with a novel CDC73 mutation. Endocr J. 62:627–32. PMID:25959515
2540. Shifrin A, LiVolsi V, Shifrin-Douglas S, et al. (2015). Primary and metastatic parathyroid malignancies: a rare or underdiagnosed condition? J Clin Endocrinol Metab. 100:E478–81. PMID:25490272
2541. Shifrin AL, LiVolsi VA, Zheng M, et al. (2013). Neuroendocrine thymic carcinoma metastatic to the parathyroid gland that was reimplanted into the forearm in patient with multiple endocrine neoplasia type 1 syndrome: a challenging management dilemma. Endocr Pract. 19:e163–7. PMID:24014011
2542. Shimada H, Ambros IM, Dehner LP, et al. (1999). Terminology and morphologic criteria of neuroblastic tumors: recommendations by the International Neuroblastoma Pathology Committee. Cancer. 86:349–63. PMID:10421272
2543. Shimada H, Ambros IM, Dehner LP, et al. (1999). The International Neuroblastoma Pathology Classification (the Shimada system). Cancer. 86:364–72. PMID:10421273
2544. Shimada H, Aoyama C, Chiba T, et al. (1985). Prognostic subgroups for undifferentiated neuroblastoma: immunohistochemical study with anti-S-100 protein antibody. Hum Pathol. 16:471–6. PMID:3886523
2545. Shimada H, Chatten J, Newton WA Jr, et al. (1984). Histopathologic prognostic factors in neuroblastic tumors: definition of subtypes of ganglioneuroblastoma and an age-linked classification of neuroblastomas. J Natl Cancer Inst. 73:405–16. PMID:6589432
2546. Shimada H, Nakagawa A, Peters J, et al. (2004). TrkA expression in peripheral neuroblastic tumors: prognostic significance and biological relevance. Cancer. 101:1873–81. PMID:15386308
2547. Shimada H, Stram DO, Chatten J, et al. (1995). Identification of subsets of neuroblastomas by combined histopathologic and N-myc analysis. J Natl Cancer Inst. 87:1470–6. PMID:7674334
2548. Shimazu S, Nagamura Y, Yaguchi H, et al. (2011). Correlation of mutant menin stability with clinical expression of multiple endocrine neoplasia type 1 and its incomplete forms. Cancer Sci. 102:2097–102. PMID:21819486
2549. Shimizu C, Koike T, Sawamura Y (2004). Double pituitary adenomas with distinct histological features and immunophenotypes. J Neurol Neurosurg Psychiatry. 75:140. PMID:14707324
2550. Shin WY, Groman GS, Berkman JI (1977). Pheochromocytoma with angiomatous features. A case report and ultrastructural study. Cancer. 40:275–83. PMID:880556
2551. Shindo K, Aishima S, Okido M, et al. (2012). A poor prognostic case of mucoepidermoid carcinoma of the thyroid: a case report. Case Rep Endocrinol. 2012:862545. PMID:22970393
2552. Shinohara M, Shitara T, Hatakeyama SI, et al. (2004). An infant with systemic hypertension, renal artery stenosis, and neuroblastoma. J Pediatr Surg. 39:103–6. PMID:14694383
2553. Shojaei-Brosseau T, Chompret A, Abel A, et al. (2004). Genetic epidemiology of neuroblastoma: a study of 426 cases at the Institut Gustave-Roussy in France. Pediatr Blood Cancer. 42:99–105. PMID:14752801
2554. Shore RE (1992). Issues and epidemiological evidence regarding radiation-induced thyroid cancer. Radiat Res. 131:98–111. PMID:1385649
2555. Shore RE, Hildreth N, Dvoretsky P, et al. (1993). Benign thyroid adenomas among persons X-irradiated in infancy for enlarged thymus glands. Radiat Res. 134:217–23. PMID:8488255
2556. Shorter NA, Glick RD, Klimstra DS, et al. (2002). Malignant pancreatic tumors in childhood and adolescence: The Memorial Sloan-Kettering experience, 1967 to present. J Pediatr Surg. 37:887–92. PMID:12037756
2557. Shuster JJ, McWilliams NB, Castleberry R, et al. (1992). Serum lactate dehydrogenase in childhood neuroblastoma. A Pediatric Oncology Group recursive partitioning study. Am J Clin Oncol. 15:295–303. PMID:1514525
2558. Sichel JY, Eliashar R, Yatsiv I, et al. (2002). A multidisciplinary team approach for management of a giant congenital cervical teratoma. Int J Pediatr Otorhinolaryngol. 65:241–7. PMID:12242140
2559. Sidorkin DV, Konovalov AN, Makhmudov UB, et al. (2009). Topographic variants of cranial chordomas. Zh Vopr Neirokhir Im N N Burdenko. (3):14–8. [Russian] PMID:20092020
2560. Silveira LG, Dias EP, Marinho BC, et al. (2008). HRPT2-related familial isolated hyperparathyroidism: could molecular studies direct the surgical approach? Arq Bras Endocrinol Metabol. 52:1211–20. PMID:19169472
2561. Silver CE, Owen RP, Rodrigo JP, et al. (2011). Aggressive variants of papillary thyroid carcinoma. Head Neck. 33:1052–9. PMID:20824810
2562. Silverberg SG, Vidone RA (1966). Adenoma and carcinoma of the thyroid. Cancer. 19:1053–62. PMID:5912322
2563. Silverberg SG, Vidone RA (1966). Carcinoma of the thyroid in surgical and postmortem material. Analysis of 300 cases at autopsy and literature review. Ann Surg. 164:291–9. PMID:5915940
2564. Silverberg SJ, Bilezikian JP (2003). "Incipient" primary hyperparathyroidism: a "forme fruste" of an old disease. J Clin Endocrinol Metab. 88:5348–52. PMID:14602772
2565. Sim SJ, Ro JY, Ordonez NG, et al. (1997). Sclerosing mucoepidermoid carcinoma with eosinophilia of the thyroid: report of two patients, one with distant metastasis, and review of the literature. Hum Pathol. 28:1091–6. PMID:9308735
2566. Simonds WF, Varghese S, Marx SJ, et al. (2012). Cushing's syndrome in multiple endocrine neoplasia type 1. Clin Endocrinol (Oxf). 76:379–86. PMID:21916912
2567. Simpson DJ, Bicknell JE, McNicol AM, et al. (1999). Hypermethylation of the p16/CDKN2A/MTSI gene and loss of protein expression is associated with nonfunctional pituitary adenomas but not somatotrophinomas. Genes Chromosomes Cancer. 24:328–36. PMID:10092131
2568. Simpson PR (1990). Adenomatoid tumor of the adrenal gland. Arch Pathol Lab Med. 114:725–7. PMID:1694656
2569. Simpson WJ, Carruthers J (1988). Squamous cell carcinoma of the thyroid gland. Am J Surg. 156:44–6. PMID:3394892
2570. Singer J, Koch CA, Kassahun W, et al. (2011). A patient with a large recurrent pheochromocytoma demonstrating the pitfalls of diagnosis. Nat Rev Endocrinol. 7:749–55. PMID:21894215
2571. Singer PA, Cooper DS, Levy EG, et al. (1995). Treatment guidelines for patients with hyperthyroidism and hypothyroidism. Standards of Care Committee, American Thyroid Association. JAMA. 273:808–12. PMID:7532241
2572. Singh Ospina N, Sebo TJ, Thompson GB, et al. (2014). Prevalence of parathyroid carcinoma in 348 patients with multiple endocrine neoplasia type 1 - case report and review of the literature. Clin Endocrinol (Oxf). EPUB 2014. PMID:25557532
2573. Singh Ospina N, Thompson GB, C Nichols F 3rd, et al. (2015). Thymic and Bronchial Carcinoid Tumors in Multiple Endocrine Neoplasia Type 1: The Mayo Clinic Experience from 1977 to 2013. Horm Cancer. 6:247–53. PMID:26070346
2574. Singh K, Sharma MC, Jain D, et al. (2008). Melanotic medullary carcinoma of thyroid–report of a rare case with brief review of literature. Diagn Pathol. 3:2. PMID:18190715
2575. Singh R, Basturk O, Klimstra DS, et al. (2006). Lipid-rich variant of pancreatic endocrine neoplasms. Am J Surg Pathol. 30:194–200. PMID:16434893
2576. Singhi AD, Chu LC, Tatsas AD, et al. (2012). Cystic pancreatic neuroendocrine tumors: a clinicopathologic study. Am J Surg Pathol. 36:1666–73. PMID:23073325
2577. Sinkre PA, Murakata L, Rabin L, et al. (2001). Clear cell carcinoid tumor of the gallbladder: another distinctive manifestation of von Hippel-Lindau disease. Am J Surg Pathol. 25:1334–9. PMID:11688471
2578. Sinnott BP, Hatipoglu B, Sarne DH (2006). Intrasellar plasmacytoma presenting as a non-functional invasive pituitary macro-adenoma: case report & literature review. Pituitary. 9:65–72. PMID:16703411
2579. Sioutos P, Yen V, Arbit E (1996). Pituitary gland metastases. Ann Surg Oncol. 3:94–9. PMID:8770309
2580. Sipos B, Sperveslage J, Anlauf M, et al. (2015). Glucagon cell hyperplasia and neoplasia with and without glucagon receptor mutations. J Clin Endocrinol Metab. 100:E783–8. PMID:25695890
2581. Skacel M, Ross CW, Hsi ED (2000). A reassessment of primary thyroid lymphoma: high-grade MALT-type lymphoma as a distinct subtype of diffuse large B-cell lymphoma. Histopathology. 37:10–8. PMID:10931213
2582. Skogseid B, Rastad J, Gobl A, et al. (1995). Adrenal lesion in multiple endocrine neoplasia type 1. Surgery. 118:1077–82. PMID:7491526
2582A. Slade I, Bacchelli C, Davies H, et al. (2011). DICER1 syndrome: clarifying the diagnosis, clinical features and management implications of a pleiotropic tumour predisposition syndrome. J Med Genet. 48:273–8. PMID:21266384
2583. Slater EP, Diehl SM, Langer P, et al. (2006). Analysis by cDNA microarrays of gene expression patterns of human adrenocortical tumors. Eur J Endocrinol. 154:587–98. PMID:16556722
2584. Slingerland J, Pagano M (2000). Regulation of the cdk inhibitor p27 and its deregulation in cancer. J Cell Physiol. 183:10–7. PMID:10699961
2585. Smallridge RC, Copland JA (2010). Anaplastic thyroid carcinoma: pathogenesis and emerging therapies. Clin Oncol (R Coll Radiol). 22:486–97. PMID:20418080
2586. Smith JM, Kirk EP, Theodosopoulos G, et al. (2002). Germline mutation of the tumour suppressor PTEN in Proteus syndrome. J Med Genet. 39:937–40. PMID:12471211
2587. Smith TG, Clark SK, Katz DE, et al. (2000). Adrenal masses are associated with familial adenomatous polyposis. Dis Colon Rectum. 43:1739–42. PMID:11156460
2588. Smith TR, Hulou MM, Huang KT, et al. (2015). Current indications for the surgical treatment of prolactinomas. J Clin Neurosci. 22:1785–91. PMID:26277642
2589. Snover DC, Foucar K (1981). Mitotic activity in benign parathyroid disease. Am J Clin Pathol. 75:345–7. PMID:7211756
2590. So JS, Epstein JI (2013). GATA3 expression in paragangliomas: a pitfall potentially leading to misdiagnosis of urothelial carcinoma. Mod Pathol. 26:1365–70. PMID:23599157
2591. Soares J, Limbert E, Sobrinho-Simões M (1989). Diffuse sclerosing variant of papillary thyroid carcinoma. A clinicopathologic study of 10 cases. Pathol Res Pract. 185:200–6. PMID:2798220
2592. Soares P, Trovisco V, Rocha AS, et al. (2004). BRAF mutations typical of papillary thyroid carcinoma are more frequently detected in undifferentiated than in insular and insular-like poorly differentiated carcinomas. Virchows Arch. 444:572–6. PMID:15095090
2593. Soares P, Trovisco V, Rocha AS, et al. (2003). BRAF mutations and RET/PTC rearrangements are alternative events in the etiopathogenesis of PTC. Oncogene. 22:4578–80. PMID:12881714
2594. Sobin LH, Gospodarowicz MK, Wittekind C, editors (2009). TNM classification of malignant tumours. 7th ed. Oxford: Wiley-Blackwell.
2595. Sobrinho-Simões M (2000). Hail to the histologic grading of papillary thyroid carcinoma? Cancer. 88:1766–8. PMID:10760750
2596. Sobrinho-Simões M, Eloy C, Magalhães J, et al. (2011). Follicular thyroid carcinoma. Mod Pathol. 24 Suppl 2:S10–8. PMID:21455197
2597. Sobrinho-Simões M, Máximo V, Castro IV, et al. (2005). Hürthle (oncocytic) cell tumors of thyroid: etiopathogenesis, diagnosis and clinical significance. Int J Surg Pathol. 13:29–35. PMID:15735852
2598. Sobrinho-Simões M, Sambade C, Fonseca E, et al. (2002). Poorly differentiated carcinomas of the thyroid gland: a review of the clinicopathologic features of a series of 28 cases of a heterogeneous, clinically aggressive group of thyroid tumors. Int J Surg Pathol. 10:123–31. PMID:12075405
2599. Sobrinho-Simões M, Stenwig AE, Nesland JM, et al. (1986). A mucinous carcinoma of the thyroid. Pathol Res Pract. 181:464–71. PMID:3020530
2600. Sobrinho-Simões MA, Nesland JM, Johannessen JV (1985). A mucin-producing tumor in the thyroid gland. Ultrastruct Pathol. 9:277–81. PMID:4090007
2601. Soga J (2005). Carcinoids of the pancreas: an analysis of 156 cases. Cancer. 104:1180–7. PMID:16104045
2602. Soga J, Tazawa K (1971). Pathologic analysis of carcinoids. Histologic reevaluation of 62 cases. Cancer. 28:990–8. PMID:4106849
2603. Soga J, Yakuwa Y (1998). Glucagonomas/diabetico-dermatogenic syndrome (DDS): a statistical evaluation of 407 reported cases. J Hepatobiliary Pancreat Surg. 5:312–9. PMID:9880781
2604. Soga J, Yakuwa Y (1998). Vipoma/diarrheogenic syndrome: a statistical evaluation of 241 reported cases. J Exp Clin Cancer Res. 17:389–400. PMID:10089056
2605. Soga J, Yakuwa Y (1999). Somatostatinoma/inhibitory syndrome: a statistical evaluation of 173 reported cases as compared to other pancreatic endocrinomas. J Exp Clin Cancer Res. 18:13–22. PMID:10374671
2606. Søkilde R, Vincent M, Møller AK, et al. (2014). Efficient identification of miRNAs for classification of tumor origin. J Mol Diagn. 16:106–15. PMID:24211363
2607. Solcia E, Capella C, Kloppel G (1997). Tumors of the pancreas. In: AFIP atlas of tumor pathology. Series 3, Fascicle 20. Washington DC: American Registry of Pathology Press.
2608. Solcia E, Capella C, Riva C, et al. (1988). The morphology and neuroendocrine profile of pancreatic epithelial VIPomas and extrapancreatic, VIP-producing, neurogenic tumors. Ann N Y Acad Sci. 527:508–17. PMID:2839087

2609. Sonabend AM, Zacharia BE, Goldstein H, et al. (2014). The role for adjuvant radiotherapy in the treatment of hemangiopericytoma: a Surveillance, Epidemiology, and End Results analysis. J Neurosurg. 120:300–8. PMID:24286142

2610. Song KB, Kim SC, Kim JH, et al. (2016). Prognostic Value of Somatostatin Receptor Subtypes in Pancreatic Neuroendocrine Tumors. Pancreas. 45:187–92. PMID:26474434

2611. Song M, Wang H, Song L, et al. (2014). Ectopic TSH-secreting pituitary tumor: a case report and review of prior cases. BMC Cancer. 14:544. PMID:25069990

2612. Song YS, Lim JA, Choi H, et al. (2016). Prognostic effects of TERT promoter mutations are enhanced by coexistence with BRAF or RAS mutations and strengthen the risk prediction by the ATA or TNM staging system in differentiated thyroid cancer patients. Cancer. 122:1370–9. PMID:26969876

2613. Song YS, Lim JA, Park YJ (2015). Mutation Profile of Well-Differentiated Thyroid Cancer in Asians. Endocrinol Metab (Seoul). 30:252–62. PMID:26435130

2614. Song Z, Yu C, Song X, et al. (2011). Primary solitary fibrous tumor of the thyroid - report of a case and review of the literature. J Cancer. 2:206–9. PMID:21509151

2615. Soon PS, Gill AJ, Benn DE, et al. (2009). Microarray gene expression and immunohistochemistry analyses of adrenocortical tumors identify IGF2 and Ki-67 as useful in differentiating carcinomas from adenomas. Endocr Relat Cancer. 16:573–83. PMID:19218281

2616. Soon PS, Tacon LJ, Gill AJ, et al. (2009). miR-195 and miR-483-5p Identified as Predictors of Poor Prognosis in Adrenocortical Cancer. Clin Cancer Res. 15:7684–92. PMID:19996210

2617. Soong CP, Arnold A (2014). Recurrent ZFX mutations in human sporadic parathyroid adenomas. Oncoscience. 1:360–6. PMID:25594030

2618. Soravia C, Sugg SL, Berk T, et al. (1999). Familial adenomatous polyposis-associated thyroid cancer: a clinical, pathological, and molecular genetics study. Am J Pathol. 154:127–35. PMID:9916927

2619. Sorbye H, Strosberg J, Baudin E, et al. (2014). Gastroenteropancreatic high-grade neuroendocrine carcinoma. Cancer. 120:2814–23. PMID:24771552

2620. Sorbye H, Welin S, Langer SW, et al. (2013). Predictive and prognostic factors for treatment and survival in 305 patients with advanced gastrointestinal neuroendocrine carcinoma (WHO G3): the NORDIC NEC study. Ann Oncol. 24:152–60. PMID:22967994

2621. Sovinz P, Urban C, Uhrig S, et al. (2010). Pheochromocytoma in a 2.75-year-old-girl with a germline von Hippel-Lindau mutation Q164R. Am J Med Genet A. 152A:1752–5. PMID:20583150

2622. Speel EJ, Richter J, Moch H, et al. (1999). Genetic differences in endocrine pancreatic tumor subtypes detected by comparative genomic hybridization. Am J Pathol. 155:1787–94. PMID:10595906

2623. Speel EJ, Scheidweiler AF, Zhao J, et al. (2001). Genetic evidence for early divergence of small functioning and nonfunctioning endocrine pancreatic tumors: gain of 9Q34 is an early event in insulinomas. Cancer Res. 61:5186–92. PMID:11431358

2624. Speisky D, Duces A, Bièche I, et al. (2012). Molecular profiling of pancreatic neuroendocrine tumors in sporadic and Von Hippel-Lindau patients. Clin Cancer Res. 18:2838–49. PMID:22461457

2625. Sponziello M, Durante C, Filetti S (2015). HABP2 Mutation and Nonmedullary Thyroid Cancer. N Engl J Med. 373:2085–6. PMID:26581004

2626. Squillaci S, Pitino A, Spairani C, et al. (2016). Mucinous Variant of Follicular Carcinoma of the Thyroid Gland: Case Report and Review of the Literature. Int J Surg Pathol. 24:170–6. PMID:26582770

2627. Srivastava A, Hornick JL (2009). Immunohistochemical staining for CDX-2, PDX-1, NESP-55, and TTF-1 can help distinguish gastrointestinal carcinoid tumors from pancreatic endocrine and pulmonary carcinoid tumors. Am J Surg Pathol. 33:626–32. PMID:19065104

2628. Stache C, Hölsken A, Fahlbusch R, et al. (2014). Tight junction protein claudin-1 is differentially expressed in craniopharyngioma subtypes and indicates invasive tumor growth. Neuro Oncol. 16:256–64. PMID:24305709

2629. Stacpoole PW (1981). The glucagonoma syndrome: clinical features, diagnosis, and treatment. Endocr Rev. 2:347–61. PMID:6268399

2630. Stanta G, Carcangiu ML, Rosai J (1988). The biochemical and immunohistochemical profile of thyroid neoplasia. Pathol Annu. 23 (Pt 1):129–57. PMID:2838792

2631. Starink TM, van der Veen JP, Arwert F, et al. (1986). The Cowden syndrome: a clinical and genetic study in 21 patients. Clin Genet. 29:222–33. PMID:3698331

2632. Starker LF, Akerström T, Long WD, et al. (2012). Frequent germ-line mutations of the MEN1, CASR, and HRPT2/CDC73 genes in young patients with clinically non-familial primary hyperparathyroidism. Horm Cancer. 3:44–51. PMID:22187299

2633. Starr JS, Attia S, Joseph RW, et al. (2015). Follicular Dendritic Cell Sarcoma Presenting As a Thyroid Mass. J Clin Oncol. 33:e74–6. PMID:24663046

2634. Steel TR, Dailey AT, Born D, et al. (1993). Paragangliomas of the sellar region: report of two cases. Neurosurgery. 32:844–7. PMID:8492863

2635. Steele SR, Royer M, Brown TA, et al. (2001). Mucoepidermoid carcinoma of the thyroid gland: a case report and suggested surgical approach. Am Surg. 67:979–83. PMID:11603557

2636. Steenbergh PH, Höppener JW, Zandberg J, et al. (1984). Calcitonin gene related peptide coding sequence is conserved in the human genome and is expressed in medullary thyroid carcinoma. J Clin Endocrinol Metab. 59:358–60. PMID:6610687

2637. Stefaneanu L, Kovacs K, Lloyd RV, et al. (1992). Pituitary lactotrophs and somatotrophs in pregnancy: a correlative in situ hybridization and immunocytochemical study. Virchows Arch B Cell Pathol Incl Mol Pathol. 62:291–6. PMID:1359702

2638. Stefaneanu L, Kovacs K, Scheithauer BW, et al. (2000). Effect of Dopamine Agonists on Lactotroph Adenomas of the Human Pituitary. Endocr Pathol. 11:341–52. PMID:12114758

2639. Steiner AL, Goodman AD, Powers SR (1968). Study of a kindred with pheochromocytoma, medullary thyroid carcinoma, hyperparathyroidism and Cushing's disease: multiple endocrine neoplasia, type 2. Medicine (Baltimore). 47:371–409. PMID:4386574

2640. Steinhagen E, Guillem JG, Chang G, et al. (2012). The prevalence of thyroid cancer and benign thyroid disease in patients with familial adenomatous polyposis may be higher than previously recognized. Clin Colorectal Cancer. 11:304–8. PMID:22425061

2641. Stenström G, Svärdsudd K (1986). Pheochromocytoma in Sweden 1958-1981. An analysis of the National Cancer Registry Data. Acta Med Scand. 220:225–32. PMID:3776697

2642. Stephan EA, Chung TH, Grant CS, et al. (2008). Adrenocortical carcinoma survival rates correlated to genomic copy number variants. Mol Cancer Ther. 7:425–31. PMID:18281524

2643. Stephens M, Williams GT, Jasani B, et al. (1987). Synchronous duodenal neuroendocrine tumours in von Recklinghausen's disease–a case report of co-existing gangliocytic paraganglioma and somatostatin-rich glandular carcinoid. Histopathology. 11:1331–40. PMID:2894342

2644. Stergiopoulos SG, Abu-Asab MS, Tsokos M, et al. (2004). Pituitary pathology in Carney complex patients. Pituitary. 7:73–82. PMID:15761655

2645. Steusloff K, Röcken C, Saeger W (1998). Basement membrane proteins, apolipoprotein E and glycosaminoglycans in pituitary adenomas and their correlation to amyloid. Virchows Arch. 433:29–34. PMID:9692822

2646. Stewart DR, Messinger Y, Williams GM, et al. (2014). Nasal chondromesenchymal hamartomas arise secondary to germline and somatic mutations of DICER1 in the pleuropulmonary blastoma tumor predisposition disorder. Hum Genet. 133:1443–50. PMID:25118636

2647. Stilling G, Sun Z, Zhang S, et al. (2010). MicroRNA expression in ACTH-producing pituitary tumors: up-regulation of microRNA-122 and -493 in pituitary carcinomas. Endocrine. 38:67–75. PMID:20960104

2648. Stojadinovic A, Brennan MF, Hoos A, et al. (2003). Adrenocortical adenoma and carcinoma: histopathological and molecular comparative analysis. Mod Pathol. 16:742–51. PMID:12920217

2649. Stojadinovic A, Hoos A, Nissan A, et al. (2003). Parathyroid neoplasms: clinical, histopathological, and tissue microarray-based molecular analysis. Hum Pathol. 34:54–64. PMID:12605367

2650. Stojic L, Mojas N, Cejka P, et al. (2004). Mismatch repair-dependent G2 checkpoint induced by low doses of SN1 type methylating agents requires the ATR kinase. Genes Dev. 18:1331–44. PMID:15175264

2651. Stone WZ, Wymer DC, Canales BK (2014). Fluorodeoxyglucose-positron-emission tomography/computed tomography imaging for adrenal masses in patients with lung cancer: review and diagnostic algorithm. J Endourol. 28:104–11. PMID:23927734

2652. Storr HL, Isidori AM, Monson JP, et al. (2004). Prepubertal Cushing's disease is more common in males, but there is no increase in severity at diagnosis. J Clin Endocrinol Metab. 89:3818–20. PMID:15292311

2653. Storr HL, Savage MO (2015). MANAGEMENT OF ENDOCRINE DISEASE: Paediatric Cushing's disease. Eur J Endocrinol. 173:R35–45. PMID:26036813

2654. Stratakis CA (2008). Cushing syndrome caused by adrenocortical tumors and hyperplasias (corticotropin- independent Cushing syndrome). Endocr Dev. 13:117–32. PMID:18493137

2655. Stratakis CA (2014). E pluribus unum? The main protein kinase A catalytic subunit (PRKACA), a likely oncogene, and cortisol-producing tumors. J Clin Endocrinol Metab. 99:3629–33. PMID:25279575

2656. Stratakis CA, Courcoutsakis NA, Abati A, et al. (1997). Thyroid gland abnormalities in patients with the syndrome of spotty skin pigmentation, myxomas, endocrine overactivity, and schwannomas (Carney complex). J Clin Endocrinol Metab. 82:2037–43. PMID:9215269

2657. Stratakis CA, Kirschner LS, Carney JA (2001). Clinical and molecular features of the Carney complex: diagnostic criteria and recommendations for patient evaluation. J Clin Endocrinol Metab. 86:4041–6. PMID:11549623

2658. Stratakis CA, Papageorgiou T, Premkumar A, et al. (2000). Ovarian lesions in Carney complex: clinical genetics and possible predisposition to malignancy. J Clin Endocrinol Metab. 85:4359–66. PMID:11095480

2659. Stratakis CA, Salpea P, Raygada M (2015). Carney complex. In: Pagon RA, Adam MP, Ardinger HH, et al., editors. GeneReviews®. Seattle: University of Washington, Seattle. PMID:20301463

2660. Stratakis CA, Tichomirowa MA, Boikos S, et al. (2010). The role of germline AIP, MEN1, PRKAR1A, CDKN1B and CDKN2C mutations in causing pituitary adenomas in a large cohort of children, adolescents, and patients with genetic syndromes. Clin Genet. 78:457–63. PMID:20507346

2661. Streubel B, Simonitsch-Klupp I, Müllauer L, et al. (2004). Variable frequencies of MALT lymphoma-associated genetic aberrations in MALT lymphomas of different sites. Leukemia. 18:1722–6. PMID:15356642

2662. Streubel B, Vinatzer U, Lamprecht A, et al. (2005). T(3;14)(p14.1;q32) involving IGH and FOXP1 is a novel recurrent chromosomal aberration in MALT lymphoma. Leukemia. 19:652–8. PMID:15703784

2663. Strong VE, Kennedy T, Al-Ahmadie H, et al. (2008). Prognostic indicators of malignancy in adrenal pheochromocytomas: clinical, histopathologic, and cell cycle/apoptosis gene expression analysis. Surgery. 143:759–68. PMID:18549892

2664. Strosberg JR, Cheema A, Weber J, et al. (2011). Prognostic validity of a novel American Joint Committee on Cancer Staging Classification for pancreatic neuroendocrine tumors. J Clin Oncol. 29:3044–9. PMID:21709192

2665. Strosberg JR, Coppola D, Klimstra DS, et al. (NANETS) (2010). The NANETS consensus guidelines for the diagnosis and management of poorly differentiated (high-grade) extrapulmonary neuroendocrine carcinomas. Pancreas. 39:799–800. PMID:20664477

2666. Stucchi CM, Vaccaro V, Magherini A, et al. (2007). Hürthle cell follicular carcinoma of the thyroid gland presenting with diffuse meningeal carcinomatosis and evolving to anaplastic carcinoma. J Clin Pathol. 60:831–2. PMID:17596549

2667. Sturiale A, Giudici F, Alemanno G, et al. (2015). Massive intrathoracic lipoma in men1 syndrome. Int J Surg Case Rep. 6C:247–50. PMID:25545711

2668. Su HC, Huang X, Zhou WL, et al. (2014). Pathologic analysis, diagnosis and treatment of adrenal myelolipoma. Can Urol Assoc J. 8:E637–40. PMID:25295136

2669. Su L, Beals T, Bernacki EG, et al. (1997). Spindle epithelial tumor with thymus-like differentiation: a case report with cytologic, histologic, immunohistologic, and ultrastructural findings. Mod Pathol. 10:510–4. PMID:9160319

2670. Subramaniam MM, Putti TC, Anuar D, et al. (2007). Clonal characterization of sporadic cribriform-morular variant of papillary thyroid carcinoma by laser microdissection-based APC mutation analysis. Am J Clin Pathol. 128:994–1001. PMID:18024325

2671. Suganuma R, Wang LL, Sano H, et al. (2013). Peripheral neuroblastic tumors with genotype-phenotype discordance: a report from the Children's Oncology Group and the International Neuroblastoma Pathology Committee. Pediatr Blood Cancer. 60:363–70. PMID:22744966

2672. Sugita R, Nomura T, Yuda F (1998). Primary schwannoma of the thyroid gland: CT findings. AJR Am J Roentgenol. 171:528–9. PMID:9694497

2673. Sugitani I, Hasegawa Y, Sugasawa M, et al. (2014). Super-radical surgery for anaplastic thyroid carcinoma: a large cohort study using the Anaplastic Thyroid Carcinoma Research Consortium of Japan database. Head Neck. 36:328–33. PMID:23729360

2674. Sugitani I, Miyauchi A, Sugino K, et al. (2012). Prognostic factors and treatment outcomes for anaplastic thyroid carcinoma: ATC Research Consortium of Japan cohort study of 677 patients. World J Surg. 36:1247–54. PMID:22311136

2675. Sujoy V, Pinto A, Nosé V (2013).

Columnar cell variant of papillary thyroid carcinoma: a study of 10 cases with emphasis on CDX2 expression. Thyroid. 23:714–9. PMID:23488912
2676. Sukov WR, Cheville JC, Giannini C, et al. (2010). Isochromosome 12p and polysomy 12 in primary central nervous system germ cell tumors: frequency and association with clinicopathologic features. Hum Pathol. 41:232–8. PMID:19801160
2677. Sun T, Wang Z, Wang J, et al. (2011). Outcome of radical resection and postoperative radiotherapy for thyroid carcinoma showing thymus-like differentiation. World J Surg. 35:1840–6. PMID:21597887
2678. Sun Y, Sun Q, Shen J, et al. (2012). Cauda equina hemangioblastoma at L5 vertebral level related to von Hippel-Lindau disease. Br J Neurosurg. 26:576–7. PMID:22133049
2679. Sundin A, Rockall A (2012). Therapeutic monitoring of gastroenteropancreatic neuroendocrine tumors: the challenges ahead. Neuroendocrinology. 96:261–71. PMID:22907438
2680. Sundin A, Vullierme MP, Kaltsas G, et al. (2009). ENETS Consensus Guidelines for the Standards of Care in Neuroendocrine Tumors: radiological examinations. Neuroendocrinology. 90:167–83. PMID:19077417
2681. Surov A, Gottschling S, Wienke A, et al. (2015). Primary Thyroid Sarcoma: A Systematic Review. Anticancer Res. 35:5185–91. PMID:26408676
2682. Suzuki A, Hirokawa M, Takada N, et al. (2015). Diagnostic significance of PAX8 in thyroid squamous cell carcinoma. Endocr J. 62:991–5. PMID:26354716
2683. Svec A, Bury Y (2010). Haemangioma of the parathyroid gland. Does it really exist? Pathol Oncol Res. 16:443–6. PMID:20063187
2684. Sweiss FB, Lee M, Sherman JH (2015). Extraventricular neurocytomas. Neurosurg Clin N Am. 26:99–104. PMID:25432188
2685. Sykes JM, Ossoff RH (1986). Paragangliomas of the head and neck. Otolaryngol Clin North Am. 19:755–67. PMID:3797012
2686. Syro LV, Horvath E, Kovacs K (2000). Double adenoma of the pituitary: a somatotroph adenoma colliding with a gonadotroph adenoma. J Endocrinol Invest. 23:37–41. PMID:10698050
2687. Syro LV, Ortiz LD, Scheithauer BW, et al. (2011). Treatment of pituitary neoplasms with temozolomide: a review. Cancer. 117:454–62. PMID:20845485
2688. Szabó J, Heath B, Hill VM, et al. (1995). Hereditary hyperparathyroidism-jaw tumor syndrome: the endocrine tumor gene HRPT2 maps to chromosome 1q21-q31. Am J Hum Genet. 56:944–50. PMID:7717405
2689. Sztal-Mazer S, Topliss DJ, Simpson RW, et al. (2008). Gonadotroph adenoma in multiple endocrine neoplasia type 1. Endocr Pract. 14:592–4. PMID:18753103
2690. Taccagni G, Sambade C, Nesland J, et al. (1993). Solitary fibrous tumour of the thyroid: clinicopathological, immunohistochemical and ultrastructural study of three cases. Virchows Arch A Pathol Anat Histopathol. 422:491–7. PMID:8333152
2691. Tadjine M, Lampron A, Ouadi L, et al. (2008). Frequent mutations of beta-catenin gene in sporadic secreting adrenocortical adenomas. Clin Endocrinol (Oxf). 68:264–70. PMID:17854394
2692. Taggart JL, Summerlin DJ, Moore MG (2013). Parathyroid carcinosarcoma: a rare form of parathyroid carcinoma with normal parathyroid hormone levels. Int J Surg Pathol. 21:394–8. PMID:23493876
2693. Taguchi R, Yamada M, Horiguchi K, et al. (2011). Haploinsufficient and predominant expression of multiple endocrine neoplasia type 1 (MEN1)-related genes, MLL, p27Kip1 and p18Ink4C in endocrine organs. Biochem Biophys Res Commun. 415:378–83. PMID:22037578
2694. Taguchi R, Yamada M, Nakajima Y, et al. (2012). Expression and mutations of KCNJ5 mRNA in Japanese patients with aldosterone-producing adenomas. J Clin Endocrinol Metab. 97:1311–9. PMID:22278422
2695. Tahara S, Kurotani R, Sanno N, et al. (2000). Expression of pituitary homeo box 1 (Ptx1) in human non-neoplastic pituitaries and pituitary adenomas. Mod Pathol. 13:1097–108. PMID:11048804
2696. Tai CM, Liang CW, Chang TC (2003). Intrathyroidal thymic carcinoma: a case report. J Formos Med Assoc. 102:109–12. PMID:12709740
2697. Takano T, Ito Y, Hirokawa M, et al. (2007). BRAF V600E mutation in anaplastic thyroid carcinomas and their accompanying differentiated carcinomas. Br J Cancer. 96:1549–53. PMID:17453004
2698. Takayama F, Takashima S, Matsuba H, et al. (2001). MR imaging of primary leiomyosarcoma of the thyroid gland. Eur J Radiol. 37:36–41. PMID:11274837
2699. Takei Y, Seyama S, Pearl GS, et al. (1980). Ultrastructural study of the human neurohypophysis. II. Cellular elements of neural parenchyma, the pituicytes. Cell Tissue Res. 205:273–87. PMID:7188885
2700. Takenaka Y, Inohara H, Yoshii T, et al. (2003). Malignant transformation of thyroid follicular cells by galectin-3. Cancer Lett. 195:111–9. PMID:12767519
2701. Takeuchi Y, Daa T, Kashima K, et al. (1999). Mutations of p53 in thyroid carcinoma with an insular component. Thyroid. 9:377–81. PMID:10319944
2702. Takizawa H, Narisawa R, Asakura H (1999). Jejunal invasion of pheochromocytoma pathologically confirmed by endoscopic biopsy. Am J Med Sci. 317:63–6. PMID:9892275
2703. Talaei A, Aminorroaya A, Taheri D, et al. (2014). Carney complex presenting with a unilateral adrenocortical nodule: a case report. J Med Case Rep. 8:38. PMID:24499519
2704. Talat N, Schulte KM (2010). Clinical presentation, staging and long-term evolution of parathyroid cancer. Ann Surg Oncol. 17:2156–74. PMID:20221704
2705. Tallini G (2011). Poorly differentiated thyroid carcinoma. Are we there yet? Endocr Pathol. 22:190–4. PMID:21969055
2706. Tallini G, Garcia-Rostan G, Herrero A, et al. (1999). Downregulation of p27KIP1 and Ki67/Mib1 labeling index support the classification of thyroid carcinoma into prognostically relevant categories. Am J Surg Pathol. 23:678–85. PMID:10366150
2707. Tallini G, Hsueh A, Liu S, et al. (1999). Frequent chromosomal DNA unbalance in thyroid oncocytic (Hürthle cell) neoplasms detected by comparative genomic hybridization. Lab Invest. 79:547–55. PMID:10334566
2708. Tallini G, Ladanyi M, Rosai J, et al. (1994). Analysis of nuclear and mitochondrial DNA alterations in thyroid and renal oncocytic tumors. Cytogenet Cell Genet. 66:253–9. PMID:7909283
2709. Tamiya H, Miyakawa M, Suzuki H, et al. (2013). A large functioning parathyroid cyst in a patient with multiple endocrine neoplasia type 1. Endocr J. 60:709–14. PMID:23386389
2710. Tamura M, Murata M, Kawafuchi J, et al. (1982). Primary cerebral neuroblastoma of the supra- and para-sellar regions: case report. Neurol Med Chir (Tokyo). 22:668–72. [Japanese] PMID:6183609
2711. Tan JN, Kroll MH, O'Hara CJ, et al. (2012). Gamma heavy chain disease in a patient with underlying lymphoplasmacytic lymphoma of the thyroid. Report of a case and comparison with other reported cases with thyroid involvement. Clin Chim Acta. 413:1696–9. PMID:22561184
2712. Tan MH, Mester JL, Ngeow J, et al. (2012). Lifetime cancer risks in individuals with germline PTEN mutations. Clin Cancer Res. 18:400–7. PMID:22252256
2713. Tan MH, Morrison C, Wang P, et al. (2004). Loss of parafibromin immunoreactivity is a distinguishing feature of parathyroid carcinoma. Clin Cancer Res. 10:6629–37. PMID:15475453
2714. Tanabe T, Yasuo M, Tsushima K, et al. (2008). Mediastinal seminoma in a patient with multiple endocrine neoplasia type 1. Intern Med. 47:1615–9. PMID:18797122
2715. Tanabeu Y, Nakahara S, Mitsuyama S, et al. (1998). Breast Cancer in a Patient with McCune-Albright Syndrome. Breast Cancer. 5:175–8. PMID:11091644
2716. Tanahashi J, Kashima K, Daa T, et al. (2006). Solitary fibrous tumor of the thyroid gland: report of two cases and review of the literature. Pathol Int. 56:471–7. PMID:16872444
2717. Tanaka T, Hiramatsu K, Nosaka T, et al. (2015). Pituitary metastasis of hepatocellular carcinoma presenting with panhypopituitarism: a case report. BMC Cancer. 15:863. PMID:26545979
2718. Tanaka Y, Notohara K, Kato K, et al. (2002). Usefulness of beta-catenin immunostaining for the differential diagnosis of solid-pseudopapillary neoplasm of the pancreas. Am J Surg Pathol. 26:818–20. PMID:12023593
2719. Tanboon J, Keskool P (2013). Leiomyosarcoma: a rare tumor of the thyroid. Endocr Pathol. 24:136–43. PMID:23729187
2720. Tanda F, Massarelli G, Bosincu L (1990). Primary mucoepidermoid carcinoma of the thyroid gland. Surg Pathol. 3:317–24.
2721. Tanda F, Massarelli G, Bosincu L, et al. (1988). Angiosarcoma of the thyroid: a light, electron microscopic and histoimmunological study. Hum Pathol. 19:742–5. PMID:3132415
2722. Tang LH, Basturk O, Sue JJ, et al. (2016). A practical approach to the classification of WHO grade 3 (G3) well-differentiated neuroendocrine tumor (WD-NET) and poorly differentiated neuroendocrine carcinoma (PD-NEC) of the Pancreas. Am J Surg Pathol. 40:1192–202. PMID:27259015
2723. Tang LH, Contractor T, Clausen R, et al. (2012). Attenuation of the retinoblastoma pathway in pancreatic neuroendocrine tumors due to increased cdk4/cdk6. Clin Cancer Res. 18:4612–20. PMID:22761470
2724. Tang LH, Untch BR, Reidy DL, et al. (2016). Well-differentiated neuroendocrine tumors with a morphologically apparent high-grade component: a pathway distinct from poorly differentiated neuroendocrine carcinomas. Clin Cancer Res. 22:1011–7. PMID:26482044
2725. Tanizaki Y, Jin L, Scheithauer BW, et al. (2007). P53 gene mutations in pituitary carcinomas. Endocr Pathol. 18:217–22. PMID:18026859
2726. Tanner HC Jr, Dahlin DC, Childs DS Jr (1961). Sarcoma complicating fibrous dysplasia. Probable role of radiation therapy. Oral Surg Oral Med Oral Pathol. 14:837–46. PMID:13775207
2727. Taskin OC, Gucer H, Mete O (2015). An Unusual Adrenal Cortical Nodule: Composite Adrenal Cortical Adenoma and Adenomatoid Tumor. Endocr Pathol. 26:370–3. PMID:25861051
2728. Tateno T, Asa SL, Zheng L, et al. (2011). The FGFR4-G388R polymorphism promotes mitochondrial STAT3 serine phosphorylation to facilitate pituitary growth hormone cell tumorigenesis. PLoS Genet. 7:e1002400. PMID:22174695
2729. Tateyama H, Tada T, Okabe M, et al. (2001). Different keratin profiles in craniopharyngioma subtypes and ameloblastomas. Pathol Res Pract. 197:735–42. PMID:11770017
2729A. Taubman ML, Goldfarb M, Lew JI. (2011). Role of SPECT and SPECT/CT in the Surgical Treatment of Primary Hyperparathyroidism. Int J Mol Imaging. 2011:141593. PMID:21776381
2730. Taweevisit M, Bunyayothin W, Thorner PS (2015). Thyroid Paraganglioma: "Naked" Nuclei as a Clue to Diagnosis on Imprint Cytology. Endocr Pathol. 26:232–8. PMID:26116097
2731. Taweevisit M, Sampatanukul P, Thorner PS (2013). Ectopic thymoma can mimic benign and malignant thyroid lesions on fine needle aspiration cytology: a case report and literature review. Acta Cytol. 57:213–20. PMID:23406665
2732. Taylor SL, Barakos JA, Harsh GR 4th, et al. (1992). Magnetic resonance imaging of tuberculum sellae meningiomas: preventing preoperative misdiagnosis as pituitary macroadenoma. Neurosurgery. 31:621–7, discussion 627. PMID:1407446
2733. TCGA Fishbein L et al. and The Cancer Genome Atlas Research Network. (2017) Comprehensive molecular characterization of pheochromocytoma and paraganglioma. Cancer Cell 31:181-193. PMID: 28162975
2734. Teears RJ, Silverman EM (1975). Clinicopathologic review of 88 cases of carcinoma metastatic to the putuitary gland. Cancer. 36:216–20. PMID:1203849
2735. Teh BT, Farnebo F, Kristoffersson U, et al. (1996). Autosomal dominant primary hyperparathyroidism and jaw tumor syndrome associated with renal hamartomas and cystic kidney disease: linkage to 1q21-q32 and loss of the wild type allele in renal hamartomas. J Clin Endocrinol Metab. 81:4204–11. PMID:8954016
2736. Teh BT, Zedenius J, Kytölä S, et al. (1998). Thymic carcinoids in multiple endocrine neoplasia type 1. Ann Surg. 228:99–105. PMID:9671073
2737. Terada T, Kovacs K, Stefaneanu L, et al. (1995). Incidence, Pathology, and Recurrence of Pituitary Adenomas: Study of 647 Unselected Surgical Cases. Endocr Pathol. 6:301–10. PMID:12114812
2738. Terada T, Matsunaga Y, Maeta H, et al. (1999). Mixed ductal-endocrine carcinoma of the pancreas presenting as gastrinoma with Zollinger-Ellison syndrome: an autopsy case with a 24-year survival period. Virchows Arch. 435:606–11. PMID:10628803
2739. Terris B, Cavard C (2014). Diagnosis and molecular aspects of solid-pseudopapillary neoplasms of the pancreas. Semin Diagn Pathol. 31:484–90. PMID:25524568
2740. Teshiba R, Kawano S, Wang LL, et al. (2014). Age-dependent prognostic effect by Mitosis-Karyorrhexis Index in neuroblastoma: a report from the Children's Oncology Group. Pediatr Dev Pathol. 17:441–9. PMID:25207821
2741. Testart J, Amiel ML (1991). Contribution of preovulatory-phase small follicles to the ovarian response in stimulated cycles. Hum Reprod. 6:823–7. PMID:1757521
2742. Teyssier JR, Liautaud-Roger F, Ferre D, et al. (1990). Chromosomal changes in thyroid tumors. Relation with DNA content, karyotypic features, and clinical data. Cancer Genet Cytogenet. 50:249–63. PMID:2265404
2743. Thakkar JP, Chew L, Villano JL (2013). Primary CNS germ cell tumors: current epidemiology and update on treatment. Med Oncol. 30:496. PMID:23436013
2744. Thakker RV (2010). Multiple endocrine neoplasia type 1 (MEN1). Best Pract Res Clin Endocrinol Metab. 24:355–70. PMID:20833329
2745. Thakker RV (2014). Multiple endocrine neoplasia type 1 (MEN1) and type 4 (MEN4). Mol Cell Endocrinol. 386:2–15. PMID:23933118
2746. Thakker RV, Newey PJ, Walls GV, et al. (2012). Clinical practice guidelines for multiple endocrine neoplasia type 1 (MEN1). J Clin Endocrinol Metab. 97:2990–3011. PMID:22723327
2747. Thakral B, Zhou J, Medeiros LJ (2015). Extranodal hematopoietic neoplasms and mimics in the head and neck: an update. Hum Pathol. 46:1079–100. PMID:26118762
2748. Thakur A, Sebag F, Micco CD, et al.

(2010). Ectopic cervical thymoma mimicking as papillary thyroid carcinoma: a diagnostic dilemma. Indian J Pathol Microbiol. 53:305–7. PMID:20551539

2749. Thannberger P, Wilhelm JM, Derragui A, et al. (2001). Von Recklinghausen's disease associated with pancreatic somatostatinoma. Presse Med. 30:1741–3. [French] PMID:11769067

2750. Thapar K, Scheithauer BW, Kovacs K, et al. (1996). p53 expression in pituitary adenomas and carcinomas: correlation with invasiveness and tumor growth fractions. Neurosurgery. 38:765–70, discussion 770–1. PMID:8692397

2751. The I, Hannigan GE, Cowley GS, et al. (1997). Rescue of a Drosophila NF1 mutant phenotype by protein kinase A. Science. 276:791–4. PMID:9115203

2752. Theodoropoulou M, Cavallari I, Barzon L, et al. (2004). Differential expression of menin in sporadic pituitary adenomas. Endocr Relat Cancer. 11:333–44. PMID:15163308

2753. Theodoropoulou M, Reincke M, Fassnacht M, et al. (2015). Decoding the genetic basis of Cushing's disease: USP8 in the spotlight. Eur J Endocrinol. 173:M73–83. PMID:26012588

2754. Thevenon J, Bourredjem A, Faivre L, et al. (2013). Higher risk of death among MEN1 patients with mutations in the JunD interacting domain: a Groupe d'etude des Tumeurs Endocrines (GTE) cohort study. Hum Mol Genet. 22:1940–8. PMID:23376981

2755. Thieblemont C, Mayer A, Dumontet C, et al. (2002). Primary thyroid lymphoma is a heterogeneous disease. J Clin Endocrinol Metab. 87:105–11. PMID:11788631

2756. Thiel AT, Huang J, Lei M, et al. (2012). Menin as a hub controlling mixed lineage leukemia. Bioessays. 34:771–80. PMID:22829075

2757. Thirlwall AS, Bailey CM, Ramsay AD, et al. (1999). Laryngeal paraganglioma in a five-year-old child–the youngest case ever recorded. J Laryngol Otol. 113:62–4. PMID:10341923

2758. Thodou E, Argyrakos T, Kontogeorgos G (2007). Galectin-3 as a marker distinguishing functioning from silent corticotroph adenomas. Hormones (Athens). 6:227–32. PMID:17724007

2759. Thodou E, Kontogeorgos G, Horvath E, et al. (1995). Asynchronous pituitary adenomas with differing morphology. Arch Pathol Lab Med. 119:748–50. PMID:7646333

2760. Thodou E, Kontogeorgos G, Scheithauer BW, et al. (2000). Intrasellar chordomas mimicking pituitary adenoma. J Neurosurg. 92:976–82. PMID:10839258

2761. Thompson LD (2002). Pheochromocytoma of the Adrenal gland Scaled Score (PASS) to separate benign from malignant neoplasms: a clinicopathologic and immunophenotypic study of 100 cases. Am J Surg Pathol. 26:551–66. PMID:11979086

2762. Thompson LD (2016). Ninety-four cases of encapsulated follicular variant of papillary thyroid carcinoma: A name change to Noninvasive Follicular Thyroid Neoplasm with Papillary-like Nuclear Features would help prevent overtreatment. Mod Pathol. 29:698–707. PMID:27102347

2763. Thompson LD, Rosai J, Heffess CS (2000). Primary thyroid teratomas: a clinicopathologic study of 30 cases. Cancer. 88:1149–58. PMID:10699906

2764. Thompson LD, Seethala RR, Müller S (2012). Ectopic sphenoid sinus pituitary adenoma (ESSPA) with normal anterior pituitary gland: a clinicopathologic and immunophenotypic study of 32 cases with a comprehensive review of the english literature. Head Neck Pathol. 6:75–100. PMID:22430769

2765. Thompson LD, Wenig BM, Adair CF, et al. (1996). Peripheral Nerve Sheath Tumors of the Thyroid Gland: A Series of Four Cases and a Review of the Literature. Endocr Pathol. 7:309–18. PMID:12114802

2766. Thompson LD, Wenig BM, Adair CF, et al. (1997). Primary smooth muscle tumors of the thyroid gland. Cancer. 79:579–87. PMID:9028371

2767. Thompson LD, Wenig BM, Adair CF, et al. (1996). Langerhans cell histiocytosis of the thyroid: a series of seven cases and a review of the literature. Mod Pathol. 9:145–9. PMID:8657721

2768. Thompson LD, Wieneke JA, Heffess CS (2005). Diffuse sclerosing variant of papillary thyroid carcinoma: a clinicopathologic and immunophenotypic analysis of 22 cases. Endocr Pathol. 16:331–48. PMID:16627920

2769. Thompson LD, Wieneke JA, Paal E, et al. (2001). A clinicopathologic study of minimally invasive follicular carcinoma of the thyroid gland with a review of the English literature. Cancer. 91:505–24. PMID:11169933

2770. Thompson NW, Dunn EL, Batsakis JG, et al. (1974). Hürthle cell lesions of the thyroid gland. Surg Gynecol Obstet. 139:555–60. PMID:4479589

2771. Thomson S, Chakrabarty A, Marks P (2001). Ependymoma of the neurohypophysis. Br J Neurosurg. 15:277–8. PMID:11478070

2772. Thorner MO, Perryman RL, Cronin MJ, et al. (1982). Somatotroph hyperplasia. Successful treatment of acromegaly by removal of a pancreatic islet tumor secreting a growth hormone-releasing factor. J Clin Invest. 70:965–77. PMID:6290540

2773. Thosani S, Ayala-Ramirez M, Román-González A, et al. (2015). Constipation: an overlooked, unmanaged symptom of patients with pheochromocytoma and sympathetic paraganglioma. Eur J Endocrinol. 173:377–87. PMID:26060051

2774. Thway K, Fisher C (2014). Malignant peripheral nerve sheath tumor: pathology and genetics. Ann Diagn Pathol. 18:109–16. PMID:24418643

2775. Tichomirowa MA, Lee M, Barlier A, et al. (2012). Cyclin-dependent kinase inhibitor 1B (CDKN1B) gene variants in AIP mutation-negative familial isolated pituitary adenoma kindreds. Endocr Relat Cancer. 19:233–41. PMID:22291433

2776. Tickoo SK, Pittas AG, Adler M, et al. (2000). Bone metastases from thyroid carcinoma: a histopathologic study with clinical correlates. Arch Pathol Lab Med. 124:1440–7. PMID:11035572

2777. Tigas S, Carroll PV, Jones R, et al. (2005). Simultaneous Cushing's disease and tuberous sclerosis; a potential role for TSC in pituitary ontogeny. Clin Endocrinol (Oxf). 63:694–5. PMID:16343106

2778. Timonera ER, Paiva ME, Lopes JM, et al. (2008). Composite adenomatoid tumor and myelolipoma of adrenal gland: report of 2 cases. Arch Pathol Lab Med. 132:265–7. PMID:18251587

2779. Tirado Y, Williams MD, Hanna EY, et al. (2007). CRTC1/MAML2 fusion transcript in high grade mucoepidermoid carcinomas of salivary and thyroid glands and Warthin's tumors: implications for histogenesis and biologic behavior. Genes Chromosomes Cancer. 46:708–15. PMID:17437281

2780. Tischler AS (2000). Divergent differentiation in neuroendocrine tumors of the adrenal gland. Semin Diagn Pathol. 17:120–6. PMID:10839612

2781. Tischler AS (2008). Pheochromocytoma and extra-adrenal paraganglioma: updates. Arch Pathol Lab Med. 132:1272–84. PMID:18684026

2782. Tischler AS (2008). Pheochromocytoma: time to stamp out „malignancy"? Endocr Pathol. 19:207–8. PMID:18991024

2783. Tischler AS, Dayal Y, Balogh K, et al. (1987). The distribution of immunoreactive chromogranins, S-100 protein, and vasoactive intestinal peptide in compound tumors of the adrenal medulla. Hum Pathol. 18:909–17. PMID:3623551

2784. Tischler AS, deKrijger RR (2015). 15 years of paraganglioma: pathology of pheochromocytoma and paraganglioma. Endocr Relat Cancer. 22:T123–33. PMID:26136457

2785. Tischler AS, Pacak K, Eisenhofer G (2014). The adrenal medulla and extra-adrenal paraganglia: then and now. Endocr Pathol. 25:49–58. PMID:24362581

2786. Tisell LE, Oden A, Muth A, et al. (2003). The Ki67 index a prognostic marker in medullary thyroid carcinoma. Br J Cancer. 89:2093–7. PMID:14647143

2787. Tissier F, Cavard C, Groussin L, et al. (2005). Mutations of beta-catenin in adrenocortical tumors: activation of the Wnt signaling pathway is a frequent event in both benign and malignant adrenocortical tumors. Cancer Res. 65:7622–7. PMID:16140927

2788. Tjörnstrand A, Gunnarsson K, Evert M, et al. (2014). The incidence rate of pituitary adenomas in western Sweden for the period 2001-2011. Eur J Endocrinol. 171:519–26. PMID:25084775

2789. Toledo RA, Maciel RM, Erlic Z, et al. (2015). RET Y791F Variant Does Not Increase the Risk for Medullary Thyroid Carcinoma. Thyroid. 25:973–4. PMID:25950813

2790. Toledo SP, Lourenço DM Jr, Sekiya T, et al. (2015). Penetrance and clinical features of pheochromocytoma in a six-generation family carrying a germline TMEM127 mutation. J Clin Endocrinol Metab. 100:E308–18. PMID:25389632

2791. Tolis G, Bertrand G, Carpenter S, et al. (1978). Acromegaly and galactorrhea-amenorrhea with two pituitary adenomas secreting growth hormone or prolactin. A case report. Ann Intern Med. 89:345–8. PMID:686546

2792. Tomasetti C, Vogelstein B (2015). Cancer etiology. Variation in cancer risk among tissues can be explained by the number of stem cell divisions. Science. 347:78–81. PMID:25554788

2793. Tömböl Z, Szabó PM, Molnár V, et al. (2009). Integrative molecular bioinformatics study of human adrenocortical tumors: microRNA, tissue-specific target prediction, and pathway analysis. Endocr Relat Cancer. 16:895–906. PMID:19546168

2794. Tomoda C, Miyauchi A, Uruno T, et al. (2004). Cribriform-morular variant of papillary thyroid carcinoma: clue to early detection of familial adenomatous polyposis-associated colon cancer. World J Surg. 28:886–9. PMID:15593462

2795. Tomsic J, Fultz R, Liyanarachchi S, et al. (2016). HABP2 G534E Variant in Papillary Thyroid Carcinoma. PLoS One. 11:e0146315. PMID:26745718

2796. Tomsic J, He H, Akagi K, et al. (2015). A germline mutation in SRRM2, a splicing factor gene, is implicated in papillary thyroid carcinoma predisposition. Sci Rep. 5:10566. PMID:26135620

2797. Tomsic J, He H, de la Chapelle A (2015). HABP2 Mutation and Nonmedullary Thyroid Cancer. N Engl J Med. 373:2086. PMID:26581005

2798. Tonelli F, Giudici F, Giusti F, et al. (2014). A heterozygous frameshift mutation in exon 1 of CDKN1B gene in a patient affected by MEN4 syndrome. Eur J Endocrinol. 171:K7–17. PMID:24819502

2799. Tonner D, Belding P, Moore SA, et al. (1992). Intracranial dissemination of an ACTH secreting pituitary neoplasm–a case report and review of the literature. J Endocrinol Invest. 15:387–91. PMID:1324266

2800. Tornóczky T, Kálmán E, Kajtár PG, et al. (2004). Large cell neuroblastoma: a distinct phenotype of neuroblastoma with aggressive clinical behavior. Cancer. 100:390–7. PMID:14716776

2801. Torpy DJ (2015). Screening for ACTH-dependent hypercortisolism in patients with pituitary incidentaloma. Eur J Endocrinol. 172:C1–4. PMID:25609777

2802. Torregrossa L, Faviana P, Camacci T, et al. (2007). Galectin-3 is highly expressed in nonencapsulated papillary thyroid carcinoma but weakly expressed in encapsulated type; comparison with Hector Battifora mesothelial cell 1 immunoreactivity. Hum Pathol. 38:1482–8. PMID:17597183

2803. Tortorelli AP, Rosa F, Papa V, et al. (2007). Retroperitoneal schwannomas: diagnostic and therapeutic implications. Tumori. 93:312–5. PMID:17679473

2804. Tóth K, Péter I, Kremmer T, et al. (1990). Lipid-rich cell thyroid adenoma: histopathology with comparative lipid analysis. Virchows Arch A Pathol Anat Histopathol. 417:273–6. PMID:2117316

2805. Tötsch M, Dobler G, Feichtinger H, et al. (1990). Malignant hemangioendothelioma of the thyroid. Its immunohistochemical discrimination from undifferentiated thyroid carcinoma. Am J Surg Pathol. 14:69–74. PMID:2294782

2806. Towfighi J, Salam MM, McLendon RE, et al. (1996). Ganglion cell-containing tumors of the pituitary gland. Arch Pathol Lab Med. 120:369–77. PMID:8619749

2807. Toyoda H, Hirayama J, Sugimoto Y, et al. (2014). Polycythemia and paraganglioma with a novel somatic HIF2A mutation in a male. Pediatrics. 133:e1787–91. PMID:24819565

2807A. Tremblay G, Pearse AG. (1960) Histochemistry of oxidative enzyme systems in the human thyroid, with special reference to Askanazy cells. J PatholBacteriol. 80:353-8. PMID 13777969

2808. Trivellin G, Daly AF, Faucz FR, et al. (2014). Gigantism and acromegaly due to Xq26 microduplications and GPR101 mutation. N Engl J Med. 371:2363–74. PMID:25470569

2809. Tronko MD, Bogdanova TI, Komissarenko IV, et al. (1999). Thyroid carcinoma in children and adolescents in Ukraine after the Chernobyl nuclear accident: statistical data and clinicomorphologic characteristics. Cancer. 86:149–56. PMID:10391575

2810. Trost BN, Koenig MP, Zimmermann A, et al. (1981). Virilization of a post-menopausal woman by a testosterone-secreting Leydig cell type adrenal adenoma. Acta Endocrinol (Copenh). 98:274–82. PMID:6270941

2811. Trouillas J, Delgrange E, Jouanneau E, et al. (2000). Prolactinoma in man: clinical and histological characteristics. Ann Endocrinol (Paris). 61:253–7. [French] PMID:10970951

2812. Trouillas J, Guigard MP, Fonlupt P, et al. (1996). Mapping of corticotropic cells in the normal human pituitary. J Histochem Cytochem. 44:473–9. PMID:8627004

2813. Trouillas J, Labat-Moleur F, Sturm N, et al. (2008). Pituitary tumors and hyperplasia in multiple endocrine neoplasia type 1 syndrome (MEN1): a case-control study in a series of 77 patients versus 2509 non-MEN1 patients. Am J Surg Pathol. 32:534–43. PMID:18300794

2814. Trouillas J, Roy P, Sturm N, et al. (2013). A new prognostic clinicopathological classification of pituitary adenomas: a multicentric case-control study of 410 patients with 8 years post-operative follow-up. Acta Neuropathol. 126:123–35. PMID:23400299

2815. Troussier B, Gaudin P, Zagala A, et al. (1989). Pulmonary rheumatoid nodules indicative of rheumatoid polyarthritis. Rev Rhum Mal Osteoartic. 56:399–402. [French] PMID:2658003

2816. Trovisco V, Vieira de Castro I, Soares P, et al. (2004). BRAF mutations are associated with some histological types of papillary thyroid carcinoma. J Pathol. 202:247–51. PMID:14743508

2817. Trülzsch B, Krohn K, Wonerow P, et al. (2001). Detection of thyroid-stimulating

hormone receptor and Gsalpha mutations: in 75 toxic thyroid nodules by denaturing gradient gel electrophoresis. J Mol Med (Berl). 78:684–91. PMID:11434721
2818. Trump D, Farren B, Wooding C, et al. (1996). Clinical studies of multiple endocrine neoplasia type 1 (MEN1). QJM. 89:653–69. PMID:8917740
2819. Truran PP, Johnson SJ, Bliss RD, et al. (2014). Parafibromin, galectin-3, PGP9.5, Ki67, and cyclin D1: using an immunohistochemical panel to aid in the diagnosis of parathyroid cancer. World J Surg. 38:2845–54. PMID:25002250
2820. Truta B, Allen BA, Conrad PG, et al. (2003). Genotype and phenotype of patients with both familial adenomatous polyposis and thyroid carcinoma. Fam Cancer. 2:95–9. PMID:14574158
2821. Tsang K, Duggan MA (1992). Vascular proliferation of the thyroid. A complication of fine-needle aspiration. Arch Pathol Lab Med. 116:1040–2. PMID:1417444
2822. Tsang RW, Brierley JD, Asa SL, et al. (2003). Malignant teratoma of the thyroid: aggressive chemoradiation therapy is required after surgery. Thyroid. 13:401–4. PMID:12804109
2823. Tsang WY, Lau MF, Chan JK (1994). Incidental Langerhans' cell histiocytosis of the thyroid. Histopathology. 24:397–9. PMID:8045533
2824. Tscholl-Ducommun J, Hedinger CE (1982). Papillary thyroid carcinomas. Morphology and prognosis. Virchows Arch A Pathol Anat Histol. 396:19–39. PMID:7123844
2825. Tsushima Y, Ishizaka H, Matsumoto M (1993). Adrenal masses: differentiation with chemical shift, fast low-angle shot MR imaging. Radiology. 186:705–9. PMID:8430178
2826. Tsutsui H, Hoshi M, Kubota M, et al. (2013). Management of thyroid carcinoma showing thymus-like differentiation (CASTLE) invading the trachea. Surg Today. 43:1261–8. PMID:23543082
2827. Tsybrovskyy O, Rössmann-Tsybrovskyy M (2009). Oncocytic versus mitochondrion-rich follicular thyroid tumours: should we make a difference? Histopathology. 55:665–82. PMID:20002768
2828. Tufano RP, Teixeira GV, Bishop J, et al. (2012). BRAF mutation in papillary thyroid cancer and its value in tailoring initial treatment: a systematic review and meta-analysis. Medicine (Baltimore). 91:274–86. PMID:22932786
2829. Tulbah A, Al-Dayel F, Fawaz I, et al. (1999). Epstein-Barr virus-associated leiomyosarcoma of the thyroid in a child with congenital immunodeficiency: a case report. Am J Surg Pathol. 23:473–6. PMID:10199478
2830. Tunio GM, Hirota S, Nomura S, et al. (1998). Possible relation of osteopontin to development of psammoma bodies in human papillary thyroid cancer. Arch Pathol Lab Med. 122:1087–90. PMID:9870857
2831. Turkova H, Prodanov T, Maly M, et al. (2016). Characteristics and outcomes of metastatic SDHB and sporadic pheochromocytoma/paraganglioma: an National Institutes of Health study. Endocr Pract. 22:302–14. PMID:26523625
2832. Turner HE, Nagy Z, Esiri MM, et al. (2000). Role of matrix metalloproteinase 9 in pituitary tumor behavior. J Clin Endocrinol Metab. 85:2931–5. PMID:10946906
2833. Twigt BA, Scholten A, Valk GD, et al. (2013). Differences between sporadic and MEN related primary hyperparathyroidism; clinical expression, preoperative workup, operative strategy and follow-up. Orphanet J Rare Dis. 8:50. PMID:23547958
2834. Tziortzioti V, Ruebel KH, Kuroki T, et al. (2001). Analysis of beta-catenin mutations and alpha-, beta-, and gamma-catenin expression in normal and neoplastic human pituitary tissues. Endocr Pathol. 12:125–36. PMID:11579678
2835. Udupa S, Usha M, Visweswara RN, et al. (2012). Left-sided giant adrenal myelolipoma secreting catecholamine. Indian J Pathol Microbiol. 55:389–91. PMID:23032842
2836. Uemura S, Yasuda I, Kato T, et al. (2013). Preoperative routine evaluation of bilateral adrenal glands by endoscopic ultrasound and fine-needle aspiration in patients with potentially resectable lung cancer. Endoscopy. 45:195–201. PMID:23299524
2837. Ueno NT, Amato RJ, Ro JJ, et al. (1998). Primary malignant teratoma of the thyroid gland: report and discussion of two cases. Head Neck. 20:649–53. PMID:9744468
2838. Ullrich NJ, Raja AI, Irons MB, et al. (2007). Brainstem lesions in neurofibromatosis type 1. Neurosurgery. 61:762–6, discussion 766–7. PMID:17986937
2839. Umeoka K, Sanno N, Osamura RY, et al. (2002). Expression of GATA-2 in human pituitary adenomas. Mod Pathol. 15:11–7. PMID:11796836
2840. Uña Orejón R, Altit Millán E, Aguar Fernández M, et al. (2016). Catecholamine-secreting paraganglioma in a patient with Eisenmenger syndrome and a single ventricle. Nitric oxide administration and minimally invasive haemodynamic monitoring. Rev Esp Anestesiol Reanim. 63:172–6. [Spanish] PMID:26235172
2841. Unger P, Hoffman K, Pertsemlidis D, et al. (1991). S100 protein-positive sustentacular cells in malignant and locally aggressive adrenal pheochromocytomas. Arch Pathol Lab Med. 115:484–7. PMID:1673596
2842. Vaccarella S, Dal Maso L, Laversanne M, et al. (2015). The Impact of Diagnostic Changes on the Rise in Thyroid Cancer Incidence: A Population-Based Study in Selected High-Resource Countries. Thyroid. 25:1127–36. PMID:26133012
2843. Vaduganathan M, Nagarur A, Kerr DA, et al. (2015). Metastatic pancreatic neuroendocrine tumor with ectopic adrenocorticotropic hormone production. Proc (Bayl Univ Med Cent). 28:46–9. PMID:25552797
2844. Vajtai I, Beck J, Kappeler A, et al. (2011). Spindle cell oncocytoma of the pituitary gland with follicle-like component: organotypic differentiation to support its origin from folliculo-stellate cells. Acta Neuropathol. 122:253–8. PMID:21590491
2845. Välimäki N, Demir H, Pitkänen E, et al. (2015). Whole-Genome Sequencing of Growth Hormone (GH)-Secreting Pituitary Adenomas. J Clin Endocrinol Metab. 100:3918–27. PMID:26280510
2846. van der Zwan JM, Mallone S, van Dijk B, et al. (2012). Carcinoma of endocrine organs: results of the RARECARE project. Eur J Cancer. 48:1923–31. PMID:22361014
2847. van Eeden S, de Leng WW, Offerhaus GJ, et al. (2004). Ductuloinsular tumors of the pancreas: endocrine tumors with entrapped nonneoplastic ductules. Am J Surg Pathol. 28:813–20. PMID:15166675
2848. van Heerden JA, Hay ID, Goellner JR, et al. (1992). Follicular thyroid carcinoma with capsular invasion alone: a nonthreatening malignancy. Surgery. 112:1130–6, discussion 1136–8. PMID:1455315
2849. van Nederveen FH, Gaal J, Favier J, et al. (2009). An immunohistochemical procedure to detect patients with paraganglioma and phaeochromocytoma with germline SDHB, SDHC, or SDHD gene mutations: a retrospective and prospective analysis. Lancet Oncol. 10:764–71. PMID:19576851
2850. van Slooten H, Schaberg A, Smeenk D, et al. (1985). Morphologic characteristics of benign and malignant adrenocortical tumors. Cancer. 55:766–73. PMID:3967172
2851. van't Sant HP, Bouvy ND, Kazemier G, et al. (2007). The prognostic value of two different histopathological scoring systems for adrenocortical carcinomas. Histopathology. 51:239–45. PMID:17593212
2852. Vanharanta S, Buchta M, McWhinney SR, et al. (2004). Early-onset renal cell carcinoma as a novel extraparaganglial component of SDHB-associated heritable paraganglioma. Am J Hum Genet. 74:153–9. PMID:14685938
2853. Vanzati A, Mercalli F, Rosai J (2013). The "sprinkling" sign in the follicular variant of papillary thyroid carcinoma: a clue to the recognition of this entity. Arch Pathol Lab Med. 137:1707–9. PMID:24283853
2854. Vasef MA, Brynes RK, Sturm M, et al. (1999). Expression of cyclin D1 in parathyroid carcinomas, adenomas, and hyperplasias: a paraffin immunohistochemical study. Mod Pathol. 12:412–6. PMID:10229506
2855. Vasilev V, Daly AF, Thiry A, et al. (2014). McCune-Albright syndrome: a detailed pathological and genetic analysis of disease effects in an adult patient. J Clin Endocrinol Metab. 99:E2029–38. PMID:25062453
2856. Vasiloff J, Chideckel EW, Boyd CB, et al. (1985). Testosterone-secreting adrenal adenoma containing crystalloids characteristic of Leydig cells. Am J Med. 79:772–6. PMID:3000178
2857. Vaziri M, Molanaei S, Tamannaei Z (2014). Solitary fibrous tumor of the intrathoracic goiter. Med J Islam Repub Iran. 28:51. PMID:25405117
2858. Vázquez Ramírez F, Otal Salaverri C, Argueta Manzano O, et al. (2000). Fine needle aspiration cytology of high grade mucoepidermoid carcinoma of the thyroid. A case report. Acta Cytol. 44:259–64. PMID:10740618
2859. Vege DS, Chinoy RF, Ganesh B, et al. (1994). Malignant peripheral nerve sheath tumors of the head and neck: a clinicopathological study. J Surg Oncol. 55:100–3. PMID:8121181
2860. Veiga LH, Neta G, Aschebrook-Kilfoy B, et al. (2013). Thyroid cancer incidence patterns in Sao Paulo, Brazil, and the U.S. SEER program, 1997-2008. Thyroid. 23:748–57. PMID:23410185
2861. Velázquez-Fernández D, Laurell C, Geli J, et al. (2005). Expression profiling of adrenocortical neoplasms suggests a molecular signature of malignancy. Surgery. 138:1087–94. PMID:16360395
2862. Venkatesh S, Ordonez NG, Ajani J, et al. (1990). Islet cell carcinoma of the pancreas. A study of 98 patients. Cancer. 65:354–7. PMID:2153046
2863. Verdi D, Pennelli G, Pelizzo MR, et al. (2011). Solitary fibrous tumor of the thyroid gland: a report of two cases with an analysis of their clinical and pathological features. Endocr Pathol. 22:165–9. PMID:21818669
2864. Verga U, Fugazzola L, Cambiaghi S, et al. (2003). Frequent association between MEN 2A and cutaneous lichen amyloidosis. Clin Endocrinol (Oxf). 59:156–61. PMID:12864791
2865. Vergès B, Boureille F, Goudet P, et al. (2002). Pituitary disease in MEN type 1 (MEN1): data from the France-Belgium MEN1 multicenter study. J Clin Endocrinol Metab. 87:457–65. PMID:11836268
2866. Vergez S, Rouquette I, Ancey M, et al. (2010). Langerhans cell histiocytosis of the thyroid is a rare entity, but an association with a papillary thyroid carcinoma is often described. Endocr Pathol. 21:274–6. PMID:20848238
2867. Verhoef S, van Diemen-Steenvoorde R, Akkersdijk WL, et al. (1999). Malignant pancreatic tumour within the spectrum of tuberous sclerosis complex in childhood. Eur J Pediatr. 158:284–7. PMID:10206124
2868. Verloes A, Stevenaert A, Teh BT, et al. (1999). Familial acromegaly: case report and review of the literature. Pituitary. 1:273–7. PMID:11081208
2869. Veronese N, Luchini C, Nottegar A, et al. (2015). Prognostic impact of extra-nodal extension in thyroid cancer: A meta-analysis. J Surg Oncol. 112:828–33. PMID:26493240
2870. Verset L, Arvanitakis M, Loi P, et al. (2011). TTF-1 positive small cell cancers: Don't think they're always primary pulmonary! World J Gastrointest Oncol. 3:144–7. PMID:22046491
2871. Vestergaard P, Mollerup CL, Frøkjaer VG, et al. (2001). Cohort study of fracture risk before and after surgery of primary hyperparathyroidism. Ugeskr Laeger. 163:4875–8. [Danish] PMID:11571864
2872. Viale G, Doglioni C, Gambacorta M, et al. (1992). Progesterone receptor immunoreactivity in pancreatic endocrine tumors. An immunocytochemical study of 156 neuroendocrine tumors of the pancreas, gastrointestinal and respiratory tracts, and skin. Cancer. 70:2268–77. PMID:1356613
2873. Viciana MJ, Galera-Davidson H, Martín-Lacave I, et al. (1996). Papillary carcinoma of the thyroid with mucoepidermoid differentiation. Arch Pathol Lab Med. 120:397–8. PMID:8619755
2874. Vidal S, Kovacs K, Bell D, et al. (2003). Cyclooxygenase-2 expression in human pituitary tumors. Cancer. 97:2814–21. PMID:12767095
2875. Vidal S, Kovacs K, Horvath E, et al. (2002). Topoisomerase IIalpha expression in pituitary adenomas and carcinomas: relationship to tumor behavior. Mod Pathol. 15:1205–12. PMID:12429800
2876. Vidal S, Kovacs K, Horvath E, et al. (2001). Microvessel density in pituitary adenomas and carcinomas. Virchows Arch. 438:595–602. PMID:11469692
2877. Vigliar E, Varone V, Pettinato G, et al. (2015). How should a follicular adenoma with papillary architecture be classified on thyroid FNA? Case report with histological correlation. Cytopathology. 26:256–8. PMID:25073478
2878. Villa A, Cervasio M, Del Basso De Caro M, et al. (2014). A rare case of ACTH-LH plurihormonal pituitary adenoma: letter to the editor. Acta Neurochir (Wien). 156:1389–91. PMID:24549526
2879. Villa C, Lagonigro MS, Magri F, et al. (2011). Hyperplasia-adenoma sequence in pituitary tumorigenesis related to aryl hydrocarbon receptor interacting protein gene mutation. Endocr Relat Cancer. 18:347–56. PMID:21450940
2880. Villano JL, Virk IY, Ramirez V, et al. (2010). Descriptive epidemiology of central nervous system germ cell tumors: nonpineal analysis. Neuro Oncol. 12:257–64. PMID:20167813
2881. Villumsen AL, Mevik K, Fjøsne HE, et al. (2013). Late onset metastases to the thyroid gland from renal carcinoma. Tidsskr Nor Laegeforen. 133:2262–5. PMID:24226333
2882. Vinayek R, Capurso G, Larghi A (2014). Grading of EUS-FNA cytologic specimens from patients with pancreatic neuroendocrine neoplasms: it is time move to tissue core biopsy? Gland Surg. 3:222–5. PMID:25493252
2883. Visone R, Pallante P, Vecchione A, et al. (2007). Specific microRNAs are downregulated in human thyroid anaplastic carcinomas. Oncogene. 26:7590–5. PMID:17563749
2884. Vivero M, Kraft S, Barletta JA (2013). Risk stratification of follicular variant of papillary thyroid carcinoma. Thyroid. 23:273–9. PMID:23025507
2885. Vodovnik A (2002). Fine needle aspiration cytology of primary thyroid paraganglioma. Report of a case with cytologic, histologic and immunohistochemical features and differential diagnostic considerations. Acta Cytol. 46:1133–7. PMID:12462095
2886. Vogels RJ, Vlenterie M, Versleijen-Jonkers YM, et al. (2014). Solitary fibrous tumor - clinicopathologic, immunohistochemical and molecular analysis of 28 cases. Diagn Pathol. 9:224. PMID:25432794
2887. Vogelstein B, Kinzler KW (2015). The Path to Cancer –Three Strikes and You're Out. N Engl J Med. 373:1895–8. PMID:26559569
2888. Volante M, Birocco N, Gatti G, et al. (2014). Extrapulmonary neuroendocrine

small and large cell carcinomas: a review of controversial diagnostic and therapeutic issues. Hum Pathol. 45:665–73. PMID:23806528

2889. Volante M, Bollito E, Sperone P, et al. (2009). Clinicopathological study of a series of 92 adrenocortical carcinomas: from a proposal of simplified diagnostic algorithm to prognostic stratification. Histopathology. 55:535–43. PMID:19912359

2890. Volante M, Brizzi MP, Faggiano A, et al. (2007). Somatostatin receptor type 2A immunohistochemistry in neuroendocrine tumors: a proposal of scoring system correlated with somatostatin receptor scintigraphy. Mod Pathol. 20:1172–82. PMID:17873898

2891. Volante M, Collini P, Nikiforov YE, et al. (2007). Poorly differentiated thyroid carcinoma: the Turin proposal for the use of uniform diagnostic criteria and an algorithmic diagnostic approach. Am J Surg Pathol. 31:1256–64. PMID:17667551

2892. Volante M, La Rosa S, Castellano I, et al. (2006). Clinico-pathological features of a series of 11 oncocytic endocrine tumours of the pancreas. Virchows Arch. 448:545–51. PMID:16491376

2893. Volante M, Landolfi S, Chiusa L, et al. (2004). Poorly differentiated carcinomas of the thyroid with trabecular, insular, and solid patterns: a clinicopathologic study of 183 patients. Cancer. 100:950–7. PMID:14983490

2894. Volante M, Papotti M, Roth J, et al. (1999). Mixed medullary-follicular thyroid carcinoma. Molecular evidence for a dual origin of tumor components. Am J Pathol. 155:1499–509. PMID:10550306

2895. Volante M, Rapa I, Gandhi M, et al. (2009). RAS mutations are the predominant molecular alteration in poorly differentiated thyroid carcinomas and bear prognostic impact. J Clin Endocrinol Metab. 94:4735–41. PMID:19837916

2896. Volante M, Terzolo M, Fassnacht M, et al. (2012). Ribonucleotide reductase large subunit (RRM1) gene expression may predict efficacy of adjuvant mitotane in adrenocortical cancer. Clin Cancer Res. 18:3452–61. PMID:22547773

2897. Vollenweider I, Hedinger C, Saremaslani P, et al. (1989). Malignant haemangioendothelioma of the thyroid, immunohistochemical evidence of heterogeneity. Pathol Res Pract. 184:376–81. PMID:2471179

2898. Volpe C, Höög A, Ogishima T, et al. (2013). Immunohistochemistry improves histopathologic diagnosis in primary aldosteronism. J Clin Pathol. 66:351–4. PMID:23436930

2899. von Dobschuetz E, Leijon H, Schalin-Jäntti C, et al. (2015). A registry-based study of thyroid paraganglioma: histological and genetic characteristics. Endocr Relat Cancer. 22:191–204. PMID:25595276

2900. von Herbay A, Sieg B, Schürmann G, et al. (1991). Proliferative activity of neuroendocrine tumours of the gastroenteropancreatic endocrine system: DNA flow cytometric and immunohistological investigations. Gut. 32:949–53. PMID:1885079

2901. Vortmeyer AO, Falke EA, Gläsker S, et al. (2013). Nervous system involvement in von Hippel-Lindau disease: pathology and mechanisms. Acta Neuropathol. 125:333–50. PMID:23400300

2902. Vortmeyer AO, Gläsker S, Mehta GU, et al. (2012). Somatic GNAS mutation causes widespread and diffuse pituitary disease in acromegalic patients with McCune-Albright syndrome. J Clin Endocrinol Metab. 97:2404–13. PMID:22564667

2903. Vortmeyer AO, Gnarra JR, Emmert-Buck MR, et al. (1997). von Hippel-Lindau gene deletion detected in the stromal cell component of a cerebellar hemangioblastoma associated with von Hippel-Lindau disease. Hum Pathol. 28:540–3. PMID:9158701

2904. Vortmeyer AO, Lubensky IA, Skarulis M,

et al. (1999). Multiple endocrine neoplasia type 1: atypical presentation, clinical course, and genetic analysis of multiple tumors. Mod Pathol. 12:919–24. PMID:10496602

2905. Voutilainen PE, Multanen M, Haapiainen RK, et al. (1999). Anaplastic thyroid carcinoma survival. World J Surg. 23:975–8, discussion 978–9. PMID:10449831

2906. Vujanić GM, Harach HR, Minić P, et al. (1994). Thyroid/cervical teratomas in children: immunohistochemical studies for specific thyroid epithelial cell markers. Pediatr Pathol. 14:369–75. PMID:8008695

2907. Vujanić GM, Kelsey A, Perlman EJ, et al. (2007). Anaplastic sarcoma of the kidney: a clinicopathologic study of 20 cases of a new entity with polyphenotypic features. Am J Surg Pathol. 31:1459–68. PMID:17895746

2908. Vujhini SK, Kolte SS, Satarkar RN, et al. (2012). Fine needle aspiration diagnosis of Rosai-Dorfman Disease involving thyroid. J Cytol. 29:83–5. PMID:22438629

2909. Vujovic S, Henderson S, Presneau N, et al. (2006). Brachyury, a crucial regulator of notochordal development, is a novel biomarker for chordomas. J Pathol. 209:157–65. PMID:16538613

2910. Vukasović A, Kuna SK, Ostović KT, et al. (2012). Diffuse sclerosing variant of thyroid carcinoma presenting as Hashimoto thyroiditis: a case report. Coll Antropol. 36 Suppl 2:219–21. PMID:23397791

2911. Vuong HG, Kondo T, Oishi N, et al. (2016). Genetic alterations of differentiated thyroid carcinoma in iodine-rich and iodine-deficient countries. Cancer Med. 5:1883–9. PMID:27264674

2912. Wachenfeld C, Beuschlein F, Zwermann O, et al. (2001). Discerning malignancy in adrenocortical tumors: are molecular markers useful? Eur J Endocrinol. 145:335–41. PMID:11517015

2913. Wada N, Duh QY, Miura D, et al. (2002). Chromosomal aberrations by comparative genomic hybridization in hürthle cell thyroid carcinomas are associated with tumor recurrence. J Clin Endocrinol Metab. 87:4595–601. PMID:12364440

2914. Wade AN, Baccon J, Grady MS, et al. (2011). Clinically silent somatotroph adenomas are common. Eur J Endocrinol. 165:39–44. PMID:21493729

2915. Wagner J, Portwine C, Rabin K, et al. (1994). High frequency of germline p53 mutations in childhood adrenocortical cancer. J Natl Cancer Inst. 86:1707–10. PMID:7966399

2916. Waguespack SG, Rich T, Grubbs E, et al. (2010). A current review of the etiology, diagnosis, and treatment of pediatric pheochromocytoma and paraganglioma. J Clin Endocrinol Metab. 95:2023–37. PMID:20215394

2917. Waguespack SG, Rich TA, Perrier ND, et al. (2011). Management of medullary thyroid carcinoma and MEN2 syndromes in childhood. Nat Rev Endocrinol. 7:596–607. PMID:21862994

2918. Waldmann J, Bartsch DK, Kann PH, et al. (2007). Adrenal involvement in multiple endocrine neoplasia type 1: results of 7 years prospective screening. Langenbecks Arch Surg. 392:437–43. PMID:17235589

2919. Wallace IR, Healy E, Cooke RS, et al. (2015). TSH-secreting pituitary adenoma: benefits of pre-operative octreotide. Endocrinol Diabetes Metab Case Rep. 2015:150007. PMID:26113979

2920. Walsh J, Griffin TP, Ryan CB, et al. (2015). A Case Report Demonstrating How the Clinical Presentation of the Diffuse Sclerosing Variant of Papillary Thyroid Carcinoma Can Mimic Benign Riedel's Thyroiditis. Case Rep Endocrinol. 2015:686085. PMID:26137328

2921. Walter T, Hervieu V, Adham M, et al. (2011). Primary neuroendocrine tumors of the main pancreatic duct: a rare entity. Virchows

Arch. 458:537–46. PMID:21431402

2922. Walter T, van Brakel B, Vercherat C, et al. (2015). O6-Methylguanine-DNA methyltransferase status in neuroendocrine tumours: prognostic relevance and association with response to alkylating agents. Br J Cancer. 112:523–31. PMID:25584486

2923. Walther MM, Herring J, Enquist E, et al. (1999). von Recklinghausen's disease and pheochromocytomas. J Urol. 162:1582–6. PMID:10524872

2924. Walther MM, Reiter R, Keiser HR, et al. (1999). Clinical and genetic characterization of pheochromocytoma in von Hippel-Lindau families: comparison with sporadic pheochromocytoma gives insight into natural history of pheochromocytoma. J Urol. 162(3 Pt 1):659–64. PMID:10458336

2925. Wan SK, Chan JK, Tang SK (1996). Paucicellular variant of anaplastic thyroid carcinoma. A mimic of Reidel's thyroiditis. Am J Clin Pathol. 105:388–93. PMID:8604680

2926. Wanebo JE, Lonser RR, Glenn GM, et al. (2003). The natural history of hemangioblastomas of the central nervous system in patients with von Hippel-Lindau disease. J Neurosurg. 98:82–94. PMID:12546356

2927. Wang C, Sun Y, Wu H, et al. (2014). Distinguishing adrenal cortical carcinomas and adenomas: a study of clinicopathological features and biomarkers. Histopathology. 64:567–76. PMID:24102952

2928. Wang EL, Qian ZR, Yamada S, et al. (2009). Clinicopathological characterization of TSH-producing adenomas: special reference to TSH-immunoreactive but clinically nonfunctioning adenomas. Endocr Pathol. 20:209–20. PMID:19774499

2929. Wang JG, Han J, Jiang T, et al. (2015). Cardiac paragangliomas. J Card Surg. 30:55–60. PMID:25331372

2930. Wang K, Diskin SJ, Zhang H, et al. (2011). Integrative genomics identifies LMO1 as a neuroblastoma oncogene. Nature. 469:216–20. PMID:21124317

2931. Wang L, Yamaguchi S, Burstein MD, et al. (2014). Novel somatic and germline mutations in intracranial germ cell tumours. Nature. 511:241–5. PMID:24896186

2932. Wang L, Yang M, Zhang Y, et al. (2015). Prognostic validation of the WHO 2010 grading system in pancreatic insulinoma patients. Neoplasma. 62:484–90. PMID:25866230

2933. Wang LL, Suganuma R, Ikegaki N, et al. (2013). Neuroblastoma of undifferentiated subtype, prognostic significance of prominent nucleolar formation, and MYC/MYCN protein expression: a report from the Children's Oncology Group. Cancer. 119:3718–26. PMID:23901000

2934. Wang LL, Teshiba R, Ikegaki N, et al. (2015). Augmented expression of MYC and/ or MYCN protein defines highly aggressive MYC-driven neuroblastoma: a Children's Oncology Group study. Br J Cancer. 113:57–63. PMID:26035700

2935. Wang N, Liu T, Sofiadis A, et al. (2014). TERT promoter mutation as an early genetic event activating telomerase in follicular thyroid adenoma (FTA) and atypical FTA. Cancer. 120:2965–79. PMID:24898513

2936. Wang O, Wang C, Nie M, et al. (2012). Novel HRPT2/CDC73 gene mutations and loss of expression of parafibromin in Chinese patients with clinically sporadic parathyroid carcinomas. PLoS One. 7:e45567. PMID:23029104

2937. Wang S, Lloyd RV, Hutzler MJ, et al. (2000). The role of cell cycle regulatory protein, cyclin D1, in the progression of thyroid cancer. Mod Pathol. 13:882–7. PMID:10955455

2938. Wang SA, Rahemtullah A, Faquin WC, et al. (2005). Hodgkin's lymphoma of the thyroid: a clinicopathologic study of five cases and review of the literature. Mod Pathol. 18:1577–84. PMID:16258502

2939. Wang TT, Zhang R, Wang L, et al. (2014). Two cases of multiple ossifying fibromas in the jaws. Diagn Pathol. 9:75. PMID:24678936

2940. Wang W, Li Y, Liang Y, et al. (2015). Primary mucinous carcinoma of thyroid gland: report of a case. Zhonghua Bing Li Xue Za Zhi. 44:289–90. [Chinese] PMID:25975920

2941. Wang W, Wang H, Teng X, et al. (2010). Clonal analysis of bilateral, recurrent, and metastatic papillary thyroid carcinomas. Hum Pathol. 41:1299–309. PMID:20471663

2942. Wang Y, Chen J, Yang W, et al. (2015). The oncogenic roles of DICER1 RNase IIIb domain mutations in ovarian Sertoli-Leydig cell tumors. Neoplasia. 17:650–60. PMID:26408257

2943. Wang Y, Hou P, Yu H, et al. (2007). High prevalence and mutual exclusivity of genetic alterations in the phosphatidylinositol-3-kinase/akt pathway in thyroid tumors. J Clin Endocrinol Metab. 92:2387–90. PMID:17426084

2944. Wang Y, Tao R, Liu B (2013). Response to: Extraventricular neurocytoma of the sellar region. Br J Neurosurg. 27:551–2. PMID:23659217

2945. Wang YF, Liu B, Fan XS, et al. (2015). Thyroid carcinoma showing thymus-like elements: a clinicopathologic, immunohistochemical, ultrastructural, and molecular analysis. Am J Clin Pathol. 143:223–33. PMID:25596248

2946. Wang YY, Kearney T, du Plessis D, et al. (2012). Extraventricular neurocytoma of the sellar region. Br J Neurosurg. 26:420–2. PMID:22122710

2947. Ward LS, Brenta G, Medvedovic M, et al. (1998). Studies of allelic loss in thyroid tumors reveal major differences in chromosomal instability between papillary and follicular carcinomas. J Clin Endocrinol Metab. 83:525–30. PMID:9467569

2948. Ward R (1960). Carcinoma of the thyroid gland: a clinical and pathologic study of 293 patients at the University of California Hospital. Calif Med. 93:261.

2949. Warnakulasuriya S, Markwell BD, Williams DM (1985). Familial hyperparathyroidism associated with cementifying fibromas of the jaws in two siblings. Oral Surg Oral Med Oral Pathol. 59:269–74. PMID:3856818

2950. Warner E, Ofo E, Connor S, et al. (2015). Mucoepidermoid carcinoma in a thyroglossal duct remnant. Int J Surg Case Rep. 13:43–7. PMID:26101054

2951. Wasniewska M, Matarazzo P, Weber G, et al. (2006). Clinical presentation of McCune-Albright syndrome in males. J Pediatr Endocrinol Metab. 19 Suppl 2:619–22. PMID:16789625

2952. Wasserman JD, Novokmet A, Eichler-Jonsson C, et al. (2015). Prevalence and functional consequence of TP53 mutations in pediatric adrenocortical carcinoma: a children's oncology group study. J Clin Oncol. 33:602–9. PMID:25584008

2953. Wassif WS, Moniz CF, Friedman E, et al. (1993). Familial isolated hyperparathyroidism: a distinct genetic entity with an increased risk of parathyroid cancer. J Clin Endocrinol Metab. 77:1485–9. PMID:7903311

2954. Watanabe N, Noh JY, Narimatsu H, et al. (2011). Clinicopathological features of 171 cases of primary thyroid lymphoma: a long-term study involving 24553 patients with Hashimoto's disease. Br J Haematol. 153:236–43. PMID:21371004

2955. Watson KJ, Shulkes A, Smallwood RA, et al. (1985). Watery diarrhea-hypokalemia-achlorhydria syndrome and carcinoma of the esophagus. Gastroenterology. 88:798–803. PMID:2981755

2956. Weber DC, Rutz HP, Pedroni ES, et al. (2005). Results of spot-scanning proton radiation therapy for chordoma and chondrosarcoma of the skull base: the Paul Scherrer Institut experience. Int J Radiat Oncol Biol Phys. 63:401–9. PMID:16168833

2957. Webster AR, Maher ER, Moore AT (1999). Clinical characteristics of ocular angiomatosis in von Hippel-Lindau disease and correlation with germline mutation. Arch Ophthalmol. 117:371–8. PMID:10088816
2958. Wei S, Baloch ZW, LiVolsi VA (2015). Pathology of Struma Ovarii: A Report of 96 Cases. Endocr Pathol. 26:342–8. PMID:26374222
2959. Wei S, LiVolsi VA, Montone KT, et al. (2015). PTEN and TP53 Mutations in Oncocytic Follicular Carcinoma. Endocr Pathol. 26:365–9. PMID:26530486
2960. Wei Z, Zhou C, Liu M, et al. (2015). MicroRNA involvement in a metastatic non-functioning pituitary carcinoma. Pituitary. 18:710–21. PMID:25862551
2961. Weiler HT, Awiszus F (2000). Differences between motion-direction perception and unspecific motion perception in the human knee joint. Exp Brain Res. 132:523–30. PMID:10912833
2962. Weinhäusel A, Behmel A, Ponder BA, et al. (2003). Long-term follow up of a "sporadic" unilateral pheochromocytoma revealing multiple endocrine neoplasia MEN2A-2 in an elderly woman. Endocr Pathol. 14:375–82. PMID:14739494
2963. Weinstein JL, Katzenstein HM, Cohn SL (2003). Advances in the diagnosis and treatment of neuroblastoma. Oncologist. 8:278–92. PMID:12773750
2964. Weinstein LS, Shenker A, Gejman PV, et al. (1991). Activating mutations of the stimulatory G protein in the McCune-Albright syndrome. N Engl J Med. 325:1688–95. PMID:1944469
2965. Weisbrod AB, Zhang L, Jain M, et al. (2013). Altered PTEN, ATRX, CHGA, CHGB, and TP53 expression are associated with aggressive VHL-associated pancreatic neuroendocrine tumors. Horm Cancer. 4:165–75. PMID:23361940
2966. Weiss LM (1984). Comparative histologic study of 43 metastasizing and nonmetastasizing adrenocortical tumors. Am J Surg Pathol. 8:163–9. PMID:6703192
2967. Weiss LM, Medeiros LJ, Vickery AL Jr (1989). Pathologic features of prognostic significance in adrenocortical carcinoma. Am J Surg Pathol. 13:202–6. PMID:2919718
2968. Weiss LM, Weinberg DS, Warhol MJ (1983). Medullary carcinoma arising in a thyroid with Hashimoto's disease. Am J Clin Pathol. 80:534–8. PMID:6688701
2969. Weissferdt A, Kalhor N, Liu H, et al. (2014). Thymic neuroendocrine tumors (paraganglioma and carcinoid tumors): a comparative immunohistochemical study of 46 cases. Hum Pathol. 45:2463–70. PMID:25294372
2970. Weissferdt A, Moran CA (2016). Ectopic primary intrathyroidal thymoma: a clinicopathological and immunohistochemical analysis of 3 cases. Hum Pathol. 49:71–6. PMID:26826412
2971. Weissferdt A, Phan A, Suster S, et al. (2013). Myxoid adrenocortical carcinoma: a clinicopathologic and immunohistochemical study of 7 cases, including 1 case with lipomatous metaplasia. Am J Clin Pathol. 139:780–6. PMID:23690121
2972. Weissferdt A, Phan A, Suster S, et al. (2014). Adrenocortical carcinoma: a comprehensive immunohistochemical study of 40 cases. Appl Immunohistochem Mol Morphol. 22:24–30. PMID:23531850
2973. Weitzner S (1964). Benign teratoma of the neck in an infant. Am J Dis Child. 107:84–5. PMID:14067461
2974. Welander J, Andreasson A, Brauckhoff M, et al. (2014). Frequent EPAS1/HIF2α exons 9 and 12 mutations in non-familial pheochromocytoma. Endocr Relat Cancer. 21:495–504. PMID:24741025
2975. Welander J, Söderkvist P, Gimm O (2013). The NF1 gene: a frequent mutational target in sporadic pheochromocytomas and beyond. Endocr Relat Cancer. 20:C13–7. PMID:23756430
2976. Wells SA Jr, Asa SL, Dralle H, et al. (2015). Revised American Thyroid Association guidelines for the management of medullary thyroid carcinoma. Thyroid. 25:567–610. PMID:25810047
2977. Wells SA Jr, Pacini F, Robinson BG, et al. (2013). Multiple endocrine neoplasia type 2 and familial medullary thyroid carcinoma: an update. J Clin Endocrinol Metab. 98:3149–64. PMID:23744408
2978. Wells SA Jr, Robinson BG, Gagel RF, et al. (2012). Vandetanib in patients with locally advanced or metastatic medullary thyroid cancer: a randomized, double-blind phase III trial. J Clin Oncol. 30:134–41. PMID:22025146
2979. Wen J, Li HZ, Ji ZG, et al. (2010). A decade of clinical experience with extra-adrenal paragangliomas of retroperitoneum: Report of 67 cases and a literature review. Urol Ann. 2:12–6. PMID:20842251
2980. Wenig BM, Adair CF, Heffess CS (1995). Primary mucoepidermoid carcinoma of the thyroid gland: a report of six cases and a review of the literature of a follicular epithelial-derived tumor. Hum Pathol. 26:1099–108. PMID:7557943
2981. Wenig BM, Thompson LD, Adair CF, et al. (1998). Thyroid papillary carcinoma of columnar cell type: a clinicopathologic study of 16 cases. Cancer. 82:740–53. PMID:9477108
2982. Wermers RA, Fatourechi V, Wynne AG, et al. (1996). The glucagonoma syndrome. Clinical and pathologic features in 21 patients. Medicine (Baltimore). 75:53–63. PMID:8606627
2983. Whalen RK, Althausen AF, Daniels GH (1992). Extra-adrenal pheochromocytoma. J Urol. 147:1–10. PMID:1729490
2984. Widder S, Guggisberg K, Khalil M, et al. (2008). A pathologic re-review of follicular thyroid neoplasms: the impact of changing the threshold for the diagnosis of the follicular variant of papillary thyroid carcinoma. Surgery. 144:80–5. PMID:18571588
2985. Wieneke JA, Thompson LD, Heffess CS (2003). Adrenal cortical neoplasms in the pediatric population: a clinicopathologic and immunophenotypic analysis of 83 patients. Am J Surg Pathol. 27:867–81. PMID:12826878
2986. Wierinckx A, Roche M, Raverot G, et al. (2011). Integrated genomic profiling identifies loss of chromosome 11p impacting transcriptomic activity in aggressive pituitary PRL tumors. Brain Pathol. 21:533–43. PMID:21251114
2987. Wild A, Langer P, Celik I, et al. (2002). Chromosome 22q in pancreatic endocrine tumors: identification of a homozygous deletion and potential prognostic associations of allelic deletions. Eur J Endocrinol. 147:507–13. PMID:12370114
2988. Will OC, Hansmann A, Phillips RK, et al. (2009). Adrenal incidentaloma in familial adenomatous polyposis: a long-term follow-up study and schema for management. Dis Colon Rectum. 52:1637–44. PMID:19690494
2989. Williams ED (2000). Guest Editorial: Two Proposals Regarding the Terminology of Thyroid Tumors. Int J Surg Pathol. 8:181–3. PMID:11493987
2990. Williams ED, Brown CL, Doniach I (1966). Pathological and clinical findings in a series of 67 cases of medullary carcinoma of the thyroid. J Clin Pathol. 19:103–13. PMID:5909693
2991. Williams ED, Morales AM, Horn RC (1968). Thyroid carcinoma and Cushing's syndrome. A report of two cases with a review of the common features of the "non-endocrine" tumours associated with Cushing's syndrome. J Clin Pathol. 21:129–35. PMID:4301476
2992. Williams VC, Lucas J, Babcock MA, et al. (2009). Neurofibromatosis type 1 revisited. Pediatrics. 123:124–33. PMID:19117870
2993. Wilson DF (1982). Pituitary carcinoma occurring as middle ear tumor. Otolaryngol Head Neck Surg. 90:665–6. PMID:6819532
2994. Winters SJ, Vitaz T, Nowacki MR, et al. (2015). Addison's Disease and Pituitary Enlargement. Am J Med Sci. 349:526–9. PMID:25004119
2995. Wiseman SM, Griffith OL, Deen S, et al. (2007). Identification of molecular markers altered during transformation of differentiated into anaplastic thyroid carcinoma. Arch Surg. 142:717–27, discussion 727–9. PMID:17709725
2996. Wiseman SM, Masoudi H, Niblock P, et al. (2007). Anaplastic thyroid carcinoma: expression profile of targets for therapy offers new insights for disease treatment. Ann Surg Oncol. 14:719–29. PMID:17115102
2997. Wiseman SM, Masoudi H, Niblock P, et al. (2006). Derangement of the E-cadherin/catenin complex is involved in transformation of differentiated to anaplastic thyroid carcinoma. Am J Surg. 191:581–7. PMID:16647341
2998. Witteveen JE, Hamdy NA, Dekkers OM, et al. (2011). Downregulation of CASR expression and global loss of parafibromin staining are strong negative determinants of prognosis in parathyroid carcinoma. Mod Pathol. 24:688–97. PMID:21240254
2999. Woenckhaus C, Cameselle-Teijeiro J, Ruiz-Ponte C, et al. (2004). Spindle cell variant of papillary thyroid carcinoma. Histopathology. 45:424–7. PMID:15469488
3000. Wohllk N, Schweizer H, Erlic Z, et al. (2010). Multiple endocrine neoplasia type 2. Best Pract Res Clin Endocrinol Metab. 24:371–87. PMID:20833330
3001. Wojcik EM (1997). Fine needle aspiration of metastatic malignant schwannoma to the thyroid gland. Diagn Cytopathol. 16:94–5. PMID:9034747
3002. Wong DD, Spagnolo DV, Bisceglia M, et al. (2011). Oncocytic adrenocortical neoplasms–a clinicopathologic study of 13 new cases emphasizing the importance of their recognition. Hum Pathol. 42:489–99. PMID:21237489
3003. Wong RL, Kazaure HS, Roman SA, et al. (2012). Simultaneous medullary and differentiated thyroid cancer: a population-level analysis of an increasingly common entity. Ann Surg Oncol. 19:2635–42. PMID:22526904
3004. Woo Young K, Young Ran K, Sang Uk W, et al. (2011). Pulmonary leiomyosarcoma metastatic to the thyroid gland: case report and review of the literature. Ann Endocrinol (Paris). 72:314–6. PMID:21784409
3005. Woo S, Cho JY, Kim SY, et al. (2014). Adrenal adenoma and metastasis from clear cell renal cell carcinoma: can they be differentiated using standard MR techniques? Acta Radiol. 55:1120–8. PMID:24252816
3006. Woo YS, Isidori AM, Wat WZ, et al. (2005). Clinical and biochemical characteristics of adrenocorticotropin-secreting macroadenomas. J Clin Endocrinol Metab. 90:4963–9. PMID:15886242
3007. Wood LD, Klimstra DS (2014). Pathology and genetics of pancreatic neoplasms with acinar differentiation. Semin Diagn Pathol. 31:491–7. PMID:25441307
3008. Wooten MD, King DK (1993). Adrenal cortical carcinoma. Epidemiology and treatment with mitotane and a review of the literature. Cancer. 72:3145–55. PMID:8242539
3009. Wray CJ, Rich TA, Waguespack SG, et al. (2008). Failure to recognize multiple endocrine neoplasia 2B: more common than we think? Ann Surg Oncol. 15:293–301. PMID:17963006
3010. Wreesmann VB, Sieczka EM, Socci ND, et al. (2004). Genome-wide profiling of papillary thyroid cancer identifies MUC1 as an independent prognostic marker. Cancer Res. 64:3780–9. PMID:15172984
3011. Wu AW, Bhuta S, Salamon N, et al. (2015). Chondroid chordoma of the sella turcica mimicking a pituitary adenoma. Ear Nose Throat J. 94:E47–9. PMID:26535833
3012. Wu D, Tischler AS, Lloyd RV, et al. (2009). Observer variation in the application of the Pheochromocytoma of the Adrenal Gland Scaled Score. Am J Surg Pathol. 33:599–608. PMID:19145205
3013. Wu G, Mambo E, Guo Z, et al. (2005). Uncommon mutation, but common amplifications, of the PIK3CA gene in thyroid tumors. J Clin Endocrinol Metab. 90:4688–93. PMID:15928251
3014. Wu MK, Sabbaghian N, Xu B, et al. (2013). Biallelic DICER1 mutations occur in Wilms tumours. J Pathol. 230:154–64. PMID:23620094
3015. Wu Q, Fu WM, Liu WG, et al. (2002). Clinical and pathological features of male pituitary prolactinoma. Zhejiang Da Xue Xue Bao Yi Xue Ban. 31:299–301. [Chinese] PMID:12601916
3016. Wu Q, Zhou P, Zhong C, et al. (2012). Sellar solitary fibrous tumor mimicking pituitary adenoma. Neurol India. 60:678–9. PMID:23287352
3017. Wu S, DeMay RM, Papas P, et al. (2012). Follicular lesions of the thyroid: a retrospective study of 1,348 fine needle aspiration biopsies. Diagn Cytopathol. 40 Suppl 1:E8–12. PMID:20954270
3018. Xekouki P, Azevedo M, Stratakis CA (2010). Anterior pituitary adenomas: inherited syndromes, novel genes and molecular pathways. Expert Rev Endocrinol Metab. 5:697–709. PMID:21264206
3019. Xekouki P, Pacak K, Almeida M, et al. (2012). Succinate dehydrogenase (SDH) D subunit (SDHD) inactivation in a growth-hormone-producing pituitary tumor: a new association for SDH? J Clin Endocrinol Metab. 97:E357–66. PMID:22170724
3020. Xekouki P, Szarek E, Bullova P, et al. (2015). Pituitary adenoma with paraganglioma/pheochromocytoma (3PAs) and succinate dehydrogenase defects in humans and mice. J Clin Endocrinol Metab. 100:E710–9. PMID:25695889
3021. Xia CX, Li R, Wang ZH, et al. (2012). A rare cause of goiter: Langerhans cell histiocytosis of the thyroid. Endocr J. 59:47–54. PMID:22019948
3022. Xiao C, Xu B, Ye H, et al. (2011). Experience with adrenal schwannoma in a Chinese population of six patients. J Endocrinol Invest. 34:417–21. PMID:20543556
3023. Xing M (2010). Genetic alterations in the phosphatidylinositol-3 kinase/Akt pathway in thyroid cancer. Thyroid. 20:697–706. PMID:20578891
3024. Xing M (2013). Molecular pathogenesis and mechanisms of thyroid cancer. Nat Rev Cancer. 13:184–99. PMID:23429735
3025. Xing M, Alzahrani AS, Carson KA, et al. (2013). Association between BRAF V600E mutation and mortality in patients with papillary thyroid cancer. JAMA. 309:1493–501. PMID:23571588
3026. Xing M, Liu R, Liu X, et al. (2014). BRAF V600E and TERT promoter mutations cooperatively identify the most aggressive papillary thyroid cancer with highest recurrence. J Clin Oncol. 32:2718–26. PMID:25024077
3027. Xu B, Gao J, Cui L, et al. (2012). Characterization of adrenal metastatic cancer using FDG PET/CT. Neoplasma. 59:92–9. PMID:22103902
3028. Xu B, Hirokawa M, Yoshimoto K, et al. (2003). Spindle epithelial tumor with thymus-like differentiation of the thyroid: a case report with pathological and molecular genetics study. Hum Pathol. 34:190–3. PMID:12612889
3029. Xu B, Wang L, Tuttle RM, et al. (2015). Prognostic impact of extent of vascular invasion in low-grade encapsulated follicular cell-derived

thyroid carcinomas: a clinicopathologic study of 276 cases. Hum Pathol. 46:1789–98. PMID:26482605
3030. Xu Z, Ellis S, Lee CC, et al. (2014). Silent corticotroph adenomas after stereotactic radiosurgery: a case-control study. Int J Radiat Oncol Biol Phys. 90:903–10. PMID:25216855
3031. Yachida S, Vakiani E, White CM, et al. (2012). Small cell and large cell neuroendocrine carcinomas of the pancreas are genetically similar and distinct from well-differentiated pancreatic neuroendocrine tumors. Am J Surg Pathol. 36:173–84. PMID:22251937
3032. Yağci B, Kandemir N, Yazici N, et al. (2007). Thyroid involvement in Langerhans cell histiocytosis: a report of two cases and review of the literature. Eur J Pediatr. 166:901–4. PMID:17443347
3033. Yakirevich E, Ali SM, Mega A, et al. (2015). A Novel SDHA-deficient Renal Cell Carcinoma Revealed by Comprehensive Genomic Profiling. Am J Surg Pathol. 39:858–63. PMID:25724004
3034. Yakoushina TV, Lavi E, Hoda RS (2010). Pituitary carcinoma diagnosed on fine needle aspiration: Report of a case and review of pathogenesis. Cytojournal. 7:14. PMID:20806088
3035. Yalcin S, Sokmensuer C, Esin E (2015). Glucagonoma. In: Yalcin S, Öberg K, editors. Neuroendocrine tumours: diagnosis and management. Berlin, Heidelberg: Springer-Verlag; pp. 233–50.
3036. Yamada S, Aiba T, Sano T, et al. (1993). Growth hormone-producing pituitary adenomas: correlations between clinical characteristics and morphology. Neurosurgery. 33:20–7. PMID:7689191
3037. Yamada S, Asa SL, Kovacs K (1988). Oncocytomas and null cell adenomas of the human pituitary: morphometric and in vitro functional comparison. Virchows Arch A Pathol Anat Histopathol. 413:333–9. PMID:3140478
3038. Yamada S, Fukuhara N, Horiguchi K, et al. (2014). Clinicopathological characteristics and therapeutic outcomes in thyrotropin-secreting pituitary adenomas: a single-center study of 90 cases. J Neurosurg. 121:1462–73. PMID:25237847
3038A. Yamada S, Inoshita N, Fukuhara N, et al. (2015). Therapeutic outcomes in patients undergoing surgery after diagnosis of Cushing's disease: a single-center study. Endocr J. 62:1115–25. PMID:26477323
3039. Yamada S, Kovacs K, Horvath E, et al. (1991). Morphological study of clinically nonsecreting pituitary adenomas in patients under 40 years of age. J Neurosurg. 75:902–5. PMID:1941118
3040. Yamada S, Ohyama K, Taguchi M, et al. (2007). A study of the correlation between morphological findings and biological activities in clinically nonfunctioning pituitary adenomas. Neurosurgery. 61:580–4, discussion 584–5. PMID:17881972
3041. Yamada S, Sano T, Takahashi M, et al. (1995). Immunohistochemical Heterogeneity Within Clinically Nonfunctioning Pituitary Adenomas. Endocr Pathol. 6:217–21. PMID:12114742
3042. Yamagishi S, Yokoyama-Ohta M (1999). A rare case of pituitary hyperplasia with suprasellar extension due to primary myxoedema: case report. J Int Med Res. 27:49–52. PMID:10417962
3043. Yamaguchi-Okada M, Inoshita N, Nishioka H, et al. (2012). Clinicopathological analysis of nonfunctioning pituitary adenomas in patients younger than 25 years of age. J Neurosurg Pediatr. 9:511–6. PMID:22546029
3044. Yamamoto Y, Maeda T, Izumi K, et al. (1990). Occult papillary carcinoma of the thyroid. A study of 408 autopsy cases. Cancer. 65:1173–9. PMID:2302665
3045. Yamamoto Y, Yamada K, Motoi N, et al. (2013). Sonographic findings in three cases of carcinoma showing thymus-like differentiation. J Clin Ultrasound. 41:574–8. PMID:23055246
3046. Yaman E, Benekli M, Coskun U, et al. (2008). Intrasellar plasmacytoma: an unusual presentation of multiple myeloma. Acta Neurochir (Wien). 150:921–4, discussion 924. PMID:18726062
3047. Yamazaki M, Fujii S, Daiko H, et al. (2008). Carcinoma showing thymus-like differentiation (CASTLE) with neuroendocrine differentiation. Pathol Int. 58:775–9. PMID:19067852
3048. Yang C, Hong CS, Prchal JT, et al. (2015). Somatic mosaicism of EPAS1 mutations in the syndrome of paraganglioma and somatostatinoma associated with polycythemia. Hum Genome Var. 2:15053. PMID:27081557
3049. Yang C, Sun MG, Matro J, et al. (2013). Novel HIF2A mutations disrupt oxygen sensing, leading to polycythemia, paragangliomas, and somatostatinomas. Blood. 121:2563–6. PMID:23361906
3050. Yang C, Zhuang Z, Fliedner SM, et al. (2015). Germ-line PHD1 and PHD2 mutations detected in patients with pheochromocytoma/paraganglioma-polycythemia. J Mol Med (Berl). 93:93–104. PMID:25263965
3051. Yang GC, Scognamiglio T, Kuhel WI (2011). Fine-needle aspiration of mucin-producing thyroid tumors. Acta Cytol. 55:549–55. PMID:22156465
3052. Yang GF, Wu SY, Zhang LJ, et al. (2009). Imaging findings of extraventricular neurocytoma: report of 3 cases and review of the literature. AJNR Am J Neuroradiol. 30:581–5. PMID:18842767
3053. Yang I, Park S, Ryu M, et al. (1996). Characteristics of gsp-positive growth hormone-secreting pituitary tumors in Korean acromegalic patients. Eur J Endocrinol. 134:720–6. PMID:8766942
3054. Yang J, Zhao N, Zhang G, et al. (2013). Clinical features of patients with non-Hodgkin's lymphoma metastasizing to the pituitary glands. Oncol Lett. 5:1643–8. PMID:23760877
3055. Yang XR, Ng D, Alcorta DA, et al. (2009). T (brachyury) gene duplication confers major susceptibility to familial chordoma. Nat Genet. 41:1176–8. PMID:19801981
3056. Yang YJ, Han JW, Youn HD, et al. (2010). The tumor suppressor, parafibromin, mediates histone H3 K9 methylation for cyclin D1 repression. Nucleic Acids Res. 38:382–90. PMID:19906718
3057. Yang Z, Tang LH, Klimstra DS (2011). Effect of tumor heterogeneity on the assessment of Ki67 labeling index in well-differentiated neuroendocrine tumors metastatic to the liver: implications for prognostic stratification. Am J Surg Pathol. 35:853–60. PMID:21566513
3058. Yantiss RK, Chang HK, Farraye FA, et al. (2002). Prevalence and prognostic significance of acinar cell differentiation in pancreatic endocrine tumors. Am J Surg Pathol. 26:893–901. PMID:12131156
3059. Yao JC, Eisner MP, Leary C, et al. (2007). Population-based study of islet cell carcinoma. Ann Surg Oncol. 14:3492–500. PMID:17896148
3060. Yao JC, Phan AT, Chang DZ, et al. (2008). Efficacy of RAD001 (everolimus) and octreotide LAR in advanced low- to intermediate-grade neuroendocrine tumors: results of a phase II study. J Clin Oncol. 26:4311–8. PMID:18779618
3061. Yart A, Gstaiger M, Wirbelauer C, et al. (2005). The HRPT2 tumor suppressor gene product parafibromin associates with human PAF1 and RNA polymerase II. Mol Cell Biol. 25:5052–60. PMID:15923622
3062. Yeh IT, Lenci RE, Qin Y, et al. (2008). A germline mutation of the KIF1B beta gene on 1p36 in a family with neural and nonneural tumors. Hum Genet. 124:279–85. PMID:18726616
3063. Yeh MW, Ituarte PH, Zhou HC, et al. (2013). Incidence and prevalence of primary hyperparathyroidism in a racially mixed population. J Clin Endocrinol Metab. 98:1122–9. PMID:23418315
3064. Yeo MK, Bae JS, Lee S, et al. (2015). The Warthin-Like Variant of Papillary Thyroid Carcinoma: A Comparison with Classic Type in the Patients with Coexisting Hashimoto's Thyroiditis. Int J Endocrinol. 2015:456027. PMID:25983754
3065. Yin L, Teng J, Zhou Q, et al. (2014). A 10-year single-center experience with surgical management of adrenal myelolipoma. J Endourol. 28:252–5. PMID:24044410
3066. Yin W, Ma C, Wu J, et al. (2010). A primary atypical solitary fibrous tumor of the sella mimicking nonfunctional pituitary adenoma: a case report. Acta Neurochir (Wien). 152:519–22. PMID:19517059
3067. Yin Z, Pringle DR, Jones GN, et al. (2011). Differential role of PKA catalytic subunits in mediating phenotypes caused by knockout of the Carney complex gene Prkar1a. Mol Endocrinol. 25:1786–93. PMID:21852354
3068. Yip L, Kelly L, Shuai Y, et al. (2011). MicroRNA signature distinguishes the degree of aggressiveness of papillary thyroid carcinoma. Ann Surg Oncol. 18:2035–41. PMID:21537871
3069. Yohe SL, Chenault CB, Torlakovic EE, et al. (2014). Langerhans cell histiocytosis in acute leukemias of ambiguous or myeloid lineage in adult patients: support for a possible clonal relationship. Mod Pathol. 27:651–6. PMID:24186134
3070. Yoon V, Treat K, Maalouf NM (2013). Ectopic atypical parathyroid lipoadenoma: a rare cause of severe primary hyperparathyroidism. J Bone Miner Metab. 31:595–600. PMID:23263783
3071. Yoshida A, Sen C, Asa SL, et al. (2008). Composite pituitary adenoma and craniopharyngioma?: an unusual sellar neoplasm with divergent differentiation. Am J Surg Pathol. 32:1736–41. PMID:18769335
3072. Yoshida A, Sugino K, Sugitani I, et al. (2014). Anaplastic thyroid carcinomas incidentally found on postoperative pathological examination. World J Surg. 38:2311–6. PMID:24687351
3073. Yoshida M, Hiroi M, Imai T, et al. (2011). A case of ACTH-independent macronodular adrenal hyperplasia associated with multiple endocrine neoplasia type 1. Endocr J. 58:269–77. PMID:21415556
3074. Yoshii T, Inohara H, Takenaka Y, et al. (2001). Galectin-3 maintains the transformed phenotype of thyroid papillary carcinoma cells. Int J Oncol. 18:787–92. PMID:11251175
3075. Yoshimoto T, Takahashi-Fujigasaki J, Inoshita N, et al. (2015). TTF-1-positive oncocytic sellar tumor with follicle formation/ependymal differentiation: non-adenomatous tumor capable of two different interpretations as a pituicytoma or a spindle cell oncocytoma. Brain Tumor Pathol. 32:221–7. PMID:25893822
3076. Young M, Kattner K, Gupta K (1999). Pituitary hyperplasia resulting from primary hypothyroidism mimicking macroadenomas. Br J Neurosurg. 13:138–42. PMID:10616581
3077. Young WF Jr, Maddox DE (1995). Spells: in search of a cause. Mayo Clin Proc. 70:757–65. PMID:7630214
3078. Yu BH, Sheng WQ, Wang J (2013). Primary paraganglioma of thyroid gland: a clinicopathologic and immunohistochemical analysis of three cases with a review of the literature. Head Neck Pathol. 7:373–80. PMID:23943066
3079. Yu CE, Oshima J, Fu YH, et al. (1996). Positional cloning of the Werner's syndrome gene. Science. 272:258–62. PMID:8602509
3080. Yu L, Yang SJ (2011). Primary follicular dendritic cell sarcoma of the thyroid gland coexisting with Hashimoto's thyroiditis. Int J Surg Pathol. 19:502–5. PMID:19448067
3081. Yu R, Nissen NN, Dhall D, et al. (2008). Nesidioblastosis and hyperplasia of alpha cells, microglucagonoma, and nonfunctioning islet cell tumor of the pancreas: review of the literature. Pancreas. 36:428–31. PMID:18437091
3082. Yu W, McPherson JR, Stevenson M, et al. (2015). Whole-exome sequencing studies of parathyroid carcinomas reveal novel PRUNE2 mutations, distinctive mutational spectra related to APOBEC-catalyzed DNA mutagenesis and mutational enrichment in kinases associated with cell migration and invasion. J Clin Endocrinol Metab. 100:E360–4. PMID:25387265
3083. Yue C, Zhang Y, Xing L, et al. (2014). Clinicopathological factors in risk prediction of lymph node metastasis in papillary thyroid carcinoma. Zhonghua Yi Xue Za Zhi. 94:3637–41. [Chinese] PMID:25622954
3084. Zaatari GS, Saigo PE, Huvos AG (1983). Mucin production in medullary carcinoma of the thyroid. Arch Pathol Lab Med. 107:70–4. PMID:6687422
3085. Zaben M, Zafar M, Bukhari S, et al. (2014). Endoscopic transsphenoidal approach for resection of malignant pituitary blastoma in an 18-month-old infant: a technical note. Neurosurgery. 10 Suppl 4:649–53. PMID:24978649
3086. Zablotska LB, Nadyrov EA, Polyanskaya ON, et al. (2015). Risk of thyroid follicular adenoma among children and adolescents in Belarus exposed to iodine-131 after the Chornobyl accident. Am J Epidemiol. 182:781–90. PMID:26443421
3087. Zacharin M, Bajpai A, Chow CW, et al. (2011). Gastrointestinal polyps in McCune Albright syndrome. J Med Genet. 48:458–61. PMID:21357941
3088. Zada G, Woodmansee WW, Ramkissoon S, et al. (2011). Atypical pituitary adenomas: incidence, clinical characteristics, and implications. J Neurosurg. 114:336–44. PMID:20868211
3089. Zambrano E, Holm I, Glickman J, et al. (2004). Abnormal distribution and hyperplasia of thyroid C-cells in PTEN-associated tumor syndromes. Endocr Pathol. 15:55–64. PMID:15067177
3090. Zamecnik J, Chanova M, Kodet R (2004). Expression of thyroid transcription factor 1 in primary brain tumours. J Clin Pathol. 57:1111–3. PMID:15452173
3091. Zantour B, Guilhaume B, Tissier F, et al. (2004). A thyroid nodule revealing a paraganglioma in a patient with a new germline mutation in the succinate dehydrogenase B gene. Eur J Endocrinol. 151:433–8. PMID:15476441
3092. Zarco-González JA, Herrera MF (2004). Adrenal incidentaloma. Scand J Surg. 93:298–301. PMID:15658671
3093. Zattoni D, Balzarotti R, Rosso R (2015). The management of bilateral myelolipoma: Case report and review of the literature. Int J Surg Case Rep. 12:31–6. PMID:25989259
3094. Zbuk KM, Eng C (2007). Cancer phenomics: RET and PTEN as illustrative models. Nat Rev Cancer. 7:35–45. PMID:17167516
3095. Zbuk KM, Eng C (2007). Hamartomatous polyposis syndromes. Nat Clin Pract Gastroenterol Hepatol. 4:492–502. PMID:17768394
3096. Zee SY, Hochwald SN, Conlon KC, et al. (2005). Pleomorphic pancreatic endocrine neoplasms: a variant commonly confused with adenocarcinoma. Am J Surg Pathol. 29:1194–200. PMID:16096409
3097. Zelger BG, Zelger B (2004). Angiomatoid metastatic melanoma. Dermatol Surg. 30(2 Pt 2):336–40. PMID:14871230
3098. Zelinka T, Musil Z, Dušková J, et al. (2011). Metastatic pheochromocytoma: does the size and age matter? Eur J Clin Invest. 41:1121–8. PMID:21692797
3099. Zeltzer PM, Marangos PJ, Evans AE, et al. (1986). Serum neuron-specific enolase in children with neuroblastoma. Relationship to stage and disease course. Cancer. 57:1230–4. PMID:3002599

3100. Zhang H, Kolb FA, Jaskiewicz L, et al. (2004). Single processing center models for human Dicer and bacterial RNase III. Cell. 118:57–68. PMID:15242644

3101. Zhang L, Lohse CM, Dao LN, et al. (2011). Proposed histopathologic grading system derived from a study of KIT and CK19 expression in pancreatic endocrine neoplasm. Hum Pathol. 42:324–31. PMID:21190722

3102. Zhang L, Smyrk TC, Oliveira AM, et al. (2009). KIT is an independent prognostic marker for pancreatic endocrine tumors: a finding derived from analysis of islet cell differentiation markers. Am J Surg Pathol. 33:1562–9. PMID:19574886

3103. Zhang W, Policarpio-Nicolas ML (2015). Aspiration cytology of primary thyroid paraganglioma. Diagn Cytopathol. 43:838–43. PMID:26178689

3104. Zhang W, Zang Z, Song Y, et al. (2014). Co-expression network analysis of differentially expressed genes associated with metastasis in prolactin pituitary tumors. Mol Med Rep. 10:113–8. PMID:24736764

3105. Zhang Y, Nosé V (2011). Endocrine tumors as part of inherited tumor syndromes. Adv Anat Pathol. 18:206–18. PMID:21490438

3106. Zhao C, Vinh TN, McManus K, et al. (2009). Identification of the most sensitive and robust immunohistochemical markers in different categories of ovarian sex cord-stromal tumors. Am J Surg Pathol. 33:354–66. PMID:19033865

3107. Zhao J, Moch H, Scheidweiler AF, et al. (2001). Genomic imbalances in the progression of endocrine pancreatic tumors. Genes Chromosomes Cancer. 32:364–72. PMID:11746977

3108. Zhao J, Roth J, Bode-Lesniewska B, et al. (2002). Combined comparative genomic hybridization and genomic microarray for detection of gene amplifications in pulmonary artery intimal sarcomas and adrenocortical tumors. Genes Chromosomes Cancer. 34:48–57. PMID:11921282

3109. Zhao J, Sun F, Jing X, et al. (2014). The diagnosis and treatment of primary adrenal lipomatous tumours in Chinese patients: A 31-year follow-up study. Can Urol Assoc J. 8:E132–6. PMID:24678351

3110. Zhao L, Sun LH, Liu DM, et al. (2014). Copy number variation in CCND1 gene is implicated in the pathogenesis of sporadic parathyroid carcinoma. World J Surg. 38:1730–7. PMID:24510244

3111. Zhao M, Li C, Zheng J, et al. (2013). Cystic lymphangioma-like adenomatoid tumor of the adrenal gland: report of a rare case and review of the literature. Int J Clin Exp Pathol. 6:943–50. PMID:23638228

3112. Zhao Z, Shen GH, Liu B, et al. (2016). Unusual adrenal and brain metastases from follicular thyroid carcinoma revealed by 131I SPECT/CT. Clin Nucl Med. 41:e53–5. PMID:26018699

3113. Zheng S, Cherniack AD, Dewal N, et al. (2016). Comprehensive pan-genomic characterization of adrenocortical carcinoma. Cancer Cell. 29:723–36. PMID:27165744

3114. Zheng WL, Zhang GS, Tan CL, et al. (2010). Diabetes insipidus as main presentation of non-Hodgkin's lymphoma with hypophyseal involvement: two case reports. Leuk Res. 34:e32–4. PMID:19747732

3115. Zheng X, Wei S, Yu Y, et al. (2012). Genetic and clinical characteristics of head and neck paragangliomas in a Chinese population. Laryngoscope. 122:1761–6. PMID:22566157

3116. Zhong Q, Yuan S (2013). Total resection of a solitary fibrous tumor of the sellar diaphragm: A case report. Oncol Lett. 5:1783–6. PMID:23833641

3117. Zhou C, Dhall D, Nissen NN, et al. (2009). Homozygous P86S mutation of the human glucagon receptor is associated with hyperglucagonemia, alpha cell hyperplasia, and islet cell tumor. Pancreas. 38:941–6. PMID:19657311

3118. Zhou J, Zhang D, Wang G, et al. (2015). Primary adrenal microcystic/reticular schwannoma: clinicopathological and immunohistochemical studies of an extremely rare case. Int J Clin Exp Pathol. 8:5808–11. PMID:26191302

3119. Zhou M, Epstein JI, Young RH (2004). Paraganglioma of the urinary bladder: a lesion that may be misdiagnosed as urothelial carcinoma in transurethral resection specimens. Am J Surg Pathol. 28:94–100. PMID:14707870

3120. Zhou P, Ma L, Cheng S, et al. (2012). Combined gangliocytoma and non-functioning pituitary adenoma of the pituitary gland. Neurol India. 60:311–3. PMID:22824692

3121. Zhou XH (2002). Primary squamous cell carcinoma of the thyroid. Eur J Surg Oncol. 28:42–5. PMID:11869012

3122. Zhu D, Kumar A, Weintraub WS, et al. (2011). A large pheochromocytoma with invasion of multiple local organs. J Clin Hypertens (Greenwich). 13:60–4. PMID:21214723

3123. Zhu Z, Gandhi M, Nikiforova MN, et al. (2003). Molecular profile and clinical-pathologic features of the follicular variant of papillary thyroid carcinoma. An unusually high prevalence of ras mutations. Am J Clin Pathol. 120:71–7. PMID:12866375

3124. Zhuang Z, Vortmeyer AO, Pack S, et al. (1997). Somatic mutations of the MEN1 tumor suppressor gene in sporadic gastrinomas and insulinomas. Cancer Res. 57:4682–6. PMID:9354421

3125. Zidan J, Karen D, Stein M, et al. (2003). Pure versus follicular variant of papillary thyroid carcinoma: clinical features, prognostic factors, treatment, and survival. Cancer. 97:1181–5. PMID:12599223

3126. Zieliński G, Maksymowicz M, Podgórski J, et al. (2013). Double, synchronous pituitary adenomas causing acromegaly and Cushing's disease. A case report and review of literature. Endocr Pathol. 24:92–9. PMID:23512282

3127. Zygourakis CC, Rolston JD, Lee HS, et al. (2015). Pituicytomas and spindle cell oncocytomas: modern case series from the University of California, San Francisco. Pituitary. 18:150–8. PMID:24823438

Subject index

List of abbreviations

3D	three-dimensional
ACTH	adrenocorticotropic hormone
AIDS	acquired immunodeficiency syndrome
ATP	adenosine triphosphate
bp	base pair
CAIX	carbonic anhydrase IX
cAMP	cyclic adenosine monophosphate
CEA	carcinoembryonic antigen
CNS	central nervous system
CRH	corticotropin-releasing hormone
CT	computed tomography
DNA	deoxyribonucleic acid
EBV	Epstein–Barr virus
EGFR	epidermal growth factor receptor
EMA	epithelial membrane antigen
ER	estrogen receptor
FDG	18F-fluorodeoxyglucose
FISH	fluorescence in situ hybridization
FSH	follicle-stimulating hormone
GAPP	Grading System for Adrenal Phaeochromocytoma and Paraganglioma
GFAP	glial fibrillary acidic protein
GH	growth hormone
GHRH	growth hormone–releasing hormone
H&E	haematoxylin and eosin
HIF	hypoxia-inducible factor
ICD-O	International Classification of Diseases for Oncology
Ig	immunoglobulin
INPC	International Neuroblastoma Pathology Classification
INRG	International Neuroblastoma Risk Group
IU/L	international units per litre
kb	kilo base pair
LH	luteinizing hormone
MAPK	mitogen-activated protein kinase
Mb	megabase
MIM number	Mendelian Inheritance in Man number
MKI	mitosis-karyorrhexis index
MRI	magnetic resonance imaging
mRNA	messenger ribonucleic acid
N:C ratio	nuclear-to-cytoplasmic ratio
NFP	neurofilament protein
NOS	not otherwise specified
PAS	periodic acid–Schiff
PASS	Phaeochromocytoma of the Adrenal Gland Scaled Score
PET	positron emission tomography
PI3K	phosphoinositide 3-kinase
PKA	protein kinase A
PRL	prolactin
PTH	parathyroid hormone
RB	retinoblastoma
RNA	ribonucleic acid
SDH	succinate dehydrogenase
SEER	Surveillance, Epidemiology, and End Results
SNP	single nucleotide polymorphism
TNM	tumour, node, metastasis
TSH	thyroid-stimulating hormone
VEGF	vascular endothelial growth factor
VIP	vasoactive intestinal peptide